AF598554

Pathology of the Gallbladder, Biliary Tract and Pancreas

OTHER MONOGRAPHS IN THE SERIES MAJOR PROBLEMS IN PATHOLOGY

VIRGINIA A. LIVOLSI, M.D.
Series Editor

Published

Azzopardi: *Problems in Breast Pathology*

Frable: *Fine Needle Aspiration Biopsy*

Wigglesworth: *Perinatal Pathology,* 2/ed

Wittels: *Surgical Pathology of Bone Marrow*

Katzenstein: *Katzenstein and Askin's Surgical Pathology of Non-Neoplastic Lung Disease,* 3/ed

Finegold: *Pathology of Neoplasia in Children and Adolescents*

Wolf and Neiman: *Disorders of the Spleen*

Fu and Regan: *Pathology of the Uterine Cervix, Vagina, and Vulva*

LiVolsi: *Surgical Pathology of the Thyroid*

Virmani, Atkinson, and Fenoglio: *Cardiovascular Pathology*

Whitehead: *Mucosal Biopsy of the Gastrointestinal Tract,* 5/ed

Mackay, Lukeman, and Ordonez: *Tumors of the Lung*

Ellis, Auclair, and Gnepp: *Surgical Pathology of the Salivary Glands*

Nash and Said: *Pathology of AIDS and HIV Infection*

Lloyd: *Surgical Pathology of the Pituitary Gland*

Henson and Albores-Saavedra: *Pathology of Incipient Neoplasia,* 2/ed

Taylor and Cote: *Immunomicroscopy,* 2/ed

Lack: *Pathology of Adrenal and Extra-Adrenal Paraganglia*

Jaffe: *Surgical Pathology of Lymph Nodes and Related Organs,* 2/ed

Striker, Striker, and d'Agati: *The Renal Biopsy,* 3/ed

Isaacs, Jr: *Tumors of the Fetus and Newborn*

Foster and Bostwick: *Pathology of the Prostate*

Neiman and Orazi: *Disorders of the Spleen,* 2/ed

Helliwell: *Pathology of Bone and Joint Neoplasms*

Forthcoming

Fu: *Pathology of the Uterine Cervix, Vagina, and Vulva,* 2/ed

Weidner: *Surgical Pathology of the Breast*

LiVolsi: *Pathology of the Thyroid,* 2/ed

DAVID A. OWEN, MB
Division of Anatomic Pathology
Vancouver General Hospital
University of British Columbia
Vancouver, BC
Canada

JAMES K. KELLY, MB
Division of Anatomic Pathology
Royal Jubilee Hospital
Victoria, BC
Canada

Pathology of the Gallbladder, Biliary Tract and Pancreas

Volume 39 in the Series
MAJOR PROBLEMS IN PATHOLOGY

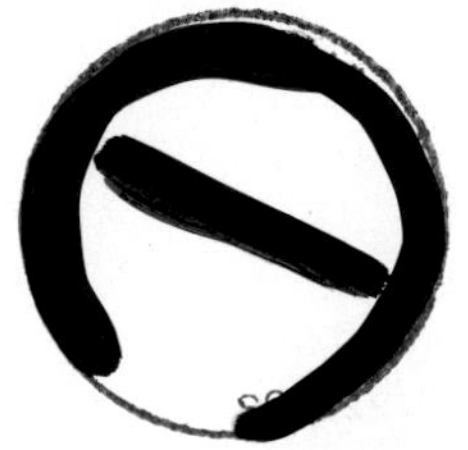

W.B. SAUNDERS COMPANY
A Harcourt Health Sciences Company
PHILADELPHIA LONDON NEW YORK ST. LOUIS SYDNEY TORONTO

W.B. SAUNDERS COMPANY
A Harcourt Health Sciences Company

The Curtis Center
Independence Square West
Philadelphia, Pennsylvania 19106

Library of Congress Cataloging-in-Publication Data

Owen, David A.

Pathology of the gallbladder, biliary tract, and pancreas / David A. Owen, James Kelly.

p. cm. — (MPP ; 39)

ISBN 0–7216–1910–X.

1. Pancreas—Diseases. 2. Gallbladder—Diseases. 3. Biliary tract—Diseases. I. Kelly, James K. II. Title. III. Major problems in pathology ; v. 39.

RC857 .O94 2001

616.3′7—dc21 00–063498

PATHOLOGY OF THE GALLBLADDER, BILIARY TRACT AND PANCREAS ISBN 0–7216–1910–X

Printed in the United States of America

Last digit is the print number: 9 8 7 6 5 4 3 2 1

Foreword

This monograph on *Pathology of the Gallbladder, Biliary Tract and Pancreas* is a welcome member of the MPP series. Doctors Owen and Kelly have produced a masterful work, including not only morphology, but related clinical, genetic, and molecular features of lesions affecting the pancreas and biliary tract.

I am convinced this book will become the standard in the field.

VIRGINIA A. LIVOLSI, M.D.
UNIVERSITY OF PENNSYLVANIA
SERIES EDITOR

Preface

Pathology of the gallbladder, biliary tract, and pancreas has, in the recent past been a relatively neglected area. The reasons for this are twofold. First there has been a perception that the pathology is mundane with little clinical significance. As we hope to show, this is incorrect. Second, until recently, surgery of the pancreas was hazardous and carried a high morbidity and mortality. Consequently, biopsies and resection specimens were rarely received in the laboratory, with the result that pathologists had little exposure to this type of material. Due to advances in surgical techniques, this situation is now changed and even radical operations such as Whipple's procedure may be carried out safely.

This volume is intended to be comprehensive and includes descriptions of congenital, degenerative, inflammatory, and neoplastic conditions. Rare and common diseases are included although it is primarily written for non-specialists. We hope the book will provide an informative, but concise text that will be of practical value to pathologists when they encounter diagnostic problems in pancreato-biliary material. In addition, we have also summarized current information about medical diseases of the pancreato-biliary tract, a topic that generally attracts scant coverage in most general pathology texts.

We acknowledge the advice and support of Charles Scudamore MD, hepato-pancreato-biliary surgeon at the University of British Columbia and Vancouver General Hospital. He has been instrumental in providing us with most of our specimen material including those used for the illustrations. In addition, working with Charles has enabled us to gain practical experience with complex diagnostic problems. We also acknowledge the dedicated secretarial support provided by Christine Kirkham.

David A. Owen, M.B.
James K. Kelly, M.B.

Contents

Chapter

1

EMBRYOLOGY, NORMAL ANATOMY, AND HISTOLOGY OF THE PANCREAS

DEVELOPMENT

The pancreas develops as two separate buds from the endoderm of the duodenum (distal foregut) during the fourth to fifth week of gestation. The dorsal bud is the first to appear when the embryo is about 3 mm in length. This arises opposite and cranial to the hepatic bud, where it grows rapidly into the mesoduodenum to the left of the vitelline veins. The ventral bud, which may be bilobed, arises later on the right side of the duodenum, just caudal to the hepatic bud, with which it shares a common orifice[1,2] (Fig. 1–1).

Later in development, during the sixth week of fetal life, the duodenum undergoes a rotation of 90°, bringing the dorsal bud to the left lateral position and the ventral bud to a posterior position below the dorsal pancreas. At this stage, the dorsal and ventral pancreas are separated by the left vitelline vein, which later in development becomes the portal vein.

As the embryo reaches the 12-mm stage at about the seventh week of fetal life, the dorsal and ventral buds fuse into a single organ. The dorsal bud forms the tail, body, and superior portion of the head of the mature pancreas. Distally, its duct persists and forms the main pancreatic duct, but the proximal portion either undergoes atrophy or persists as an accessory duct, the duct of Santorini. If present, the duct of Santorini empties into the duodenum at its own separate orifice, proximal to the main pancreatic duct on the medial duodenal wall. The ventral bud forms the lower portion of the head of the adult pancreas. Its duct, called the duct of Wirsung, connects the ampulla with the distal portion of the dorsal pancreatic duct, thus forming the terminal portion of the main pancreatic duct.

As the pancreas grows, the main ducts branch to form ductules and develop luminal spaces. Both acinar and islet cells are derived from these ductules[3] and may be recognized morphologically at about the second to third month of intrauterine life, although endocrine cells are generally identified somewhat earlier. The lobules of the pancreas form as acinar units aggregated around terminal ductules. The lobules are separated from each other by thin septae of mesenchyme (Fig. 1–2). The theory that endocrine cells of the pancreas are derived from the neural crest is now considered to be incorrect.[3] At about the fourth month, cytoplasmic granulation of acinar cells may be identified. Initially, the granules are elongated, angular, and somewhat fibrillar in appearance and may resemble granules present in adult acinar neoplasms. Enzymatic activity is not detected in the elongated granules.[4] By mid-term, fetal acini come to more closely resemble adult acinar cells.

Endocrine cell granulation is usually identifiable after 12 weeks' gestation. The cells bud off from interlobular and intralobular ductules and form small aggregates surrounding capillaries. When compared with an adult pancreas, the fetal endocrine cells are more dispersed and the islets of Langerhans are less well de-

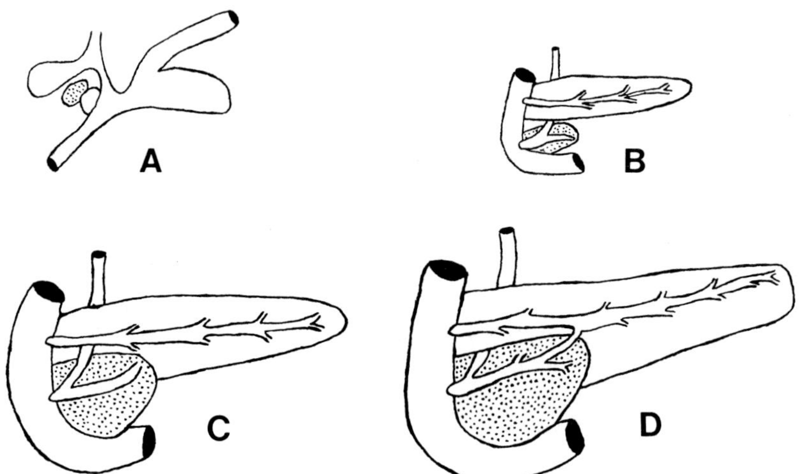

Figure 1–1. Embryologic development of the pancreas. *A,* The ventral primordium is located to the right of the primitive duodenum. *B,* As the bowel rotates, the ventral primordium now lies to the left of the duodenum and inferior to the dorsal primordium. The bile duct accompanies it and lies partly behind the dorsal primordium. *C,* The parenchyma of the two pancreatic primordia has fused. *D,* Anastamosis of the ductal systems. (From Kozu T, Suda K, Toki F: Pancreatic development and anatomical variation. Gastrointest Endosc Clin North Am 5:1–30, 1995.)

fined (Fig. 1–2). At 16 weeks' gestation, fetal endocrine granules can be readily identified and separated into A cells and B cells, located at opposite ends of the islets. Only later in fetal life do they assume the adult distribution, with a central core of B cells, surrounded by a rim of A cells.

Mesenchymal cells are prominent in the fetal pancreas. The interlobular connective tissue may be highly compact and may resemble ovarian stroma.

GROSS ANATOMY

The normal pancreas lies on the posterior wall of the abdominal cavity, behind the stomach and transverse colon, but anterior to the aorta and vena cava.[5] Normally, it is between 15 and 20 cm in length, but it can be up to 27 cm. The head is inserted into the curve of the duodenum and the tip of the tail reaches to the hilum of the spleen. Peritoneum of the posterior wall of the lesser sac covers its anterior

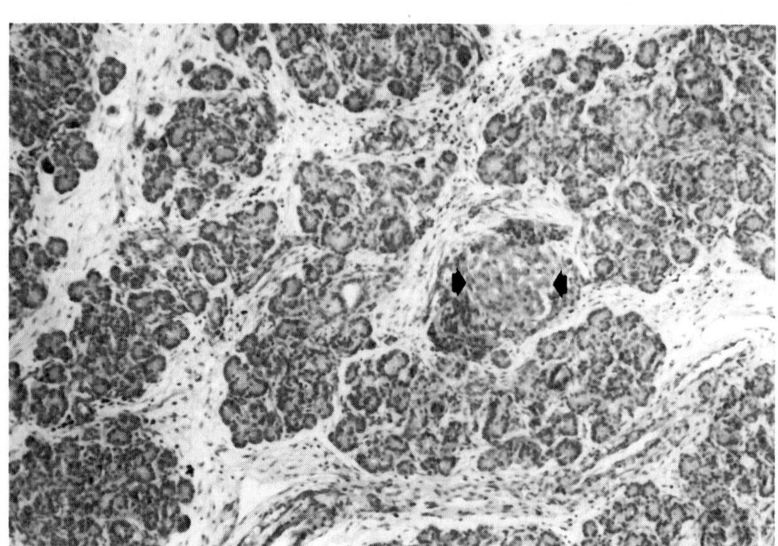

Figure 1–2. Fetal pancreas: Note the widely spaced lobules and ill-defined islets (*arrows*).

surface. The weight of the adult gland at autopsy is 41–182 g (average, 92 g),[6–8] which decreases in the elderly (average, 70 g). At birth, an infant's pancreas weighs only 2 to 3 g but increases in size to 7 g at 1 year of age.

Four anatomic regions are recognized: head, neck, body, and tail; however, the exact anatomic demarcation of these is blurred. The uncinate process is part of the lower pole of the head, which projects upward and medially behind the superior mesenteric artery and vein. In cross-section, the head and body are triangular in shape; the tail is flattened. By gross inspection, the gland is light tan to yellowish in color and has a lobulated appearance. There is no discrete capsule and, particularly in obese individuals, its outer margin may be difficult to distinguish from the surrounding fat. The cut surface of the pancreas shows well-demarcated lobules, separated by thin connective-tissue septae. In the center of the gland, the main duct runs longitudinally, with an average diameter of 4.8 mm in the head, 3.5 mm in the body, and 2.4 mm in the tail. Secondary ducts enter the main duct in a herringbone fashion. These are placed alternately on each side. As the main pancreatic duct enters the head of the pancreas, it becomes sharply angulated inferiorly at the site of fusion with the accessory duct of Santorini (Fig. 1–3). The anatomy of the ampulla of Vater and the junction between common bile duct and main pancreatic duct is variable. This is discussed fully in Chapter 14.

Blood supply to the head, neck, and body is from branches of the superior mesenteric artery and celiac artery via the anterior and posterior pancreaticoduodenal arteries, the dorsal pancreatic artery, and the inferior pancreatic artery. Branches of the splenic artery (itself a branch of the celiac artery) supply the tail.[9] The venous drainage is to the portal vein. The pancreatic veins parallel the arteries and are generally superficial to them. Lymphatics follow the course of the vessels and regional lymph nodes may be present along the upper and lower margins of the gland, or around the common bile duct, the hilum of the spleen, and in the celiac axis.[10] Occasionally, lymph nodes may be embedded within the substance of the gland. Nerves to the pancreas include sympathetic supply from the splanchnic nerves and parasympathetic supply from the vagus. These nerves are generally to be found alongside vessels.

HISTOLOGIC APPEARANCES

Three main histologic components are present within the pancreas: the acini, the islets of Langerhans, and the duct system.

The exocrine secretory acini comprise over 80% of the organ. Acini may be spherical or tubular.[11] They have a small central lumen, surrounded by a single layer of triangular-shaped secretory cells. No myoepithelial layer is present. Most acini are present as the terminal unit of the ductular system, but they may occasionally bud from the side of ductules.[9] There may also be anastamoses between adjacent acini.[11] The nucleus of the acinar cells is basally located and is rounded and contains an even distribution of chromatin with small nucleoli. The nuclear membrane may be prominent, with attached small chromatin clumps. The cytoplasm is packed with organelles, giving it a granular appearance. In general, the basal granules are basophilic because they consist predominately of ribosomes (RNA), whereas the luminal granules are eosinophilic and contain protein (zymogen granules) within secretory

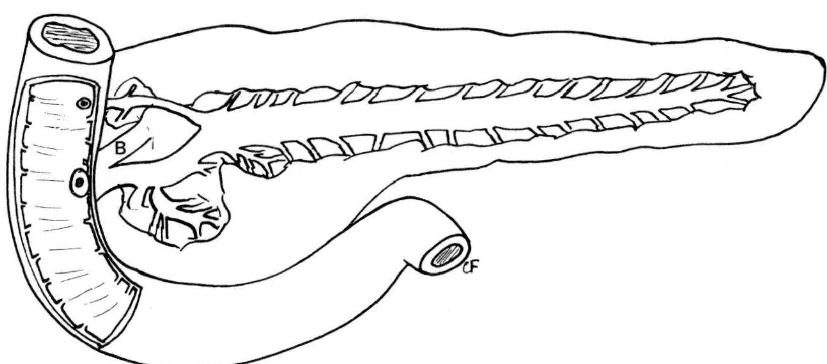

Figure 1–3. Mature adult pancreas showing location of duodenal papillae and bile duct (*B*).

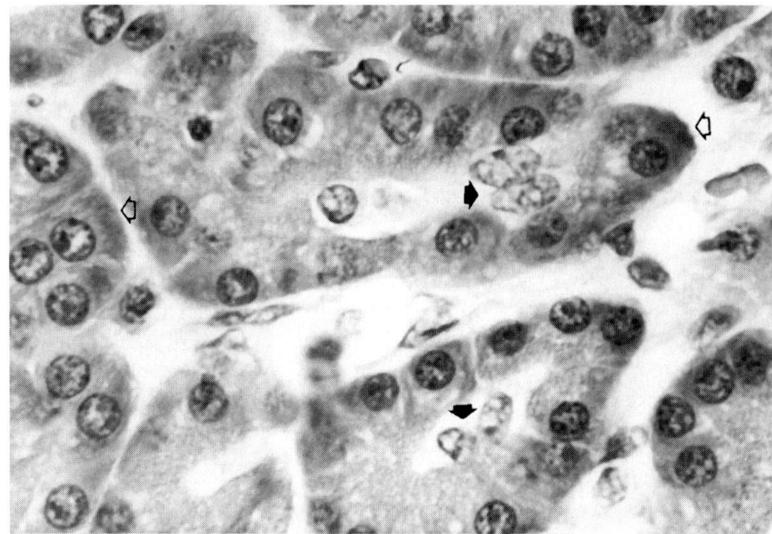

Figure 1–4. Exocrine acinus, showing centrilobular cells (*solid arrows*) and basal basophilic granularity (*open arrows*).

vacuoles (Fig. 1–4). In some cells, there is a clear Golgi zone, superficial to the nucleus. The numbers of basal and apical granules within individual cells and also within acini may, however, vary, depending on the current stimulation and secretory activity.

Ultrastructural examination of acinar cells reveals that the basal cytoplasm contains parallel stacks of rough endoplasmic reticulum, free polyribosomes, and occasional mitochondria. The Golgi apparatus is located on the luminal side of the nucleus; from this originate the zymogen granules. Mature zymogen granules, located in the apical cytoplasm, are typically large (250–1,000 nm), dense, and rounded, with a closely apposed limiting membrane.[9] When the pancreas is stimulated, the membrane of these granules merges with the apical plasma membrane and discharges their contents into the lumen. Stunted microvilli containing microfilaments are present on the luminal surface.

Zymogen granules stain positively with diastase/periodic acid–Schiff (PAS) stains (Fig. 1–5). However, as they do not contain mucus, negative staining will be obtained with mucicarmine and alcian blue techniques. Stains for butyrate esterase are also positive.[9] Immunohistochemical stains for amylase, lipase, trypsin, and chymotrypsin are positive. Keratin positivity is shown with Cam 5.2 but not with AE1, AE3,

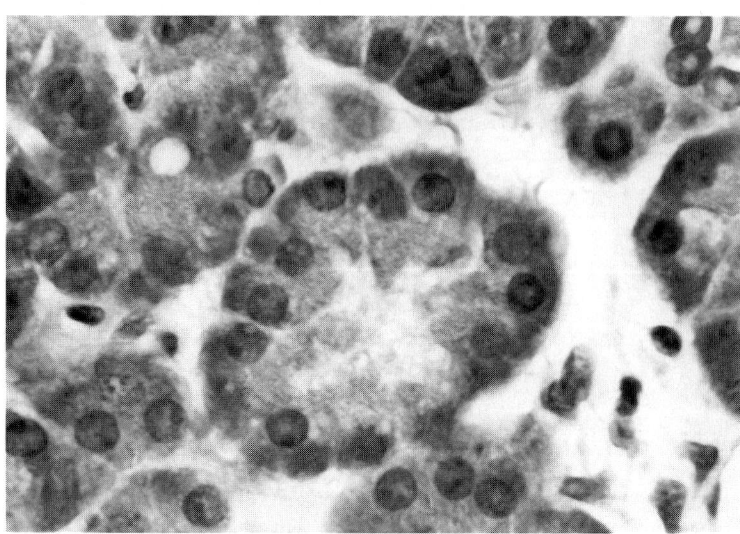

Figure 1–5. Exocrine acinus with periodic acid–Schiff (PAS) staining to optimally demonstrate secretory granules in the luminal portion of the cells.

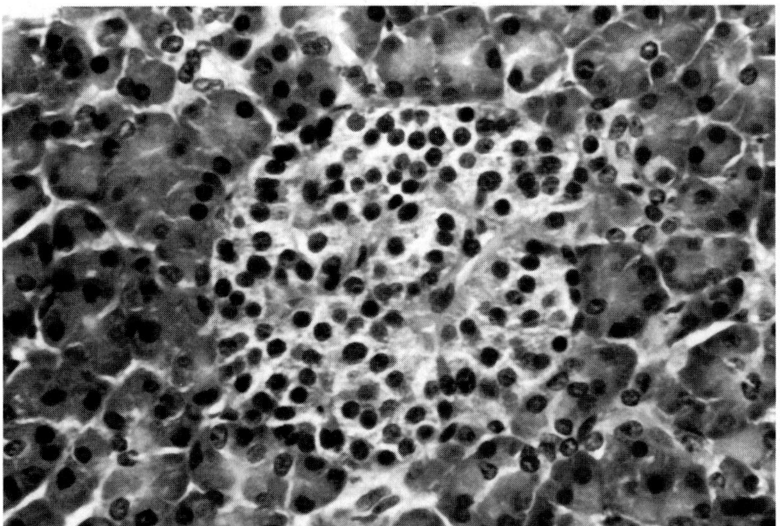

Figure 1–6. Compact islet with well-defined borders.

or cytokeratins 7 and 20.[9] Stains for Ca 19.9 and DUPAN-2 are also negative.

Endocrine cells of the pancreas account for 1% to 2% of the volume of the gland in adults and approximately 10% of the volume in neonates.[12] The overwhelming majority of these cells are present within the islets of Langerhans, but small numbers of dispersed cells are present also. These are located along the main duct and major interlobular ducts interspersed with the duct lining cells. Islets are present throughout the pancreas, although they are most frequent in the tail. Two types of islets occur: compact and diffuse. Compact islets occur in the body and tail of the pancreas, as well as in the superior portion of the head, which constitute the parts of the pancreas derived from the dorsal pancreatic bud. The compact islets comprise 90% of the total and generally measure 75 to 225 μm, although occasionally they may be as small as 50 μm or as large as 280 μm[13] (Fig. 1–6). The diffuse islets occur in the inferior portion of the pancreatic head, which is derived from the ventral bud. Diffuse islets measure up to 450 μm in diameter and, as their name implies, they are less well circumscribed than the compact islets (Fig. 1–7). Compact islets are composed of intertwined polygonal cells

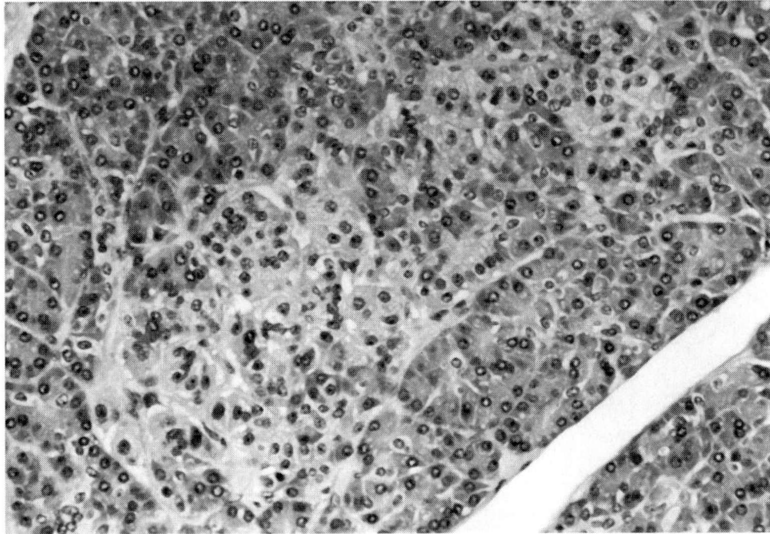

Figure 1–7. Diffuse islet with ill-defined borders.

with nuclei that have a coarsely clumped chromatin pattern and small nucleoli. The cytoplasm is palely amphophilic. Diffuse islets are trabecular in appearance and, because of their ill-defined border, may appear to infiltrate adjacent acini. Most cells are cuboidal, although occasional columnar cells are present. Their cytoplasm is generally basophilic in appearance. The nuclei commonly have a conspicuous hyperchromatism, with occasional prominent nucleoli. Both types of islet are richly vascular, with an extensive capillary network, which is in contact with every islet cell. These capillaries have a fenestrated endothelium. Islets have no true capsule separating them from the adjacent acinar tissue, although they may be surrounded by a thin rim of connective tissue.[9] Mitotic figures are only rarely seen within the acini.[14]

Functionally and morphologically, four types of cell may be identified within the islets. Each cell produces only a single hormone. Silver stains and aldehyde fuchsin stains for different cell types are now obsolete and have been replaced by immunohistochemical techniques. Within compact islets, B cells, which produce insulin, are the most numerous and comprise 60% to 70% of cells.[13] They tend to be located at the center of the islets (Fig. 1–8). Occasional B cells have markedly enlarged nuclei and are tetraploid, or even octoploid. Ultrastructurally, B cells contain granules measuring 225 to 375 nm, with irregularly shaped crystalline cores and a broad halo beneath the limiting membrane[15] (Fig. 1–9). There is considerable pleomorphism of cores. Cytoplasmic ceroid bodies (lipid inclusions) may also be seen. A cells (alpha cells), which make up most (15% to 20%) of the remainder of the compact islets, are concentrated around the periphery (Fig. 1–10). They secrete glucagon. Ultrastructurally, the granules measure 200 to 300 nm and contain an eccentrically located dense core, a less dense outer region, and a narrow halo (Fig. 1–9). D cells (delta cells), which secrete somatostatin, are almost always located in close contact with A cells. They are relatively rare, comprising < 10% of cells in both the compact and diffuse islets. Ultrastructurally, the D cells are about 170 to 220 nm in diameter and have a uniformly dense core, with only a very thin halo (Fig. 1–9). D cells have ultrastructurally identifiable thin cytoplasmic processes that extend toward the A and B cells and presumably facilitate release of somatostatin in a paracrine role.[13] The compact islets also contain small numbers of PP (pancreatic polypeptide) cells. Within the diffuse islets, PP secreting cells predominate and account for approximately 70% of the total. Twenty percent of the cells are B cells, 5% are A cells, and 5% are D cells. By ultrastructural examination, the granules of diffuse islet PP cells measure 120 to 220 nm in diameter. They are quite pleomorphic, with considerable variation in shape and density (Fig. 1–9). In the compact islets, the PP cells are smaller (120 to 150 nm in diameter) and demonstrate less variability.[16,17]

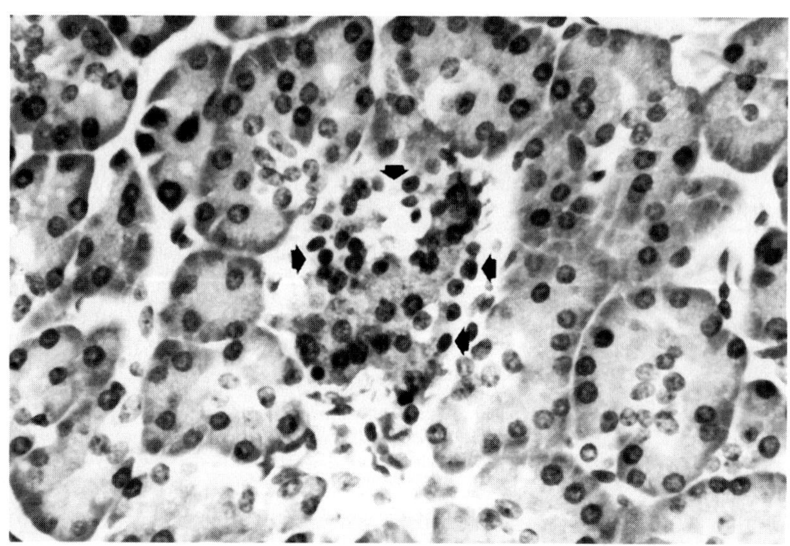

Figure 1–8. Immunohistochemical stain for insulin. Note the positive-staining cells at the center of the islet. Immunonegative cells are present at the periphery (*arrows*).

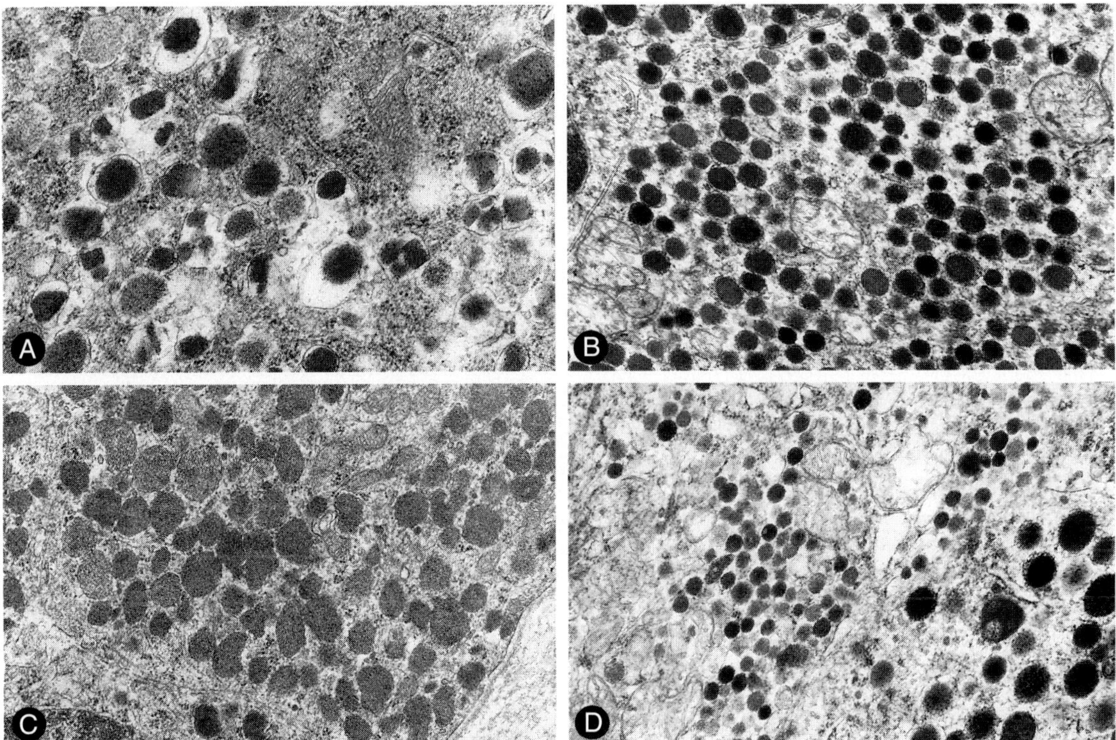

Figure 1–9. Various types of normal islet cells granule. *A,* B-cell granules with large, finely granular insulin granules and dense angular crystalloids, with an empty space separating core from limiting membrane. (× 29,250.) *B,* A-cell granules, showing a dense core with less dense periphery. (× 16,350.) *C,* D cell showing somatostatin granules that are irregular in shape and are larger and less dense than glucagon granules. (× 20,480.) *D,* PP cell. The granules are small and uniformly dense, with a closely applied membrane. (× 16,350.) (Illustration courtesy of Ron Jaffe, MD, Children's Hospital of Pittsburgh. From Wigglesworth JS, Singer DB: Textbook of Fetal and Perinatal. Pathology. Malden, MA: Blackwell Science, 1998.)

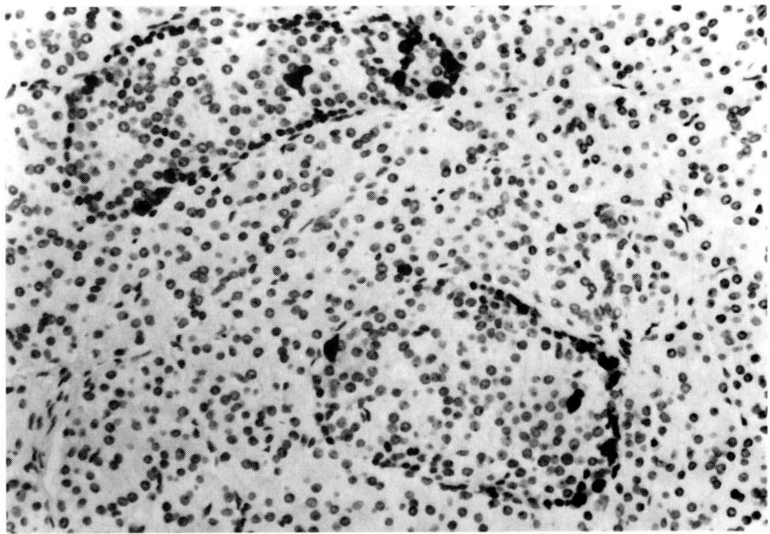

Figure 1–10. Immunostain for glucagon with positive cells present at the periphery of the acinus.

A wide variety of scattered single endocrine cells may be detected outside of the islets in ductal epithelium and occasionally within acini. These are sparse and comprise < 10% of the total complement of adult pancreatic endocrine cells.[9] Most of these dispersed endocrine cells are present within the larger ducts. They may be located either between adjacent ductular cells or between the ductal cells and the basement membrane. Secretion products of these cells may be detected within secreted pancreatic fluid.[18] Most secrete either insulin, somatostatin, or pancreatic polypeptide[18,19]; however, a small minority produce serotonin and presumably represent the precursors of true pancreatic carcinoid tumors.[20]

Five subdivisions of pancreatic ducts are recognized: main pancreatic ducts, interlobular ducts, intralobular ducts, intracalated ducts, and centroacinar ducts.[21] The main ducts (ducts of Wirsung and Santorini) receive numerous tributaries from interlobular ducts and are lined by a simple flattened epithelium, except in the ampulla, where the epithelium is typically thrown into papillary projections. The individual lining cells are columnar, with regular basally located nuclei. The cytoplasm contains a mixture of sialomucin and neutral mucin, with only small amounts of sulfomucin.[22] The interlobular ducts are similar in morphology to the main ducts, but tend to have more obvious cytoplasmic mucin, which contains greater quantities of sulfomucin. Both main and interlobular ducts are surrounded by a thick collagen layer, that may contain multiple lobulated aggregates of mucus-secreting ductules within the wall. These closely resemble aggregations of ductules found alongside the major extra- and intrahepatic bile ducts (the ductules of Beale) (Fig. 1–11).

The major intralobular ducts are histologically similar to interlobular ducts and are lined by a low columnar epithelium with rounded nuclei. The cytoplasm also contains mucus, predominantly sulfomucin. The larger ducts are therefore most rich in neutral mucin and contain only traces of sulfomucin. The reverse is true of the smaller ducts. The intercalated ducts and the centroacinar ducts are also lined by a single layer of cells. However, these are flattened, with an oval nucleus and cytoplasm that is nonsecretory (Fig. 1–12). The centroacinar cells form an incomplete acinar lining, being attached by tight junctions to acinar secretory cells. All duct-lining cells, including centroacinar cells, are easily demonstrated immunohistochemically, by their positivity for keratins AE1, AE3, Cam 5.2, and CK7. They are negative for CK20.[9] Immunohistochemical staining of ductal cells also reveals positivity for CA 19-9 and DUPAN-2.[23,24]

CONNECTIVE TISSUE

The lobules of the adult pancreas are separated only by thin strands of loose connective tissue (Fig. 1–13). This represents a considerable reduction from the situation present in the neonatal pancreas, where 30% of the organ may

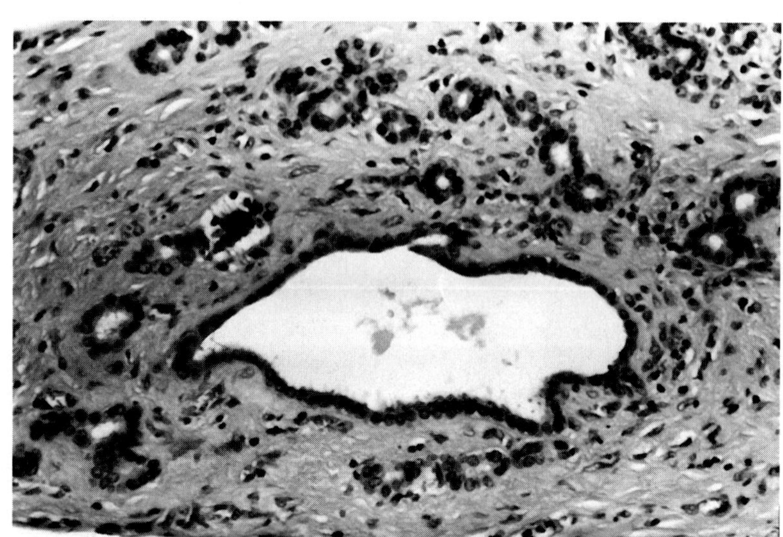

Figure 1–11. Major duct with fibrous coat and surrounding ductular structures resembling the ductules of Beale.

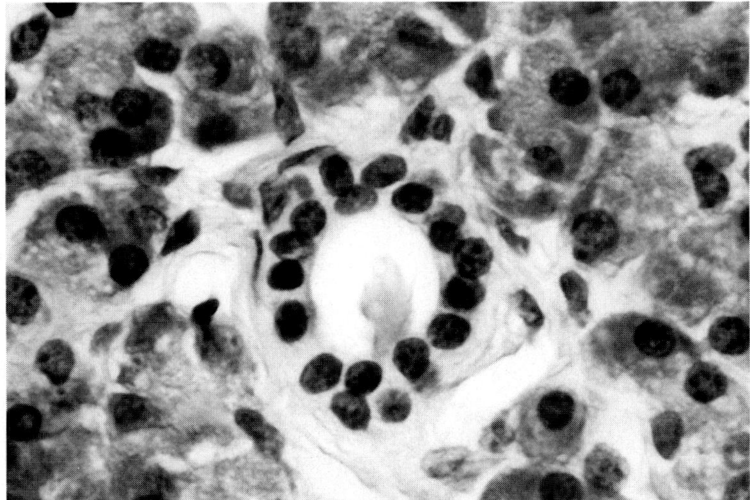

Figure 1–12. Intralobular duct with only a thin, fibrous tissue covering.

be composed of mesenchymal tissue[12] (Fig. 1–2). Children progressively lose this excess connective tissue as they get older. In adults, there is a little loose connective tissue between lobules but very little at intralobular sites.

The pancreas is richly vascular and innervated. Most of the larger nerves and vessels are present within the fibrous septae, although smaller nerves and vessels may be found in an intralobular location. Islets have both a sympathetic and parasympathetic nerve supply. These nerves may contain neuropeptide Y, substance P, cholecystokinin, and calcitonin gene-related peptide.[9,25] Also present within the pancreatic capsule is varying amounts (3% to 20% of gland weight) of adipose tissue, depending on the nutritional status of the individual.[9] The amount of fat also increases with age, but for unexplained reasons, the dorsal pancreas may contain more fat than does the ventral lobe.[26]

VARIANTS OF NORMAL

Minor abnormalities considered to be variants of normal may involve the acini, the islets, or the ductal collecting system. These probably are a reflection of physiologic differences, minor injuries, or the effects of aging.

The two most common acinar alterations that are encountered are centroacinar ectasia and differences in acinar cell cytoplasmic stain-

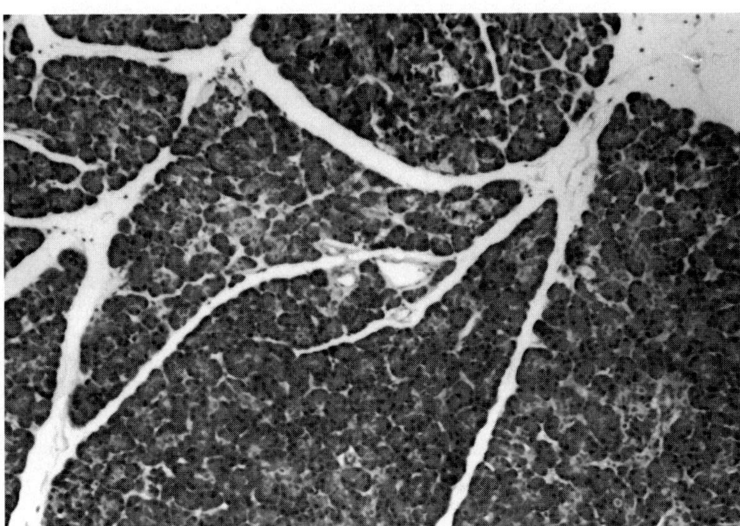

Figure 1–13. At low power, the pancreas is divided up into a lobular architecture.

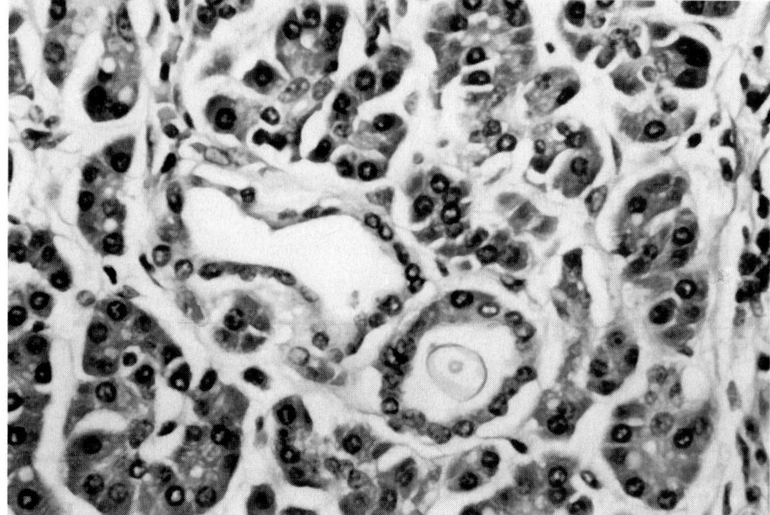

Figure 1–14. Centroacinar dilation (acinar ectasia).

ing intensity. Acinar ectasia, or dilation, is a relatively common finding, particularly at autopsy.[6,27,28] Typically, this involves acini throughout a whole lobule, rather than single isolated acini. It may be the result of major duct obstruction, uremia, septicemia, or dehydration and is a relatively common finding at autopsy. Microscopically, the acinar cells are flattened and have reduced numbers of zymogen granules. The lumen may contain inspissated secretions (Fig. 1–14). Alterations in cytoplasmic staining intensity also tend to involve entire lobules[29–31] and appear as nodules on low-power microscopic examination (Fig. 1–15). Most commonly, there is a loss in staining intensity and cells appear more eosinophilic than those in the surrounding lobules. This alteration, which is the result of loss of basophilia, occurs secondary

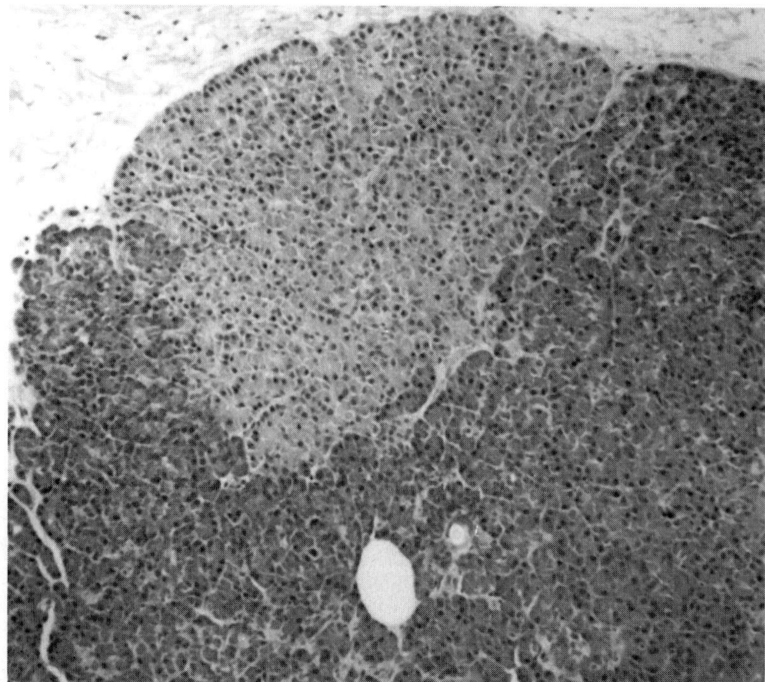

Figure 1–15. Pale eosinophilic cluster of acini (focal acinar transformation).

to dilation of rough endoplasmic reticulum.[29] The cause is unknown, but it is acquired, not congenital. Conversely, hyperintense acinar staining may occur after a loss of cytoplasmic zymogen granules. This results in acinar cell basophilia and an increased nuclear-to-cytoplasmic ratio. For unknown reasons, there may be accompanying nuclear enlargement and hyperchromasia. Lobular staining alterations have been referred to previously as acinar cell dysplasia, or atypical nodules; however, there is no convincing evidence that they are in any way connected to the subsequent development of malignancy.

Abnormalities of islet cells include hyperplasia, nesidioblastosis, peliosis, and amyloidosis. Islet cell hyperplasia has been described in association with the Beckwith–Wiedemann syndrome [exophthalmos, macroglossia, and gigantism (somatic and visceral)], diabetes mellitus, erythroblastosis, and both childhood and adult hyperinsulinemia.[9,32] Hyperplasia may be recognized by the presence of increased ($>$ 250 μm) size of islets as well as increased numbers of islets.[33] The enlarged islets contain an increased population of B cells, some of which may actually be hypertrophic.[9] The term *nesidioblastosis* refers to growth and budding off of endocrine cells from pancreatic ducts (Fig. 1–16). It frequently accompanies islet cell hyperplasia, especially in hyperinsulinemic hypoglycemia.[33,34] Some studies,[12,33] in which comparisons were made between the pancreas of normal infants and those with hyperinsulinemic hypoglycemia, have, however, suggested that nesidioblastosis is, at least to some extent, a normal finding (see Chapter 3). Nesidioblastosis may also occur in the pancreas of adult patients with chronic pancreatitis. *Peliosis insulis* may be defined as the presence of blood filled spaces within islets. It is regarded as a normal finding of no clinical significance, although in one case it has been associated with multiple islet cell neoplasms occurring in the multiple endocrine neoplasia type I syndrome.[35] Insular amyloid deposition is a relatively common finding in elderly patients. It is probably never normal, however, and its presence should raise the possibility of type 2 diabetes. Islet amyloid is not related to systemic amyloidosis.

A large number of minor alterations have been recognized within pancreatic ducts. For the most part, these are metaplastic and reflect alterations secondary to chronic pancreatitis. Hyperplastic lesions may also be encountered with or without epithelial atypia: These are discussed in Chapter 6. Mucinous metaplasia, also called *pyloric gland metaplasia,* is the most common lesion (Fig. 1–17). This may occur in ducts of any size.[36] It is seen in up to 90% of pancreata, particularly in the head region.[37] It consists of replacement of the normal duct-lining cells by tall columnar mucus-containing cells, resembling gastric surface epithelium. However, unlike the stomach, this mucus is histochemically a mixture of neutral mucin and sialomucin, with an absence of sulfomucin. Proliferation may occasionally be so great that small papillae with fibrovascular cores are present. Downward proliferation may give rise to glandlike struc-

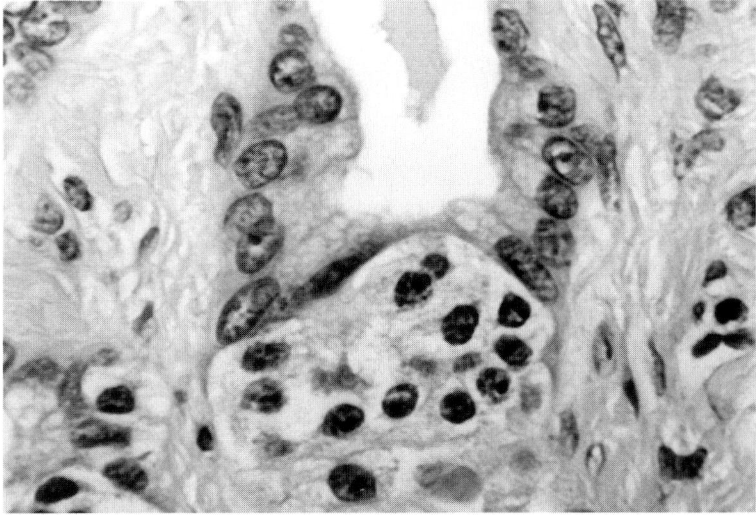

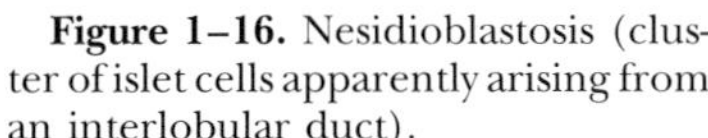

Figure 1–16. Nesidioblastosis (cluster of islet cells apparently arising from an interlobular duct).

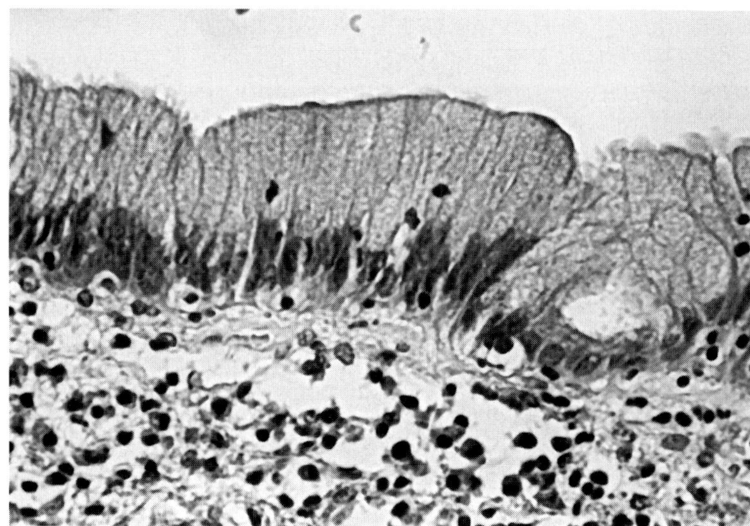

Figure 1–17. Mucinous metaplasia involving the main pancreatic duct.

tures alongside ducts that resemble the gastro pyloric mucus glands. Single ducts, or groups of ducts, may be involved in this process.

Squamous metaplasia is reported in up to 47% of pancreata, where it is generally associated with chronic pancreatitis.[9,27] It may be encountered in ducts of any size but is most frequently seen in the small intercalated and centroacinar ducts. Keratinization and the presence of keratohyaline granules is rare and the squamous change is usually confined to the presence of a multilayered epithelium.[27] Oncocytic metaplasia is also relatively common and is characteristically found in association with chronic pancreatitis.[38] It also is most common in the smaller, more proximal ducts and resembles oncocytic change encountered at other locations. In contrast, goblet cell metaplasia is a change found most frequently in the larger ducts near the ampulla of Vater.[22] The metaplastic cells resemble goblet cells of the small and large intestines. Acinar metaplasia is a recently described lesion.[9] As the name implies, it consists of exocrine secretory cells within the epithelium-lining proximal ductules. It has no known clinical associations.

REFERENCES

1. Kozu T, Suda K, Toki F: Pancreatic development and anatomical variation. Gastrointest Endoscop Clin North Am 5:1–30, 1995.
2. Bock P, Abdel-Moneim M, Egerbacher M: Development of the pancreas. Microsc Res Tech 37:374–383, 1997.
3. Debas HT: Molecular insights into the development of the pancreas. Am J Surg 174:227–231, 1997.
4. Chong JM, Fukayama M, Shiozawa Y, et al.: Fibrillary inclusions in neoplastic and fetal acinar cells of the pancreas. Virchows Arch [A] 428:261–266, 1996.
5. Skandalakis LJ, Rowe JS, Gray SW, et al.: Surgical embryology and anatomy of the pancreas. Surg Clin North Am 73:661–697, 1993.
6. Stamm BH: Incidence and diagnostic significance of minor pathologic changes in the adult pancreas at autopsy: A systematic study of 112 autopsies in patients without known pancreatic disease. Hum Pathol 15:677–683, 1984.
7. Innes JT, Carey LC: Normal pancreatic dimensions in the human adult. Am J Surg 167:261–263, 1994.
8. Innes JT, Carey LC: Normal pancreatic dimensions in the adult human. Am J Surg 167:261–263, 1994.
9. Klimstra DS: Pancreas. *In* Sternberg SS (ed): Histology for Pathologists, 2nd ed. Philadelphia: Lippincott-Raven, 1997, pp 613–647.
10. O'Morchoe CC: Lymphatic system of the pancreas. Microsc Res Tech 37:456–477, 1997.
11. Akao S, Blockman DE, Ledune de la Porte P, et al.: Three-dimensional pattern of ductulo-acinar associations in normal and pathological human pancreas. Gastroenterology 90:661–668, 1986.
12. Rahier J, Wallon J, Henquin JC: Cell populations in the endocrine pancreas of human neonates and infants. Diabetologia 20:540–546, 1981.
13. Grube D, Bohn R: The microanatomy of human islets of Langerhans, with special reference to somatostatin (D-) cells. Arch Histol Jpn 46:327–353, 1983.
14. Le Compte PM, Merriam JC: Mitotic figures and enlarged nuclei in the islands of Langerhans in man. Diabetes 11:35–39, 1962.
15. Pelletier G: Identification of four cell types in human endocrine pancreas by immune electron microscopy. Diabetes 26:749–756, 1977.
16. Bommer G, Friedl U, Heitz PU, et al.: Pancreatic PP cell distribution and hyperplasia. Immunocytochemical distribution in the normal human pancreas, in chronic pancreatitis and pancreatic carcinoma. Virchows Arch [A] 387:319–331, 1980.

17. Orci L, Malaisse-Lagae F, Baetens D: Pancreatic-polypeptide rich regions in the human pancreas. Lancet 2:1200–1201, 1978.
18. Bendayan M: Presence of endocrine cells in pancreatic ducts. Pancreas 2:393–397, 1987.
19. Chen J, Baithun SI, Pollock DJ, et al.: Argyrophilic and hormone immunoreactive cells in normal and hyperplastic pancreatic ducts and exocrine pancreatic carcinoma. Virchows Arch [A] 413:399–405, 1988.
20. Wilson RW, Gal AA, Cohen C, et al.: Serotonin immunoreactivity in pancreatic endocrine neoplasms (carcinoid tumors). Mod Pathol 4:727–732, 1991.
21. Kodama T: A light and electron microscopic study on the pancreatic ductal system. Acta Pathol Jpn 33:297–321, 1983.
22. Roberts PF, Burns J: A histochemical study of mucins in normal and neoplastic pancreatic tissue. J Pathol 107:87–94, 1972.
23. Haglund C, Lindgren J, Roberts PJ, et al.: Gastrointestinal cancer-associated antigen CA 19-9 in histological specimens of pancreatic tumor and pancreatitis. Br J Cancer 53:189–195, 1986.
24. Borowitz MJ, Tuck FL, Sindelar WF, et al.: Monoclonal antibodies against human pancreatic adenocarcinoma: Distribution of DU-PAN 2 antigen on glandular epithelia and adenocarcinomas. J Natnl Cancer Inst 72:999–1003, 1984.
25. Adeghate E, Donath T: Distribution of neuropeptide Y and vasoactive intestinal polypeptide immunoreactive nerves in normal and transplanted pancreatic tissue. Peptides 11:1087–1092, 1990.
26. Orci L, Stefan Y, Malaisse-Lagae F, et al.: Pancreatic fat. N Engl J Med 301:1292, 1979.
27. Oertel JE: The pancreas. Non-neoplastic alterations. Am J Surg Pathol 13(Suppl1):50–65, 1989.
28. Walters MN: Studies on the exocrine pancreas. I. Non-specific pancreatic ductular ectasia. Am J Pathol 89:569–572, 1965.
29. Kodama T, Mori W: Atypical acinar nodules of the human pancreas. Acta Pathol Jpn 33:701–714, 1983.
30. Shinozuka H, Lee RE, Dunn JL, et al.: Multiple atypical acinar cell nodules of the pancreas. Hum Pathol 11:389–390, 1980.
31. Tanaka T, Mori H, Williams GM: Atypical and neoplastic acinar cell lesions of the pancreas in an autopsy study of Japanese patients. Cancer 61:2278–2285, 1988.
32. Longnecker DS, Shinozuka H, Dekker A: Focal acinar cell dysplasia in human pancreas. Cancer 45:534–540, 1980.
33. Jaffe R, Hashida Y, Yunis EJ: Pancreatic pathology in hyperinsulinemic hypoglycemia of infancy. Lab Invest 42:356–365, 1980.
34. Gossens A, Gepts W, Saudubray JM, et al.: Diffuse and focal nesidioblastosis; a clinicopathological study of 24 patients with persistent neonatal hyperinsulinemic hypoglycemia. Am J Surg Pathol 13:766–775, 1989.
35. Kovacs K, Horvath E, Asa SL, et al.: Microscopic peliosis of pancreatic islets in a woman with MEN-1 syndrome. Arch Pathol Lab Med 110:607–610, 1986.
36. Roberts PF: Pyloric gland metaplasia of the human pancreas: A comparative histochemical study. Arch Pathol 97:92–95, 1974.
37. Allen-Mersh TG: Pancreatic ductal mucinous hyperplasia: Distribution within the pancreas and effect of variation in ampullary and pancreatic duct anatomy. Gut 29:1392–1396, 1988.
38. Frexinos J, Ribet A: Oncocytes in human chronic pancreatitis. Digestion 7:294–301, 1972.

Chapter

2

DEVELOPMENTAL ANOMALIES OF THE PANCREAS

The principal developmental anomalies of the pancreas are listed in Table 2–1.

Table 2–1. Developmental Anomalies of the Pancreas

Agenesis
Hypoplasia
Shwachman syndrome
Pearson syndrome
Annular pancreas
Pancreas divisum
Pancreaticobiliary maljunction
Heterotopic pancreas
Dysgenetic cysts and other cysts

AGENESIS AND CONGENITAL SHORT PANCREAS

Agenesis of the pancreas is rare. It constitutes the embryonic failure of both pancreatic anlagen to develop. Agenesis has been described in stillborn infants, or infants who have died soon after birth with multiple malformations, some of whom have a trisomy syndrome, acardia, or anencephaly.[1,2] These infants may lack that portion of the intestine from which the liver and pancreas are derived. Pancreatic agenesis may also be accompanied by aplasia of the intrahepatic bile ducts and other malformations, such as a common arterial trunk and ventricular septal defect.[3] Agenesis of the exocrine pancreas also implies absence of the islets of Langerhans and diabetes mellitus. An infant affected by pancreatic agenesis is growth retarded, because insulin functions as the antenatal growth hormone and the placenta is impermeable to maternal insulin. The developing fetus, therefore, has to depend on its own supply. If imaging studies suggest pancreatic aplasia, blood should be collected at autopsy for measurement of the insulin level. This would be expected to be zero. Other features of pancreatic aplasia are meconium ileus and steatorrhea.[1,4] Pancreatic agenesis can also be a manifestation of the autosomal-recessive condition, type III shortrib-polydactyly syndrome.[5]

Agenesis of one of the pancreatic buds is also a rare occurrence.[6–12] Only 13 cases of agenesis of the dorsal primordium had been reported to 1993.[9,10] The dorsal duct, accessory papilla, body, and tail of pancreas are lacking. Early reports of this abnormality were based on autopsy findings, but recent cases have been diagnosed by imaging studies in patients presenting with diabetes mellitus or chronic pancreatitis. Pancreatography displays no duct of Santorini. Because most of the islets of Langerhans are located in the tail of the pancreas, the absence of the body and tail likely contributes to the development of diabetes in these individuals. One report documents dorsal bud agenesis in a woman and her two sons, conceived of different fathers. This finding suggests an autosomal or X-linked dominant inheritance.[10] A single case of agenesis of the ventral pancreas has been reported.[13]

The term *pancreatic defect* is used to indicate clinical uncertainty as to reason for absence of the body and tail of the gland, whether resulting from aplasia, hypoplasia, malformation, or acquired conditions.[6] Defects are detected by pancreatography, and when the duct of Santorini is present, a defect of the body and tail of the gland suggests that either defective development or secondary obliteration has occurred.[6]

Congenital short pancreas is a term that has been applied to a short pancreas that contains both dorsal and ventral ducts but lacks a body and tail. It is believed to represent a partial agenesis of the dorsal pancreas.[14–17] The duct of Santorini is present and typically fuses with the duct of Wirsung to form a horseshoe shape that may be demonstrated on pancreatography. The ductal system images suggest congenital rather than acquired disease.[14] This rare condition may be discovered on pancreatography, or computed tomography (CT) in adults, most of whom have diabetes mellitus and who present with abdominal pain of uncertain cause. The symptoms of diabetes may relate to the distribution of islets within the normal pancreas. There is a relative abundance of islets in the pancreatic tail. These are therefore absent in congenital short pancreas. No significant abnormality of exocrine pancreatic function has been described in this condition. Congenital short pancreas has been described in association with vaginal atresia, autoimmune gastritis, and duodenal papillary dysfunction.[16] The abnormality may also result in polysplenia.[18,19] The major differential diagnosis of congenital short pancreas is distal pancreatic atrophy, secondary to an obstructed duct. This distinction can be clinically subtle,[14] but no evidence of pancreatitis is found in patients with congenital disease who undergo open biopsy.[11,17,20]

Congenital absence of the islets of Langerhans throughout an otherwise normal pancreas has been described in male siblings, resulting in intrauterine growth retardation and neonatal death. It has been suggested that this condition has a recessive mode of inheritance.[21]

HYPOPLASIA

Hypoplasia of the pancreas is a rare condition in which glandular pancreatic tissue is present in the normal location but is greatly reduced in size. The major ducts are intact but reduced in number, and there is diminished duct branching. There is, thus, a generalized reduction in pancreatic volume, but there is no localized defect as in pancreatic agenesis. Neither inflammation of islets nor fibrosis is present. Malabsorption and failure to thrive are the main symptoms.[22,23] There are two well-characterized syndromes in which pancreatic hypoplasia is a feature—Shwachman syndrome and Pearson syndrome—although isolated hypoplasia has also been described. A report described two infant brothers who were small in size at birth and had early-onset insulin-dependent diabetes with pancreatic exocrine insufficiency.[24] In contrast to the findings in pancreatic aplasia, the twins' serum C-peptide and glucagon levels were low but measurable. Another case report describes a man who had type I diabetes since childhood and a severely hypoplastic pancreas at autopsy.[25] There has been a report of a family in which hereditary pancreatic hypoplasia, diabetes mellitus, and congenital heart disease were apparently inherited as an autosomal-dominant trait. This is in contrast to the autosomal-recessive inheritance of the Shwachman syndrome (congenital hypoplasia with lipomatous atrophy).[26] A review of the English-language literature on pancreatic hypoplasia from 1966 to 1993 found 30 cases. Fourteen of these were not associated with other congenital anomalies. Polysplenia was the most common associated anomaly. Most cases were sporadic, but there were two other reports of familial cases. Twelve patients had diabetes mellitus and one had glucose intolerance, undoubtedly as a result of insufficient endocrine tissue. The mechanism of the diabetes may be similar to that of adult-onset non–insulin-dependent diabetes mellitus.[26]

Isolated absence of pancreatic acinar cells has been described in conjunction with clinical features of *leprechaunism*[27] and *Ivemark's syndrome* (dysplasia of the pancreas, with dysplasia of liver and kidneys).[28] Pancreatic exocrine insufficiency is also a manifestation of the *Johanson–Blizzard syndrome,* an autosomal-recessive disease, in which there is congenital aplasia of the alae nasi, deafness, hypothyroidism, dwarfism, absent permanent teeth, and malabsorption. Deficiency of the exocrine pancreas is the major cause of growth failure[29] and there is virtually complete replacement of the pancreas with adipose tissue.[30] Hypoplasia of the islets of Langerhans and of the B cells has been described in small-for-date infants.[31]

The differential diagnosis of pancreatic hypoplasia includes various acquired conditions. Pancreatic fibrosis and atrophy mimicking hypoplasia can be found in *Jeune's syndrome,* an autosomal inherited disease characterized by bone dysplasia, as well as renal and hepatic malformations of variable expressivity.[32] Ductal dilation and fibrosis of the pancreas are found in 30% of cases of *Meckel's syndrome.*[33] Acquired pancreatic fibrosis may be a manifestation of *neonatal asphyxiating thoracic dystrophy,* an autosomal-recessive disorder characterized by an abnormally small thorax, variable shortening of the extremities, and pelvic anomalies. Most children with the disorder die in infancy of respiratory failure.[34]

Shwachman syndrome (see also Chapter 4) is the main cause of pancreatic hypoplasia. The hypoplasia is distinctive because although the overall size of the gland is normal, the acinar tissue is extensively replaced by fat. Shwachman syndrome is a condition of childhood, characterized by a widely variable phenotype affecting multiple organ systems. Virtually all patients have maldigestion, due to exocrine pancreatic hypoplasia, and bone marrow dysfunction.[35–38] Neutropenia is the most common hematologic abnormality (88% of patients), but leukopenia, thrombocytopenia, and anemia are also encountered.[35] Forty-four percent of patients have hypoplasia of all three bone marrow cellular lines, and these individuals have the worst prognosis, with near 50% mortality, as a result of sepsis or acute myelogenous leukemia.[35]

The overall size and shape of the pancreas in Shwachman syndrome are normal. Histologic examination of the pancreas reveals hypoplasia of the exocrine acini, with fatty replacement. The excretory ducts persist but may be diminished in number and are not dilated. The few surviving acinar cells are enlarged, with cytoplasmic vacuolization, nuclear enlargement, and intranuclear inclusions.[35,36] The islets of Langerhans survive. The proportion of cases of infantile pancreatic hypoplasia that are examples of Shwachman syndrome is unclear and awaits the advent of a definitive genetic test.

Pearson syndrome, a refractory sideroblastic anemia with exocrine pancreatic insufficiency, was first described in 1979, as a syndrome in four unrelated children, consisting of severe transfusion-dependent macrocytic anemia, with variable neutropenia and thrombocytopenia.[39] The bone marrow showed vacuolated erythroid and myeloid precursors, hemosiderosis, and ringed sideroblasts. One child had clinical malabsorption, and this child and one other had extensive pancreatic fibrosis demonstrated at autopsy. The other two children had findings consistent with malabsorption.[39] This disease is now recognized to result from deletions of mitochondrial DNA.[40] The manifestations of the disease vary; there are patients without marrow involvement,[41] patients whose disease progresses to the Kearns–Sayre syndrome (encephalopathy with ophthalmoplegia, retinal degeneration, ataxia, and endocrine abnormalities),[42] and patients with normal pancreatic function.[43] Insulin-dependent diabetes mellitus has been described in the neonatal period.[44] At autopsy, the exocrine pancreas shows fibrosis and acinar atrophy.[44] At present, it is not clear whether Pearson syndrome is a true hypoplasia or an acquired atrophy with secondary fibrosis.

ANNULAR PANCREAS

Annular pancreas is a rare anomaly in which a ring of pancreatic tissue, including ducts, encircles the duodenum. The ring is in continuity with the head of pancreas and may be complete or incomplete. The ring is usually proximal to the ampulla of Vater, in the second part of the duodenum (85%), but in 15% of patients with the anomaly, it encircles the first or third parts of the duodenum.[6,45–47] The duodenal lumen is either normal, greatly narrowed, or entirely obliterated, and duodenal obstruction may be caused by a diaphragm, distal to the annulus.[45,48,49] Annular pancreas is believed to result either from fixation of the tip of the ventral anlage, so that it persists in its rotational pathway around the duodenum, or from a persistent left lobe of the ventral pancreatic bud. The embryonic ventral pancreatic bud is bilobed and normally the left lobe atrophies before rotation. Annular pancreas has the same distribution of pancreatic polypeptide cells as the normally located ventral primordium.[50] The islets have the irregular outlines of the normal ventral pancreatic islets and the acinar cells have morphologic attributes of normal ventral pancreatic acinar cells.[51] At pancreatography, annular pancreas displays a ringlike duct, surrounding the duodenum, that drains into the duct of Wirsung. Multiple smaller ducts are sometimes present, instead of one large duct.

The prevalence of annular pancreas is not accurately determined. Three instances of annular pancreas were found among 20,000 autopsies at Johns Hopkins Hospital.[52] Annular pancreas accounts for 30% of cases of intrinsic duodenal obstruction in children, and an incidence rate of 1 symptomatic case per 20,000 births is estimated from the data of Irving and

Rickham.[45] However, this figure does not include cases diagnosed in adults, where there has been no history of infantile duodenal obstruction. Some individuals with annular pancreas remain asymptomatic throughout their life and the abnormality is first detected at autopsy.

Annular pancreas is the single most common cause of duodenal obstruction in infancy, although when the obstruction manifests in the first week of life, it is usually accompanied by duodenal atresia or stenosis.[45,53] The plain film of the abdomen shows a "double bubble" sign, which is large air bubbles in the stomach and first part of the duodenum. With contrast medium, the dilated first part of duodenum and constricted second part are recognized.[54] The double bubble sign has been identified antenatally by ultrasonography.[55] Maternal hydramnios may be present when the duodenum is obstructed.

About one quarter of pediatric cases of annular pancreas are associated with Down syndrome.[56–59] Other congenital malformations that are often associated with annular pancreas are malrotation, abnormalities of the heart and great vessels, esophageal atresia, imperforate anus, Meckel's diverticulum, and unilateral absence of kidney.[45,54] It has also been described in the Rothmund–Thomson syndrome (poikiloderma, short stature, sparse hair, juvenile cataracts, small hands and feet, bone defects, photosensitivity, hypogonadism, defective dentition, onychodystrophy, and hyperkeratosis).[60] Familial occurrences of annular pancreas have been recorded.[45]

More than half of those patients with symptomatic, annular pancreas present in adulthood, most often in the fourth or fifth decade of life, with partial or complete obstruction of the duodenum due to pancreatitis of the annulus,[51,56,57] a complication that occurs in 13% of patients.[56] Episodic abdominal pain is the most frequent symptom.[56,57] The annulus may be diagnosed on ultrasound, barium study, endoscopy, or CT. Annular pancreas is one cause of retention of small foreign objects in the stomach or duodenum.[61] Rarely, it may be a cause of extrahepatic biliary obstruction and jaundice.[62] Microscopically, the pancreatic tissue not only surrounds the duodenum but actually grows into the muscle coat, in most cases. The usual treatment for annular pancreas is surgical bypass, because mechanical division of the ectopic tissue is not effective.

VARIATIONS OF PANCREATIC DUCTAL ANATOMY AND PANCREAS DIVISUM

Pancreatography has given us new insight into the variations of pancreatic ductal anatomy and their relationships with disease states (Fig. 2–1). The most common arrangement, in about 71% to 90% of people, is that the main pancreatic duct (of Wirsung) drains the tail, body, and part of the head of pancreas through the ampulla of Vater, whereas in 10% to 29% of individuals, the dorsal duct (duct of Santorini) is the major pancreatic duct.[6] The diameters of pancreatic ducts have been measured in pancreatograms and show a progressive decline in caliber from head to tail. The mean diameter of the lumen in the head is 3.6 mm; in the body, 2.7 mm; and in the tail, 1.6 mm.[63] Embryologically, the main duct is derived from fusion of the ventral pancreatic duct with the dorsal pancreatic duct, so that the main channel runs through what was originally ventral duct. The downstream (proximal) part of the dorsal duct becomes the accessory duct of Santorini and drains part of the embryonic dorsal pancreas into the duodenum through the minor papilla, 2 cm proximal to the ampulla of Vater. Normally, the accessory duct communicates with the main duct. Anomalies can be divided into two main types—those involving the accessory duct and those involving the main duct[6,64,65] (Fig. 2–1). The accessory duct may empty in a retrograde fashion into the main duct, there being no minor papilla. It may fail to communicate with the main duct but may empty normally through a minor papilla, or it may be absent altogether. Similarly, the dorsal duct may follow its original embryonic course and empty through the minor papilla while communicating with the ventral duct, which remains a lesser duct and empties with the bile duct through the ampulla of Vater. Rarely, the accessory duct atrophies entirely and the only drainage is through the minor papilla. Lastly, the ducts may remain as separate entities.

Complete failure of the two pancreatic primordia to fuse is rare. The term *pancreas divisum* is nowadays used to describe failure of fusion of the dorsal and ventral pancreatic ducts, despite normal fusion of the parenchymal tissue. The larger dorsal pancreas, including the neck, body, and tail, drains through the minor papilla and the ventral pancreas through the papilla of Vater. Pancreas divisum has been called a variety of other names, including *dominant dor-*

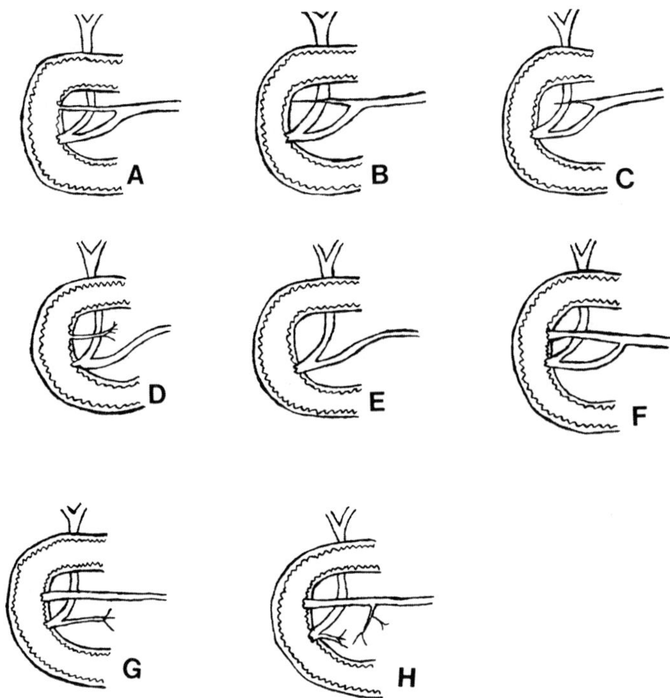

Figure 2–1. Variations in the anatomy of the pancreatic duct. *A,* Both ducts open separately into the duodenum (60% of individuals). *B,* The duct of Santorini ends blindly in the duodenal wall. *C,* The duct of Santorini ends blindly before reaching the duodenum. *D,* The ducts of Santorini and Wirsung are not connected. *E,* Absent duct of Santorini. *F,* Usual anatomy, but the duct of Santorini is the same size as or larger than the duct of Wirsung. *G,* The ducts are not connected and the duct of Wirsung is short and narrow. *H,* The duct of Santorini drains almost the whole pancreas. (From Skandalakis JE, Gray SW, Rowe JS, et al.: Anatomical complications of pancreatic surgery. Contemporary Surgery 15:17–50, 1979.)

sal duct syndrome. Pancreas divisum usually occurs without other anomalies but has been seen in association with annular pancreas, duodenal web, and duodenal atresia. A familial occurrence of pancreas divisum with pancreatitis has been described.[66] The family in question was not investigated for trypsinogen mutations, which are the main cause of hereditary pancreatitis. Other studies report an incidence of pancreas divisum occurring in children with pancreatitis in the range of 12% to 25%.[64,67–69]

Pancreas divisum is found by endoscopic retrograde cholangiopancreatography (ERCP) or by magnetic resonance cholangiopancreatography in between 1% and 9% of patients, depending on the population studied,[70] with an average figure being between 3.6%, reported by Axon et al.,[63] and 5.5% in patients with no clinical pancreatic disease, reported by Delhaye et al.[71]

Pancreas divisum is thought by some to be a cause of abdominal pain and pancreatitis, arising from inadequate drainage of the dorsal pancreas through the narrow minor papilla. However, studies are contradictory and some large series did not find an increased incidence of pancreas divisum in patients presenting with pancreatitis, either acute or chronic.[71,72] The 5% of French patients with chronic calcifying pancreatitis who have pancreas divisum show no difference in disease behavior from those patients with normal pancreatic anatomy.[73] However, Cotton found that among 78 patients with recurrent pancreatitis unexplained by other causes, the incidence of pancreas divisum was 25.6%.[69] In addition, there are several recorded cases in which chronic pancreatitis was confined to the part of the pancreas drained by the dorsal duct, supporting the idea that the anatomic abnormality predisposes to pancreatitis.[69,74,75] Sphincterotomy of the minor papilla effectively prevents relapse of acute pancreatitis in patients with pancreas divisum but has no effect in patients with other causes for chronic pancreatitis.[76] It is proposed that high pressures in the dorsal duct, combined with narrowing of the accessory papillae, may account for clinical symptoms and induce pancreatitis. A variety of therapeutic procedures, aimed at correcting what is perceived as an excessively narrow minor papilla or duct of Santorini, have been proposed. These include papillotomy, stenting, and sphincteroplasty. The results are hard to compare from one series to another, because of different diagnostic indications, differences in procedures, and the variety of added procedures, such as cholecystectomy.

PANCREATOBILIARY MALJUNCTION

The ventral pancreas develops as a bud or branch off the common bile duct, and thus in most people (85%), the ventral pancreatic duct and common bile duct fuse to form a common distal channel. Variations of normal include a short common channel, separate openings of both ducts at the ampulla, and pancreaticobiliary maljunction (PBM), in which the union of the pancreatic and biliary ducts occurs proximal to the duodenal wall. This malformation results in a common channel that is abnormally long. PBM may be seen alone or in combination with choledochal cysts,[77] congenital biliary dilation,[78] congenital biliary atresia,[79] and intrahepatic choledocholithiasis.[78] Because fluid pressure in the pancreatic duct is higher than in the biliary tract, pancreatic juice may flow into the biliary tree and gallbladder. This is the likely cause of the dilation of the biliary tract[80] and results in elevated amylase levels within choledochal cysts. Direct cholangiography in patients with this abnormality also shows that bile refluxes into the pancreatic duct.[81] Carcinoma of the bile ducts frequently complicates choledochal cysts but also occurs in cases of PBM without cyst formation. Carcinoma of the gallbladder also complicates maljunction in cases with or without bile duct cysts. In one study, 8 of 18 patients with PBM developed a carcinoma.[82] In another study, 12% of gallbladder cancers occurred in association with PBM.[83] Experiments reveal that exposure of the biliary tree to pancreatic juice results in epithelial damage and accelerated cell turnover, conditions known to favor neoplasia.[6] Prophylactic cholecystectomy is now recommended for patients with anomalous pancreatobiliary junction. The anomaly also predisposes to acute pancreatitis.[84,85] Cases of PBM have been described in which the anomaly was accompanied by an abnormally located papilla in the fourth portion of the duodenum.[86] The relationship of PBM to carcinomas of the gallbladder and extrahepatic biliary tree is further described in Chapters 13 and 15.

HETEROTOPIC PANCREAS

Heterotopic pancreas is generally defined as pancreatic tissue present outside its usual location and not connected to the pancreas proper. Heterotopia may result from aberrant contact between the ventral pancreatic anlage and other tissues during rotation of the anlage in embryonic life. It may also be the result of anomalous differentiation by embryonic endoderm. Heterotopic pancreas is most often found in the stomach, duodenum, or proximal jejunum but also occurs in the ileum, colon, ampulla of Vater, mesentery, Meckel's diverticulum, other diverticula, gallbladder, liver, omentum, and spleen.[6,87–90] Other rare sites include the umbilicus, fallopian tube,[91] mediastinum,[92] gastric duplication,[93] ileal duplication,[94] rectal duplication,[95] and intralobular pulmonary sequestration.[96] Most heterotopias contain pancreatic acini, but some merely consist of ducts and ductules without acinar cells. As these are usually intermingled with the fibers of the muscularis propria or muscularis mucosae, they have been termed *adenomyomas.* Brunner-type glands may be present, too. Benign teratomas of the anterior mediastinum often contain pancreas.[97]

Heterotopic pancreas is more often an incidental finding at surgery or autopsy (56% of cases) than a cause of symptoms (44%).[98] In the small bowel or stomach, it forms a mural or submucosal nodule or a polypoid outgrowth and can undergo ulceration, intussusception, obstruction, and cyst formation.[98–102] It can be complicated by inflammation, "pancreatitis," pseudocyst, or pseudotumor.[99] Cystic change and inflammation ("cystic dystrophy") in heterotopic pancreas located in the duodenal or gastric wall can cause abdominal pain and luminal stenosis and can mimic carcinoma on imaging studies. This has sometimes resulted in Whipple's operation being carried out inappropriately.[103] Heterotopia with dilated ducts and mucus retention can mimic mucinous carcinoma of the stomach,[104] and if islets predominate, it may mimic carcinoid tumor.[105] Heterotopic pancreas at the ampulla of Vater can cause biliary obstruction.[106] In the stomach, heterotopic pancreas may present as a mural mass or polyp. Most heterotopias are located in the prepyloric antrum; the remainder, in the proximal antrum. Less than half have a central punctum, often large in relation to the mass, simulating a gastric ulcer or ulcerated neoplasm.[107]

Grossly, heterotopic pancreas is usually a nodule of variable size, between 2 mm and 4 cm in diameter, that drains to the mucosa through a central punctum, which may give a bull's-eye image on barium radiography. The bulk of the heterotopia is most often located in submucosa but may also be found in the muscle coat, or serosa. The cut surface is yellowish, firm, and faintly lobulated. Microscopically, the elements of normal pancreas, acini, ductules, ducts, and islets of Langerhans are usually present in normal proportions, although in about one third of patients with heterotopic pancreas, islets are absent (Fig. 2–2). Carcinoma may occasionally arise in heterotopic pancreas, especially in the wall of the stomach,[108] but rarely in the jejunum.[109] Nesidioblastosis has also been described in the islets of Langerhans in ectopic pancreas.[110] A single example of solid-cystic-papillary neoplasm that arose in ectopic pancreas located in the mesocolon has been reported.[111]

Table 2–2. Cysts of the Pancreas

True congenital cysts
Simple cyst
Enterogenous cyst
Dermoid cyst
Polycystic conditions
Isolated polycystic disease of the pancreas
Polycystic disease of pancreas with von Hippel–Lindau disease
Polycystic disease of pancreas with polycystic kidney disease
Pancreatic macrocysts with cystic fibrosis
Acquired cysts
Pseudocyst: acute and chronic
Retention cyst
Parasitic cyst: *Echinococcus, Taenia solium*
Lymphoepithelial cyst and cyst in ectopic spleen
Neoplastic cysts
Serous cystadenoma
Mucinous cystadenoma and cystadenocarcinoma
Cystic degeneration in a ductal adenocarcinoma
Cystic acinar cell carcinoma
Papillary-cystic neoplasm
Cystic islet cell tumor
Cystic teratoma and cystic choriocarcinoma
Other cysts
Cystic angiomas
Multicystic pancreatic hamartoma
Endometriotic cyst
Cysts of uncertain type

CYSTS OF THE PANCREAS

There are a variety of cystic developmental lesions of the pancreas. These need to be distinguished from cystic neoplasms and pseudocysts, as the prognosis and treatment is quite different. True cysts are lined by epithelium, whereas pseudocysts are lined by granulation tissue and connective tissue. A classification of pancreatic cysts is given in Table 2–2.

SIMPLE CONGENITAL CYST

Congenital cysts are derived from the ductal system; they may be solitary or multiple and are usually unilocular. They are lined by a single layer of flattened or cuboidal epithelium, although rarely, there may be squamous metaplasia. The majority of congenital cysts are small and asymptomatic, although, in infants, rare examples have been so large that they pre-

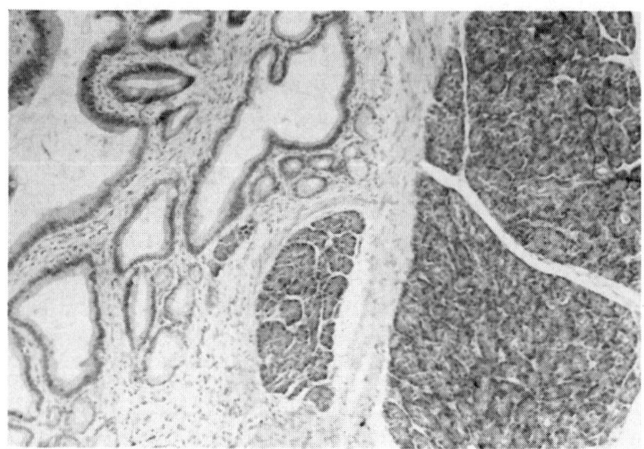

Figure 2–2. Heterotopic pancreas in the wall of the stomach. The tissue is lobulated and, in this example, contains only ducts and acini without islets.

sented with abdominal distension.[112–114] Solitary cysts are usually not associated with cysts in other organs. One 15-cm cyst in a 50-year-old woman was associated with splenic vein thrombosis and bleeding esophageal varices.[115] Multiple congenital malformations, in conjunction with pancreatic cysts, were seen in one infant.[116] Pancreatitis has been attributed to a large cyst.[117] This patient was a girl who presented with repeated episodes of widespread osteolysis, subcutaneous fat necrosis, and periarticular fat necrosis mimicking arthritis. Her symptoms persisted for 4 years, after an initial episode of severe abdominal pain.[117] The differential diagnosis of congenital cysts from cystic neoplasms is based on their bland histologic features, lack of mucin secretion, and absence of epithelial papillary tufts. There is no evidence that congenital cysts are premalignant. Rarely, unilocular true cysts have been reported in adults.[118]

The rare *multilocular congenital pancreatic cyst* is most often seen in infant girls, although it has been demonstrated in utero by ultrasound examination. Conventional radiographic signs and clinical symptoms primarily reflect mass effects, whereas imaging modalities demonstrate the cystic nature of the mass. Although rare, this cyst should be considered in the differential diagnosis of fetal and pediatric cystic abdominal masses.[119]

ENTEROGENOUS CYST

Ciliated cysts of foregut origin, equivalent to bronchogenic cysts and *enteric duplication cysts* (enterogenous cysts), are rarely found within the pancreas itself, either in adults or in children, but are more likely to be located on the surface of the pancreas.[120–125] They arise from gastric or intestinal tissue that was displaced in embryonic life. Enterogenous cysts are recognized by the specific characteristics of their lining epithelium and the presence of a muscle coat. The epithelium may be gastric or intestinal or may be a pseudostratified ciliated epithelium with goblet cells. The muscularis of enterogenous cysts is thin and composed of the usual two distinct layers, characteristic of bowel wall. Enteric duplication cysts are otherwise found most commonly in the distal ileum, the posterior mediastinum, and the third part of the duodenum. In one described case, the cyst fluid revealed elevated carcinoembryonic antigen (CEA) and carbohydrate antigen (CA) 125 with increased fluid viscosity, features otherwise typical of a mucinous cystic neoplasm.[121] The term *alimentary duplication* has been used for congenital malformations that are connected to, and share the same blood supply as, their enteric origin. They may have a communication with one of the pancreatic ducts. Typically, these duplications are lined by gastric-type epithelium and have ectopic pancreatic tissue within their walls.[121,126,127] They commonly present in childhood with pancreatitis.

POLYCYSTIC DISEASE

Polycystic disease of the pancreas may be an isolated condition or a manifestation of one of three hereditary diseases: von Hippel–Lindau disease, cystic fibrosis, or polycystic kidney disease.[128–130] A full clinical and family history, including documentation of the presence or absence of tumors of the central nervous system or retina, together with imaging of the kidneys and liver, will clarify the type of cyst. Histologically, in all the above disorders, the multiple cysts are lined by a single layer of epithelium and cannot be distinguished morphologically. Von Hippel–Lindau disease should be suspected if there is a family history of any of its main manifestations. This includes hemangioblastomas of the cerebellum or of other parts of the central nervous system, including the retina, multiple renal cysts, renal cell carcinoma, pheochromocytoma, epididymal cystadenoma, pancreatic cysts, pancreatic cystadenocarcinoma, or islet cell tumor.[131]

Pancreatic cysts are uncommon in adult polycystic kidney disease but are nearly always present, along with hepatic cysts, in the infantile type of polycystic kidney disease. Unlike the renal lesions, the pancreatic cysts are not clinically important. Pediatric cases of kidney, hepatic, and pancreatic cysts fall into Potter types I and II polycystic disease.[128] Most children with polycystic kidney disease who also have pancreatic cysts do not survive into adulthood.[128] Pancreatic cysts can also occur in association with congenital hepatic fibrosis.

Fibrocystic disease of the pancreas (see Chapter 4) commonly gives rise to microcysts, but only rarely does it produce macroscopic cysts. The cysts generally contain characteristic inspissated eosinophilic secretions. The remainder of the pancreas is atrophic and fibrotic.[128] A case of CHARGE syndrome has been associated with fibrocystic disease of the pancreas. This syndrome is characterized by colobomatous malformation, heart defect, atresia choanae, growth and mental deficiency, genital hypoplasia, and ear anomalies with or without deafness. Any four of these defects are sufficient to establish the diagnosis.[132]

Patients with trisomy 13 may develop pancreatic microcysts, along with focal proliferation of small ductules. In about half of these patients, there is intrapancreatic splenic tissue.[133]

Polycystic disease of the pancreas may very rarely occur as an isolated finding. In these instances, the lesion at surgery has been described as resembling a cluster of grapes.

DERMOID CYSTS

These unusual lesions are seen in children more often than in adults. In common with ovarian and mediastinal dermoid cysts, they are benign cystic teratomas that exude thick, greasy sebum when opened. They present with abdominal mass, sometimes in the left upper quadrant. The lining epithelium is squamous and may incorporate sebaceous and sweat glands. Mesenchymal components include adipose tissue and cartilage. Teethlike structures are often present. Fine-needle aspiration (FNA) in one patient yielded cyst fluid containing numerous benign mature squamous cells, keratin, and inflammatory cells.[134]

EPIDERMOID CYSTS AND ECTOPIC SPLEEN WITHIN THE PANCREAS

The rare entity of epidermoid cysts and ectopic spleen within the pancreas was first reported in the tail of pancreas of a 40-year-old man who presented with abdominal pain, nausea, and vomiting.[131] A similar instance was discovered in a 32-year-old Japanese woman. The cyst wall consisted of three components: an inner lining of mature squamous epithelium with keratinization, a middle layer consisting of splenic pulp with a sinus structure, and a peripheral layer of dense fibrous connective tissue in which some involutional pancreatic ducts and islets were recognized.[136] The histogenesis of this anomaly is undetermined.

LYMPHOEPITHELIAL CYSTS

Lymphoepithelial cysts, which are uncommon, resemble branchial cleft cysts and are lined by stratified squamous epithelium that is surrounded by lymphoid tissue[137–140] (Fig. 2–3). The lymphoid tissue merges into compressed pancreatic tissue. Numerous lymphocytes, mainly T cells, are present in the lining epithelium, and germinal centers can be present. The cysts are well circumscribed and commonly about 6 cm in diameter. Epithelial cords, continuous with the squamous epithelium lining the cyst, may radiate out through the lymph-

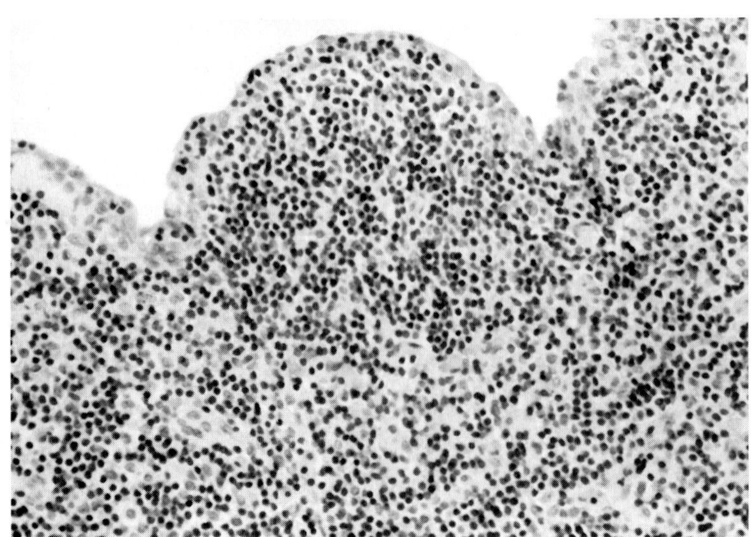

Figure 2–3. Lymphoepithelial cyst of the pancreas.

oid tissue toward the pancreatic parenchyma.[139] The histogenesis is uncertain. They may arise from benign epithelial inclusions in peripancreatic or intrapancreatic lymph nodes, followed by squamous metaplasia of the epithelial inclusion,[140] or they may arise directly from pancreatic ducts.[139] One example has shown sebaceous differentiation within the squamous epithelium.[141]

Most lymphoepithelial cysts are discovered by abdominal imaging studies in young adults, presenting with various symptoms that may include backache and weight loss. Some patients are asymptomatic. Lymphoepithelial cysts may resemble pseudocysts or cystic neoplasms on imaging studies. They are usually unilocular.[142] FNA cytology may confirm a benign preoperative assessment.[143] The cyst contains fluid with keratin debris and exfoliated squames. Fluid aspirated from one lymphoepithelial cyst showed elevated CEA and CA 19.9, erroneously pointing to a diagnosis of cystic pancreatic carcinoma.[139]

MULTICYSTIC PANCREATIC HAMARTOMA

The term *multicystic pancreatic hamartoma* has been used to describe a unique anomaly.[144,145] One well-described case involved a 20-month-old girl who presented with abdominal distension and tenderness. The hamartoma consisted of a 9-cm–diameter encapsulated cystic mass located in the lower aspect of the head of the pancreas. The cut surface demonstrated numerous cysts filled with clear yellow fluid, ranging from 0.3 to 1.2 cm in diameter. Solid areas were present and composed of fleshy, tan-pink tissue. Histologically, the mass was composed of large, irregular lobules of well-formed pancreatic acini, admixed with fat, fibrous tissue, and cystically dilated ducts. Islets of Langerhans were absent, but insulin-producing cells, and other endocrine cells, were dispersed throughout the exocrine tissue as single cells or small groups.[144] A second case of pancreatic hamartoma was described in a 25-year-old man who presented with a nontender mass in the upper right quadrant of his abdomen. All laboratory findings were normal. A solid and cystic mass, 10.6 cm in maximum diameter, was excised. Histologically, the cystic areas represented dilated ducts, which were surrounded by dense fibrous tissue. The solid areas represented lobules of acinar tissue. Islets were present alongside the dilated ducts.[145] This mixture of mature cell types in abnormal proportions fulfills the criteria for a hamartoma, or malformation, rather than a neoplasm.

OTHER CYSTS

Endometriotic cysts of the pancreas have been recorded.[146–148] These occur in women in the third and fourth decades of life and patients present with abdominal pain resembling pancreatitis. The lesion is frequently cystic[145,146] and is located in the tail of the pancreas. In one example, the mass was large enough to be confused, preoperatively, with a renal neoplasm.[147]

Solitary cysts of the head of pancreas, demonstrable on pancreatography, have been reported in adults. These have been termed *retention cysts* but are likely to be pseudocysts, not congenital cystic abnormalities.[149]

CONGENITAL ANOMALIES IN ADULTS

Congenital abnormalities of the pancreaticobiliary tree may go undetected until adulthood. In adult patients with persistent and unexplained signs and symptoms, such as cholangitis, pancreatitis, jaundice, recurrent abdominal pain, nausea, and vomiting, a congenital anomaly of the pancreatic or bile duct must be considered. Confirmation of the diagnosis may be obtained by performing cholangiopancreatography. The most common congenital pancreaticobiliary abnormalities encountered in adults are choledochal cyst, anomalous junction of the pancreatic and common bile ducts, aberrant biliary ducts, and pancreas divisum. More rarely, choledochoceles, multiple communicating intra- and extrahepatic duct cysts, Caroli's disease, pancreaticobiliary abnormalities associated with situs anomalies, annular pancreas, and aberrant pancreatic ducts associated with enteric duplication cysts are encountered. Cholangiopancreatography usually allows confirmation of diagnosis and may demonstrate associated abnormalities, such as choledocholithiasis or neoplasms. In some instances, confusion with acquired pseudocysts may occur. Accurate diagnosis of congenital anomalies will aid in surgical planning and prevent inadvertent ductal injury. Although congenital pancreaticobiliary abnormalities are relatively uncommon, the increased prevalence of cholangitis, gallstones and cholangiocarcinoma that occurs with the various types of biliary cystic disease and junctional anomalies and the association of pancreatitis with pancreatic anomalies make recognition of variant anatomy clinically important.[150]

REFERENCES

1. Lemons JA, Ridenour R, Orsini EN: Congenital absence of the pancreas and intrauterine growth retardation. Pediatrics 64:255–257, 1979.
2. Warkany J, Passarge E, Smith LB: Congenital malformations in autosomal trisomy syndromes. Am J Dis Child. 112:502–517, 1966.
3. Wockel W, Scheibner K: Aplasie des Pankreas mit Diabetes mellitus, intrahepatische Gallengangsaplasie und weitere Missbildungen bei einem hypotorophen Neugeborenen. (Aplasia of the pancreas with diabetes mellitus, aplasia of the intrahepatic bile ducts, and additional malformations in a small-for-date baby). Zentralbl Allg Pathol 121:186–194, 1977.
4. Voldsgaard P, Kryger-Baggesen N, Lisse I: Agenesis of the pancreas. Acta Paediatr 83:791–793, 1994.
5. Habeck JO, Kunzel W, Muller D, et al.: Kurzrippen-Polydaktylie-Syndrom Typ III (Verma-Naumoff) mit Zeichen einer ektodermalen Dysplasie. (Type III shortrib-polydactyly syndrome (Verma-Naumoff) in concomitance with ectodermal dysplasia). Zentralbl Gynakol 104:568–575, 1982.
6. Kozu T, Suda K, Toki F: Pancreatic development and anatomical variation. Gastrointest Endosc Clin N Am 5:1–30, 1995.
7. Leese T, Cliche L, Bismuth H: Pancreatitis caused by congenital anomalies of the pancreatic ducts. Surgery 105:125–130, 1989.
8. Klein WA, Dabesies MA, Freidman AC, et al.: Agenesis of the dorsal pancreas in a patient with weight loss and diabetes mellitus. Dig Dis Sci 39:1708–1713, 1994.
9. Soler R, Rodriguez E, Comesana ML, et al.: Agenesis of the dorsal pancreas with polysplenia syndrome: CT features. J Comput Assist Tomogr 16:921–923, 1992.
10. Wildling R, Schnedl WJ, Reisinger EC, et al.: Agenesis of the dorsal pancreas in a woman with diabetes mellitus and in both of her sons. Gastroenterology 104:1182–1186, 1993.
11. Lechner GW, Read RC: Agenesis of the dorsal pancreas in an adult diabetic presenting with duodenal ileus. Ann Surg 163:311–314, 1966.
12. Deignan RW, Nizzero A, Malone DE: Case report: Agenesis of the dorsal pancreas: A cause of diagnostic error on abdominal sonography. Clin Radiol 51:145–147, 1996.
13. Theodor F. Angeborene aplasie der gallenwege verbunden mit Lebercirrhose, durch Operation behandelt. Arch Kinderheilkd 49:358, 1909 (Cited by Wilding [reference 10]).
14. Gilinski NH, delFavero G, Cotton PB, et al.: Congenital short pancreas: A report of two cases. Gut 26:304–310, 1985.
15. Shimizu T, Kakitsubata Y, Watanabe K, et al.: A case of aplasia of the pancreatic body and tail accidentally detected on computed tomography. Rinsho Hoshasen 35:1443–1445, 1990.
16. Nishimori I, Okazaki K, Morita M, et al.: Congenital hypoplasia of the dorsal pancreas: With special reference to duodenal papillary dysfunction. Am J Gastroenterol 85:1029–1033, 1990.
17. Morita M, Otsubo C, Kozu T, et al.: Aplasia of the body and tail of the pancreas—a report to two cases. Nippon Shokakibyo Gakkai Zasshi 77:102–106, 1980.
18. Herman TE, Siegel MJ: Polysplenia syndrome and congenital short pancreas. AJR Am J Roentgenol 156:799–800, 1991.
19. Wainwright H, Nelson M: Polysplenia syndrome and congenital short pancreas. Am J Med Genet 47:318–320, 1993.
20. Suda K, Matsumoto Y, Fujii H, et al.: Clinicopathologic differentiation of atrophy of the pancreatic body and tail aplasia. Int J Pancreatol 24:227–235, 1998.
21. Dodge JA, Laurence KM: Congenital absence of islets of Langerhans. Arch Dis Child 52:411–413, 1977.
22. Durie PR: Inherited causes of exocrine pancreatic dysfunction. Can J Gastroenterol 11:145–152, 1997.
23. Lumb G, Bequtyman W: Hypoplasia of the exocrine tissue of the pancreas. J Pathol Bacteriol 94:679–686, 1952.
24. Winter WE, MacLaren NK, Riley WJ, et al.: Congenital pancreatic hypoplasia: A syndrome of exocrine and endocrine pancreatic insufficiency. J Pediatr 109:465–468, 1986.
25. Carroll PB, Finegold DN, Becker DJ, et al.: Hypoplasia of the pancreas in a patient with type I diabetes mellitus. Pancreas 7:21–25, 1992.
26. Yorifuji T, Matsumura M, Okuno T, et al.: Hereditary pancreatic hypoplasia, diabetes mellitus and congenital heart disease: A new syndrome? J Med Genet 31:331–333, 1994.
27. Szilagyi PG, Corsetti J, Callahan CM, et al.: Pancreatic exocrine aplasia, clinical features of leprechaunism and abnormal gonadotropin regulation. Pediatr Pathol 7:51–61, 1987.
28. Strayer DS, Kissane JM: Dysplasia of the kidneys, liver and pancreas: Report of a variant of Ivemark's syndrome. Hum Pathol 10:228–234, 1979.
29. Townes PL, White MR: Identity of two syndromes. Proteolytic, lipolytic and amylolytic deficiency of the exocrine pancreas with congenital anomalies. Am J Dis Child 135:248–250, 1981.
30. Daentl DL, Frias JL, Gilbert EF, et al.: The Johanson-Blizzard syndrome: Case report and autopsy findings. Am J Med Genet 3:129–135, 1979.
31. Van Assche FA, Prins F, Aerts L, et al.: The endocrine pancreas in small-for-dates infants. Br J Obstet Gynaecol 84:751–753, 1977.
32. Harms K, Klinge O, Speer CP: Variability of the Jeune syndrome. Lung hypoplasia, renal failure and direct hyperbilirubinemia in a newborn infant. Monatsschr Kinderheilkd 141:868–873, 1993.
33. Rapola J, Salonen R: Visceral anomalies in the Meckel syndrome. Teratology 31:193–201, 1985.
34. Turkel SB, Diehl EJ, Richmond JA: Necropsy findings in neonatal asphyxiating thoracic dystrophy. J Med Genet 22:112–118, 1985.
35. Shwachman H, Diamond LK, Oski FA, et al.: The syndrome of pancreatic insufficiency and bone marrow dysfunction. J Pediatr 65:645–663, 1964.
36. Bodian M, Sheldon W, Lightwood R: Congenital hypoplasia of the exocrine pancreas. Acta Pediatr Scand 53:282–293, 1964.
37. Aggett PJ, Cavanagh NPC, Matthew DJ, et al.: Shwachman's syndrome. Arch Dis Child 55:331–437, 1980.

38. Mack DR, Forstner GG, Wilschanski M, et al.: Shwachman syndrome: Exocrine pancreatic dysfunction and variable phenotypic expression. Gastroenterology 111:1593–1602, 1996.
39. Pearson HA, Lobel JS, Kocoshis SA, et al.: A new syndrome of refractory sideroblastic anemia with vacuolization of marrow precursors and exocrine pancreatic dysfunction. J Pediatr 95:976–984, 1979.
40. Rotig A, Cormier V, Koll F, et al.: Site-specific deletions of the mitochondrial genome in the Pearson marrow-pancreas syndrome. Genomics 10:502–504, 1991.
41. Morris AA, Lamont PJ, Clayton PT: Pearson's syndrome without marrow involvement. Arch Dis Child 77:56–57, 1997.
42. Simonsz HJ, Barlocher K, Rotig A: Kearns-Sayre's syndrome developing in a boy who survived Pearson's syndrome caused by mitochondrial DNA deletion. Doc Ophthalmol 82:73–79, 1992.
43. Sansone G, Masera G, Terzoli S, et al.: Congenital refractory anaemia with vacuolisation of bone marrow precursors, sideroblastosis and growth failure in a girl with normal endocrine pancreatic function. Haematologica 74:587–590, 1989.
44. Morikawa Y, Matsuura N, Kakudo K, et al.: Pearson's marrow/pancreas syndrome: A histological and genetic study. Virchows Arch A Pathol Anat Histopathol 423:227–231, 1993.
45. Irving IM, Rickham PP: Duodenal atresia and stenosis: Annular pancreas. *In* Lister J, Irving IM (eds): Neonatal Surgery, 3rd ed. London: Butterworth, pp 355–370, 1990.
46. Urayama S, Kozarek R, Ball T, et al.: Presentation and treatment of annular pancreas in an adult population. Am J Gastroenterol 90:995–999, 1995.
47. England RE, Newcomer MK, Leung JW, et al.: Case report: annular pancreas divisum—a report of two cases and a review of the literature. Br J Radiol 68:324–328, 1995.
48. Elliott B, Kliman MR, Elliott KA: Pancreatic annulus: A sign or a cause of duodenal obstruction? Can J Surg 11:357–364, 1968.
49. Fantoni PA, Kaluso G, Sequenzia S, et al.: Duodenal stenosis from intramural cystic annular pancreas. Hepatogastroenterology 43:776–778, 1996.
50. Suda K: Immunohistochemical and gross dissection studies of annular pancreas. Acta Pathol Jpn 40:505–508, 1990.
51. Rode J, Dowsett J, Russell RCG: The annular pancreas derives from the ventral primordium (abstract). J Pathol 155:351A, 1988.
52. Ravitch MM: Anomalies of the pancreas. *In* Carey LC (ed): The Pancreas. St Louis: Mosby, pp 404–427, 1973.
53. Synn AY, Mulvihill SJ, Fonkalsrud EW: Surgical disorders of the pancreas in infancy and childhood. Am J Surg 156:201–205, 1988.
54. Warkany J: The Pancreas. *In* Congenital Malformations, Notes and Comments. Chicago: Year Book Medical Publishers, pp. 729–731, 1971.
55. Pachi A, Maggi E, Giancotti A, et al.: Ultrasound diagnosis of fetal annular pancreas. J Perinatal Med 17:361–364, 1989.
56. Yogi Y, Shibue T, Hashimoto S: Annular pancreas detected in adults, diagnosed by endoscopic retrograde cholangiopancreatography: Report of four cases. Gastroenterol Japn 22:92–99, 1987.
57. Lloyd-Jones W, Mountain JC, Warren KW: Annular pancreas in the adult. Ann Surg 176:163–170, 1972.
58. Akhtar J, Guiney EJ: Congenital duodenal obstruction. Br J Surg 79:133–135, 1992.
59. Kallen B, Mastroiacouo P, Robert E: Major congenital malformations in Down syndrome. Am J Med Genet 65:160–166, 1996.
60. Blaustein HS, Stevens AW, Stevens PD, et al.: Rothmund-Thomson syndrome associated with annular pancreas and duodenal stenosis: a case report. Pediatr Dermatol 10:159–163, 1993.
61. Kassner EG, Rose JS, Kottmeier PK, et al.: Retention of small foreign objects in the stomach and duodenum. A sign of partial obstruction caused by duodenal anomalies. Radiology 114:683–686, 1975.
62. Benger JR, Thompson MH: Annular pancreas and obstructive jaundice. Am J Gastroenterol 92:713–714, 1997.
63. Axon ATR, Classen M, Cotton PB, et al.: Pancreatography in chronic pancreatitis: International definitions. Gut 25:1107–1112, 1984.
64. Lindstrom E, Ihse I. Pancreatic disease caused by pancreas divisum. Eur J Surg 160:385–387, 1994.
65. Lehman GA, Sherman S: Pancreas divisum. Diagnosis, clinical significance and management alternatives. Gastrointest Endosc Clin N Am 5:145–170, 1995.
66. Muzaffar AR, Moyer MS, Dobbins J, et al.: Pancreas divisum in a family with hereditary pancreatitis. J Clin Gastroenterol 22:16–20, 1996.
67. Wagner CW, Golladay ES: Pancreas divisum and pancreatitis in children. Am Surg 54:22–26, 1988.
68. Richter JM, Schapiro RH, Mulley AG, et al.: Association of pancreas divisum and pancreatitis and its treatment by sphincteroplasty of the accessory ampulla. Gastroenterology 81:1104–1110, 1981.
69. Cotton PB: Congenital anomaly of pancreas division as cause of obstructive pain and pancreatitis. Gut 21:105–114, 1980.
70. Bret PM, Reinhold C, Taourel P, et al.: Pancreas divisum: Evaluation with MR cholangiopancreatography. Radiology 199:99–103, 1966.
71. Delhaye M, Engelholm L, Cremer M: Pancreas divisum: Congenital variant or anomaly? Gastroenterology 89:951–958, 1985.
72. Mitchell CJ, Lintott DJ, Ruddell WSJ, et al.: Clinical relevance of an unfused pancreatic duct system. Gut 20:1066–1077, 1979.
73. Barthet M, Valantin V, Spinosa S, et al.: Clinical course and morphological features of chronic calcifying pancreatitis associated with pancreas divisum. Eur J Gastroenterol Hepatol 7:993–998, 1995.
74. Rusnak CH, Hosie RT, Kuechler PM, et al.: Pancreatitis associated with pancreas divisum: Results of surgical intervention. Am J Surg 155:641–643, 1988.
75. Blair AJ, Russell CG, Cotton PB: Resection for pancreatitis in patients with pancreas divisum. Ann Surg 200:590–594, 1984.
76. Keith RG, Shapero TF, Saibil FG, et al.: Dorsal duct sphincterotomy is effective long-term treatment of acute pancreatitis associated with pancreas divisum. Surgery 106:660–666, 1989.
77. Babbitt DP: Congenital choledochal cysts: New etiological concept based on anomalous relationships of common bile duct and pancreatic bulb. Ann Radiol 12:231–240, 1969.
78. Kimura K, Ohto M, Ono T, et al.: Congenital cystic dilatation of the common bile duct: Relationship to anomalous pancreaticobiliary ductal union. Am J Roentgenol 128:571–577, 1977.

79. Suda K, Miyano T, Hashimoto K: The choledochopancreatico-ductal junction in infantile obstructive jaundice diseases. Acta Pathol Japn 30:187–194, 1980.
80. Lilly JR, Stellin GP, Karrer FM: Forme fruste choledochal cyst. J Pediatr Surg 20:449–451, 1985.
81. Kimura K, Tsugawa C, Ogawa K, et al.: Choledochal cyst. Etiological considerations and surgical management in 22 cases. Arch Surg 113:159–163, 1978.
82. Kimura K, Ohto M, Saisho H, et al.: Association of gallbladder carcinoma and anomalous pancreatobiliary ductal union. Gastroenterology 89:1258–1265, 1985.
83. Sugiyama M, Atomi Y: Anomalous pancreatobiliary junction without congenital choledochal cyst. Br J Surg 85:911–916, 1998.
84. Mori K, Nagakawa T, Ohta T, et al.: Acute pancreatitis associated with anomalous union of the pancreaticobiliary ductal system. J Clin Gastroenterol 13:673–677, 1991.
85. Mori K, Nagakawa T, Ohta T, et al.: Pancreatitis and anomalous union of the pancreaticobiliary ductal system in childhood. J Pediatr Surg 28:67–71, 1993.
86. Doty J, Hassell E, Fonkalsrud EW: Anomalous draining of the common bile duct into the fourth portion of the duodenum. Clinical sequelae. Arch Surg 120:1077–1079, 1985.
87. Taylor RH, Owen DA: Acute inflammation of pancreatic tissue in a Meckel's diverticulum. Can J Surg 25:656–657, 1982.
88. Qizilbash AH: Acute pancreatitis occurring in heterotopic pancreatic tissue in the gallbladder. Can J Surg 19:413–414, 1976.
89. Duphare H, Nijhawan S, Rana S, et al.: Heterotopic gastric and pancreatic tissue in large bowel. Am J Gastroenterol 85:68–71, 1990.
90. Dolan RV, ReMine WH, Dockerty MB: The fate of heterotopic pancreatic tissue. A study of 212 cases. Arch Surg 109:762–765, 1974.
91. Mason TE, Quagliarello JR: Ectopic pancreas in the fallopian tube. Report of a first case. Obstet Gynecol 48(suppl):70S–75S, 1976.
92. Carr MJ, Deiraniya AK, Judd PA: Mediastinal cyst containing mural pancreatic tissue. Thorax 32:512–516, 1977.
93. Ueda D, Taketazu M, Itoh S, et al.: A case of gastric duplication cyst with aberrant pancreas. Pediatr Radiol 21:379–380, 1991.
94. Sato T, Oyamada M, Chiba H, et al.: Ileal duplication cyst associated with heterotopic pancreas: Report of a case and literature review. Acta Pathol Japn 43:597–602, 1993.
95. Narasimharao KL, Patel RV, Malik AK, et al.: Chronic perianal fistula: Beware of rectal duplication. Postgrad Med J 63:213–214, 1987.
96. Corrin B, Danel C, Allaway A, et al.: Intralobar pulmonary sequestration of ectopic pancreatic tissue with gastropancreatic duplication. Thorax 40:637–638, 1985.
97. Suda K, Mizaguchi K, Hebisawa A, et al.: Pancreatic tissue in teratoma. Arch Pathol Lab Med 108:835–837, 1984.
98. Pang LC: Pancreatic heterotopia: A reappraisal and clinicopathologic analysis of 32 cases. South Med J 81:1264–1275, 1988.
99. Green PHR, Barratt PJ, Percy JP, et al.: Acute pancreatitis occurring in gastric aberrant pancreatic tissue. Am J Dig Dis 22:734–740, 1977.
100. Moen J, Mack E: Small bowel obstruction caused by heterotopic pancreas in an adult. Am Surg 55:503–504, 1989.
101. Claudon M, Verain AL, Bigard MA, et al.: Cyst formation in gastric heterotopic pancreas: report of two cases. Radiology 169:659–660, 1988.
102. Anseline P, Grundfest S, Carey W, et al.: Pancreatic heterotopia—a rare cause of bowel obstruction. Surgery 90:110–113, 1981.
103. Flejou J-F, Potet F, Molas G, et al.: Cystic dystrophy of the gastric and duodenal wall developing in heterotopic pancreas: an unrecognized entity. Gut 34:343–347, 1993.
104. Nopajaroonsri C: Mucus retention in heterotopic pancreas of the gastric antrum. Am J Surg Pathol 18:953–957, 1994.
105. Padberg B-C, Schroder S: Letter. Am J Surg Pathol 19:1445–1446, 1995.
106. Laughlin EH, Keown ME, Jackson JE. Heterotopic pancreas obstructing the ampulla of Vater. Arch Surg 118:979–980, 1983.
107. Kilman WJ, Berk RN: The spectrum of radiographic features of aberrant pancreatic tests involving the stomach. Radiology 123:291–296, 1977.
108. Barbosa J, Dockerty MB, Waugh JM: Pancreatic heterotopia: surgical cases. Proc Mayo Clin 21:246–255, 1946.
109. Persson GE, Boiesen PT: Cancer of aberrant pancreas in jejunum. Case report. Acta Chir Scand 154:599–601, 1988.
110. Seki S, Ikenoue T, Murakami N, et al.: Ectopic nesidioblastosis. Acta Paed Japn 32:308–310, 1990.
111. Ishikawa O, Ishiguor S, Ohhigashi H, et al.: Solid and papillary neoplasm arising from an ectopic pancreas in the mesocolon. Am J Gastroenterol 85:597–601, 1990.
112. Miles RM: Pancreatic cyst in the newborn; a case report. Ann Surg 149:576–581, 1959.
113. Power WH: Pancreatic cyst in infancy. Br Med J 5252:625–626, 1961.
114. Kalani BP, Broadhead RL, Bhargav RK: Giant congenital pancreatic cyst in a child. Ann Trop Pediatr 2:47–49, 1982.
115. Wolloch Y, Chaimoff C, Lukin E, et al.: Splenic vein thrombosis, segmental portal hypertension and bleeding esophageal varices produced by congenital pancreatic cyst. Isr J Med Sci 10:670–673, 1974.
116. De Lange C, Janssen TAE: Large solitary pancreatic cyst and other developmental errors in a premature infant. Am J Dis Child 75:587–594, 1948.
117. Hollingworth P, Isaacs D, Bydder G: Recurrent osteolytic lesions and subcutaneous fat necrosis in association with a developmental pancreatic cyst. Arch Dis Child 54:790–792, 1979.
118. Mao C, Greenwood S, Wagner S, et al.: Solitary true cyst of the pancreas in an adult. Int J Pancreatol 12:181–186, 1992.
119. Auringer ST, Ulmer JL, Sumner TE, et al.: Congenital cyst of the pancreas. J Pediatr Surg 28:1570–1571, 1993.
120. Kohzaki S, Fukuda T, Fujimoto T, et al.: Case report: Ciliated foregut cyst of the pancreas mimicking teratomatous tumour. Br J Radiol 67:601–604, 1994.
121. Pins MR, Compton CC, Southern JF, et al.: Ciliated enteric duplication cyst presenting as a pancreatic cystic neoplasm: Report of a case with cyst fluid analysis. Clin Chem 38:1501–1503, 1992.

122. Pilcher CS, Bradley EL 3rd, Majmudar B: Enterogenous cyst of the pancreas. Am J Gastroenterol 77:576–577, 1982.
123. Martin DF, Haboubi NY, Tweedle DE: Enteric cyst of the pancreas. Gastrointest Radiol 12:35–36, 1987.
124. D'Amato A, Montesani C, Narilli P, et al.: Enterogenous reduplication cyst of the pancreas. A case report. Ital J Surg Sci 14:337–340, 1984.
125. Johnstone DW, Forde KA, Markowitz D, et al.: Gastric duplication cyst communicating with the pancreatic duct: A rare cause of recurrent abdominal pain. Surgery 109:97–100, 1991.
126. Black PR, Welch KJ, Eraklis AJ: Juxtapancreatic intestinal duplications with pancreatic ductal communication: A cause of pancreatitis and recurrent abdominal pain in childhood. J Pediatr Surg 21:257–261, 1986.
127. Green PH, Barratt PJ, Percy JP, et al.: Acute pancreatitis occurring in gastric aberrant pancreatic tissue. Am J Dig Dis 22:734–740, 1977.
128. Howard JM: Cystic neoplasms and true cysts of the pancreas. Surg Clin North Am 69:651–665, 1989.
129. McGeogh JE, Darmady EM: Polycystic disease of kidney, liver and pancreas: A possible pathogenesis. J Pathol 119:221–228, 1976.
130. Neumann H, Dinkel E, Brambs H, et al.: Pancreatic lesions in von Hippel–Lindau syndrome. Gastroenterology 101:465–471, 1991.
131. Lamiell JM, Salazar FG, Hsia YE: Von Hippel–Lindau disease affecting 43 members of a single kindred. Medicine 68:1–29, 1989.
132. Giorgetti R, Gelso C, Riganti G, et al.: Un caso di associazione CHARGE e fibrosi cistica del pancreas. [A case of CHARGE with fibrocystic disease of the pancreas]. Minerva Pediatr 44:451–454, 1992.
133. Hashida Y, Jaffe R, Yunis EJ: Pancreatic pathology in trisomy 13: Specificity of the morphologic lesion. Pediatr Pathol 1:169–178, 1983.
134. Markovsky V, Russin VL: Fine-needle aspiration of dermoid cyst of the pancreas: A case report. Diagn Cytopathol 9:66–69, 1993.
135. Davidson ED, Campbell WG, Hersh T. Epidermoid splenic cyst occurring in an intrapancreatic accessory spleen. Dig Dis Sci 25:964–967, 1980.
136. Morohoshi T, Hamamoto T, Kunimura T, et al.: Epidermoid cyst derived from an accessory spleen in the pancreas. A case report with literature survey. Acta Pathol Jpn 41:916–921, 1991.
137. DiCorato MP, Schned AR: A rare lymphoepithelial cyst of the pancreas. Am J Clin Pathol 98:188–191, 1992.
138. Gafa R, Grandi E, Cavazzini L: Lymphoepithelial cyst of the pancreas. J Clin Pathol 50:794–795, 1997.
139. Kaiserling E, Seitz KH, Rettenmaier G, et al.: Lymphoepithelial cyst of the pancreas. Clinical, morphological and immunohistochemical findings. Zentralbl Pathol 137:431–438, 1991.
140. Kisaoka M, Haratake J, Horie A, et al.: Lymphoepithelial cyst of the pancreas in a 65-year-old man. Hum Pathol 22:924–926, 1991.
141. Fitko R, Kampmeier PA, Batti FH, et al.: Lymphoepithelial cyst of the pancreas with sebaceous differentiation. Int J Pancreatol 15:145–147, 1994.
142. Truong LD, Rangdaeng S, Jordan PH Jr: Lymphoepithelial cyst of the pancreas. Am J Surg Pathol 11:899–903, 1987.
143. Cappellari JO: Fine-needle aspiration cytology of a pancreatic lymphoepithelial cyst. Diagn Cytopathol 9:77–81, 1993.
144. Flaherty MJ, Benjamin DR: Multicystic pancreatic hamartoma. A distinctive lesion with immunohistochemical and ultrastructural study. Hum Pathol 23:1309–1312, 1992.
145. Izbicki JR, Knoefel WT, Müller-Höcker J, et al.: Pancreatic hamartoma: A benign tumor of the pancreas. Am J Gastroenterol 89:1261–1262, 1994.
146. Marchevsky AM, Zimmerman MJ, Aufses AH Jr, et al.: Endometrial cyst of the pancreas. Gastroenterology 86:1589–1591, 1984.
147. Verbeke C, Harle M, Sturm J: Cystic endometriosis of the upper abdominal organs. Report on three cases and review of the literature. Pathol Res Pract 192:300–304, 1996.
148. Goswami AK, Sharma SK, Tandon SP, et al.: Pancreatic endometriosis presenting as a hypovascular renal mass. J Urol 135:112–113, 1986.
149. Nardi GL, Lyon DC, Sheiner HJ, et al.: Solitary occult retention cysts of the pancreas. N Engl J Med 280:11–15, 1969.
150. Rizzo RJ, Szucs RA, Turner MA: Congenital abnormalities of the pancreas and biliary tree in adults. Radiographics 15:49–68, 1995.

Chapter

3

DIABETES AND ABNORMALITIES OF INSULIN PRODUCTION

DIABETES MELLITUS

Diabetes mellitus may be defined as a heterogeneous group of metabolic diseases, characterized by hyperglycemia, resulting from defects in insulin secretion, insulin action, or both.[1] Insulin deficiency may be absolute or relative. Modern criteria for a diagnosis require fulfillment of at least one of the following: (1) symptoms of diabetes, plus a random plasma glucose concentration > 200 mg/dL (11.1 mmol/L); (2) fasting plasma glucose > 126 mg/dL (7.0 mmol/L); (3) a plasma glucose > 200 mg/dL (11.1 mmol/L) obtained 2 hours following a glucose load of 75 g of anhydrous glucose given orally.[1] Typical symptoms of untreated diabetes include polyuria, polydipsia, and unexplained weight loss.

A number of causes of diabetes and types of diabetes exist. These are detailed in Table 3–1, which is a simplified version of a scheme devised by an international expert committee working under the sponsorship of the American Diabetes Association.[1,2] The terms *insulin-dependent diabetes mellitus* (*IDDM*) and *non–insulin-dependent diabetes mellitus* (*NIDDM*) have been dropped because it is no longer considered appropriate to base a classification on treatment parameters. The terms *type 1* and *type 2* have replaced *IDDM* and *NIDDM,* respectively. The current classification is modified from one first developed in 1979,[2] and subsequently endorsed by the World Health Organization.[3]

The regulation of blood glucose depends on three major mechanisms: insulin secretion by B cells in the islets of Langerhans, glucose production in the liver, and uptake of glucose by peripheral tissues. Within the islets, proinsulin is synthesized in the rough endoplasmic reticulum, cleaved into mature insulin and C peptide, then stored in secretory granules until release. The major stimulus to insulin release is an increase in blood glucose. In addition, if hyperglycemia persists, this will also cause an increase in insulin synthesis. Insulin acts on peripheral tissues, particularly skeletal muscle, by increasing transmembrane transport of glucose. This is accomplished by first binding to an insulin receptor on the cell surface. Receptor activation then triggers various cellular responses, resulting in activation of DNA synthesis, protein synthesis, and anabolic metabolic pathways. It also triggers GLUT 4, a membrane protein, that has the ability to transport glucose into the cell. When blood sugar levels start to fall, glucose may be transported back into the blood from the liver. This process is non–insulin dependent.

Type 1 Diabetes

Type 1 diabetes is characterized by an absolute insulin deficiency and is the most commonly occurring form of diabetes in children of Caucasian origin. However, the disease can first present at any age, with about 50% of cases developing after the patient is 21 years old.[4] Ultimately, the prevalence may reach 1% of the

Table 3–1. Current Scheme Used to Classify Diabetes Mellitus

Type 1 diabetes
Type 2 diabetes
Other specific types
Genetic defects of B-cell function
Genetic defects in insulin action
Diseases of the exocrine pancreas
Endocrinopathies
Drug- or chemical-related diabetes
Infections
Uncommon forms of immune-related diabetes
Rare genetic syndromes sometimes associated with diabetes
Gestational diabetes

general population.[5] Clinically, in children, the disease is usually of rapid onset, with the development of ketoacidosis. Exogenous insulin is required to sustain life. In adults, however, the onset may be slower, with a longer symptomatic period before diagnosis.[6] Sufficient B-cell function may be preserved to prevent ketoacidosis for many years.[7] Ultimately, however, most adult-onset type 1 diabetes will require exogenous insulin.

Type 1 diabetes appears to have two subtypes: one in which there is some evidence of an autoimmune cause and one in which the cause is unknown (idiopathic diabetes).[1] The predominant form in Caucasians is autoimmune, whereas the idiopathic type is much more common in individuals of African and Asian origin. The autoimmune form appears to be triggered by external factors but requires a background of genetic susceptibility. Evidence for the presence of autoimmunity in patients with diabetes includes the finding of serum islet cell autoantibodies (ICA), insulin autoantibodies (IAA), antibodies to glutamic acid decarboxylase (GAD_{65}), and antibodies to tyrosine phosphatases IA-2 and IA-2β.[1,8] These antibodies occur in 85% to 90% of Caucasian individuals with type 1 diabetes when fasting hyperglycemia is first detected. Recent studies suggest that GAD-reactive T cells are implicated in the pathogenesis of the disease and their presence precedes the development of clinical diabetes. The histologic features of the pancreas in type 1 diabetes occurring in Caucasians are also consistent with a cellular immune reaction. These include a lymphocyte-rich infiltrate, in which CD8 T cells are predominant. It is postulated that two mechanisms of B-cell damage occur. The first is a classic autoimmune reaction, in which B cells are targeted for destruction by cytotoxic T lymphocytes. The other postulated mechanism suggests that B-cell destruction is primarily a cytokine-mediated macrophage and T-helper-cell–dependent process.

Factors that predispose to autoimmune damage are incompletely understood at the present time. Type 1 diabetes tends to run in families. For the siblings of affected individuals, the risk is between 6% and 10%,[4] and for human leukocyte antigen (HLA)-identical siblings, the risk is 15%.[9] Both HLA- and non–HLA-linked genetic factors appear to be important and probably operate in concert.[10,11] HLA class II alleles located on chromosome 6 (especially HLA-DR3 and -DR4) show the strongest association and individuals bearing the HLA-DQ3.2 gene have a risk of developing type 1 diabetes that is eight times normal. The mechanisms controlling how class II molecules regulate the immune response are not clear. An earlier view that regulation was mediated via their control of antigen presentation to mature T lymphocytes does not fully explain the situation. Regulation may, however, also relate either to the role of the class II molecules in controlling the T-cell repertoire or to the specific binding of certain proteins with gene products. Alterations in the genes DQA, DQB, and DRB may be responsible and changes may be predisposing or protective (HLA-DQ1.2).[12,13] Interest in non-HLA genetic factors has centered on the insulin gene (INS) and a region termed IDDM2 situated upstream on chromosome 11.[14,15] Population studies of those with type 1 diabetes and controls without diabetes demonstrate a positive association between certain alleles and the development of diabetes.[16] However, early linkage analyses have failed to confirm this finding. The discrepancy has not entirely been explained but may be the result of maternal imprinting or an interaction between HLA and INS gene loci.[17] The cellular mechanism by which the INS genes impart susceptibility to type 1 diabetes is not known.

Environmental risk factors that may be important in the triggering of type 1 diabetes include the early introduction of cow's milk into a child's diet,[18] the presence of various viral infections, and certain chemical toxins. A recently performed metanalysis[18] demonstrated an increased risk for childhood type 1 diabetes of 1.57 (confidence interval, 1.19–2.07) in infants exposed to cow's milk before 4 months of age. Such children have an increased incidence of bovine serum albumin (BSA) antibodies. Possible mechanisms of pathogenesis remain speculative. It has, however, been suggested that BSA acts via a process of molecular mimicry, in which it creates antibodies directed not only at itself but also against a B-cell protein (p69).

Viral infections have long been thought of as a cause of type 1 diabetes. Candidate viruses include retroviruses, mumps, rubella, morbilli, cytomegalovirus (CMV), Epstein–Barr virus, and Coxsackie B.[19,20] The evidence for this association consists of studies of maternal infections during pregnancy, studies of viral specific antibodies in the serum of patients with type 1 diabetes, and single-case reports. It seems possible that a number of viruses have the ability to damage genetically susceptible B cells, provoking cytokine production and inducing surface expression of p69.

Chemical factors that have been associated with type 1 diabetes include the drugs streptozotocin, Alloxan, and pentamidine, as well as Vacor, a type of industrial rodenticide. These chemicals may also have the ability to damage B cells, thus triggering an autoimmune reaction.

As the name indicates, idiopathic diabetes type 1 has no known cause and demonstrates no evidence of autoimmunity.[1] Most patients are of African or Asian origin and the disease is not HLA associated, although there is a strong familial pattern of inheritance. Those with idiopathic diabetes have a permanent deficiency of insulin and are prone to periodic ketoacidosis. They have a variable requirement for insulin therapy.[21]

Pathology of the Pancreas in Type 1 Diabetes

In type 1 diabetes of recent onset, the pancreas is generally normal in size, weight, and consistency. In long-standing diabetes, however, there may be loss of size and weight by up to 50%. In addition, the organ has a firmer consistency than normal, owing to the presence of a diffuse fine fibrosis. The loss of pancreatic bulk is more extreme than is usually encountered in type 2 diabetes.[22]

Histologic appearances in the pancreas are variable, depending on the duration of the disease. Differences also exist in morphologic findings documented in various published accounts. This is hardly surprising, given that reliance has to be placed on scarce autopsy material.[10,23–25] Because of advances in the treatment of diabetes, deaths in the early stages are quite uncommon and only a few pathologists are in a position to acquire sufficient autopsy tissue and gain wide personal experience.

In general terms, it is possible to divide the histologic findings into those encountered early in the course of the disease (typically in the first 6 months) and those that appear later on in the course (typically after 1 year). One of the earliest findings noted is a difference in size and shape between islets. Some islets are of normal size and some appear shrunken. Small numbers of islets may actually appear enlarged and hypertrophic with the usual smooth outline becoming irregular. Immunohistochemical staining reveals that the shrunken islets have a reduced or even absent population of B cells. High-power examination of residual B cells reveals patchy degranulation and mildly pleomorphic nuclei, some of which are pyknotic.

The second major finding in the early stages of the disease is insulitis. This is most typical of children with diabetes and is relatively rare in adults. Insulitis consists of an infiltrate of inflammatory cells, occurring mainly at the periphery of the islets but also, to a lesser extent, percolating into the islets along the sinusoids (Fig. 3–1). The infiltrate is predominately lymphocytic in composition, with smaller numbers of macrophages and neutrophils. Plasma cells are not encountered. Insulitis is of variable extent, not all islets are affected, and those that are affected usually constitute only a minority. Not all individuals with type 1 diabetes have insulitis and, at the present time, it is not clear whether this finding reflects a fundamental difference in the nature of the disease or simply represents a difference in the stage of disease.

Chronic type 1 diabetes (disease present for longer than 1 year) is characterized by a diffuse interlobular and interacinar fibrosis, often accompanied by progressively more severe atrophy of the exocrine acini. As fibrosis and atrophy occurs in individuals with and without diabetic angiopathy, it is presumed to be a primary event, rather than a complication of ischemia. This finding of exocrine atrophy has given rise to speculation that in some way, either insulin is trophic for exocrine acini[26] or B cell and exocrine damage are the result of a common immunologic pathogenesis.[27] In late-stage disease, the islets are quite variable in size and distribution and may be hard to distinguish from the surrounding acini. Immunohistochemical staining reveals a complete or near complete absence of B cells. The presence of residual functional islets can be determined in

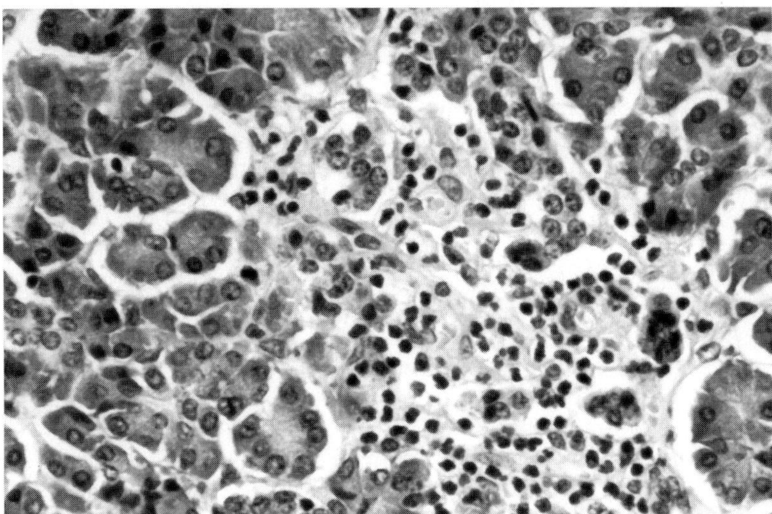

Figure 3–1. Early-stage type I diabetes. The islet is infiltrated by lymphocytes. Obvious atrophy of islet cells is noted.

vivo by serologic tests measuring C-peptide production.

Specific degenerative changes within the islets, such as fibrosis, amyloidosis,[28] and calcification,[29] are distinctly uncommon in type 1 diabetes.

Type 2 Diabetes

Type 2 diabetes, which was formerly referred to as *adult-onset diabetes* or *NIDDM,* occurs in individuals who have a relative rather than an absolute insulin deficiency.[30] Most persons with type 2 diabetes do not need insulin to survive and seldom experience ketoacidosis. Type 2 diabetes does not appear to be mediated by autoimmunity, and the cause is considered to be a combination of peripheral resistance to insulin action with an inadequate compensatory insulin secretory response by the pancreas.[1] Hyperglycemia may be present for many years prior to the onset of specific symptoms and may give rise to complications, such as macro- and microangiopathy. Many patients are obese and control of their diabetic state may be achieved simply by weight reduction and dietary modifications. Exactly how obesity is pathogenetically related to type 2 diabetes is not clear. Abdominal obesity is more significant than is subcutaneous fat deposition and the diabetes may be related to the release of free fatty acids by catabolized abdominal fat.

Measurement of insulin levels in those with type 2 diabetes may reveal normal or even elevated levels. This finding is most commonly observed in the early stages of the disease or in individuals who do not yet have glucose intolerance but are at risk of developing diabetes. This hyperinsulinemia is attributed to hyperresponsiveness of B cells to blood glucose elevations. As diabetes becomes established, insulin levels may remain normal but do not show the normal fluctuations expected with changes in blood sugar levels. Later in the course of the disease, insulin levels become low but are never as low as those encountered in type 1 diabetes. This is considered to represent cell exhaustion, possibly a manifestation of premature cell aging. Thus, for all states of type 2 diabetes, insulin secretion is still regarded as defective, as it is inadequate to compensate for the effects of peripheral resistance.

Insulin resistance may be defined as a situation in which insulin is no longer able to exert a normal biologic effect in its target tissues.[31] The target tissues include skeletal muscle, adipose tissue, and liver. Insulin resistance can involve metabolism of glucose, free fatty acids, and protein, although it is customary to confine use of the term to glucoregulatory effects.[31] Skeletal muscle consumes most of the body's energy and is correspondingly the most important organ for the development of insulin resistance. In contrast, adipose tissue takes up $< 5\%$ of glucose to be metabolized. The effects of insulin resistance include defects in glucose storage as glycogen and increased liver gluconeogenesis. The exact biochemical mechanisms of insulin resistance have yet to be defined. It is postulated, however, that there may be a deficiency of GLUT (membrane protein responsible for transporting glucose into the cell).

Worldwide, about 3% of the population has type 2 diabetes, although there are large geographic and racial differences. It is particularly common in North America and western Europe, where it has been related to lifestyle, particularly the presence of obesity and a lack of exercise. Genetic influences are multifactorial. Family clustering is observed, with a lifetime risk of 40% in children with one parent affected, or 70% if both parents have diabetes. It seems possible that transmission occurs in an autosomal-dominant fashion but that in most families there is low penetrance. No HLA linkage is described. A different mode of inheritance appears to operate in certain non-Caucasian populations. The groups most extensively studied are the Pima Indians of the southwestern United States and the inhabitants of Nauru, an island in the Pacific Ocean. In both groups, the prevalence of diabetes in the general population may reach 40%. In the Pima Indians, the FABP-2 gene, located on chromosome 4, may play a role in the inheritance of insulin resistance.[32]

Pathology of the Pancreas in Type 2 Diabetes

Changes that occur in the pancreas of those with type 2 diabetes are difficult to distinguish from the effects of aging. Recent work, however, has now identified four characteristic features: overall reduction in size, fibrosis, quantitative changes in the density of islet cells, and islet amyloidosis.[33]

When assessed by ultrasound examination, the size of the pancreas is reduced.[22,34] This finding has also been confirmed by autopsy studies, which have shown not only a reduction in the average weight but also that the weight can be highly variable, predominantly because of the amount of fatty infiltration that may be present.[35] The weight range usually quoted is between 50 and 120 g. Those with diabetes—whatever the type—also have decreased pancreatic exocrine function.[26,27,36] Part of the reason for this may be that insulin acts as a trophic factor for exocrine growth. In those with longstanding type 2 diabetes, however, it is equally plausible that the exocrine atrophy is the result of macro- and microvascular disease occurring as a complication of the diabetes.

Reduction in acinar volume is frequently accompanied by fibrosis. Generally, this occurs in a fine perilobular and intra-acinar pattern, although there may also be small areas of denser collagen deposition. Fine fibrosis may extend into the islets, where it spreads from the outside along capillaries. The larger areas of fibrosis can be accompanied by foci of ductular proliferation.[37] This pattern of fibrosis is not specific to type 2 diabetes, but also occurs, to a lesser extent, simply as a result of aging.

Careful observation and measurement of the number and distribution of islets demonstrates that they are reduced in both number and density by approximately 50%.[38] However, the size of each individual islet remains unchanged. This makes it difficult to appreciate any reduction in numbers, unless strict measurements are performed. Within each individual islet there is also a reduction in the numbers of B cells and an increase in both absolute numbers and percentage of other cell types, particularly A cells.[38,39] In those without diabetes, the usual ratio of B cells to A cells is 3:1, whereas in those with type 2 diabetes, this becomes 1:1.[40,41] Despite this very considerable reduction in number of B cells, morphologic abnormalities of individual cells are difficult to appreciate. The cells are of normal size and only occasionally demonstrate cytoplasmic degranulation. Degranulation appears to be confined to those cases where diabetes is out of control and the patients die in a diabetic coma.[42]

Amyloid deposition within islets is characteristic of type 2 diabetes. The prevalence and density of amyloid deposition increases with age, so that although those with diabetes who are younger than age 40 years show no amyloidosis, it is found in 50% of individuals over the age of 70.[43] The highest prevalence of amyloid is noted in those with the most severe diabetes and in those treated with insulin.[44] However, amyloidosis of the islets is not diagnostic of clinical diabetes and is also present in 4% to 23% of elderly people without diabetes,[40,44] although it has been suggested that at least some of these individuals may be prediabetic. Amyloid is deposited within the perisinusoidal spaces, where it forms cords and nodules (Fig. 3–2). In general, the extent of deposition within individual islets parallels the number of islets affected, so that when most islets are involved, they tend to be involved extensively. In persons with the

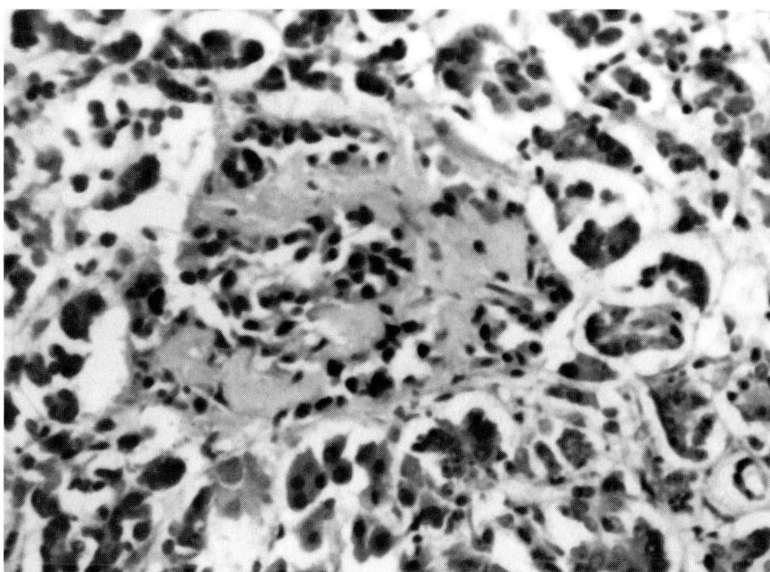

Figure 3–2. Amyloid deposition in an islet from an individual who had type II diabetes. Note the sinusoidal distribution.

most extensive amyloidosis, the number of B cells may be reduced by 75%, although the cells are still readily identifiable, especially with appropriate immunohistochemical stains.[45] By ultrastructural examination, amyloid fibrils, made up of thin and often wavy units, are noted to be arranged perpendicular to the plasma membrane of B cells, occasionally being located within deep cytoplasmic invaginations.[46,47] Morphologically, this is different from the appearances in systemic amyloid, which tends to have thicker nonbranching units.

The nature and significance of islet amyloid deposition has been the subject of considerable research activity.[48–54] There is now general agreement that the islet amyloid deposits are derived from a substance cosecreted by B cells termed *islet amyloid polypeptide* (*IAPP*) or *amylin*.[49,52] Amyloid represents a concentrated and highly polymerized form of IAPP, which is a highly conserved and carboxy–terminally amidated 37–amino acid polypeptide.[2,52] In individuals without diabetes, IAPP production is only 1% of the amount of insulin secreted. These levels increase in response to hyperglycemia.[52] As well as acting at a local level, IAPP may also function as a hormone that antagonizes the effects of insulin on peripheral tissues.[54] It has been postulated that deposition of IAPP may contribute to the development of type 2 diabetes by either destroying B cells, or disrupting the passage of insulin and glucose to and from the islets.[49] However, at present, this work simply suggests that IAPP production is a result, rather than a cause, of diabetes. It is quite possible that islet amyloid deposition exacerbates established diabetes but the pattern of its distribution is not an adequate explanation for the initial onset of hyperglycemia. This hypothesis is in accordance with the finding that individuals with the most extensive amyloid deposition tend to be more severely diabetic, often requiring insulin. Amyloid may act by impairing nutrition simply as a result of the physical barrier created by perivascular deposits or by a direct toxic effect of fibrils developing at intracellular or extracellular sites.[55] Therefore, the cellular mechanisms responsible for type 2 diabetes remain to be elucidated. Its cause may be regarded as being a complex interaction of genetic predisposition, B-cell dysfunction, and insulin resistance.

GENETIC DEFECTS AFFECTING B-CELL FUNCTION

Genetic defects that affect B-cell function are listed in Table 3–2. They were formerly referred to collectively as *maturity-onset diabetes of the young* (*MODY*). This group of conditions is characterized clinically by the onset of mild hyperglycemia before age 25 years, with deficient insulin secretion but no insulin resistance. They are all inherited in an autosomal-dominant pattern. Currently, abnormalities have been detected at loci on chromosomes 7, 12, and 20.[56–62] In two of these conditions, there are defects in hepato-

Table 3–2. Genetic Defects of B-Cell Function

Hepatocyte nuclear factor 1α defect (MODY* type 3)
Hepatocyte nuclear factor 4α defect (MODY type 1)
Glucokinase deficiency (MODY type 2)
Mitochondrial DNA defects
Impaired proinsulin conversion
Mutant insulin production

* MODY, maturity-onset diabetes of the young.

cyte nuclear factors (HNFs). The 4α gene on chromosome 20*q* (HNF-4α) regulates the expression of the *k* gene on chromosome 12 (HNF-1α). Either gene may be mutated with the most common mutation (MODY type 3) affecting chromosome 12.[56–59] Less commonly, the 4α gene is mutated (MODY type 1). The second type of mutation involves the glucokinase gene on chromosome 7*p*[60,61] (MODY type 2). Glucokinase is involved in metabolizing glucose to glucose-6-phosphate, which, in turn, has the ability to stimulate insulin secretion. If glucokinase is defective, blood glucose levels rise before insulin is secreted.

Rarer examples of genetic defects affecting B-cell function include point mutations in mitochondrial DNA, which are associated with diabetes mellitus and deafness[63,64]; inability to convert proinsulin to insulin[65]; and the production mutant insulin molecules with impaired receptor binding.[66]

GENETIC DEFECTS IN INSULIN ACTION

A list of genetic defects in insulin action, which are unusual conditions, is given in Table 3–3. Type A insulin resistance in women may be associated with virilization and polycystic ovaries.[67,68] Older patients may develop acanthosis nigricans. Leprechaunism is diagnosed by the presence of elfinlike facial features with retrusion of the nose, thick lips, low-set ears, and prominent external genitalia. Patients usually die in early childhood. In the Rabson–Mendenhall syndrome, individuals have abnormalities of teeth and nails, together with pineal gland hyperplasia. In both leprechaunism and the Rabson–Mendenhall syndrome, there is extreme insulin resistance, due to mutations in the insulin receptor gene, with subsequent alterations in insulin receptor function.[67–70]

Table 3–3. Genetic Defects in Insulin Action

Type A insulin resistance
Leprechaunism
Rabson–Mendenhall syndrome
Lipoatrophic diabetes
Prader–Willi syndrome
Porphyria cutanea tarda
Acute intermittent porphyria
Ataxia-telangiectasia
Fanconi's anemia
Xeroderma pigmentosum
Common variable immunodeficiency
Severe combined immunodeficiency

Total or generalized lipoatrophy is also termed the *Seip–Lawrence syndrome,* or *lipoatrophic diabetes mellitus.* As well as diabetes, those with the syndrome may have hypertrichosis, acanthosis nigricans, hypertriglyceridemia, and liver disease with cirrhosis. Subcutaneous fat is lost, although breast fat is retained. High insulin plasma levels are recorded. Recent work suggests that the insulin receptor gene is not involved and that there is another mechanism of insulin resistance.[71]

In Prader–Willi syndrome, the patients may become morbidly obese and develop diabetes. This appears to occur on the basis of (1) a reduced B-cell response to glucose stimulation, (2) increased hepatic insulin extraction, and (3) a dissociation of obesity and insulin resistance.[72] Diabetes mellitus has also been described in various types of porphyria: porphyria cutanea tarda[73] and acute intermittent porphyria.[74] In porphyria cutanea tarda, there is insulin resistance, with the metabolic defect appearing to be postreceptor in location.[73] In acute intermittent porphyria, it has been postulated that insulin resistance is due to a heme deficiency involving the cytochrome enzymes.[74]

Diabetes mellitus is also associated with ataxia-telangiectasia, Fanconi's anemia, xeroderma pigmentosum, common variable immune deficiency, and severe combined immunodeficiency.[75] In ataxia-telangiectasia, there may be extreme insulin resistance.[74]

DISEASES OF THE EXOCRINE PANCREAS

Diseases of the exocrine pancreas are more fully discussed in Chapters 4 and 5. Basically, any disease that causes injury to the pancreas may result in diabetes. However, for this to occur, extensive damage has to take place, because the normal pancreas has considerable functional reserve and destruction of islets will reduce both insulin- and glucagon-secreting cells. Examples of conditions that can damage the pancreas sufficiently to cause diabetes include pancreatitis,[76,77] trauma, infections, cystic fibrosis (CF)[78,79] hemochromatosis,[80] and fibrocalcific pancreatopathy[81] (Table 3–4).

Diabetes occurring secondary to chronic pancreatitis is relatively common.[77] Frank diabetes occurs in 10% to 30% of individuals with chronic pancreatitis, and impaired glucose tolerance is present in an additional 10% to 30%. The diagnosis may be difficult, however, because clinical evidence of malabsorption may not become manifest until after the onset of hyperglycemia. Patients in whom this syndrome has arisen because of chronic pancreatitis typically have low glucagon levels that respond abnormally to physiologic stimuli, blunted adrenaline responses to insulin-induced hyperglycemia, and malabsorption. Many examples of chronic pancreatitis occur secondary to alcoholism and may be accompanied by liver disease.[76] In advanced pancreatitis, the whole organ is fibrotic, with duct scarring and dilation. Inspissated proteinaceous material may be found within cystlike structures and may show early calcification. Apparent budding of endocrine cells from surviving ducts can be observed (nesidioblastosis).[82] Islets become closely aggregated, because of the loss of acinar tissue. These aggregates are frequently irregular in shape and come to resemble microadenomas. Ultimately, bland fibrous tissue predominates and islets are appreciably reduced in number, with dense bands of fibrous tissue extending into and separating the islet aggregates. Measurements that have been made of the numbers of different types of islet cells have shown a decrease in the B cells relative to the number of A cells.[37] D cells are well preserved, but PP cells, particularly those in the portion of pancreas derived from the ventral lobe, are markedly reduced. Throughout the course of chronic pancreatitis, the morphology of individual islet cells on both light microscopy and electron microscopy is little changed.

Table 3–4. Diseases of the Exocrine Pancreas Associated with Diabetes

Acute and chronic pancreatitis
Trauma/pancreatectomy
Cystic fibrosis
Hemochromatosis
Fibrocalculous pancreatopathy
Carcinoma of the pancreas

In its most extreme forms, acute pancreatitis carries a high degree of morbidity and mortality. Many of these individuals develop hyperglycemia and glycosuria, but in most instances, if they survive the acute attack, blood sugar levels return to normal. Permanent islet cell damage occurs in $<$ 10% of patients with acute pancreatitis. Histologic examination of the pancreas at autopsy in patients dying of acute pancreatitis is difficult, because of accelerated autolysis. In areas of pancreatitis, the islets are destroyed by autodigestive necrosis; outside of these areas, however, they may survive intact.

Diabetes complicating CF is now being encountered more commonly as individuals with this condition survive into adulthood. There seems to be general agreement that the follow-up care of CF patients should include screening for diabetes.[78] When it occurs, the diabetes generally cannot be adequately controlled by diet alone and insulin is commonly required.[79] The mechanism of chronic pancreatic damage in CF is essentially ongoing inflammation, similar to chronic pancreatitis of other causes. The histologic features are parallel, with ductal dilation and inspissation of secretion seen in the early stages, which later progresses to acinar atrophy, islet clustering, and fibrosis. Ultimately, dense fibrosis starts to dissect the islet aggregates, with obvious global reduction of islet cells. Quantitation of the different types of islet cell reveal diminution of B cells, with relative abundance of A cells, so that the normal beta–to–A cell ratio becomes inverted.

Primary or genetic hemochromatosis is a rare cause of diabetes mellitus, accounting for $<$ 1% of cases.[80] Conversely, however, diabetes (so-called *bronze diabetes* because of the color of the skin and other organs) occurs to a greater or lesser extent in over half the patients with hemochromatosis. Diabetes may also occur, but less frequently, in individuals who accumulate iron, secondary to other conditions. These include thalassemia[83] and Bantu hemosiderosis.[84] Morphologic examination of the pancreas reveals that iron is deposited mainly within acinar cells. Smaller amounts are seen in ductular epithelial cells and stromal cells. Islet cells contain only small quantities of iron; this is confined to B cells, with sparing of the A cells.[85] Late in the course of hemochromatosis, the pancreas may show considerable fibrosis, with tongues of fibrous tissue extending into and dissecting the islets. The mechanism by which hemochromatosis causes diabetes is somewhat controversial. It was formerly considered that diabetes arose simply as a complication of islet cell failure, secondary to iron deposition. However, this is hard to reconcile with the known distribution of iron within the pancreas and with the fact that exocrine failure in hemochromatosis is rare. It has been suggested that genetic factors may play a role and it has been pointed out that 25% of patients with hemochromatosis plus diabetes have a relative who has diabetes, whereas only 4% of patients with hemochromatosis and no diabetes have an affected relative.[86] Another factor predisposing to diabetes is the known insulin resistance[87] and hyperglucagonemia[88] associated with the development of cirrhosis. At the present time, it appears likely that three mechanisms contribute to the development of diabetes: direct pancreatic damage by iron, familial predisposition to develop diabetes, and diminished insulin sensitivity due to the presence of cirrhosis.

Fibrocalculous pancreatic diabetes is a unique condition that occurs secondary to fibrocalculous pancreatopathy (tropical calcific pancreatitis).[81,89–92] The relationship between the pancreatic damage and development of diabetes is unclear,[89] as some individuals with fibrocalculous pancreatopathy develop only exocrine insufficiency without diabetes mellitus. It has been suggested that a genetic predisposition exists in those individuals with the disease who develop diabetes.[93] Fibrocalculous pancreatopathy is a disease occurring predominately in Third World countries. Most reports are from India, but cases have also been described in West Africa, South Africa, and Papua New Guinea. The condition appears to be the result of either overt protein-calorie malnutrition, or a more subtle deficiency of micronutrients, especially antioxidants.[81] It tends to affect young adults and, in a majority of cases, causes pancreatic fibrosis and calcification, exocrine insufficiency, and diabetes mellitus. Detailed reports of the pathology findings at autopsy are not available.

There is a well-established association between diabetes mellitus and pancreatic carcinoma. What is not completely clear, however, is whether the carcinoma precedes the development of diabetes or vice versa. There is evidence for both types of relationship. The traditional view, and one that applies in the majority of instances, is that diabetes is not a risk factor for the development of cancer but is a complication.[94–96] This is supported by the finding that when large groups of patients are studied, a statistical association between the diseases exists only for those patients in whom diabetes developed within 3 years prior to the diagnosis of cancer.[94,95] The disease present in these patients is atypical for type 2 diabetes and is characterized by an absence of a family history of diabetes, absence of obesity, and rapid progression to insulin dependence.[96] The mechanism of diabetes development is not known. The possibilities exist of ectopic hormone production by the tumor[97] or destruction of the distal pancreas secondary to blockage of ducts by intraductal tumor and papillary hyperplasia.[98] The alternative hypothesis, however, is supported by studies that have established a strong familial predisposition to pancreatic cancer. Of patients with pancreatic cancer, 7.8% report a positive family history of carcinoma, compared with 0.6% of controls—a 13-fold difference.[99] A linkage of diabetes and pancreatic cancer has been shown by a study of a large pedigree in which pancreatic cancer was inherited in an autosomal-dominant fashion. In this family, both diabetes and exocrine insufficiency were present, often existing for many years before the development of cancer.[100] Presence of the allele for cancer could be reliably predicted by testing for diabetes.

NONPANCREATIC ENDOCRINE DISORDERS CAUSING DIABETES

There are several hormones that antagonize insulin actions. The syndromes associated with their overproduction are listed in Table 3–5. In most instances, once the primary hormonal disturbance is corrected, the diabetic state is

Table 3–5. Nonpancreatic Endocrine Disorders Causing Diabetes

Acromegaly (growth hormone)
Cushing's syndrome (glucocorticoids)
Pheochromocytoma (adrenaline and nonadrenaline)
Glucagonoma
Hyperthyroidism
Somatostatinoma
Conn's syndrome (aldosterone)
Carcinoid syndrome (serotonin)

reversed. The pancreas is typically unremarkable in all these syndromes.

In acromegaly,[101] excess production of growth hormone causes overt diabetes in between 10% and 20% of individuals and impaired glucose tolerance in a further 40%. This is likely the result of peripheral resistance to insulin that is not overcome by hyperinsulinemia.

In Cushing's disease and Cushing's syndrome, there is an excess of glucocorticoids, which are either of endogenous or exogenous origin.[102] Depending on the level of overproduction, about 20% of patients develop fasting hyperglycemia. The mechanism of action is considered to be a change in the affinity of insulin receptors, causing peripheral insulin resistance.

In pheochromocytoma,[103] glucagonoma, and Conn's syndrome, the diabetic state is usually only manifest as impaired glucose tolerance. It is thought to be produced either by an inhibition of insulin secretion or by insulin-antagonistic effects. The mechanisms of glucose intolerance in hyperthyroidism are considered to consist of increased hexose intestinal absorption, decreased responsiveness to insulin, and increased glucose production.[104] More than 80% of patients with the carcinoid syndrome have glucose intolerance.[105] Serotonin appears to exert this effect by impairing insulin secretion.

DRUG-INDUCED DIABETES MELLITUS

A large number of drugs and toxins may cause diabetes. These can be divided into those that impair insulin secretion and those that impair insulin action. Extreme examples of impaired insulin secretion are provided by the drug pentamidine[106] and the rodenticide Vacor,[107] which may permanently destroy B cells. Other drugs may be less toxic and their effects may become evident only in individuals who already have a degree of insulin resistance.[108–110] Drugs that may impair insulin action include corticosteroids and nicotinic acid.[108,109]

INFECTIONS CAUSING DIABETES MELLITUS

Viral infectious agents have been implicated in the causation of type 1 diabetes. It is postulated that in genetically susceptible individuals, B-cell destruction may be induced either by direct damage by viruses or by the triggering of an autoimmune reaction. Viruses implicated include retroviruses, mumps, rubella, morbilli, CMV, Epstein–Barr virus and Coxsackie B.[19,20] In the majority of cases, however, direct evidence of a viral etiology is weak and relies on epidemiologic associations and animal models. In rare instances, however, there is clear evidence of virus-induced pancreatic damage. Congenital rubella is the best example.[111]

UNCOMMON CAUSES OF DIABETES

A wide variety of conditions may be grouped under this heading. They include diabetes with an autoimmune cause and those with a genetic basis. The most clearly defined autoimmune condition is the stiff-man (or -person) syndrome, also known as the *Moersch–Woltman syndrome.*[112,113] This is a rare neurologic condition characterized by stiffness of axial muscles with superimposed painful muscle spasms. Antibodies directed against GAD and pancreatic islet cells are present in the serum.[114]

In other disease with an autoimmune basis, such as lupus erythematosus,[115,116] mixed connective tissue disease, and systemic sclerosis,[117] diabetes may arise as a result of the presence of antibodies binding to insulin receptors. These antibodies block insulin binding and immunoprecipitate solubilized insulin receptors. Secretion of insulin receptor antibodies by lymphocytes may be demonstrated by immunologic techniques.[118] This pattern of insulin resistance has been termed *type B* and, for unknown reasons, is commonly found in association with acanthosis nigricans.

A number of syndromes in which there are abnormalities in chromosome number may be associated with diabetes. These include Down syndrome,[119,120] Klinefelter's syndrome,[121,122] and Turner's syndrome.[123,124] In Down syndrome, the prevalence of diabetes is between 1.4% and 10.6%, which is considerably higher than in the general population.[119] Patients have typical type 1 diabetes and require insulin for its control. In Turner's syndrome, diabetes is the result of insulin resistance. Results suggest that this is a metabolic defect, restricted to the nonoxidative pathways of intracellular glucose metabolism.[123] The Wolfram syndrome is characterized by diabetes insipidus, diabetes mellitus, optic atrophy, and deafness (DIDMOAD).[125,126] It is an autosomal-recessive genetic disorder, with a frequency of 1 in 770,000 in the United Kingdom.[126] Nonautoimmune insulin-deficient diabetes develops at an average age of 6 years, followed by optic atrophy at age 11. Those with the syndrome usually die at 30 years of age (average, 25–49 years). The molecular mechanism of diabetes causation in DIDMOAD appears to be an absence of B cells within the islets.[126]

Friedreich's ataxia is known to be associated with diabetes mellitus in up to 20% of patients.[127] The molecular defect present has been difficult to characterize, with some investigators showing a loss of islet cells[127] but others demonstrating insulin resistance.[128] It seems probable, however, that there is a membrane abnormality altering the binding function of the insulin receptor,[128] but this does not exclude the possibility of an islet cell defect also. Insulin resistance of undetermined mechanisms is also the explanation for the higher incidence of diabetes encountered in myotonic dystrophy[129] and Huntington's chorea.[130,131] Diabetes has also been described in acute intermittent porphyria,[74] porphyria cutanea tarda,[73] Prader–Willi syndrome,[72] ataxia-telangiectasia,[74,75] and Wolcott–Rallison syndrome.[132]

GESTATIONAL DIABETES

Gestational diabetes may be defined as any degree of glucose intolerance with onset or first recognition during pregnancy.[1] This includes women who may have had unrecognized glucose intolerance before pregnancy and those in which glucose intolerance is reversed 6 weeks after pregnancy terminates.[133] The term *gestational diabetes* includes glucose intolerance of all types and causes, irrespective of whether insulin is required for control, but after delivery, the disease should be reclassified as listed in Table 3–1.

Gestational diabetes complicates approximately 4% of all pregnancies.[134] The criteria developed for diagnosis include the finding of two or more plasma glucose values of four tests that are ≥ 2 SD above the mean.[135]

PERSISTENT HYPERINSULINEMIC HYPOGLYCEMIA OF INFANCY

Persistent hyperinsulinemic hypoglycemia of infancy (PHHI) is an excessively rare but interesting condition. Its prevalence in the general population of North America and western Europe is approximately 1 per 50,000.[136] It is, however, more common in some Arabic communities, where an autosomal-recessive familial form of the disease has been identified (1 in 2,500).[137] PHHI accounts for slightly less than half of all cases of infantile hypoglycemia. Other causes include pituitary disease, Addison's disease, hypothyroidism, and various glycogen storage diseases. The clinical course of PHHI is rather uniform and consists of somnolence, ataxia, seizures, and coma.[137] These are the result of excessive and inappropriate secretion of insulin by the pancreas. Symptoms may commence with a few hours of birth or, rarely, they may be delayed to later infancy, or even early childhood. If appropriate treatment is not instituted, permanent brain damage may occur, secondary to severe hypoglycemia. Medical treatment, consisting of frequent feeding and glucose infusions, may be temporarily effective, but ultimately, some form of surgical pancreatic resection is required.

Studies of pancreatic morphology in patients with PHHI have subdivided cases into those that involve tumorlike lesions and those that do not.[138,139] The tumorlike lesions may be further subdivided into those with an established adenoma and those with adenoma-like hyperplasia. The nontumorous forms of the disease have a diffuse lesion. This has been variously termed *diffuse nesidioblastosis,*[137,138] *endocrine cell dysplasia,*[140] and *nesidiodysplasia.*[141]

Nesidioblastosis, as originally defined by Laidlaw in 1938, described the budding off of endocrine cells from pancreatic ducts.[142] Yakovac et al., in 1971, were the first to recognize this lesion in hypoglycemic infants.[143] Since these reports were originally published, the term *diffuse nesidioblastosis* has been expanded and used somewhat differently by various authors. In addition to the budding off of endocrine cells from ductular structures (ductulo-insular complexes) (Fig. 3–3D), lesions described include hyperplasia of the islets, irregularly shaped and poorly delineated islets (Fig. 3–3), hypertrophied islet cells, and the presence of giant nuclei[137] (Fig. 3–4). In addition, small groups of endocrine cells, usually numbering between 2 and 25 cells, may be scattered throughout the acinar tissue, quite separate from the islets (Fig. 3–3C). These small clusters of endocrine cells have a tendency to be located toward the periphery of the pancreatic lobules, in contrast to the normal islets, which are more centrally

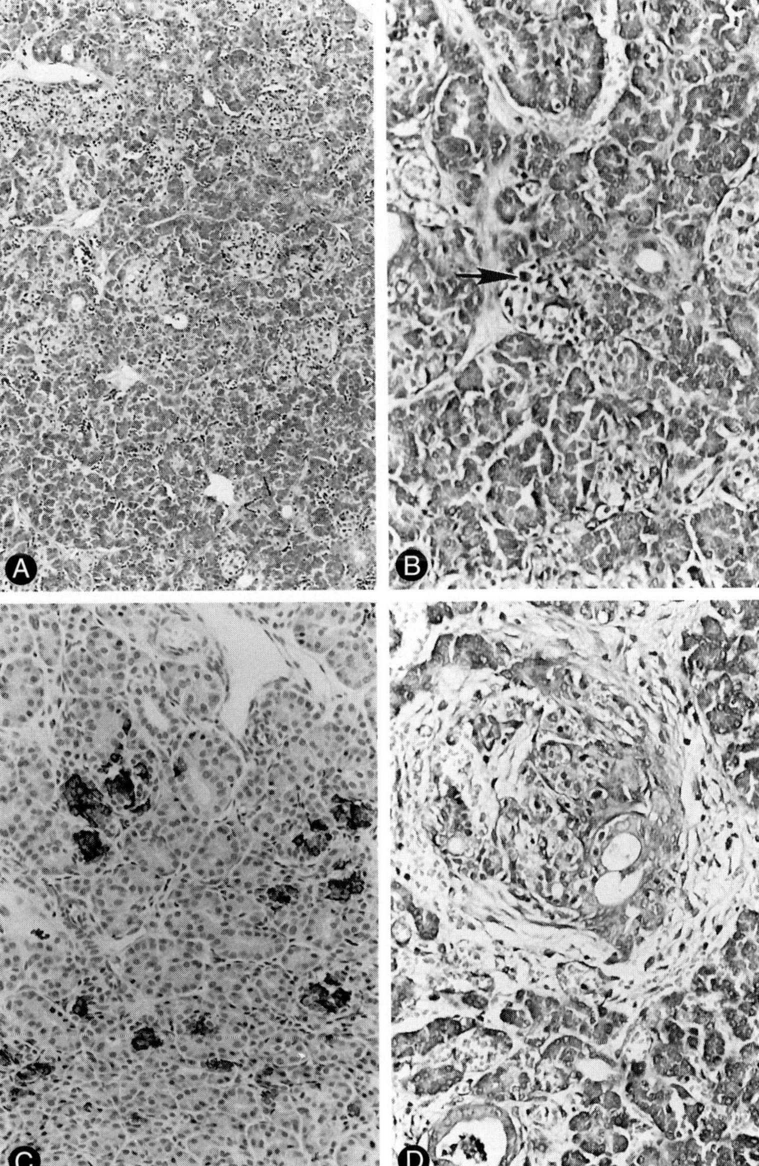

Figure 3–3. Diffuse nesidioblastosis. The routine histologic sections (*A* and *B*) are not impressive, but islets of Langerhans are poorly formed with clusters of endocrine cells scattered throughout the acinar tissue, *B,* Nucleomegaly is present (*arrow*). *C,* Immunostaining for insulin highlights the small packages of insulin-containing cells throughout the acinar elements. *D,* Ductulo-insular complex. (All photomicrographs courtesy of Ron Jaffe, MD, Children's Hospital of Pittsburgh.)

distributed. Studies on the relative numbers of the different types of islet cells in PHHI have been disappointing. Although B cells are prominent, other cell types are also present. Earlier reports of a relative deficiency of D cells and A cells have not been confirmed. All these histologic features may be found, to a greater or lesser extent, in the pancreata of children with PHHI.[137–140] It has now been realized, however, that diffuse nesidioblastosis is not specific for a diagnosis of PHHI and may be found in the pancreata of normoglycemic children dying from causes unrelated to pancreatic dysfunction.[137,144,145] Furthermore, recent studies of the rate of proliferation of B cells in PHHI have demonstrated that this is normal, both in the islets and in the ectopic clusters of diffuse nesidioblastosis.[139] Most authors have concluded that diffuse nesidioblastosis is more striking in infants with PHHI but that the histologic features are heterogeneous, with considerable overlap between features in individual patients. In addition, the histologic appearances vary from area to area, so that multiple histologic

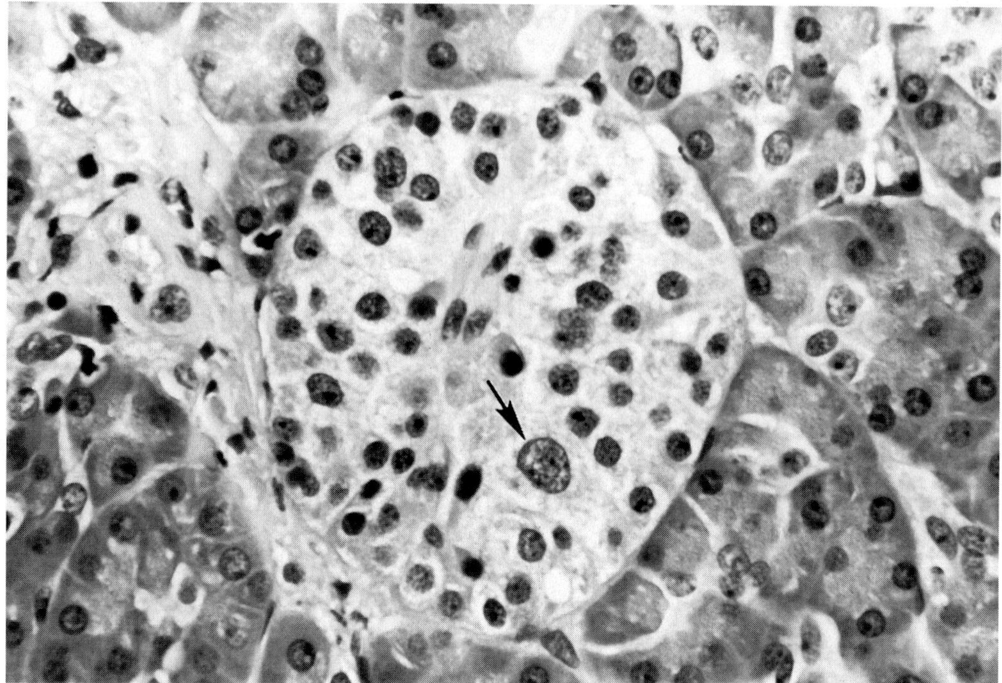

Figure 3–4. Giant islet cell nucleus from a patient with persistent hyperinsulinemic hypoglycemia of infancy.

sections must be examined to give a true impression of the extent of diffuse nesidioblastosis. In one series,[137] budding of islet cells from ducts was observed only in infants with PHHI and was not encountered in normal infants. This has not, however, been confirmed. It seems reasonable to conclude, therefore, that nesidioblastosis itself is not the structural basis for hyperinsulinemia and its presence may not be a useful tool for the definitive diagnosis of PHHI. Nevertheless, infants with PHHI and no focal lesion present will benefit from a partial pancreatectomy.

Instances of PHHI involving tumorlike lesions are approximately as common as those of diffuse nesidioblastosis.[137] Conventionally, they are divided into cases in which multiple nodules are present (these are termed *adenomatous hyperplasia* or *focal nesidioblastosis*) and those with a solitary lesion (termed *adenoma*—that is, insulinoma). However, even within these two groups, variations in morphology have been described. In focal nesidioblastosis,[137,138,144] some patients have a grossly recognizable nodule, typically 5 mm in diameter and generally located within the head or body of the pancreas. In the remainder of patients, the pancreas is grossly normal. Microscopically, all cases show focal endocrine hyperplasia, characterized by the presence of multiple ill-defined nodules that consist of partly confluent expanded islets (Fig. 3–5A and B). Lesions may consist of a single group of nodules, or several groups, located in various parts of the pancreas. However, nodularity is not generalized. Between the nodules, the pancreas is generally normal. The nodules push aside acinar tissue but are not bounded by a fibrous capsule. Within the nodules, there is considerable variation in cell size, but many cells are 50% larger than normal, with macronuclei occasionally double normal size (Fig. 3–4). Immunohistochemical analysis reveals all normal types of endocrine cell present with a normal localization (A cells and D cells at the periphery, B cells located centrally) (Fig. 3–5C and D). Quantitative analysis reveals a predominance of B cells (70% to 90% of cells, versus 50% present in normal neonates).[137]

Adenomas of the pancreas are rare in children. They may resemble the adenomas of adults and appear as rounded, relatively homogeneous nodules, with a thin, fibrous capsule. Sometimes, however, they may appear multilobated and, in such cases, it is not clear whether the lesions represent a true benign neoplasm or a single hyperplastic nodule. Prob-

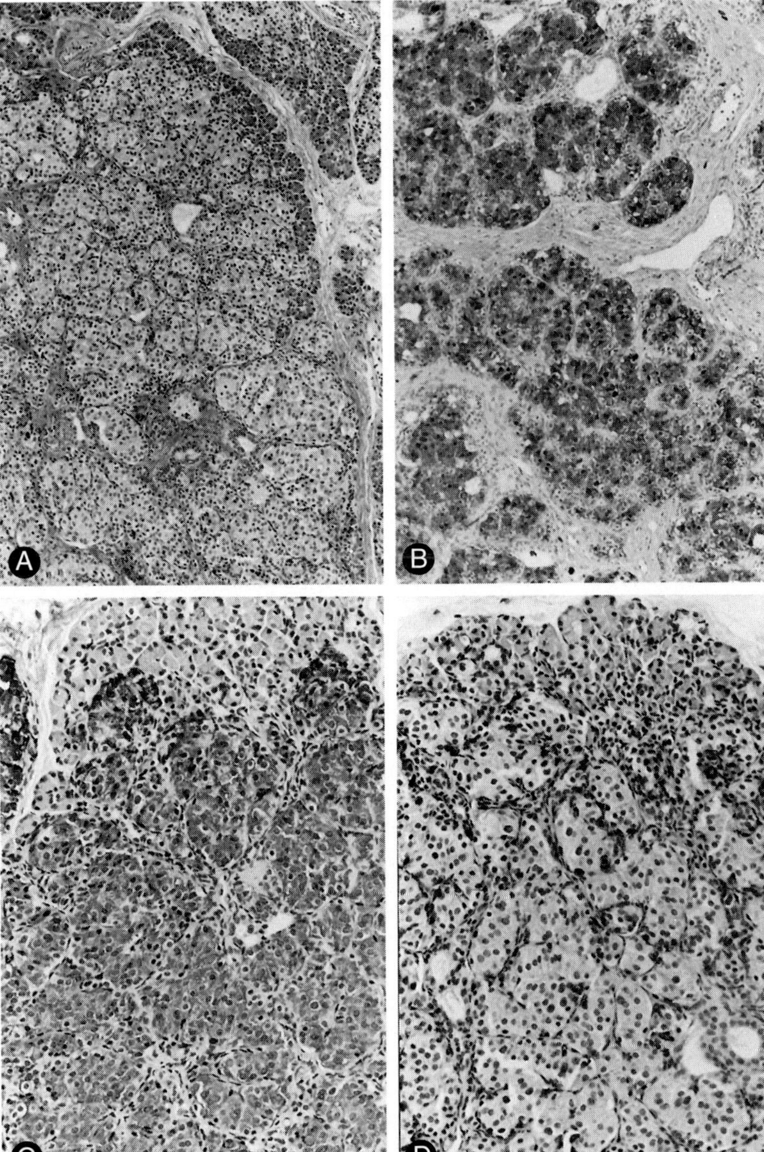

Figure 3–5. Focal nesidioblastosis (adenomatosis). *A,* Low power demonstrates that most of the field is occupied by confluent insular tissue with a small peripheral rim of acini. *B,* Immunostain with anti-PgP 9.5 reveals extensive endocrine overgrowth. (PgP 9.5 [protein growth product] is a marker for hyperplastic and neoplastic B cells of the islets.) *C,* Immunostain for insulin demonstrating that most insular cells are positive. *D,* Immunostain for somatostatin showing the D cells lying peripherally in the islet cell proliferation, recapitulating the pattern in the normal islet. (All photomicrographs courtesy of Ron Jaffe, MD, Children's Hospital of Pittsburgh).

ably this distinction has little practical importance. Theoretically, however, hyperplastic islets should retain a multihormonal immunoprofile, with the usual central distribution of B cells and peripheral localization of A and D cells. True adenomas may also be multihormonal but do not retain this normal physiologic distribution. Studies of cellular proliferation in the two tumorlike forms of PHHI have also demonstrated significant differences, suggesting that they are truly separate conditions rather than morphologic variants. In focal nesidioblastosis, proliferation as measured by nuclear Ki-67 positivity is three times greater than in adenomas.[139]

Genetic abnormalities responsible for PHHI are now becoming recognized. The adenosine triphosphate (ATP)-sensitive potassium (K_{ATP}) channel, located in the plasma membrane of pancreatic B cells, appears to have a pivotal role in the regulation of insulin secretion. Closure of the channel induced by glucose initiates depolarization of the B-cell membrane and opening of the calcium channels results in an increase of calcium, thus triggering the secretion of insulin.[136] K_{ATP} channels are formed from two proteins: the sulfonylurea receptor SUR1 and Kir6.2.[146] Abnormalities of both these proteins have been associated with PHHI. Genes coding for the SUR1 receptor are located on chromosome 11 and mutations have been detected in both familial and sporadic forms of the disease.[136,147] Numerous SUR1 mutations may be identified and are distributed throughout the molecule.[146] This genetic heterogeneity may account for the multiple phenotypic variations encountered in PHHI, but at present, specific gene abnormalities have not been linked to a distinct morphology.

Medical treatment of PHHI may consist of frequent feeding with a low-protein diet and the drug diazoxide (a hyperglycemic agent). Surgical treatment consists of excision of nodular lesions, if they can be identified, or subtotal pancreatectomy, if the diffuse form of the disease is present.

PANCREAS TRANSPLANTATION

Pancreas transplantations are usually performed in individuals with type 1 diabetes complicated by renal failure.[148,149] They may provide better control of blood sugar levels than does exogenous insulin and they avoid the problem of insulin reactions. In addition, a reduction in some of the long-term complications of diabetes, particularly microvascular and diabetic neuropathy, have been recognized.[149] Although not as frequently performed as kidney and liver transplantations, pancreatic transplantations are becoming much more common. As of December 31, 1996, a total of 9,012 pancreas transplantations had been reported to the International Pancreas Transplant Registry.[150] Most of these (75%) were performed in the United States, where currently there are over 1,000 pancreas transplantations per year.[150]

Most pancreas transplantations are performed simultaneously with renal transplantations in patients with diabetes and end-stage renal failure (simultaneous pancreas–kidney, or SPK). Smaller numbers of solitary transplantations are performed, following renal transplantation (pancreas after kidney, or PAK). At present, solitary pancreas transplantation performed on its own without concurrent or subsequent renal transplantation (known as pancreas transplantation alone, or PTA) is uncommon. This is because the potential benefits of glucose regulation have to be weighed against the disadvantages of prolonged immunosuppression. Currently, the 1-year survival of pancreas grafts (cadaveric) performed simultaneously with renal transplantation (SPK) is ≥ 82%, depending on the transplantation center. For other types of pancreas transplantations (PAK and PTA), 1-year graft survival is significantly less (70%–74%).[150] The surgical technique of pancreas transplantation varies somewhat from center to center.[151] Most commonly, the pancreas is transplanted whole, along with a segment of duodenum. Usually, the bowel is anastamosed to the urinary bladder, which drains the exocrine secretions. This system has the advantage of permitting subsequent studies of pancreatic function by urinary amylase measurement. It also has been found to result in fewer postoperative septic complications. Less commonly, the pancreas and duodenal segment may be anastamosed to a loop of small bowel, either directly or via a Roux-en-Y arrangement. With either drainage system, the pancreas is placed in an intra-abdominal location, so that direct monitoring of causes of dysfunction in a solitary transplantation (PAK or PTA) requires a needle biopsy.[152] An adequate biopsy consists of a fragment of tissue measuring 3 mm^2 or larger.[152] In the case of SPK transplantation both organs are taken from the same donor, so that monitoring of kidney function in the usual way simplifies follow-up. It may be assumed that rejection present in a renal biopsy indicates a similar grade of rejection within the transplanted pancreas.

Histologic examination of pancreas grafts before they are transplanted not uncommonly reveals minor ischemic damage, with saponification of peripancreatic fat.[153] In addition, small numbers of T lymphocytes, macrophages, and dendritic reticulum cells may be found within the exocrine and endocrine components. The complications associated with pancreas transplantation are listed in Table 3–6. These are considerably less frequent now than they used to be, because of improved surgical technique

Table 3–6. Complications of Pancreas Transplantation

Acute rejection
Chronic rejection
Pancreatitis
Thrombosis/infarction
Infections
Insulitis
Silastic duct destruction
Lymphoproliferative disorders

and postoperative management.[154] Rejection is a major complication of pancreas transplantation but is not the most common cause of graft loss. Pancreas rejection, as with rejection of other transplanted organs, may be divided into hyperacute, acute, and chronic phases. Hyperacute rejection is distinctly uncommon. The histologic findings include extensive fibrin thrombosis of small and medium arteries, veins, and capillaries, with margination of polymorphonuclear leukocytes in the small vessels.[153] Acute rejection has been extensively studied and systems of grading the histopathologic findings are in place.[152,155,156] In solitary transplantations, biopsy of the transplanted pancreas is usually prompted by a rise in urinary amylase (bladder-drained grafts) or hyperglycemia (enteric-drained grafts).[155] Five grades of acute rejection are established: grade 0, normal; grade 1, rare lymphocytes in septae, normal acini (borderline rejection); grade 2, mixed inflammatory septal infiltrates, with focal acinar involvement and ductulitis or venulitis (mild rejection); grade 3, septal inflammation, with multifocal acinar involvement and acinar cell dropout (moderate rejection); grade 4, moderate rejection, plus arterial endotheliitis or vasculitis; grade 5, extensive inflammatory infiltrates, with confluent acinar necrosis (severe).[152] Pancreatic biopsy and grading of the histopathologic changes of acute rejection has been found useful in the postoperative management of transplantation.[152]

Chronic rejection is less commonly encountered. This clinical diagnosis may be made only in instances where there has been either clear clinical evidence of an episode of prior acute rejection or biopsy evidence of chronic rejection. Chronic rejection of the transplanted pancreas has morphologic features similar to those encountered in chronic rejection of other organs. It consists of a variable concentric narrowing of the lumen of arteries by fibroproliferative endarteritis.[153] In advanced chronic rejection, the transplant may be shrunken and fibrous, with acini and islets being hard to identify.

Acute pancreatitis is an extremely common early complication of pancreatic transplantation. It may manifest, in the first few days after surgery, as raised serum amylase levels. Biopsy, if performed at this time, may reveal typical foci of acute pancreatitis and fat necrosis. Recovery from this initial episode of acute pancreatitis is usual. Chronic pancreatitis is an almost inevitable complication of duct obstruction, which may occur irrespective of the method employed for the draining of secretions. Histologic examination, performed in the early stages, may show duct ectasia, with periductular fibrosis and chronic inflammation. The parenchyma shows acinar atrophy and perilobular fibrosis. Later in the course of the disease, there may be more extensive parenchymal acinar atrophy and fibrosis. Islets are preserved but may coalesce. B cells in the islets are generally well preserved, even in extensive chronic pancreatitis.[153] Only rarely does chronic pancreatitis progress to islet cell failure.

Thrombosis and infarction are complications of pancreas transplantation most likely to be encountered within the first month after surgery, often with the first few days.[153,154] In most instances, thrombosis is considered to be a surgical problem related to vascular anastamotic techniques. Thrombosis may affect either arteries or veins. Arterial thrombosis produces a pale infarct, with coagulative necrosis, which ultimately may develop a fibrotic and "gritty" texture.[153] Venous infarcts produce more of a hemorrhagic appearance and are softer in texture.

Infectious complications of pancreas transplantation are of two types: intra-abdominal abscess formation, usually developing as a surgical complication, and CMV infection, occurring as a direct result of prolonged immunosuppression. CMV infection is rather common and occurs in up to 10% of patients. Although it may cause graft loss, it is rarely fatal.[153] As is usual with posttransplantation CMV infection, the capillary endothelial cells are the most extensively affected. Resulting vascular damage leads to shallow ulceration, particularly of the transplanted cuff of duodenal mucosa. The consequent hemorrhage may be extensive and difficult to treat.

Recurrent insulitis has been described in the transplanted pancreata of occasional patients with type 1 diabetes.[153,154,155] This implies a recurrence of autoimmunity and is characterized by a selective B-cell destruction, just like de novo type 1 diabetes.[157] The frequency of insulitis in transplanted pancreata is unknown but is probably in the region of 1.5%.[157] This low figure is probably explained by the suppression of autoimmunity, as well as alloimmunity, by the usual immunosuppressive drugs used after organ transplantation.[158] Why some transplants but not others are affected is presently unclear.

In the early days of pancreatic transplantation, problems were encountered with appropriate drainage of the main pancreatic duct and many individuals lost their grafts because of surgical leaks. To counteract this problem, a technique of injecting the ductal system with neoprene or silicone material was developed. This obliterated the ductal system and destroyed the acinar component of the pancreas while preserving functional islets. The injection procedure has now been largely abandoned, as surgical graft procedures have improved. However, the pathologic appearances produced by these injections are most interesting.[153] In the acute phase, there is edema, fat necrosis, necrotizing pancreatitis, and neutrophil exudation. Later, the reaction becomes fibrotic and chronic inflammation predominates. The extravasated injected material causes a marked foreign-body reaction, with giant cell formation. Adjacent vessels may show thrombotic occlusion.

Post-transplantation lymphoproliferative disorder (PTLD) is a rare complication of pancreas grafting.[159] Characteristic features of PTLD in needle biopsies and resected grafts are the presence of nodular and expansile infiltrates, consisting of 40% to 70% of atypical plasmacytoid B lymphocytes, some of which may resemble Reed–Sternberg cells. These infiltrates occur in a random fashion throughout the pancreatic parenchyma and are not specifically focused on acinar tissue. Involvement of the peripancreatic adipose tissue is common. In contrast, the changes of florid acute rejection are distributed more evenly throughout the tissue but particularly target the exocrine acini. Small lymphoid cells predominate in rejection, with a minor (< 10%) population of larger lymphoid cells and smaller numbers of plasma cells and eosinophils.[159]

ISLET TRANSPLANTATION

Islet transplantation is still in its early phase of development.[148,149] Approximately 300 transplantations have been performed to date, with a clinical success rate of 8% (providing exogenous insulin independence after 1 year.)[160] However, in 20% of individuals, some graft function could be identified after 1 year. Theoretically islet transplantation should be preferred over pancreas transplantation because it is easier and has few surgical complications. However, numerous technical problems and the high prevalence of graft failure have meant that the technique has yet to fulfill its promise.[161–163]

Islets chosen for engraftment may be salvaged from the patient's native pancreas (autotransplant), from pooled cadaveric islets (allotransplant), or from animal species, usually a pig (xenotransplant). They are separated from the remainder of the pancreas by a process involving selective enzyme digestion, usually using collagenases. The isolated islets are then collected, purified, and injected into the recipient. A variety of sites have been used, including subcutaneous tissues of the forearm, subserosal locations within the abdomen, and directly into the portal vein, so that they engraft within the liver sinusoids. Little is known as to why the grafts fail, as, in most instances, obtaining serial biopsies for histologic examination is not practical. Studies that have been performed have provided variable results. Some have shown recurrent autoimmunity (type 1 diabetes),[157,164] B-cell degranulation and loss,[165] and rejection.[158]

REFERENCES

1. Expert Committee on the Diagnosis and Classification of Diabetes Mellitus: Report of the expert committee on the diagnosis and classification of diabetes mellitus. Diabetes Care 20:1183–1197, 1997.
2. National Diabetes Data Group: Classification and diagnosis of diabetes mellitus and other categories of glucose intolerance. Diabetes 28:1039–1057, 1979.
3. World Health Organization: Diabetes mellitus: Report of a WHO study group. Geneva, World Health Org., 1985 (Tech Rep Ser, 727).
4. Lorenzen T, Pociot F, Hongaard P, et al.: Long term risk of IDDM in first degree relatives of patients with IDDM. Diabetologia 37:321–327, 1994.
5. Moelback AG, Christan B, Marner B, et al.: Incidence of insulin-dependent diabetes mellitus in age groups over 30 years in Denmark. Diabet Med 11:650–655, 1994.
6. Karjalainen J, Salmela P, Ilonen J, et al.: A comparison of childhood and adult type 1 diabetes mellitus. N Engl J Med 320:881–886, 1989.
7. Zimmet PZ, Tuomi T, Mackay R, et al.: Latent autoimmune diabetes mellitus in adults (LADA): The role of antibodies to glutamic acid decarboxylase in diagnosis and prediction of insulin dependency. Diabet Med 11:299–303, 1994.
8. Sepe V, Lai M, Shattock M, et al.: Islet related autoantigens and the pathogenesis of insulin dependent diabetes mellitus. *In* Leslie RGD (ed): Molecular Pathogenesis of Diabetes Mellitus. Basel: S Karger AG, 1997, pp 68–89.
9. Thomson G, Robison WP, Kuhner MK, et al.: Genetic heterogeneity, modes of inheritance and risk estimates for a joint study of Caucasians with insulin-dependent diabetes mellitus. Am J Hum Genet 43:799–816, 1988.
10. Scherbaum WA: Etiology and pathogenesis of type 1 diabetes. Horm Metab Res 26[suppl 1]:111–116, 1992.

11. Foulis AK: The pathogenesis of beta-cell destruction in type 1 (insulin-dependent) diabetes. J Pathol 152:141–181, 1987.
12. Hoover ML, Marta RT: Molecular modelling of HLA-DQ suggests mechanisms of resistance in type 1 diabetes. Scand J Immunol 45:193–202, 1997.
13. Huang W, Connor E, De la Rosa T, et al.: Although DR3-DQB1* may be associated with multiple component diseases of the autoimmune polyglandular syndromes, the human leukocyte antigen DB+ DQB11302 haplotype is implicated only in beta-cell autoimmunity. J Clin Endocrinol Metab 81:1–5, 1996.
14. Bui MM, Luo DF, She JY, et al.: Paternally transmitted IDDM2 influences diabetes susceptibility despite biallelic expression of the insulin gene in human pancreas. J Autoimmun 9:97–103, 1996.
15. Vifiadis P, Bennett ST, Colle E, et al.: Imprinted and genotype-specific expression of genes at the IDDM2 locus in pancreas and leukocytes. J Autoimmun 9:397–403, 1996.
16. Bain SC, Barnett AH, Gough SCL: Genetic factors associated with insulin-dependent diabetes. *In* Leslie RGD (ed): Molecular Pathogenesis of Diabetes Mellitus, Basel: S Karger AG, 1997, pp 23–45.
17. Julier C, Hyer RN, Davies J, et al.: Insulin-IGF2 region on chromosome 11*p* encodes a gene implicated in HLA-DR4–dependent diabetes susceptibility. Nature 354:155–159, 1991.
18. Gerstein H: Cow's milk exposure and type 1 diabetes. Diabetes Care 17:13–19, 1994.
19. Szopa T, Titchener P, Portwood N, et al.: Diabetes mellitus due to viruses: Some recent developments. Diabetologia 36:687–695, 1993.
20. Yoon J-W: A new look at viruses in type 1 diabetes. Diab Metab Rev 11:83–107, 1995.
21. Banerji M, Lebovitz H: Insulin sensitive and insulin resistant variants in IDDM. Diabetes 38:784–792, 1989.
22. Alzaid A, Aideyan O, Nawaz S: The size of the pancreas in diabetes mellitus. Diabet Med 10:759–763, 1993.
23. Gepts W, Lecompte PM: The pancreatic islands in diabetes. Am J Med 70:105–115, 1981.
24. Lohr M, Kloppel G: Residual insulin positivity and pancreatic atrophy in relation to duration of chronic type 1 (insulin-dependent) diabetes mellitus and microangiopathy. Diabetologia 30:757–762, 1987.
25. Waguri M, Hanafusa T, Itoh N: Histopathologic study of the pancreas shows a characteristic lymphocytic infiltration in Japanese patients with IDDM. Endocr J 44:23–33, 1997.
26. Williams JA, Goldfine ID: The insulin-pancreatic acinar axis. Diabetes 34:980–986, 1985.
27. Groger G, Layer P: Exocrine pancreatic function in diabetes mellitus. Eur J Gastroenterol Hepatol 7:740–746, 1995.
28. Maloy AL, Longnecker DS, Greenberg ER: The relation of islet amyloid to the clinical type of diabetes. Hum Pathol 12:917–922, 1981.
29. Colelingam JD, Hellstrom R: Selective calcification of pancreatic islets of Langerhans. An unusual association with hypercalcemia and diabetes mellitus. Diabetes 27:620–624, 1978.
30. Reaver GM, Bernstein R, Davis B, et al.: Non ketotic diabetes mellitus: Insulin deficiency or insulin resistance? Am J Med 60:80–88, 1976.
31. Groop LC: Etiology of non-insulin dependent diabetes mellitus. *In* Leslie RGD (ed): Molecular Pathogenesis of Diabetes Mellitus. Basel: S Karger AG, 1997, pp 131–156.
32. Prochazka M, Lillioja S, Tait JF, et al.: Linkage of chromosomal markers on 4*q* with a putative gene determining maximal insulin action in Pima Indians. Diabetes 42:514–519, 1993.
33. Anonymous: Pancreatic abnormalities in type 2 diabetes mellitus. Lancet 2:1497–1498, 1987.
34. Fonseca V, Berger LA, Beckett AG, et al.: Size of the pancreas in diabetes mellitus: A study based on ultrasound. Br Med J 291:1240–1241, 1985.
35. Olsen TS: Lipomatosis of the pancreas in autopsy material and its relation to age and overweight. Acta Pathol Microbiol Scand A 86:367–373, 1978.
36. Dandona P, Freedman DB, Foo Y, et al.: Exocrine pancreatic function in diabetes mellitus. J Clin Pathol 37:302–306, 1984.
37. Kloppel G, Bommer G, Commandeur G, et al.: The endocrine pancreas in chronic pancreatitis: Immunocytochemical and ultrastructural studies. Virch Arch A Path Anat 377:157–174, 1978.
38. MacLean N, Ogilvie RF: Quantitative estimation of the pancreatic islet tissue in diabetic subjects. Diabetes 4:367–376, 1955.
39. Kloppel G, Drenck CR, Carstensen A, et al.: Ultrastructure and immunocytochemistry of the endocrine pancreas in diabetes. Medicina 2:299–308, 1982.
40. Seifert G: Die pathologische Morphologie der Langerhansschen Inselen besonders beim Diabetes Mellitus des Menschen. Verb Dtsch Ges Pathol 18:50–84, 1959.
41. Clark A, Wells CA, Buley D, et al.: Abnormal proportions of three pancreatic endocrine cell types and islet amyloid deposition in type-2 (non-insulin dependent) diabetes. Diabetologia 26:528A, 1986.
42. Bell ET: The incidence and significance of degranulation of the beta cells in the islets of Langerhans in diabetes mellitus. Diabetes 2:125–129, 1953.
43. Kloppel G: Islet histopathology in diabetes mellitus. *In* Kloppel G, Heitz PU (eds): Pancreatic Pathology. Edinburgh: Churchill Livingstone, 1984, pp 154–192.
44. Maloy AL, Longnecker DS, Greenberg ER: The relation of islet amyloid to the clinical type of diabetes. Hum Pathol 12:917–922, 1981.
45. Westermark P, Wilander E: The influence of amyloid deposits on the islet volume in maturity onset diabetes. Diabetologia 15:417–421, 1978.
46. Westermark P: Fine structure of islets of Langerhans in insular amyloidosis. Virchows Arch A Pathol Anat 359:1–18, 1973.
47. Westermark P: Amyloid of human islets of Langerhans. II. Electron microscopic analysis of isolated amyloid. Virchows Arch A Pathol Anat Histol 373:161–166, 1977.
48. Westermark P, Wilander E: Islet amyloid in Type 2 (non-insulin dependent) diabetes is related to insulin. Diabetologica 24:342–346, 1983.
49. Johnson KH, O'Brien TD, Betsholtz C, et al.: Islet amyloid, islet-amyloid polypeptide and diabetes mellitus. N Engl J Med 321:513–518, 1989.
50. Porte D Jr, Kahn SE: Hyperproinsulinemia and amyloid in NIDDM. Clues to etiology of islet beta-cell dysfunction. Diabetes 38:1333–1336, 1989.
51. Porte D Jr: Banting lecture 1990. Beta-cells in diabetes mellitus. Diabetes 40:166–180, 1991.
52. Johnson KH, O'Brien TD, Betsholtz C, et al.: Islet amyloid polypeptide: Mechanisms of amyloidogenesis in the pancreatic islets and potential roles in diabetes mellitus. Lab Invest 66:522–535, 1992.
53. Rocken C, Linke RP, Saeger W: Immunohistochemistry of islet amyloid polypeptide in diabetes mellitus:

Semi-quantitative studies in a post-mortem series. Virchows Arch A Pathol Anat Histopathol 421:339–344, 1992.
54. Westermark P: Islet pathology of non-insulin-dependent diabetes mellitus (NIDDM). Diabet Med 13[9suppl 6]:546–548, 1996.
55. Lorenzo A, Rozzaboni B, Weir GC, et al.: Pancreatic islets cell toxicity of amylin associated with type 2 diabetes mellitus. Nature 368:756–760, 1994.
56. Herman WH, Fajans SS, Oritz FJ, et al.: Abnormal insulin secretion, not insulin resistance is the primary genetic defect of MODY in the RW pedigree. Diabetes 43:40–46, 1994.
57. Yamagata K, Oda N, Kaisaki PJ, et al.: Mutations in the hepatic nuclear factor-1α gene in maturity onset diabetes of the young (MODY3). Nature 384:455–458, 1996.
58. Bell GI, Xiang K, Newman MV, et al.: Gene for non-insulin-dependent diabetes (maturity-onset diabetes of the young subtype) is linked to DNA polymorphism on human chromosome 20*q*. Proc Natl Acad Sci 88:1484–1488, 1991.
59. Yamagata K, Furuta H, Oda N, et al.: Mutations in the hepatocyte factor-4α gene in maturity onset diabetes of the young (MODY1). Nature 384:458–460, 1996.
60. Clement K, Pueyo ME, Vaxillaire M, et al.: Assessment of insulin sensitivity in glucokinase-deficient subjects. Diabetologia 39:82–90, 1996.
61. Froguel P, Vaxillaire M, Sun F, et al.: Close linkage of glucokinase locus on chromosome 7*p* to early-onset non-insulin dependent diabetes mellitus. Nature 356:162–164, 1992.
62. Hattersley AT: Maturity onset diabetes of the young: Clinical heterogeneity explained by genetic heterogeneity. Diabet Med 15:15–24, 1998.
63. Reardon W, Ross RJM, Sweeney MG: Diabetes mellitus associated with a pathogenic point mutation in mitochondrial DNA. Lancet 340:1376–1379, 1992.
64. Johns DR: Mitochondrial DNA and disease. N Engl J Med 333:638–644, 1995.
65. Gruppuso PA, Gorden P, Kahn CR, et al.: Familial hyperproinsulinemia due to a proposed defect in conversion of proinsulin to insulin. N Engl J Med 311:629–634, 1984.
66. Given BD, Mako ME, Tager HS, et al.: Diabetes due to secretion of an abnormal insulin. N Engl J Med 302:129–135, 1980.
67. Takahashi Y, Kadowaki H, Momomura K, et al.: A homozygous kinase-defective mutation in the insulin receptor gene in a patient with leprechaunism. Diabetologia 40:412–420, 1997.
68. Kaplowitz JN, Furlanetto RW: Homozygous nonsense mutation in the insulin receptor gene of a patient with severe congenital insulin resistance: Leprechaunism and the role of the insulin-like growth factor receptor. Clin Endocrinol 45:229–235, 1996.
69. Desbois-Mouthon C, Magre J, Duprey J, et al.: Major circadian variations of glucose homeostasis in a patient with Rabson–Mendenhall syndrome and primary insulin resistance due to a mutation (Cys284-Tyr) in the insulin receptor alpha-subunit. Pediatr Res 42:72–77, 1997.
70. Taylor SI: Lilly Lecture: Molecular mechanisms of insulin resistance: Lessons from patients with mutations in the insulin receptor gene. Diabetes 41:1473–1490, 1992.
71. Desbois-Mouthon C, Magre J, Amselem S, et al.: Lipoatrophic diabetes: Genetic exclusion of the insulin receptor gene. J Clin Endocrinol Metab 80:314–319, 1995.
72. Schuster DP, Osei K, Zipf WB: Characterization of alterations in glucose and insulin metabolism in Prader–Willi subjects. Metabolism 45:1514–1520, 1996.
73. Calcinaro F, Basta G, Lisi P, et al.: Insulin resistance in porphyria cutanea tarda. J Endocrinol Invest 12:393–399, 1989.
74. Robinson S, Kessling A: Diabetes secondary to genetic disorders. Baillieres Clin Endocrinol Metab 6:867–898, 1992.
75. Morrell D, Chase CL, Kupper LL, et al.: Diabetes mellitus in ataxia-telangiectasia, Fanconi anemia, xeroderma pigmentosum, common variable immunodeficiency and severe combined immune deficiency families. Diabetes 35:143–147, 1986.
76. Sjoberg RJ, Kidd GS: Pancreatic diabetes mellitus. Diabetes Care 12:715–724, 1989.
77. Nakasugi H, Funakoshi A, Iguchi H: Clinical assessment of pancreatic diabetes caused by chronic pancreatitis. J Gastroenterol 33:254–259, 1998.
78. Hodson ME: Diabetes mellitus and cystic fibrosis. Ballieres Clin Endocrinol Metab 6:797–805, 1992.
79. Allen HF, Gay EC, Klingensmith GJ, et al.: Identification and treatment of cystic fibrosis–related diabetes. A survey of current medical practice in the U.S. Diabetes Care 21:943–948, 1998.
80. Turnbull AJ, Mitchison HC, Peaston RT, et al.: The prevalence of hereditary hemochromatosis in a diabetic population. Q J Med 90:271–275, 1997.
81. Mohan V, Nagalotimath SJ, Yajnik CS: Fibrocalculous pancreatic diabetes. Diabetes Metab Rev 14:153–170, 1998.
82. Bartow SA, Mukai K, Rosai J: Pseudoneoplastic proliferation of endocrine cells in pancreatic fibrosis. Cancer 47:2627–2633, 1981.
83. Saudek CD, Hemm RM, Peterson CM: Abnormal glucose tolerance in β-thalassemia major. Metabolism 26:43–52, 1977.
84. Seftel HC, Keeley KJ, Isaacson MB, et al.: Siderosis in the Bantu: The clinical incidence of hemochromatosis in diabetic subjects. J Lab Clin Med 58:837–844, 1961.
85. Gepts W: Islet cell changes in human diabetes. *In* Cooperstein SJ, Watkins D (eds): The Islets of Langerhans: Biochemistry, Physiology, and Pathology. New York: Academic Press, 1981, pp 321–356.
86. Dymock IW, Cassar J, Pyke DA, et al.: Observations on the pathogenesis, complications and treatment of diabetes in 115 cases of haemochromatosis. Am J Med 52:203–210, 1972.
87. Megyesi C, Samols E, Marks V: Glucose tolerance and diabetes in chronic liver disease. Lancet 2:1051–1056, 1967.
88. Sherwin R, Joshi P, Hendler R, et al.: Hyperglucagonemia in Laennec's cirrhosis. The role of portal-systemic shunting. N Engl J Med 290:239–242, 1974.
89. Khan AA, Ali L: Tropical calcific pancreatitis and fibrocalculus pancreatic diabetes in Bangladesh. J Gastroenterol Hepatol 12:548–552, 1997.
90. Yajnik CS, Shelgikar KM, Naik SS, et al.: The ketoacidosis resistance in fibro-calculous-pancreatic diabetes. Diabetes Res Clin Prat 15:149–156, 1992.
91. Yajnik CS, Shelgikar KM: Fibrocalculous pancreatic diabetes in Pune, India. Clinical features and follow up for 7 yr. Diabetes Care 16:916–921, 1993.
92. Sidhu SS, Shah P, Prasanna BM, et al.: Chronic calcific pancreatitis of the tropics (CCPT): Spectrum and cor-

relates of exocrine and endocrine pancreatic dysfunction. Diabetes Res Clin Pract 27:127–132, 1995.
93. Kambo PK, Hitman GA, Mohan V, et al.: The genetic predisposition to fibrocalculous pancreatic diabetes. Diabetologia 32:45–51, 1989.
94. Gullo L, Pezzilli R, Morselli-Labate AM: Diabetes and the risk of pancreatic cancer. Italian Pancreatic Cancer Study Group. N Engl J Med 331:81–84, 1994.
95. La Vecchia C, Negri E, Franceschi S, et al.: A case-control study of diabetes mellitus and cancer risk. Br J Cancer 70:950–953, 1994.
96. Noy A, Bilezikian JP: Clinical review 63: Diabetes and pancreatic cancer: Clues to the early diagnosis of pancreatic malignancy. J Clin Endocrinol Metab 79:1223–1231, 1994.
97. Permert J, Larssen J, Fruin AB, et al.: Islet hormone secretion in pancreatic cancer patients with diabetes. Pancreas 15:60–68, 1997.
98. Ishikawa O, Ohhigashi H, Wada T, et al.: Morphologic characteristics of pancreatic carcinoma with diabetes mellitus. Cancer 64:1107–1112, 1989.
99. Ghadirian P, Boyle P, Simard A, et al.: Reported family aggregation of pancreatic cancer within a population-based case-control study in the Francophone community in Montreal, Canada. Int J Pancreatol 10:183–196, 1991.
100. Evans JP, Burke W, Chen R, et al.: Familial pancreatic adenocarcinoma: Association with diabetes and early molecular diagnosis. J Med Genet 32:330–335, 1995.
101. Jadresic A, Banks LM, Child DF, et al.: The acromegaly syndrome. Q J Med 202:189–204, 1982.
102. Soffer LJ, Iannaccone A, Gabrilore JL: Cushing's syndrome. Am J Med 30:129–146, 1961.
103. Stenstrom G, Sjostrom L, Smith U: Diabetes in phaeochromocytoma. Fasting blood glucose levels before and after surgery in 60 patients with phaeochromocytoma. Acta Endocrinologica 106:511–515, 1984.
104. Mouradian M, Abourizk N: Diabetes mellitus and thyroid disease. Diabetes Care 6:512–520, 1983.
105. Feldman JM, Plonk JW, Bivens CH, et al.: Glucose intolerance and the carcinoid syndrome. Diabetes 24:664–671, 1975.
106. Bouchard P, Sai P, Reach G, et al.: Diabetes mellitus following pentamidine-induced hypoglycemia in humans. Diabetes 31:40–45, 1982.
107. Esposti MD, Ngo A, Myers MA: Inhibition of mitochondrial complex I for IDDM induced by intoxication with rodenticide Vacor. Diabetes 45:1531–1534, 1996.
108. Pandit MK, Burke J, Gustafson AB, et al.: Drug induced disorders of glucose tolerance. Ann Int Med 118:529–540, 1993.
109. O'Bryne S, Feely J: Effects of drugs on glucose tolerance in non-insulin-dependent diabetes (parts I and II). Drugs 40:203–219, 1990.
110. Chan JC, Cockram CS, Critchley JA: Drug-induced disorders of glucose metabolism. Mechanisms and management. Drug Saf 15:135–157, 1996.
111. Menser MA, Forrest JM, Bandsby RD: Rubella infection and diabetes mellitus. Lancet 1:57–60, 1978.
112. McEvoy KM: Stiff man syndrome. Mayo Clin Proc 66:300–304, 1991.
113. Tarsy D, Miyawaki EK: Stiff man syndrome. Report of a case. Arch Intern Med 154:1285–1288, 1994.
114. Solimena M, Folli F, Denis-Donini S, et al.: Antibodies to glutamic acid decarboxylase in a patient with stiff-man syndrome, epilepsy and type 1 diabetes. N Engl J Med 318:1012–1020, 1988.
115. Kellett HA, Collier A, Taylor R, et al.: Hyperandrogenism, insulin resistance, acanthosis nigricans and systemic lupus erythematosus associated with insulin receptor antibodies. Metabolism 37:656–659, 1988.
116. Baird JS, Johnson JL, Elliott-Mills D, et al.: Systemic lupus erythematosus, with acanthosis nigricans, hyperpigmentation and insulin receptor antibody. Lupus 6:275–278, 1997.
117. Bloise W, Wajchenberg BL, Moncada VY, et al.: Atypical insulin receptor antibodies in a patient with type B insulin resistance and scleroderma. J Clin Endocrinol Metab 68:227–231, 1989.
118. Di Paolo S, Lattanzi V, Guastamacchia E, et al.: Extreme insulin resistance due to anti-insulin receptor antibodies: A direct demonstration of autoantibody secretion by peripheral lymphocytes. Diabetes Res Clin Pract 9:65–73, 1990.
119. Van Goor JC, Massa GG, Hirasing R: Increased incidence and prevalence of diabetes mellitus in Down's syndrome. Arch Dis Child 77:186, 1997.
120. Anwar AJ, Walker JD, Frier BM: Type 1 diabetes mellitus and Down's syndrome: Prevalence, management and complications. Diabet Med 15:160–163, 1998.
121. Burch PR: Klinefelter's syndrome, dizygotic twinning and diabetes mellitus. Nature 221:175–177, 1969.
122. Esmann V, Nielsen J, Petersen GB: A case of Klinefelter's syndrome with 48,XXXY and diabetes mellitus. Acta Med Scand 186:27–33, 1969.
123. Caprio S, Boulware S, Diamond M, et al.: Insulin resistance: An early metabolic defect of Turner's syndrome. J Clin Endocrinol Metab 72:832–836, 1991.
124. Kumon Y, Hisatake K, Suehiro T, et al.: Insulin resistance in a patient with diabetes mellitus associated with Turner's syndrome. Intern Med 33:560–563, 1994.
125. Najjar SS, Saikaly MG, Zaytoun GM, et al.: Association of diabetes insipidus, diabetes mellitus, optic atrophy and deafness. The Wolfram or DIDMOID syndrome. Arch Dis Child 60:823–838, 1985.
126. Barrett TG, Bundey SE, Macleod AF: Neurodegeneration and diabetes: UK nationwide study of Wolfram (DIDMOID) syndrome. Lancet 346:1458–1463, 1995.
127. Schoente EJ, Boltshauser EJ, Baekkeskov S, et al.: Preclinical and manifest diabetes mellitus in young patients with Friedreich's ataxia: No evidence of immune process behind the islet cell destruction. Diabetologia 32:378–391, 1989.
128. Fantus IG, Seni MH, Andermann E: Evidence for abnormal regulation of insulin receptors in Friedrich's ataxia. J Clin Endocrinol Metab 76:60–63, 1993.
129. Tevaarwerk GJ, Hudson AJ: Carbohydrate metabolism and insulin resistance in myotonia dystrophica. J Clin Endocrinol Metab 44:491–498, 1977.
130. Podolsky S, Leopold NA, Sax DS: Increased frequency of diabetes mellitus in patients with Huntington's chorea. Lancet 24:1356–1358, 1972.
131. Farrer LA: Diabetes mellitus in Huntington disease. Clin Genet 27:62–67, 1985.
132. Thornton CM, Carson DJ, Stewart FJ: Autopsy findings in the Wolcott–Rallison syndrome. Pediatr Pathol Lab Med 17:487–496, 1997.
133. Metzger BE, Organizing Committee: Summary and recommendations of the Third International Workshop-Conference on Gestational Diabetes Mellitus. Diabetes 40:197–201, 1991.
134. Engelgan MM, Herman WH, Smith PJ, et al.: The epidemiology of diabetes and pregnancy in the US, 1988. Diabetes Care 18:1029–1033, 1995.

135. Anon: Diabetes and pregnancy. *In* ACOG Technical Bulletin 200, 1994.
136. Dunne MJ, Kane C, Shepherd RM: Familial persistent hyperinsulinemic hypoglycemia of infancy and mutations in the sulfonylurea receptor. N Engl J Med 336:703–706, 1997.
137. Gossens A, Gepts W, Saudubray J-M, et al.: Diffuse and focal nesidioblastosis: A clinicopathological study of 24 patients with persistent neonatal hyperinsulinemic hypoglycemia. Am J Surg Pathol 13:766–775, 1989.
138. Dahms BB, Landing BH, Blaskovics M, et al.: Nesidioblastosis and other islet cell abnormalities in hyperinsulinemic hypoglycemia of infancy. Hum Pathol 11:641–649, 1980.
139. Sempoux C, Guiot Y, Dubois D, et al.: Pancreatic B-cell proliferation in persistent hyperinsulinemic hypoglycemia of infancy: An immunohistochemical study of 18 cases. Mod Pathol 11:444–449, 1998.
140. Jaffe R, Hashida Y, Yunis J: Pancreatic pathology in hyperinsulinemic hypoglycemia of infancy. Lab Invest 42:356–365, 1980.
141. Gould VE, Memoli VA, Dardi LE, et al.: Nesidiodysplasia and nesidioblastosis of infancy: Ultrastructural and immunohistochemical analysis of islet cell alterations with and without associated hyperinsulinemic hypoglycemia. Scand J Gastroenterol 16[suppl 70]:129–142, 1981.
142. Laidlaw GF: Nesidioblastoma, the islet cell tumor of the pancreas. Am J Pathol 14:125–134, 1938.
143. Yakovac WC, Baker L, Hummeler K: Beta-cell nesidioblastosis in idiopathic hypoglycemia of infancy. J Ped 79:226–231, 1971.
144. Witte DP, Greider MH, DeSchryver-Kecskemeti K, et al.: The juvenile human endocrine pancreas: Normal v idiopathic hyperinsulinemic hypoglycemia. Semin Diagn Pathol 1:30–42, 1984.
145. Gondswaard WB, Houthoff HJ, Koudstaal J, et al.: Nesidioblastosis and endocrine hyperplasia of the pancreas: A secondary phenomenon. Hum Pathol 17:46–53, 1986.
146. Shyng SL, Ferrigni T, Shepherd JB, et al.: Functional analysis of novel mutations in the sulfonylurea receptor 1 associated with persistent hyperinsulinemic hypoglycemia of infancy. Diabetes 47:1145–1151, 1998.
147. Verkarre V, Fournet JC, de Lonlay P, et al.: Paternal mutation of the sulfonylurea receptor (SUR1) gene and maternal loss of 11*p*15 imprinted genes lead to persistent hyperinsulinism in focal adenomatous hyperplasia. J Clin Invest 102:1286–1291, 1998.
148. Kendall DM, Robertson RP: Pancreas and islet transplantation in humans. Diabetes Metab 22:157–163, 1996.
149. Sutherland DE, Gruessner AC, Gruessner RW: Pancreas transplantation: A review. Transplant Proc 30:1940–1943, 1998.
150. Gruessner AC, Sutherland DER, Gruessner RWG: Report of the international transplant registry. Transplant Proc 30:242–243, 1998.
151. Di Carlo V, Castoldi M, Cristallo G, et al.: Techniques of pancreas transplantation throughout the world: An IPITA center survey. Transplant Proc 30:231–241, 1987.
152. Kuo PC, Johnson LB, Schweitzer EJ, et al.: Solitary pancreas allografts. The role of percutaneous biopsy and standardized histologic grading of rejection. Arch Surg 132:52–57, 1997.
153. Sibley RK: Pancreas transplantation. *In* Sale GE (ed): The Pathology of Organ Transplantation. Boston: Butterworth Publishers, 1990, pp 179–216.
154. Sibley RK, Sutherland DER: Pancreas transplantation: An immunohistologic and histopathologic examination of 100 grafts. Am J Pathol 128:151–170, 1987.
155. Nakhleh RE, Sutherland DER: Pancreas rejection. Significance of histopathologic findings with implications for classification of rejection. Am J Surg Pathol 16:1098–1107, 1992.
156. Drachenberg CB, Papadimitriou JC, Klassen DK, et al.: Evaluation of pancreas transplant needle biopsy: Reproducibility and revision of histologic grading system. Transplantation 63:1579–1586, 1997.
157. Tydén G, Reinholt FP, Sundkvist G, et al.: Recurrence of autoimmune diabetes mellitus in recipients of cadaveric pancreas grafts. N Engl J Med 335:860–863, 1996.
158. Eisenbarth GS, Stegall M. Islet and pancreatic transplantation—Autoimmunity and alloimmunity. N Engl J Med 335:888–889, 1996.
159. Drachenberg CB, Abruzzo LV, Klassen DK, et al.: Epstein–Barr virus–related posttransplantation lymphoproliferative disorder involving pancreas allografts: Histological differential diagnosis from acute allograft rejection. Hum Pathol 29:569–577, 1998.
160. Cretin N, Bhler L, Fournier B, et al.: Human islet allotransplantation: World experience and current status. Dig Surg 15:656–662, 1998.
161. Brunicardi FC, Atiya A, Stock P, et al.: Clinical islet transplantation experience at the University of California Islet Transplant Consortium. Surgery 118:967–921, 1995.
162. London NJ: Clinical studies of islet transplantation. Ann R Coll Surg Engl 77:263–269, 1995.
163. Bretzel RG, Hering BJ, Federlin KF: Islet cell transplantation in diabetes mellitus—from bench to bedside. Exp Clin Endocrinol Diabetes 103[suppl 2]:143–159, 1995.
164. Stegall MD, Lafferty KJ, Kam I, et al.: Evidence of recurrent autoimmunity in human allogenic islet transplantation. Transplantation 61:1272–1274, 1996.
165. Sever CE, Demitris AJ, Zeng Y, et al.: Islet cell autotransplantation in diabetic patients. Histologic findings in four adults simultaneously receiving kidney or liver transplants. Am J Pathol 140:1255–1260, 1992.

Chapter

4

DEGENERATIVE DISEASES OF THE PANCREAS

Included in this chapter are the various forms of pancreatic atrophy, not primarily caused by an inflammatory process. In many instances, these conditions result in the pancreatic parenchyma's being replaced by adipose tissue (so-called lipomatous atrophy and lipomatosis). Also included here, for the sake of convenience, is a discussion of pancreatic morphology in hemochromatosis and cystic fibrosis (mucoviscidosis).

SHWACHMAN SYNDROME

This condition is also known as the Shwachman–Diamond syndrome, lipomatous atrophy, or congenital hypoplasia of the exocrine pancreas.[1–5] It occurs in between 1 in 20,000 and 1 in 200,000 live births and is the second most common cause of exocrine pancreatic insufficiency in children after cystic fibrosis (CF). At present, it is considered to be the result of an autosomal-recessive disorder, although the gene mutation has yet to be identified. Classically, the syndrome affects small children and is characterized by atrophy of exocrine pancreatic elements, reduced ductular elements, normal islets, and a replacement of the acini by adipose tissue. Not surprisingly, affected infants present clinically with maldigestion and a failure to thrive.

Apart from the pancreatic abnormalities, infants with the Shwachman syndrome may also develop skeletal abnormalities and bone marrow dysfunction. The skeletal abnormalities are found in 30% to 50% of cases.[6,7] Clinically, they present with dwarfism. Radiologically, the changes are predominately localized in the metaphysis of the femoral neck and consist of an irregular configuration of the growth zone, with amorphous precipitates of calcium salts in the opening zones (metaphyseal dysostosis).[7] The skeletal abnormalities do not appear to be purely a consequence of malnourishment and are not reversed when supplementary digestive enzymes are provided.

Bone marrow dysfunction in the Shwachman syndrome consists of overall hypocellularity, resulting in anemia, neutropenia, and thrombocytopenia.[8,9] Neutropenia is present in 88% of patients with Shwachman syndrome and sometimes, the bone marrow abnormality is confined to neurophil production with a maturation arrest, leading to peripheral blood neutropenia.[6,10] In addition, the neutrophils may show defects in chemotaxis and surface adhesion properties. Complications arising from the bone marrow defect include an increased susceptibility to infection and to juvenile acute myelogenous leukemia.[11,12] The overall risk of leukemia is estimated to be approximately 25%.[12]

Examples of idiopathic exocrine pancreatic abnormalities have also been described in adults.[3,13–15] Some of these cases have occurred in conjunction with hematologic abnormalities and fulfill the criteria for Shwachman syndrome.[16] In two other cases, exocrine pancreatic atrophy and fatty replacement occurred in conjunction with cirrhosis[13] and Parkinson's disease.[14] These examples, labeled lipomatous pseudohypertrophy, were not accompanied by clinical evidence of exocrine failure, or marrow hypoplasia, so they cannot be considered as a true Shwachman syndrome.

In the normal newborn infant, the exocrine pancreas is functionally immature. Protease secretion is generally adequate, but lipase activity is only 5% to 10% that of an adult.[17] This low level of lipase activity persists throughout the first few years of life. In Shwachman syndrome, measurements of duodenal lipase vary. In individuals without clinical steatorrhea, they are between 3.7% and 13.6% of normal. In individuals with steatorrhea, they may be as low as 2% of normal.[1] The natural history of the disease is for a gradual improvement in symptoms and increase in lipase secretion, most of which occurs before 4 years of age.[1]

Few detailed morphologic descriptions of the pancreas in Shwachman syndrome exist.[6,11,18] Grossly, the organ is enlarged, with obvious replacement of the parenchyma by adipose tissue. Histologic examination reveals preservation of the islets, which appear normal in numbers and in cytologic appearance. Small amounts of exocrine acini and ducts may remain, but the organ otherwise is extensively infiltrated by adipose tissue. The ducts are not dilated and do not contain inspissated secretions. Inflammatory cells are not present and there is no fibrosis.

JOHANSON–BLIZZARD SYNDROME

Johanson–Blizzard syndrome is characterized by pancreatic exocrine insufficiency, hypothyroidism, sensorineural deafness, aplastic alae nasi, dental anomalies, developmental delay, and growth retardation.[19–23] It is thought probable that it is inherited as an autosomal-recessive disorder.[24] The pancreatic abnormality is very similar to the one described in Shwachman syndrome, with extensive acinar atrophy and replacement by adipose tissue.[24,25] The islets are not involved and patients do not develop diabetes. Stool fat losses represent about 30% of intake.

Not all children with primary pancreatic acinar atrophy are readily classified into Shwachman or Johanson–Blizzard syndromes. Intermediate examples exist, which may also have features of leprechaunism.[26]

LIPOMATOSIS

The term *pancreatic lipomatosis* is appropriately applied to cases in which there is marked fatty infiltration of the pancreas, without exocrine insufficiency or islet cell abnormality.[27] The condition is one that affects adults and is related to age and obesity.[28] Individuals with pancreatic lipomatosis may also develop type 2 diabetes. This is not surprising, as they are both related to obesity, although not directly to each other.

Detailed studies in unselected individuals of the pancreas at autopsy[27–30] have shown that the weight of the whole organ is correlated with age and body weight. Any enlargement that occurs is entirely due to an increase in adipose tissue, which comprises 10% of the weight at age 30 years and 35% of the weight at age 80 years.[27] In contrast, the weight of the pancreatic parenchyma is unchanged by age and obesity.[27] Fatty infiltration in lipomatosis is diffusely distributed throughout the dorsal pancreatic anlage, where involvement tends to be maximal. The ventral anlage is less severely affected.[27] Radiologic studies of pancreata affected by lipomatosis show a diffuse overall enlargement of the organ, often accompanied by an elongation of the main duct. In one example, multiple pancreatic cysts were identified.[30]

Lipomatosis, therefore, represents an exaggeration of the normal pancreatic response to aging and obesity. There is no clear point of demarcation between "normal" and "abnormal." As lipomatosis is entirely benign clinically, there seems little purpose in creating artificial boundaries for a "nondisease." Some cases documented in the literature[13,14] as "lipomatous pseudohypertrophy" of the pancreas are probably lipomatosis as defined above.

INFLAMMATORY BOWEL DISEASE

A variety of pancreatic abnormalities have been described in inflammatory bowel disease. Crohn's disease and ulcerative colitis have been implicated, although, in the majority of instances, Crohn's disease is present. As might be anticipated, most of the relevant data has been gathered by clinical observation, with only rare documentation of pancreatic morphology. Abnormalities may be grouped under three major headings: pancreatitis leading to pancreatic insufficiency, granulomatous pancreatitis, and pancreatic ductal changes resembling primary sclerosing cholangitis.

It has been apparent for some time that idiopathic pancreatitis may accompany long-standing Crohn's disease in individuals who do not have coincident duodenal involvement by Crohn's disease or classical sclerosing cholangitis.[31–38] The disease may be painless or may be accompanied by moderately severe atypical upper abdominal pain.[36] Persistent pancreatitis may lead to malabsorption and measurement of enzyme activity in duodenal aspirates may reveal significantly reduced levels of both amylase and lipase.[33] The prevalence of pancreatitis and malabsorption in unselected patients with Crohn's disease is not accurately known but has been estimated to be in the range of 1% to 2%.[35] Impaired pancreatic function is most severe in those individuals who have extensive and severely active disease but is not correlated with duration of disease or a history of prior bowel resection.[33]

The cause of pancreatitis and pancreatic malfunction in Crohn's disease is not firmly established but may be related to the presence of pancreatic autoantibodies (PABs).[36,37] These autoantibodies are of two types: subtype I, characterized by a droplike fluorescence when tested against pancreatic acini (includes immunoglobulin G [IgG] 1 and IgG 2 subclasses), and subtype II, characterized by a fine speckled acinar positivity and consisting of IgG 1 subclass.[33] Overall, PABs may be found in 27% to 40% of patients with Crohn's disease but are absent in control tissues originating from patients with ulcerative colitis. However, antibodies are also detected in 2.5% of asymptomatic first-degree relatives of patients with Crohn's disease. In patients with Crohn's disease, PAB positivity is divided equally between type I and type II antibodies. PAB-positive and -negative patients are clinically indistinguishable with regard to such characteristics as age, sex, disease activity, drug treatment, and prior surgical resections. In one study, 27% of antibody-positive patients had pancreatic dysfunction, in contrast to only 8% of antibody-negative patients with dysfunction.[36] However, conflicting results were obtained in a study of patients with Crohn's disease who also had chronic pancreatitis, where the incidence of autoantibodies was the same as in a control group of patients with Crohn's disease but without pancreatitis.[35] By themselves, therefore, these serologic findings do not establish a direct cause–effect relationship.

Abnormal results on liver function tests are the case for 16% of patients with idiopathic inflammatory bowel disease.[34] Abnormalities are more commonly encountered in individuals with Crohn's disease than in those with ulcerative colitis (30.4% versus 11.2%). When patients with sclerosing cholangitis are examined by endoscopic retrograde cholangiopancreatography, pancreatic ductal abnormalities may be detected in 48%.[38] In a study by Heikius et al., 4.6% of all patients with idiopathic inflammatory bowel disease had radiographic abnormalities in both the pancreatic duct and the bile duct.[38] Microscopic evaluation of the pancreas in these patients may reveal focal or diffuse pancreatic ductal dilation, acinar atrophy, and periductular inflammation with fibrosis.[39]

Direct involvement of the pancreas by Crohn's disease is exceptionally uncommon.[40,41] Duodenal Crohn's disease may extend directly into the head of the pancreas and produce fistulas of various types, which may be complicated by duodenopancreatic reflux.[41] Isolated inflammatory masses may also occur.[40] These may be granulomatous and histologically resemble Crohn's disease at other locations. The mass may cause obstructive jaundice by impinging on the distal common bile duct.

PANCREATIC DYSFUNCTION IN MALNUTRITION

It is probably not surprising that pancreatic exocrine insufficiency may occur in children with an inadequate dietary intake of protein. Pancreatic secretion is protein rich (enzymes) and cannot be produced properly in situations of malnutrition.[42,43] Pancreatic abnormalities are more commonly encountered in kwashiorkor and marasmic kwashiorkor than in marasmus (pure caloric malnutrition).[44] In malnourished children, measurement of pancreatic enzymes in duodenal secretions after stimulation by secretin and cholecystokinin reveals reduced amounts.[43] Feeding such children with a well-balanced diet may restore pancreatic function in some, but not all, individuals.

Morphologic studies of the pancreas in children dying from malnutrition reveal a number of changes.[42,44] Grossly, there is atrophy and fibrosis. Microscopically, there is atrophy and degranulation of the acinar cells. The ducts may be dilated and there is increased intra- and interlobular fibrous tissue. Ultrastructurally, there may be disorganization of the endoplasmic reticulum, with intracisternal sequestration.[44]

CYSTIC FIBROSIS

CF is an inherited disorder of epithelial chloride transport. Clinical manifestations are predominantly in the pancreas, lungs, gut, liver, and endocrine glands.[45] The basic abnormality is a defect in a gene located on the long arm of chromosome 7, which encodes a protein of about 1,480 amino acids. This is termed the *cystic fibrosis transmembrane conductance regulator (CFTR)*.[46] CFTR contains two ATP binding folds termed *NDB 1* and *NDB 2*, two membrane-spanning domains, and one central domain. In excess of 200 different mutations of the CFTR gene have been described. In North America, the most common mutation, which is present in 70% of CF patients, consists of a deletion of three nucleotides coding for phenylalanine at position F508[47] (class II mutation).

In CF, a chloride secretory defect is present in all epithelial cells. This was first recognized in cutaneous sweat glands, and the detection of abnormally high levels of sodium and chloride in sweat is still widely used as a diagnostic test. The primary defect is located in apical chloride channels, which are unresponsive to normal regulation by cyclic adenosine monophosphate (cAMP).[48] Affected cells exhibit abnormal chloride conductance, with secondary disruption of water transport. CF mutations may affect CFTR function through four possible mechanisms.[49] Class I mutations may produce premature termination signals, resulting in little or no full-length CFTR protein and no CFTR function. Class II mutations, such as F508, produce an abnormal CFTR protein, which does not mature to its fully glycosylated form and is degraded, rather than being inserted into the cell membrane. In class III mutations, the CFTR protein is processed correctly, but the chloride channel does not respond normally to adenosine triphosphate, because of defects in the NDB region. Class IV mutations produce abnormalities in the membrane-spanning domain, resulting in altered chloride channels. The extent of organ dysfunction in CF is related to the class of mutation present, with the most severe dysfunction being encountered in class I and II mutations. The biologic effect of CF is the production of concentrated and dehydrated secretions containing highly viscous mucus. Because of this facet of the disease, the term *mucoviscidosis* has been used in the past, synonymously with *CF*. By immunohistochemical analysis and in situ hybridization of pancreatic tissue, it appears probable that a significant proportion of the inspissated mucus is MUC6. The MUC6 gene also shows a very similar pattern of expression to that of CFTR in the fetal pancreas.[50,51]

Abnormal CF genes are inherited in a simple autosomal-recessive fashion. Homozygotes develop frank clinical features of CF; heterozygotes, especially those with the F508 mutation, may (72%) develop pancreatic insufficiency and malabsorption.[52] CF is most frequent in Caucasians but does occur rarely in African and southeast Asian populations. Among Caucasians, CF gene defects are present in between 4% and 5% of the general population. Most individuals are heterozygotes. Homozygosity and, hence, full effect in individuals, occurs in between 1 in 1,500 to 1 in 3,000 live births.[53] A small number of patients with CF are compound heterozygotes.

Formerly, CF was a highly lethal condition and few sufferers survived to adult life. Advances in treatment have now significantly improved the prognosis and over 70% of individuals affected live beyond the age of 20 years. In the majority of patients, symptoms are so severe that the diagnosis is made in infancy or childhood. In only 3% of instances is the diagnosis established after age 18 years. Clinical suspicion of CF occurs when a child develops meconium ileus, malabsorption due to pancreatic insufficiency, unexplained chronic pulmonary or liver disease, and failure to thrive. A sweat test is positive in 98% of affected individuals, if it is performed by experienced personnel. A finding of sweat sodium and chloride levels each above 60 mEq/L is considered diagnostic (normal, 10–15 mEq/L). Techniques for the prenatal diagnosis of CF are in the process of development.

CF is a disease with multisystem involvement. Major organs affected include lung, gut, liver, and pancreas. In males, there may be aspermia and hypoplastic epididymal ducts. Lung involvement is manifest by hyperplasia of the mucosal glands and epithelial goblet cells of the trachea and bronchi. An exceptionally viscous mucus is secreted, which effectively occludes air passages, leading to infection and pneumonia. Repeated infections, which are slow to resolve, lead to bronchiectasis and emphysema. Intestinal tract involvement may be characterized by accumulation of thick, densely adherent plugs of mucus, especially in the distal ileum and proximal colon. Obstruction of the bowel in the neonatal period results in the syndrome of meconium ileus. If untreated, this leads ultimately to intestinal perforation. Accumulation of thick mucus is not, however, confined to the neonatal period and may occasionally occur in young adults (meconium ileus equivalent). Liver involvement is secondary to biliary disease. Within the liver itself, disease is manifest by ductular dilation, ductular proliferation, and periductal inflammation with fibrosis. Eventually, secondary biliary cirrhosis develops.

Clinical features of pancreatic involvement may be divided into those indicating exocrine dysfunction and those associated with endocrine dysfunction. Approximately 85% of CF patients have exocrine insufficiency, characterized by protein and fat maldigestion with fecal loss. In two thirds of affected children, deficiency is evident at birth. The remainder develop problems during the first few years of life.[54] Clinically, this is characterized by passage of frequent and bulky stools. The stools may be gray, oily, and foul smelling. In small infants, the caloric loss leads to a failure to gain weight, with loss of subcutaneous fat and decreased muscle mass, leading to hypotonia. Vitamin K deficiency can produce a coagulopathy. Vitamin A deficiency leads to irritability, lethargy, and pseudotumor cerebri with sixth-nerve palsy. Laboratory testing demonstrates hypoalbuminemia and a severe normochromic, normocytic anemia. By 3 years of age, approximately 20% of untreated CF children will have a rectal prolapse. This appears to be precipitated by poor nutrition, frequent bulky bowel movements, and persistent coughing.

In individuals who do not have complete loss of enzyme activity, periodic pancreatic duct obstruction may lead to episodes of acute pancreatitis. This occurs in approximately 1% of patients with CF, especially adults. CF testing should be considered in patients who have otherwise unexplained pancreatitis. The presentation is typical, with repeated episodes of acute abdominal pain, vomiting, upper abdominal tenderness, and elevations of serum amylase and lipase. An individual may experience between one and seven attacks before the correct diagnosis is made.[55]

Glucose intolerance is the major manifestation of endocrine dysfunction in CF. This is present in between 30% and 40% of patients with the disease. Frank diabetes mellitus is present in approximately 5% of children and may develop in up to 15% of individuals over 18 years of age.[56,57] Diabetes in these patients is accompanied by insulinopenia, presumably reflecting the ongoing destruction of islet cells within the pancreas.

The basic pathogenetic mechanism of pancreatic damage in CF is the accumulation of mucoid material within the duct system.[52,58,59] This has the effect of plugging of the ducts, so that enzyme-containing secretions cannot be expressed into the duodenum. Plugging also causes acinar atrophy, periductal inflammation, and fibrosis. Abnormalities of fluid secretion primarily involve the duct-lining cells and centroacinar cells. CFTR is not localized to acinar cells themselves. The defect in chloride production promotes water and bicarbonate secretion from the centroacinar cells, resulting in reduced apical trafficking of zymogen granules and reduced solubilization of secretory proteins in zymogen granule–rich proximal ductules.[60]

Findings on macroscopic examination of the pancreas in affected neonates are usually unremarkable, apart from a firmer pancreatic consistency than normal.[61] After 2 to 3 years of age, the pancreas in patients with CF develops increased lobular markings and becomes noticeably firmer in texture. In advanced disease, the pancreas is generally scarred, with intervening cyst formation and patchy fatty infiltration. In occasional examples, fatty infiltration may become so prominent that lipomatosis may be suggested. Cysts present are generally multiple and may measure up to 3 cm in diameter, although they are most frequently less than 1 cm. They contain turbid, mucoid material.

The earliest histologic changes of cystic fibrosis may be detected in the pancreas after 32 to 38 weeks' gestation but become more marked after birth.[61] They consist of a lack of normal acinar maturation, degenerative acinar changes, and, most particularly, a dilation of interlobular and centroacinar ducts. Initially, these qualitative changes are subtle and accurate diagnosis depends on a quantitative approach, using normal controls.[61] In addition to these findings, the pancreas in newborns may show an increase in the ratio of connective tissue to acinar parenchyma. This ratio continues to increase as the child becomes older. In the first 2 years of life, the characteristic qualitative finding of duct dilation and mucoid plugging may be seen but is highly variable in extent.

A detailed histologic study of the autopsy appearances of the pancreas in CF has been conducted in adults.[62] Four patterns of abnormality are recognized and may be predominant in different areas of the pancreas. The suggestion has been made that there is a progression from

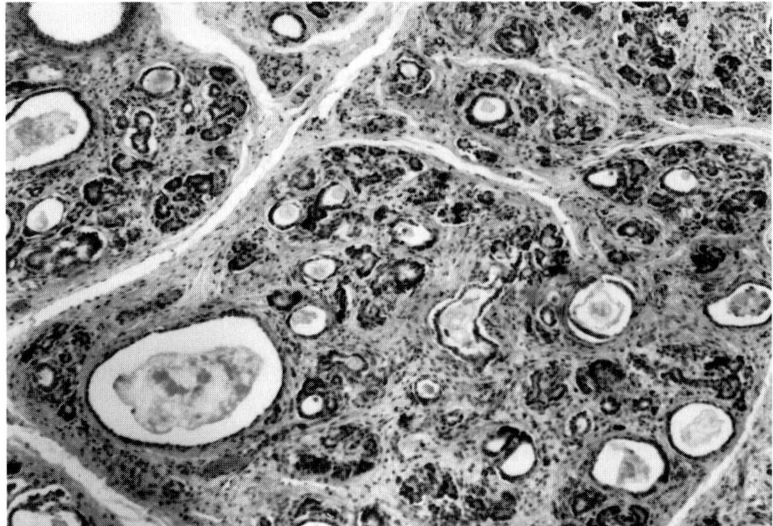

Figure 4–1. The earliest lesion of cystic fibrosis, which consists of acinar luminal dilation with mucus plugging.

type I to type IV lesions. Type I abnormality is primarily intralobular and consists of a loss of intracellular zymogen granules, with intralumenal dilation and inspissated eosinophilic material plugging the smallest radicals. Fig. 4–1 Type II abnormality consists of exocrine atrophy, with intra- and perilobular fibrosis. The segmental ductal system is ectatic and microcysts may be present (Fig. 4–2). Both may contain laminated eosinophilic material. In type III abnormalities, there is severe acinar atrophy, fibrosis, and fatty infiltration. Ruptured ducts (mucoceles) may be encountered. Type IV changes consist of total acinar loss with periductal sclerosis and central obliteration. Liposclerotic tissue may contain surviving islets of Langerhans. Surviving ducts are dilated and contain calcium-rich (hematoxophilic) mucus or concretions. The duct-lining epithelium may show goblet cell metaplasia or may be lined by a single flattened layer of cells. Inflammatory infiltrates are generally scanty and, if present, are located around dilated acini and small ducts. Rarely encountered and nonspecific changes include fat necrosis, conspicuous chronic inflammation, neuronal hyperplasia, and atherosclerotic lesions.[62] In adult pancreata, fatty tissue may account for 25% of the weight of the

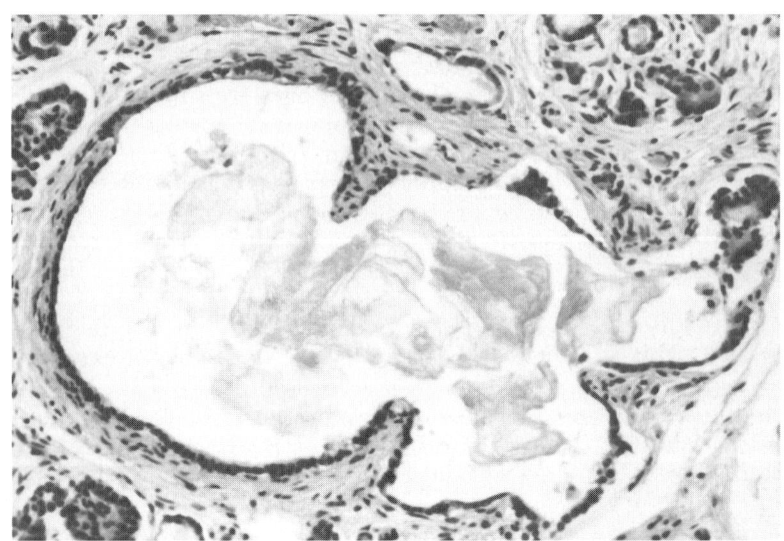

Figure 4–2. Moderately advanced lesion in cystic fibrosis. The segmental ductal system is ectatic and forms microcysts.

organ.[63] In the terminal stages of CF, the pancreas may be indistinguishable from examples of chronic sclerosing pancreatitis (38% of patients),[55,63] thus suggesting the prior occurrence of repeated localized episodes of acute pancreatitis.

The morphology of the islets of Langerhans in CF has been extensively studied.[64–67] In advanced disease, it is generally agreed that there is a reduction in both the number of islets and the number of B cells within the islets.[65,66] For example, in normal individuals, insulin-producing cells occupy 64% of islet surface area, whereas in patients with CF and diabetes, this was found to fall to 34%.[66] In another study, the B-cell area was found to be 53% in normal individuals, 47% in normoglycemic patients with CF, and 22% in diabetic patients with CF.[64] With the decrease in percentage of B cells, there is a corresponding relative increase in A cells, D cells, and PP cells.[64] Nesidioblastosis (see Chapter 3) may be prominent in the pancreas patients with CF who do not have diabetes, but is not found in CF patients with diabetes.[64] Nesidioblastosis may therefore be an adaptive mechanism to protect patients from glucose intolerance. Other histologic findings include fibrous disorganization of the islets and islet amyloidosis. Interestingly, amyloidosis is present in 69% of patients with CF and frank diabetes and in 17% of patients with CF and borderline diabetes, but is uniformly absent in controls.[67]

Radiologic evaluation of the pancreas in CF is best performed by computed tomography or magnetic resonance imaging (MRI). The correlation with radiologic changes and functional abnormalities is poor. Three MRI patterns are described: complete fatty replacement, an atrophic pancreas with partial fatty replacement usually at the rim, and diffuse atrophy without fatty replacement.[68,69]

HEMOCHROMATOSIS

The term *hemochromatosis* implies the presence within the body of iron in sufficient quantities to produce tissue damage. The term *hemosiderosis* (sometimes referred to simply as *siderosis*) implies the presence of increased quantities of iron unassociated with tissue damage. Hemosiderosis is, therefore, a usual precursor to hemochromatosis. Total body iron accumulation in established hemochromatosis is in the range of 20 to 40 g present at the time of diagnosis.

Iron overload may be due to a variety of causes. Primary hemochromatosis, usually called hereditary hemochromatosis (HHC), idiopathic hemochromatosis, or genetic hemochromatosis, is the result of a genetic mutation giving rise to an inborn error of metabolism. Secondary hemochromatosis may occur after repeated blood transfusion, especially in cases of refractory hypoplastic anemia. Anemias in which there is a hyperplastic bone marrow but ineffective erythropoiesis, for example, β-thalassemia, will lead to a considerable rise in absorption of dietary iron and its tissue accumulation.

The gene responsible for HHC has recently been discovered and named the HFE gene.[70] It is located on the short arm of chromosome 6 (6*p*21.23), close to the human leukocyte antigen locus. The most common mutation is termed C282Y, which appears to account for the majority of cases of HHC in all populations studied.[71–74] The C282Y mutation substitutes tyrosine for cysteine at amino acid 282. This is a missense mutation and appears to act by disrupting the binding of β_2-microglobulin to the heterodimeric HFE protein, with the result that the mutant molecule is not expressed on the cell surface.[73] Another mutation, termed H63D, has also been identified. This substitutes aspartate for histidine at amino acid 63 and is not associated with the same degree of iron loading as C282Y.[75,76] Reports from North America, western Europe, and Australia indicate that the genetic makeup of individuals with HHC is 84% homozygous for C282Y, 2% heterozygous for C282Y, 3.5% heterozygous for C282Y/H63D, 1% homozygous for H63D, and 3% heterozygous for H63D. The remaining 6% of individuals have no detectable mutation.[77] At the present, patients with iron overload who are not C282Y homozygotes or compound heterozygotes should be considered to have HHC, only if they have no other contributing cause for iron accumulation and have a family history of iron overload.[77]

HHC is an autosomal-recessive disorder. The HFE gene is mutated in about 10% of individuals, who are of European extraction.[76,78] Because most of these are heterozygous, they do not develop HHC, although they may have measurable abnormalities of iron metabolism and may accumulate iron. Men are particularly at risk if there are associated diseases, such as cirrhosis or alcoholism.[79] Homozygotes comprise 0.3% to 0.5% of Caucasian populations.

Clinical HHC will not usually be manifest in patients before the age of 40 years and its development is influenced by other factors, including dietary iron content and blood loss. The HFE mutation is less common in Asian and African populations and does not appear to be responsible for hemochromatosis occurring in South Africa (Bantu hemochromatosis). The HFE gene is also not implicated in iron overload in infants or children.[77]

A healthy adult man's body contains 3 to 4 g of iron, mainly present in hemoglobin or myoglobin. About one third of this amount is stored, either as a soluble fraction called *ferritin* or as an insoluble fraction termed *hemosiderin*. Hemosiderin is a degraded form of ferritin in which the iron aggregates are not associated with a protein shell. Most iron stores are located within the liver. In HHC, total iron content of the body is 5 to 10 times greater than normal. The excess iron is in storage, so that the stores are 20 to 50 times greater than normal. Maintenance of iron balance is normally achieved through regulation of absorption in the gut. A maximum of 3 to 5 mg is absorbed per day and obligatory losses are in the region of 1.0 mg/d. In women, 0.5 mg is lost with each menstrual period and about 1 g is needed for each pregnancy. Because of menstruation- and pregnancy-associated loss, tissue damage, secondary to iron accumulation, is less common in women than in men and occurs later in life. The mechanisms controlling cellular iron metabolism and iron absorption are complex.[77,80] It appears that iron absorption is regulated in cells at the base of intestinal crypts, where the HFE receptor, bound to a transferrin receptor, modulates uptake of diferric transferrin.[77] HHC is the result of inappropriately high degrees of absorption and retention of iron from the gut.[71]

Hemochromatosis involves a variety of organs within the body. Major manifestations may affect liver, pancreas, spleen, bone marrow, heart, joints, endocrine organs, and skin. Continuous iron deposition in the liver ultimately results in cirrhosis. Symptoms are often nonspecific and may include cachexia, weight loss, and weakness. Hepatic function is often well maintained, even after cirrhosis has developed, provided that alcoholism is not a cofactor in liver damage. Portal hypertension and splenomegaly may be present. Approximately 50% of HHC cases are now diagnosed in the precirrhotic phase, and repeated venesection may adequately deplete iron stores, so that a normal life expectancy may be anticipated. If individuals with HHC do develop cirrhosis, approximately 30% will develop hepatocellular carcinoma.[81] This complication does not occur in HHC without cirrhosis.

Iron accumulation in the heart may result in a congestive cardiomyopathy. This produces both congestive cardiac failure and dysrhythmias, particularly ventricular extrasystoles. At autopsy examination, the weight of the heart is two to three times normal, with biventricular hypertrophy. Microscopic examination demonstrates hemosiderin deposition within muscle fibers. The cells themselves may show degenerative features, including necrosis and fragmentation with interstitial edema and fibrosis.[82]

Endocrine involvement in HHC affects a variety of glands, in addition to the pancreas. There may be adrenal, thyroid, and parathyroid damage. Loss of libido and impotence in men and amenorrhea in women are probably secondary to damage to the anterior pituitary.

Joint involvement is common in HHC. The small joints of the hand, particularly the metacarpophalangeal joints and proximal interphalangeal joints, are the ones characteristically involved. The knees are the most common large joints affected. Microscopically, synovial cells are heavily laden with hemosiderin and there is nonspecific synovial thickening. Calcification of fibrocartilage and hyaline cartilage may be observed.

Skin pigmentation is a prominent clinical feature in $> 90\%$ of patients with HHC. It is most pronounced in light-exposed areas of the body, especially the face. In addition, ichthyosis-like changes, koilonychia, and hair loss are common. Histologic examination of affected skin shows that most of the increased pigmentation results from melanin present within the basal layer of the epidermis. Hemosiderin granules are present in the dermis around blood vessels, around sweat glands, and within the basement membrane zone of the sweat glands. It is thought that iron stimulates melanocytic activity, either by increasing oxidation or by blocking sulfhydryl groups' inhibitory effects on enzyme systems regulating melanin synthesis.

Pancreatic damage in HHC may affect exocrine and endocrine functions. At the time of diagnosis of HHC, most adult individuals will have impaired enzyme secretion, demonstrable by specific testing of duodenal aspirates. Clinical evidence of exocrine malfunction is rare, however. Endocrine malfunction is much more common and may be manifest either by impaired glucose tolerance or by frank diabetes mellitus. It appears that three mechanisms may be involved in the generation of diabetes: a familial predisposition to develop diabetes, diminished insulin sensitivity secondary to cirrhosis, and direct islet cell damage with hypoinsulinemia. Between 53% and 80% of patients with hemochromatosis will develop diabetes.[83] Furthermore, in individuals without overt HHC, even modestly increased iron stores, as assessed by elevated serum ferritin levels, are a risk factor for the subsequent development of diabetes.[84,85]

Some controversy exists about a genetic linkage between HHC and type II diabetes. It has been observed[86] that in HHC patients with diabetes, 25% of their non-HHC first-degree relatives also have diabetes, whereas in HHC patients without diabetes, only 4% of their first-degree relatives are diabetic. With the discovery of the HFE gene, it has become possible to screen those with diabetes for the presence of C 282Y and H63D mutations. Some investigators have found a mutation prevalence among those with diabetes of more than two times that of the general population.[87,88] Other investigators have found no difference.[89,90] The reasons for this discrepancy are unclear but may relate to differences in the populations screened.

Insulin resistance and hyperglucagonemia occur in patients with cirrhosis of all types. Iron overload, however, may by itself directly produce insulin resistance.[91] Insulin resistance is lowered when body iron stores are depleted by phlebotomy.[92] Low levels of insulin have been detected in some HHC patients with diabetes, indicating that islet cell destruction may also contribute to abnormal glucose metabolism.[86,92]

The diagnosis of hemochromatosis may initially be suspected by serologic determinations of iron and iron binding capacity (IBC). In normal subjects, serum iron is between 80 and 120 μg/dL and the IBC is approximately 200 μg/dL. In hemochromatosis, the serum iron is generally in excess of 200 μg/dL and the residual IBC is 30 to 40 μg/dL. The diagnosis may be further strengthened by obtaining a liver biopsy. As well as demonstrating excess iron storage and providing tissue for biochemical measurements of iron content, the biopsy will provide information about the presence of fibrosis or cirrhosis. The hepatic iron index (HII) is defined as the hepatic iron concentration measured in micromoles (μmol) of ferrous iron per gram of dry liver, divided by the patient's age in years.[71,93] Values in excess of 1.9 are regarded as highly reliable for a positive diagnosis of homozygous HHC in clinical situations, when there is an absence of hematologic disorders, such as thalassemia and dyserythropoietic conditions. The HII correlates well with serologic measurements of serum ferritin. No doubt in the future, detection of mutations of the HFE gene will simplify the diagnostic workup. Detection of the C282Y mutation cannot be used in isolation for screening purposes, as it is present in only 80% of patients with apparent HHC.[94] However, in the presence of homozygosity for C282Y, a confident diagnosis of HHC can be made if there is an elevation of transferrin saturation (low residual IBC), elevation of ferritin, or a family history of hemochromatosis.[70] Significant liver fibrosis is present in 50% of homozygous C282Y individuals, who have serum ferritin > 1,000 μg/L or elevated serum aspartate aminotransferase levels or hepatomegaly.[77]

In advanced HHC, the pancreas is a distinct rusty brownish color. The consistency is firmer than normal and the pancreas may be larger in size. There may be advanced fibrosis (Fig. 4–3). At histologic examination, hemosiderin deposition is noted within the acinar cells, duct cells, and islet cells. It is most obvious within acinar cells[95] (Fig. 4–4). Smaller amounts of hemosiderin may be encountered within interstitial cells. Fibrosis is often extensive at autopsy, with increased amounts present in inter- and intralobular locations[96] (Fig. 4–5). Routine staining generally reveals islets that are normal in shape and size.[95] Islet amyloid and atrophic islets are not encountered. Immunostaining of the islets reveals significant abnormalities in numbers of B cells. In patients with HHC and glucose intolerance, there is a 37% reduction, and in patients with HHC and diabetes, there is an 89% reduction.[95] Ultrastructural examination of the islets reveals that iron deposition is restricted to the cytoplasm of B cells and is associated with progressive loss of endocrine granules.[95]

Hemochromatosis, occurring in juvenile patients, is a separate entity from adult HHC.[97,98] It also is inherited as an autosomal-recessive disorder but is not related to the HFE gene on chromosome 6. The molecular abnormality has not yet been elucidated. Affected individuals present between the ages of 15 and 30 years with severe iron overload and heart failure.[99] Hypogonadism is also common, although liver disease tends to be milder than in adult HHC.[98]

A third type of hemochromatosis has been identified in infants and neonates.[100-104] This is

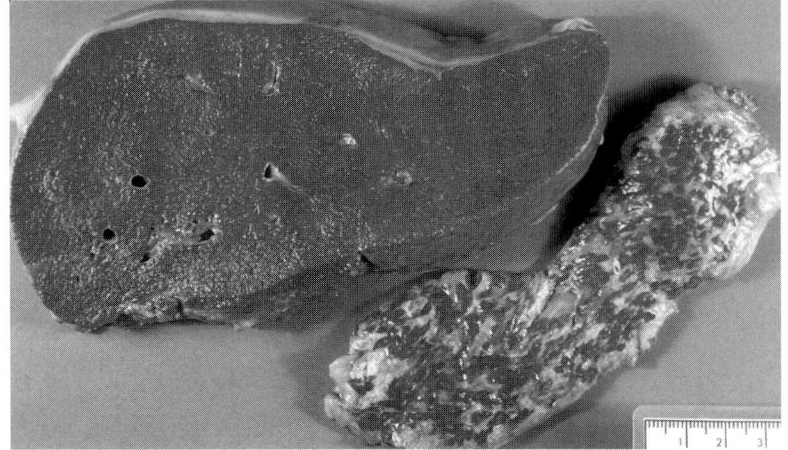

Figure 4–3. Gross appearances of the liver and pancreas from a case of hemochromatosis coming to autopsy. The liver demonstrates micronodular cirrhosis. The pancreas shows a profound coarse fibrosis, in which the appearance is accentuated by the pigmentation of residual parenchyma.

also unrelated to adult HHC and is not the result of HFE gene mutations. The condition may be familial in some individuals, but the biochemical defect is unknown. Sporadic cases and affected siblings have been reported, giving rise to suggestions of both autosomal-recessive and autosomal-codominant modes of inheritance.[104,105] Patients present at birth with severe liver disease and heavy iron deposition in all internal organs. Findings include hypoglycemia, hypoalbuminemia, edema, ascites, thrombocytopenia and bleeding. The fetus may be characterized by immaturity and growth retardation and the pregnancy, by oligohydramnios. There is a high mortality, usually within a few weeks of birth, from progressive hepatic failure.[93] Autopsy findings include cirrhosis or severe fibrosis, cholestasis, and giant cell transformation. Although iron deposition within hepatocytes can be prominent, Kupffer's cells and bile duct epithelium are relatively spared.[104]

Extremely rare examples of adult HHC, with a possible autosomal-dominant inheritance, have been described.[106] These have been described in Melanesian families of the South Pacific region. Again, any relationship to the HFE gene is not known.

It is known that men with an elevated store of body iron are at a greater risk of developing benign colonic neoplasms.[107] Studies of male heterozygotes for HHC have revealed an increased risk for both colon cancer and hematologic malignancies.[108] Female heterozygotes have an increased risk for the development of colonic adenomas and gastric cancer.[108] These

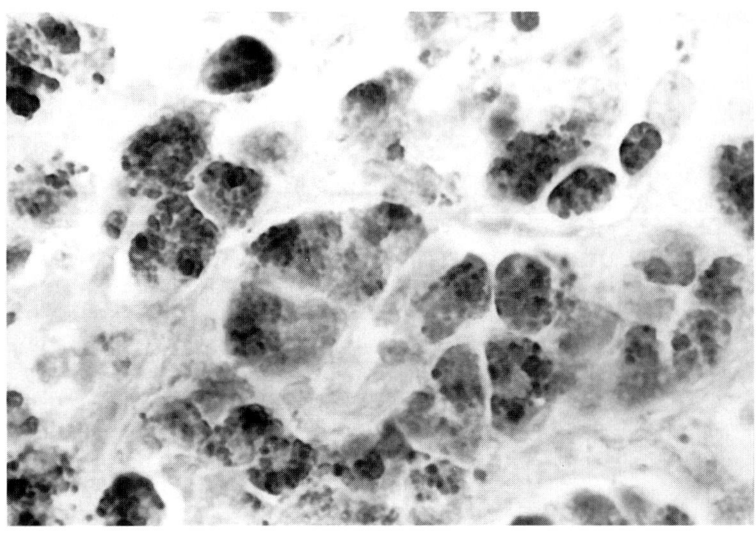

Figure 4–4. Hemochromatosis with advanced iron deposition within acinar cells. (Perl's Prussian blue stain.)

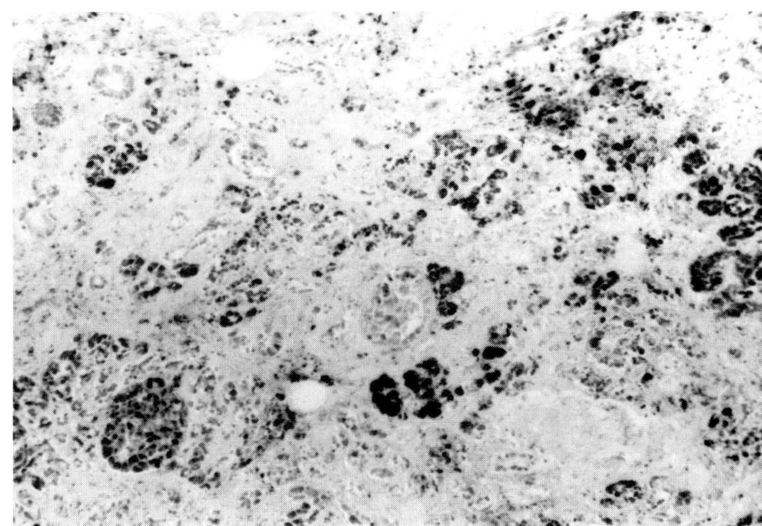

Figure 4–5. Advanced pancreatic fibrosis in hemochromatosis. (Perl's Prussian blue stain.)

risks are relatively small, however, in the order of 1.1 to 1.4 times normal. In contrast, in HHC with cirrhosis, hepatocellular carcinoma develops in approximately 30% of individuals.[81]

It is not generally appreciated that individuals with increased stores of body iron are at an increased risk of developing infections by *Yersinia* organisms, both *Y. enterocolitica* and *Y. pseudotuberculosis*. This is because *Yersinia* thrive best in an iron-rich environment. They lack the siderophores necessary to capture iron from the environment and are thus dependent on deriving it from external sources. Individuals with HHC may develop life-threatening infections, such as liver abscesses[109] or spontaneous bacterial peritonitis.[110] Infections with *Yersinia* organisms should always lead to clinical suspicion that disordered iron metabolism is present and should prompt relevant investigations.[111]

REFERENCES

1. Hill RE, Durie PR, Gaskin KJ, et al.: Steatorrhea and pancreatic insufficiency in Shwachman syndrome. Gastroenterology 83:22–27, 1982.
2. Danovich SH, Paley R, Mann O, et al.: Lipomatous infiltration of the pancreas. JAMA 253:1442–1443, 1985.
3. Lozano M, Navarro S, Perez-Ayuso R, et al.: Lipomatosis of the pancreas: An unusual cause of massive steatorrhea. Pancreas 3:580–582, 1988.
4. Robberecht E, Nachtegaele P, Van Rattinghe R, et al.: Pancreatic lipomatosis in the Shwachman–Diamond syndrome. Identification by sonography and CT-scan. Pediatr Radiol 15:348–349, 1985.
5. Mack D, Forstner G, Wilchanski M, et al.: Shwachman syndrome: Exocrine pancreatic dysfunction and variable phenotypic expression. Gastroenterology 111: 1593–1602, 1996.
6. Burke V, Colebatch JH, Anderson SM, et al.: Association of pancreatic insufficiency and chronic neutropenia in childhood. Arch Dis Child 42:147–157, 1967.
7. Giedion A, Prader A, Hadorn B, et al.: Metaphysäre Dysostose und angeborene Pankreas insuffizienz [metaphyseal dysostosis and pancreatic insufficiency]. Fortsch Geb Rontgenstr Nuklearmed 108:51–57, 1968.
8. Lebenthal E, Shwachman H: The pancreas—development, adaption and malfunction in infancy and childhood. Clin Gastroenterol 6:397–413, 1977.
9. Hadorn B: Diseases of the pancreas in children. Clin Gastroenterol 1:51–57, 1972.
10. Smith O, Hann I, Chessells J, et al.: Haematological abnormalities in Shwachman–Diamond syndrome. Br J Hematol 94:279–284, 1996.
11. Caselitz J, Kloppel G, Delling G, et al.: Shwachman's syndrome and leukemia. Wirchows Arch A Pathol Pathol Anat 385:109–116, 1979.
12. Woods W, Roloff J, Lukens J, et al.: The occurrence of leukemia in patients with the Shwachman syndrome. J Pediatr 99:425–428, 1981.
13. Sasaki M, Nakanuma Y, Ando H: Lipomatous pseudohypertrophy of the pancreas in a patient with cirrhosis due to chronic hepatitis B. Pathol Int 48:566–568, 1998.
14. Yoshimura N, Hayashi S, Fukushima Y: Diffuse Mallory bodies in the liver, diffuse Lewy bodies in the brain and diffuse fat replacement (lipomatous pseudohypertrophy) of the pancreas in a patient with juvenile Parkinson's disease. Acta Pathol Jpn 42:826–831, 1992.
15. Bom EP, van der Sande FM, Rjon RT, et al.: Shwachman syndrome: CT and MR diagnosis. J Comput Assist Tomogr 17:474–476, 1993.
16. MacMaster SA, Cummings TM: Computed tomography and ultrasonography findings for an adult with Shwachman syndrome and pancreatic lipomatosis. Can Assoc Radiol J 44:301–303, 1993.
17. Durie PR: Inherited causes of exocrine pancreatic dysfunction. Can J Gastroenterol 11:145–152, 1997.

18. Shwachman H, Diamond LK, Oski FA, et al.: The syndrome of pancreatic insufficiency and bone marrow dysfunction. J Pediatr 65:645–663, 1964.
19. Hurst JA, Baraitser M: Johanson-Blizzard syndrome. J Med Genet 26:45–48, 1989.
20. Gould NS, Paton JB, Bennett AR: Johanson–Blizzard syndrome: Clinical and pathological findings in 2 sibs. Am Med Genet 33:194–199, 1989.
21. Sandhu BK, Brueton MJ: Concurrent pancreatic and growth hormone insufficiency in Johanson–Blizzard syndrome. J Pediatr Gastroenterol Nutr 9:535–538, 1989.
22. Gershoni-Baruch R, Lerner A, Braun J, et al.: Johanson–Blizzard syndrome: Clinical spectrum and further delineation of the syndrome. Am J Med Genet 35:546–551, 1990.
23. Jones NL, Hofley PM, Durie PR: Pathophysiology of the pancreatic defect in Johanson–Blizzard syndrome: A disorder of acinar development. J Pediatr 125:406–408, 1994.
24. Daentl DL, Frias JL, Gilbert EF, et al.: The Johanson–Blizzard syndrome: Case report and autopsy findings. Am J Med Genet 3:129–135, 1979.
25. Moeschler JB, Polak MJ, Jenkins JJ 3rd, et al.: The Johanson–Blizzard syndrome: A second report of full autopsy findings. Am J Med Genet 26:133–138, 1987.
26. Szilagyi PG, Corsetti J, Callahan CM, et al.: Pancreatic exocrine aplasia, clinical features of leprechaunism and abnormal gonadotrophin regulation. Pediatr Pathol 7:51–61, 1987.
27. Schmitz-Moorman P, Pittner PM, Heinze W: Lipomatosis of the pancreas. A morphometrical investigation. Pathol Res Pract 173:45–53, 1981.
28. Stamm BH: Incidence and diagnostic significance of minor pathologic changes in the adult pancreas at autopsy: A systematic study of 112 autopsies in patients without known pancreatic disease. Hum Pathol 15:677–683, 1984.
29. Olsen TS: Lipomatosis of the pancreas in autopsy material and its relation to age and overweight. Acta Pathol Microbiol Scand [A] 86:367–373, 1978.
30. Nakamura M, Katada N, Sakakibara A, et al.: Huge lipomatous pseudohypertrophy of the pancreas. Am J Gastroenterol 72:171–174, 1979.
31. Seyrig JA, Jian R, Modigliani R, et al.: Idiopathic pancreatitis associated with inflammatory bowel disease. Dig Dis Sci 30:1121–1126, 1985.
32. Meyers S, Greenspan J, Greenstein AJ, et al.: Pancreatitis coincident with Crohn's ileocolitis. Report of a case and review of the literature. Dis Colon Rectum 30:119–122, 1987.
33. Hegnhoj J, Hansen CP, Rannem T, et al.: Pancreatic function in Crohn's disease. Gut 31:1076–1079, 1990.
34. Piontek M, Hengels KJ, Strohmeyer G: Crohn's disease: What about the pancreas? J Clin Gastroenterol 12:491–493, 1990.
35. Weber P, Seibold F, Jenss H: Acute pancreatitis in Crohn's disease. J Clin Gastroenterol 17:286–291, 1993.
36. Seibold F, Scheurlen M, Muller A, et al.: Impaired pancreatic function in patients with Crohn's disease with and without pancreatic autoantibodies. J Clin Gastroenterol 22:202–206, 1996.
37. Seibold F, Mork H, Tanza S, et al.: Pancreatic autoantibodies in Crohn's disease. Gut 40:481–484, 1997.
38. Heikius B, Niemela S, Lehtola J, et al.: Hepatobiliary and co-existing pancreatic duct abnormalities in patients with inflammatory bowel disease. Scand J Gastroenterol 32:153–161, 1997.
39. Ball WP, Baggenstoss AH, Bargen JA: Pancreatic lesions associated with chronic ulcerative colitis. Arch Pathol 50:347–358, 1950.
40. Gschwantler M, Kogelbauer G, Klose W, et al.: The pancreas as a site of granulomatous inflammation in Crohn's disease. Gastroenterology 108:1246–1249, 1995.
41. Legge DA, Hoffman HN, Carlson HC: Pancreatitis as a complication of regional enteritis of the duodenum. Gastroenterology 61:834–837, 1971.
42. Blackburn WR, Vinijchaikul K: The pancreas in kwashiorkor. An electron microscopic study. Lab Invest 20:305–318, 1960.
43. Sauniere JF, Sarles H: Exocrine pancreatic function and protein-caloric malnutrition in Dakar and Abidjan (West Africa): Silent pancreatic insufficiency. Am J Clin Nutr 48:1233–1238, 1988.
44. Brooks SE, Golden MH: The exocrine pancreas in kwashiorkor and marasmus. Light and electron microscopy. West Indian Med J 41:56–60, 1992.
45. Milla PJ: Cystic fibrosis: present and future. Digestion 59:579–588, 1998.
46. Riordan JR, Rommens JM, Kerem B, et al.: Identification of the cystic fibrosis gene: Cloning and characterization of complementary DNA. Science 245:1066–1073, 1989.
47. Consortium, CFGA: Worldwide survey of the delta-F508 mutation-report from the Cystic Fibrosis Genetic Analysis consortium. Am J Hum Genet 47:354–359, 1990.
48. Hyde K, Reid CJ, Tebbutt SJ, et al.: The cystic fibrosis transmembrane conductance regulator as a marker of human pancreatic duct development. Gastroenterology 113:914–919, 1997.
49. Welsh M: Cystic fibrosis: Approaches to therapy. Am J Gastroenterol 89:97–105, 1994.
50. Reid CJ, Hyde K, Ho SB, et al.: Cystic fibrosis of the pancreas: Involvement of MUC6 mucin in obstruction of pancreatic ducts. Mol Med 3:403–411, 1997.
51. Harris A: The duct cell in cystic fibrosis. Ann NY Acad Sci 880:17–30, 1999.
52. Kerem E, Corey M, Kerem BS, et al.: The relationship between genotype and phenotype in cystic fibrosis—analysis of the most common mutation (delta F508). N Engl J Med 323:1516–1522, 1990.
53. Best TF, Welsh MJ, Beaudet AL: Cystic fibrosis. *In* Scriver CR, Beaudet AC, Sly WS, Valle D (eds): The Metabolic Basis of Inherited Disease. New York: McGraw-Hill, 1989, p 2649.
54. Bronstein M, Sokol R, Abman S, et al.: Pancreatic insufficiency growth and nutrition in infants identified by newborn screening as having cystic fibrosis. J Pediatr 120:533–540, 1992.
55. Shwachman H, Lebenthal E, Khaw K-T: Recurrent acute pancreatitis in patients with cystic fibrosis and normal pancreatic enzymes. Pediatrics 55:86–95, 1975.
56. Moran A, Diem P, Klein DJ, et al.: Pancreatic endocrine function in cystic fibrosis. J Pediatr 118:715–723, 1991.
57. Rodman HM, Doershuk CF, Roland JM: The interaction of two diseases: Diabetes mellitus and cystic fibrosis. Medicine 65:389–397, 1986.
58. Durie PR: The pathophysiology of the pancreatic defect in cystic fibrosis. Acta Pediatr Scand Suppl 363:41–44, 1989.

59. Sinaasappel M, Veeze JH, De Jonge HR: New insights into the pathogenesis of cystic fibrosis. Scand J Gastroenterol Suppl 178:17–25, 1990.
60. Scheele G, Fukuoka S, Kern H, et al.: Pancreatic dysfunction in cystic fibrosis occurs as a result of impairments in luminal pH, apical trafficking of zymogen membrane granules, and solubilization of secretory enzymes. Pancreas 12:1–9, 1996.
61. Sturgess JM: Structural and developmental abnormalities of the exocrine pancreas in cystic fibrosis. J Pediatr Gastroenterol Nutr 3[suppl I]:S55–S66, 1984.
62. Vawter GF, Shwachman H: Cystic fibrosis in adults: An autopsy study. Pathol Annu 14(pt 2):357–382, 1979.
63. Kopito LE, Shwachman H, Vawter GF, et al.: The pancreas in cystic fibrosis. Chemical composition and comparative morphology. Pediatr Res 10:742–749, 1976.
64. Iannucci A, Mukai K, Johnson D, et al.: Endocrine pancreas in cystic fibrosis: An immunohistochemical study. Hum Pathol 15:278–284, 1984.
65. Abdul-Karim FW, Dahms BB, Velasco ME, et al.: Islets of Langerhans in adolescents and adults with cystic fibrosis. A quantitative study. Arch Pathol Lab Med 110:602–606, 1986.
66. Lohr M, Goertchen P, Nizze H, et al.: Cystic fibrosis associated islet changes may provide a basis for diabetes. An immunocytochemical and morphological study. Virchows Arch A Pathol Anat Histopathol 414:179–185, 1989.
67. Couce M, O'Brien TD, Moran A, et al.: Diabetes mellitus in cystic fibrosis is characterized by islet amyloidosis. J Clin Endocrinol Metab 81:1267–1272, 1996.
68. Murayama S, Robinson AE, Muluhill DM, et al.: Imaging of the pancreas in cystic fibrosis. Pediatr Radiol 20:536–539, 1990.
69. Tham RT, Heyerman HG, Falke TH, et al.: Cystic fibrosis: MR imaging of the pancreas. Radiology 179:183–186, 1991.
70. Feder JN, Gnirke A, Thomas W, et al.: A novel MHC class I-like gene is mutated in patients with hereditary hemochromatosis. Nat Genet 13:399–408, 1996.
71. Bonkovsky HL, Ponka P, Bacon BR, et al.: An update on iron metabolism: Summary of the Fifth International Conference on Disorders of Iron Metabolism. Hepatology 24:718–729, 1996.
72. Camaschella C, Piperno A: Hereditary hemochromatosis: Recent advances in molecular genetics and clinical management. Hematologica. 82:77–84, 1997.
73. Jazwinska EC: Hemochromatosis: A genetic defect in iron metabolism. Bioessays 20:562–568, 1998.
74. Walker EM Jr, Wolfe MD, Norton ML, et al.: Hereditary hemochromatosis. Ann Clin Lab Sci 28:300–312, 1998.
75. Worwood M: Hemochromatosis. Clin Lab Hematol 20:65–75, 1998.
76. Nielsen P, Carpinteiro S, Fischer R, et al.: Prevalence of the C 282Y and H63D mutations in the HFE gene in patients with hereditary hemochromatosis and in control subjects from Northern Germany. Br J Hematol 103:842–845, 1998.
77. Bacon BR, Powell LW, Adams PC, et al.: Molecular medicine and hemochromatosis: At the crossroads. Gastroenterology 116:193–207, 1999.
78. Bothwell TH, MacPhail AP: Hereditary hemochromatosis: Etiologic, pathologic and clinical aspects. Semin Hematol 35:55–71, 1998.
79. Piperno A, Vergani A, Malosio I, et al.: Hepatic iron overload in patients with chronic viral hepatitis: Role of HFE gene mutations. Hepatology 28:1105–1109, 1998.
80. Klausner RD, Rovault T, Harford JB: Regulating the fate of mRNA: The control of cellular iron metabolism. Cell 72:19–28, 1993.
81. Fargion S, Mandelli C, Piperno A, et al.: Survival and prognostic factors in 212 Italian patients with genetic hemochromatosis. Hepatology 15:655–659, 1992.
82. Buja LM, Roberts WC: Iron in the heart: Etiology and clinical significance. Am J Med 51:209–221, 1971.
83. Witte DL, Crosby WH, Edwards CQ, et al.: Practice Guideline Development Task Force of the College of American College of Pathologists: Hereditary hemochromatosis. Clin Chem Acta 245:139–200, 1996.
84. Salonen JT, Tuomainen T-P, Nyyssönen K, et al.: Relation between iron stones and non–insulin dependent diabetes in men: Case control study. Br Med J 317:727, 1998.
85. Hramiak IM, Finegood DT, Adams PC: Factors affecting glucose tolerance in hereditary hemochromatosis. Clin Invest Med 20:110–118, 1997.
86. Dymock IW, Cassar J, Pyke DA, et al.: Observations on the pathogenesis, complications and treatment of diabetes in 115 cases of hemochromatosis. Am J Med 52:203–210, 1972.
87. Conte D, Manachino D, Colli A, et al.: Prevalence of genetic hemochromatosis in a cohort of Italian patients with diabetes mellitus. Ann Intern Med 128:370–373, 1998.
88. Kwan T, Leber B, Ahuja S, et al.: Patients with type 2 diabetes have a high frequency of the C 282Y mutation of the hemochromatosis gene. Clin Invest Med 21:251–257, 1998.
89. Frayling T, Ellard S, Grove J, et al.: C 282Y mutation in HFE (haemochromatosis) gene and type 2 diabetes. Lancet 351:1933–1934, 1998.
90. Dubois-Laforgue D, Caillat-Zucman S, Djilali-Saiah I, et al.: Mutations in HFE, the hemochromatosis candidate gene, in patients with NIDDM. Diabetes Care 21:1371–1372, 1998.
91. Niederau C, Berger M, Stemmel W, et al.: Hyperinsulinemia in non-cirrhotic haemochromatosis: Impaired hepatic insulin degradation? Diabetologia 26:441–444, 1984.
92. Stremmel W, Niederau C, Berger M, et al.: Abnormalities in estrogen, androgen and insulin metabolism in idiopathic hemochromatosis. Ann NY Acad Sci 526:209–223, 1988.
93. Summers K, Halliday J, Powell L: Identification of homozygous hemochromatosis subjects by measurement of biochemical hepatic iron index. Hepatology 12:20–25, 1990.
94. Shahien NJ, Bacon BR, Grimm IS: Clinical characteristics of hereditary hemochromatosis patients who lack the C 282Y mutation. Hepatology 28:526–529, 1998.
95. Rahier J, Loozen S, Goebbels RM, et al.: The haemochromatotic human pancreas: A quantitative immunohistochemical and ultrastructural study. Diabetologia 30:5–12, 1987.
96. Suda K: Hemosiderin deposition in the pancreas. Arch Pathol Lab Med 109:996–999, 1985.
97. Camaschella C, Roetto A, Cicilano M, et al.: Juvenile and adult hemochromatosis are distinct genetic disorders. Eur J Hum Genet 5:371–375, 1997.
98. Camaschella C: Juvenile hemochromatosis. Baillieres Clin Gastroenterol 12:227–235, 1998.
99. Kaltwasser JP, Schalk K, Werner E: Juvenile hemochromatosis. Ann NY Acad Med 526:339–341, 1988.

100. Blisard KS, Bartow SA: Neonatal hemochromatosis. Hum Pathol 17:376–383, 1986.
101. Colletti RB, Clemmons JJ: Familial neonatal hemochromatosis with survival. J Pediatr Gastroenterol Nutr 7:39–45, 1988.
102. Witzleben CL, Uri A: Perinatal hemochromatosis: Entity or end result. Hum Pathol 20:335–340, 1989.
103. Moerman P, Panwels P, Vandenberghe K, et al.: Neonatal hemochromatosis. Histopathology 17:345–351, 1990.
104. Barnard JA 3rd, Manci E: Neonatal iron-storage disease. Gastroenterology 101:1420–1427, 1991.
105. Knisely AS: Neonatal hemochromatosis. Adv Pediatr 39:383–403, 1992.
106. Eason RJ, Adams PC, Aston CE, et al.: Familial iron overload with possible autosomal dominant inheritance. Aust N Z J Med 20:226–230, 1990.
107. Nelson RL, Davis F, Sutter E, et al.: Body iron stores and the risk of colonic neoplasia. J Natl Cancer Inst 86:455–460, 1994.
108. Nelson RL, Davis FG, Persky V, et al.: Risk of neoplastic and other diseases among people with heterozygosity for hereditary hemochromatosis. Cancer 76:875–879, 1995.
109. Oleson LL, Ejlertsen T, Paulsen SM, et al.: Liver abscesses due to *Yersinia enterocolitica* in patients with hemochromatosis. J Intern Med 225:351–354, 1989.
110. de Cuenca-Moron B, Solis-Herruzo JA, Moreno D, et al.: Spontaneous bacterial peritonitis due to *Yersinia enterocolitica* in secondary alcoholic hemochromatosis. J Clin Gastroenterol 11:675–678, 1989.
111. Muench KH: Hemochromatosis and infection: Alcohol and iron, oysters and sepsis. Am J Med 87:40(N)–43(N), 1989.

Chapter

5

PANCREATITIS

CLASSIFICATION OF PANCREATITIS

Pancreatitis is traditionally classified into acute and chronic forms. The Marseilles symposium in 1963 added acute relapsing and chronic relapsing forms.[1] However, these subsequently fell into disuse when it became apparent that to distinguish relapse of acute pancreatitis from exacerbation of chronic pancreatitis was often difficult.[2–4] The 1984 Marseilles–Rome classification of pancreatitis introduced a third category—obstructive pancreatitis that is evenly distributed throughout the pancreas but is not accompanied by either ductal plugs or calcification.[5,6] In 1992, the Atlanta international consensus meeting agreed on a set of working definitions of acute pancreatitis and its complications that is supported by short clinical descriptions.[7]

ACUTE PANCREATITIS

Acute pancreatitis is an autodigestive and inflammatory process ranging in severity from interstitial edema and minimal necrosis (mild acute pancreatitis) to confluent necrosis and hemorrhage (severe pancreatitis).[8,9] Most attacks are self-limited, but in severe cases, the condition progresses to shock, respiratory failure, renal failure, and death. Clinically, acute pancreatitis most often has a rapid onset, with upper abdominal pain associated with variable abdominal findings that range from mild to rebound tenderness. Acute pancreatitis is often accompanied by vomiting, fever, tachycardia, leukocytosis, and elevated pancreatic enzyme levels in the blood and/or urine.[7]

Most often, acute pancreatitis is mild, although one case in five is severe. Mild acute pancreatitis is associated with minimal organ dysfunction and uneventful recovery. There is no necrosis demonstrated on dynamic computed tomography (CT). Mild acute pancreatitis responds to appropriate fluid administration with prompt normalization of physical signs and laboratory values.[7] Severe acute pancreatitis is recognized by substantial pancreatic necrosis on contrast-enhanced CT, or clinical organ failure, Ranson score of 3 or more[10] (Table 5–1), or by APACHE II (acute physiology, age, chronic health evaluation) score of ≥ 8.[11,12] Severe disease is often complicated by necrosis, abscess, or pseudocyst. The clinical manifestations include abdominal tenderness, rebound, distension, and underactive or absent bowel sounds. An epigastric mass may be present. Rarely, flank ecchymosis (Grey Turner's sign) or periumbilical ecchymosis (Cullen's sign) may be seen. Organ failure may occur and is defined as shock (systolic blood pressure <90 mm Hg), pulmonary insufficiency (Pa_{O_2} ≤ 60 mm Hg), renal failure (creatinine level >177 μmol/L after rehydration), or gastrointestinal bleeding (>500 mL per 24 hours). Systemic complications, such as disseminated intravascular coagulation (platelets $\leq 100{,}000/mm^3$ fibrinogen <1.0 g/L, and fibrin split products >80 μg/mL) or severe metabolic disturbances (calcium level ≤ 1.87 mmol/L [7.5 mg/dL]), may also be seen.[7] The sex of the patient is not an independent risk factor for severe acute pancreatitis.[13] The overall mortality in severe acute pancreatitis is about 30%. Early deaths, occurring within 1 to 2 weeks, are due to multisystem organ failure, caused by inflammatory mediators and cytokines. Late deaths result from local or systemic infection.[14] The mortality rate triples if there is infected necrosis and is greatly increased if there is multisystem organ failure.[14]

Contrast-enhanced dynamic sequential CT is the single most important imaging modality in

Table 5–1. Ranson's Score* for Severe Acute Pancreatitis

At admission:
Age > 55 y
White blood cell count > 16,000/mm^3
Blood glucose > 200 mg/dL (11.1 mmol/L)
Serum lactate dehydrogenase > 350 IU/L
Serum aspartate aminotransferase > 250 IU/L
During initial 48 hours:
Absolute decrease in hematocrit > 10%
Increase in blood urea nitrogen > 5mg/dL (1.8 mmol/L)
Serum calcium < 8mg/dL (2 mmol/L)
Arterial Pa_{O_2} < 60 mm Hg
Base deficit > 4 mmol/L
Fluid sequestration > 6 L

* Score 1 point for each feature. A score of ≥3 is severe.

the diagnosis of pancreatitis. The CT signs of pancreatitis are swelling, peripancreatic mixed-attenuation collections, and necrosis.[15] Pancreatic necrosis is recognized on CT as lack of enhancement of all or a portion of the gland, owing to loss of the microcirculation. Necrosis is diagnosed if there is a focal or diffuse, well-marginated zone of nonenhanced pancreatic parenchyma >3 cm in diameter or involving >30% of the area of the pancreas.[16] The extent of peripancreatic fat necrosis cannot be reliably determined with CT. Patients with necrosis at first or subsequent CT have a 23% mortality and an 82% complication rate, whereas patients without necrosis have zero mortality and only 6% morbidity. Serious complications occur in patients who develop > 30% necrosis.[15,16]

There is considerable geographic variation in the incidence of acute pancreatitis. In Western countries, the incidence is 5 to 10/100,000 per annum. This incidence is rising, likely due to increased alcohol consumption.[17–20] Men are affected slightly more than women and pancreatitis occurs at an earlier age in men than in women.[17,21] The alcohol-related form is most common in young men and the gallstone-related forms are most common in older women. The peak incidence occurs in the third to fifth decades of life in men and in the fifth to sixth decades in women.[9]

The causes of acute pancreatitis are listed in Table 5–2 and the main causes by country are listed in Table 5–3. Gallstone disease and chronic alcohol abuse together account for 60% to 70% of cases.[13,17–19,22] Alcoholism is the most common cause in the United States, and the incidence of alcoholism as a cause is increasing in Europe and elsewhere.[17–20] More than one causative factor may be present in the same patient—for instance, chronic alcoholism with gallstone disease.[19] In Sweden, gallstone disease is the main cause in first attacks, but alcohol is the main cause when relapses are included.[17] Eighteen percent to 23% of cases of acute pancreatitis are of unknown cause.[13,17–19,23] Postoperative pancreatitis looms larger in autopsy studies than in clinical series, being as high as 9.1% to 14%.[19,23] Some drugs may cause acute pancreatitis (Table 5–4). The risk of pancreatitis relapse by cause is given in Table 5–5.[17]

Associated Conditions

Alcoholism

Chronic alcoholism, but not isolated alcoholic binges, is associated with both acute and chronic pancreatitis.[24] In France, the average duration of alcohol consumption before the appearance of symptoms is 18 years for men and 11 years for women.[25] As the majority of heavy drinkers do not develop pancreatitis, there is clearly an element of individual suscep-

Table 5–2. Causes of Acute Pancreatitis

Alcohol
Ductal obstruction
Gallstones
Neoplasms
Parasites
Pancreas divisum
Anomalous union of the pancreaticobiliary ducts
Ascaris lumbricoides or *Clonorchis sinensis*
Endoscopic retrograde cholangiopancreatography
Trauma and surgery
Hyperlipidemia, types I, IV, and V
Hypercalcemia
Hyperparathyroidism
Calcium infusions during cardiac surgery
Ischemia
Penetrating duodenal ulcer
Drugs and toxins (see Table 5–4)
Infections
Tuberculosis
Cytomegalovirus
Hepatitis viruses
Hydatid disease
Mumps
Toxoplasmosis
Congenital syphilis
Other
Systemic lupus erythematosus
Behçet's disease
Bone marrow transplantation
Liver disease (?)

Table 5–3. Frequency of the Main Attributed Causes of Acute Pancreatitis[13,17–19]

	Great Britain (%)	Germany (%)	Sweden (%)	United States (%)
Idiopathic	23	22.1	23	19.2
Alcohol	8	29.4	45	60.9
Gallstones	50	37.7	25.5	≥ 6.2
Other	19	10.8	7.5	

tibility[26] and therefore genetic factors are thought to play a role. For example, an increased frequency of HLA Bw39 has been found in alcoholics with pancreatitis.[27] The mechanism of alcohol-induced injury to the pancreas is still uncertain. Ethanol is not directly toxic to the pancreas, but cytochrome P4502E1, which is present in the pancreas, metabolizes ethanol, producing oxygen free radicals. These are thought to contribute to the state of oxidative stress in the pancreas.[28] Ethanol is metabolized to acetaldehyde by alcohol dehydrogenase and acetaldehyde can serve as a substrate for xanthine oxidase, also resulting in free radical generation. Free radicals have been demonstrated to initiate acute pancreatitis in animals[29] and there is considerable evidence that free radicals are often part of the final pathway of damage in pancreatitis. Inhibitors of free radicals have the potential to limit the injury in animal models of pancreatitis.[30–32] Ethanol ingestion may cause pancreatic exocrine hypersecretion through increased secretin production and sensitization to cholecystokinin (CCK). Recently, ethanol has been found to sensitize the acinar cell to CCK, so that the effect of ethanol plus CCK is similar to that of CCK hyperstimulation.[33] The mechanism of sensitization is unclear. Ethanol also evokes the release of CCK from the intestine.[34] However, a variety of therapies designed to diminish pancreatic secretion do not improve the clinical course of acute pancreatitis. These include cimetidine, nasogastric suction, glucagon, and somatostatin.[35–38] There is no demonstrated nutritional deficiency in alcoholic pancreatitis. The suggestion that alcohol causes deposition of protein plugs in the pancreatic ducts, resulting in obstructive pancreatitis,[5] is unproven. Protein plugs seem to follow, rather than to precede, pancreatitis of various causes. The pancreatic juice of patients with chronic pancreatitis displays decreased volume, normal bicarbonate concentration, increased protein concentration, increased calcium concentration, and normal citrate concentration.[5] Ethanol increases the permeability of the pancreatic duct,[39] and this, too, may incite pancreatitis.

Table 5–4. Drugs That May Cause Acute Pancreatitis

Acetaminophen (overdose)	Isotretinoin
Aminosalicylic acid	Lovastatin
Angiotensin-converting enzyme inhibitors	Maprotiline
Asparaginase	Mercaptopurine
Azathioprine	Mesalazine (Mesasal)
Cimetidine	Methyldopa
Codeine	Metronidazole
Corticosteroids	Nitrofurantoin
Cytarabine	Olsalazine
Danazol	Oxyphenbutazone
Dideoxyinosine	Pentamidine
Diphenoxylate	Piroxicam
Ergotamine (overdose)	Procainamide
Estrogens	Ranitidine
Ethacrynic acid	Rifampin
Furosemide	Sulfasalazine
Gemfibrozil	Sulfonamides
Gold	Sulindac
Ibuprofen	Tetracycline
Interferon-α	Thiazides
Interleukin-2	Valproic acid

Table 5–5. Risk of Relapse After a First Attack of Acute Pancreatitis

Etiology	Risk (%)
Alcohol	48.3
Gallstones	21.0
Unknown	18.7
Other	5.7
Total	28.2

From Appelros S, Borgstrom A: Incidence, aetiology and mortality rate of acute pancreatitis over 10 years in a defined urban population in Sweden. Br J Surg 86:465–470, 1999.

Gallstone Pancreatitis

Gallstone pancreatitis is more common in women than men and is caused by gallstones migrating down the bile duct and transiently obstructing the main pancreatic duct at or near the ampulla.[40] Gallstones can be recovered from the feces of 84% to 94% of patients with acute pancreatitis associated with gallstones, compared with only 9% to 11% of controls with gallstones but without pancreatitis.[41,42] The gallstones recovered are small; the mean size of stones that impact at the ampulla is 3.1 mm,[43] and small gallstones are significantly more common in gallbladders from patients with gallstone pancreatitis.[43] The cystic ducts are typically wider in patients with pancreatitis than in controls.[43,44] Men with gallstones are significantly more likely to develop pancreatitis than are women.[44] Gallstones measuring 1 to 3 mm in diameter are usually not detected on gallbladder imaging studies, but microscopic crystals or microliths in bile (biliary sludge) predict the presence of small gallstones.[45] Seventy-three percent of patients with acute or relapsing acute pancreatitis of apparently idiopathic type have occult biliary microlithiasis or "sludge," consisting of calcium bilirubinate granules, cholesterol monohydrate crystals, or calcium carbonate microspheres.[45–49] Calcium bilirubinate sludge is often detectable on ultrasonography, but cholesterol monohydrate crystals are not. In patients with cholesterol crystals, recurrence of pancreatitis can be prevented by cholecystectomy, papillotomy, or ursodeoxycholic acid therapy.[45,49] Whether sludge itself can cause pancreatitis is unclear, but sludge alone is capable of elevating pancreatic duct pressures.[50] The mechanism by which transient pancreatic duct obstruction, with or without reflux, induces pancreatitis is not yet fully elucidated. In the isolated perfused canine pancreas, partial obstruction of the pancreatic duct, combined with secretin stimulation, produces pancreatitis, and this may mimic the transient impaction of a gallstone. Obstruction at the ampulla may increase ductal pressure, but factors other than pressure are likely needed to produce full-blown pancreatitis. One of these factors could be infection. Patients with biliary tract infection present with more severe pancreatitis.[40] The role of bile reflux into the pancreatic duct is controversial. Maximal duct pressures are higher in the pancreatic duct than in the biliary tract,[51] suggesting that reflux of bile into the pancreatic ducts is unlikely to occur physiologically. However, the common bile duct and main pancreatic duct form a common channel in three of every four people[52] and bile reflux has been demonstrated by intraoperative cholangiography in between 50% and 79% of patients with gallstone pancreatitis, compared with only 18% of controls.[42,43,53] Bile alone is not capable of activating pancreatic proteases. In animals, injection of sterile bile at physiologic pressures does not provoke pancreatitis, but injection of bacterially contaminated bile does.[54,55] There is bacterial contamination of the bile in 25% to 50% of patients with chronic cholecystitis and in close to 100% of patients with acute cholecystitis.[40,56] Thus, gallstone pancreatitis may sometimes be due to reflux of bacterially contaminated bile, although proof of this is lacking in many cases. Treatment of patients with acute biliary pancreatitis is supportive in the short term, but papillotomy and/or cholecystectomy are often performed after recovery. Early endoscopic retrograde cholangiopancreatography (ERCP) and sphincterotomy are not beneficial, unless there is jaundice.[57]

Obstructive Pancreatitis

Obstructive pancreatitis is due to obstruction of the main pancreatic duct by scar, stricture, neoplasm, parasite, or congenital abnormality, such as pancreas divisum or anomalous union of the pancreaticobiliary ducts.[58–60] It is regarded as a variant of typical acute pancreatitis described above. The obstruction of the main pancreatic duct occurs gradually before the development of the pancreatitis. Neoplasms that may present with obstructive pancreatitis are carcinomas of the pancreas, overt or occult,[61,62] and ampullary tumors including adenomas, carcinoids, and carcinomas.[63–66] Pancreatic carcinoma is the cause of 1.4% of cases of acute pancreatitis.[21,67] Rarely, metastatic tumors in the pancreas or lymphomas that enlarge the peripancreatic lymph nodes are associated with pancreatitis.[68] There is debate about the role, if any, of pancreas divisum (failure of the dorsal and ventral ducts to fuse) in causing obstructive pancreatitis[69] (see Chapter 2). This is the most common congenital anomaly of the pancreas, and although most studies have found no statistical relationship with pancreatitis, individual case reports keep the concept alive. By contrast, *anomalous union of the pancreaticobiliary ductal system (AUPBD)*, the condition in which the common bile duct and main pancreatic duct join one another outside the duodenal wall and form a long common channel, does have a high rate of associated acute pancreatitis. Obstructive pancreatitis was present in 13 of 48 patients with AUPBD described in one Japanese study.[59] The pancreatitis may be caused by a rise in pressure in the pancreatic duct, which is caused by bile reflux into the pancreatic duct in situations in which the abnormally long channel is blocked by a gallstone, protein plug, or sphincter of Oddi dysfunction (SOD). Four of these Japanese patients were children younger than 13 years of age; AUPBD thus appears to be an important cause of pancreatitis in children.[60] Gastrointestinal duplications are a rare cause of relapsing pancreatitis and can be treated surgically.[70] Obstruction by *Ascaris lumbricoides* occurs when the worm enters the bile duct or pancreatic duct at the ampulla of Vater. Most commonly, the bile duct is involved, because it is wider. In one report, 8 of 25 patients with wandering *Ascaris* presented with acute pancreatitis and the others with cholangitis, biliary colic, or painless obstructive jaundice. The worms were in the extrahepatic ducts in 15 patients, in the intrahepatic ducts in 9, in the pancreatic duct in 3, and in the gallbladder in 1.[71]

Acute Pancreatitis After Endoscopic Retrograde Cholangiopancreatography

Pancreatitis is the main complication of ERCP and of endoscopic sphincterotomy of the bile duct. Unless there is a common channel, biliary sphincterotomy has little effect on the pancreatic duct sphincter. The incidence varies according to the definition of pancreatitis, the more common figures quoted being between 5% and 12% of all cases,[72,73] though a much lower figure (2.5%) is reported from specialist centers.[74] Although the pathogenesis of the pancreatitis is not fully understood, the injection of contrast medium under pressure appears to disrupt ductal and acinar epithelium.[53] Hyperamylasemia is found in up to 70% of patients after ERCP, indicating some degree of acinar cell leakage. Patients who have difficult bile duct cannulations and a greater number of injections into the pancreatic ducts have a higher incidence of pancreatitis.[75] Spasm and edema of the sphincter of Oddi, resulting in pancreatic sphincter hypertension, are now believed to be important. Male sex is a protective factor (odds ratio, 0.38), whereas female sex, cannulation of the pancreatic duct, and repeated unsuccessful attempts to cannulate the bile duct are positively associated.[74] The spectrum of pancreatitis that follows ERCP is the same as with other causes, the majority being mild but a proportion being severe and infected[76] with rare fatalities. Pancreatic duct stenting protects significantly against post-ERCP pancreatitis in patients with pancreatic sphincter hypertension undergoing biliary sphincterotomy.[77] Further, pancreatic sphincter of Oddi manometry identifies which high-risk patients may benefit from stenting.[77]

Theoretically, corticosteroids might decrease ampullary inflammation and thus the risk of pancreatitis. One study showed a decreased rate of pancreatitis after ERCP in patients pretreated with corticosteroids for iodine allergy (4.6% versus 7.4%),[72] but a prospective study showed no significant effect of methylprednisolone pretreatment.[73] A broad-spectrum enzyme inhibitor, gabexate, which inhibits the proteases and phospholipase A_2, reduces the rate of pancreatitis after ERCP and endoscopic sphincterotomy to 2% (from 8%) of cases. It also reduces both the rate of abdominal pain after the procedure and the level, but not the incidence, of hyperamylasemia. Trypsin is the enzyme that is likely inhibited by gabexate.[78]

Postoperative Pancreatitis

Postoperative pancreatitis is most often the result of direct injury during operations in the vicinity of the gland, but it can also occur after operations outside the region. Calcium chloride infusions and hypotension or ischemia have been implicated in these cases. About 23% of patients do not have local trauma.[79] A prospective study found that the incidence of pancreatic injury after cardiopulmonary bypass surgery was 27%, when injury was defined as elevated amylase and either lipase or isoamylase, but only 8% of patients had abdominal signs or symptoms and only 1% had severe pancreatitis.[80] The single most important risk factor for pancreatic injury was perioperative infusion of calcium chloride, and administration of >800 mg of calcium chloride per square meter of body surface area is an independent predictor of pancreatic injury.[80] By contrast, a retrospective study found that the incidence of clinical pancreatitis was only 0.44% after cardiopulmonary bypass in 5,621 patients (25 cases),[81] but the mortality rate was extremely high—11 of 25 cases—which suggests that only severe cases were detected. The reported data on calcium infusion in this study were not complete enough to draw general conclusions.[81] Hypotension is a recognized complication of cardiopulmonary bypass and cardiac surgery that may result in hypoperfusion (ischemia) of the pancreas, acinar cell injury, and hyperamylasemia. Patients who undergo cross-clamping of the aorta during aortic surgery may also suffer injury to the pancreas and sometimes acute necrotizing pancreatitis.[82]

Hyperlipidemia

Hyperlipidemia has a complex relationship with pancreatitis. When patients present with acute pancreatitis, almost 50% of them have serum lipid abnormalities and about 10% have severe hyperlipidemia, as defined by the presence of serum triglycerides >20 mmol/L,[83] a level that is probably a risk factor for developing acute pancreatitis. Hyperlipidemia may precede the pancreatitis and exacerbate it.[83] However, a marked elevation of serum lipid should not be invariably considered the cause of the pancreatic disease, even if other potential causes are not immediately evident.[84] In the rat, hyperlipidemia intensifies the course of acute edematous and acute necrotizing pancreatitis.[85] Primary hyperlipidemias types I and V and hyperlipidemia secondary to kidney failure predispose to pancreatitis. It is proposed that in these cases, pancreatic lipase hydrolyzes triglycerides to glycerol and free fatty acids and that the released free fatty acids are toxic to the pancreas once albumin binding is saturated. The rare type I hyperlipidemia is inherited as an autosomal-dominant characteristic and manifests as pancreatitis in childhood, lipemia retinalis, hyperchylomicronemia, hepatosplenomegaly, and eruptive xanthomas. Either lipoprotein lipase activity is absent and apo C-II levels are normal or the converse is the case. The more common type V hyperlipidemia is seen in adults, who are often obese, diabetic, and hyperuricemic, and these patients may have attacks of pancreatitis. Chylomicrons and very-low-density lipoproteins (VLDLs) are increased, clearance of triglyceride is reduced, and lipoprotein lipase activity is normal. It is suggested that patients who have had previous acute pancreatitis have defective catabolism of chylomicrons, which may have predisposed them to pancreatitis.[86] Severe hypertriglyceridemia (levels >2,000 mg%) is often complicated by pancreatitis, but the mechanism is unknown. Most cases of severe hypertriglyceridemia are a result of hereditary defects in apoprotein C-II or lipoprotein lipase. A circulating lipoprotein lipase inhibitor has also been identified.

Hypercalcemia

Hypercalcemia causing pancreatitis has been reported in association with primary hyperparathyroidism; immobilization; multiple myeloma; adult T-cell lymphoma; renal carcinoma; malignancies metastatic to bone, including breast carcinoma and small cell undifferentiated carcinoma; vitamin D poisoning; total parenteral nutrition; thyrotoxic hypercalcemia; renal transplantation; and thiazide diuretics. Pancreatitis after cardiopulmonary bypass is significantly related to calcium infusion.[80] Several mechanisms by which hypercalcemia induces pancreatitis are postulated. In human volunteers, intravenous infusions of calcium chloride increase output of pancreatic enzymes and of gastric acid. Hypercalcemia also enhances cholecystokinin-stimulated pancreatic enzyme secretion and gallbladder contraction.[87] In cultured rat pancreatic acini, elevated calcium levels accelerate trypsinogen activation only when the acini are maximally stimulated by cerulein (a cholecystokinin analogue) or carbachol.[88] The greater difficulty in inducing acute pancreatitis in animals than humans may be a function of the quantity and properties of human cationic trypsinogen. In humans, the ratio of cationic to anionic trypsinogen (2:1) is high, compared with animals. Cationic trypsinogen autoactivates more easily than does anionic trypsinogen, and cationic trypsin is more resistant to self-destruction in the presence of hypercalcemia.[89] Hypercalcemia induces inappropriate trypsinogen activation[90] and inhibits the autohydrolysis of trypsin (in a manner analogous with the hereditary R117H defect).[89] Affected acinar cells display an arrest of exocrine secretion, accumulation of secretory proteins, and increased autophagocytosis.[91] In animal models, hypercalcemia also increases the permeability of the pancreatic ducts to molecules the size of pancreatic enzymes.[92]

Hypothermia

The pancreatitis of hypothermia is poorly understood but has been reproduced in animals and can complicate therapeutic hypothermia used in surgery. One hypothesis is that it may be due to ischemia, secondary to venous thrombosis, or to the "microcirulatory shock" of hypothermia.[93,94] However, both hypothermia and pancreatitis may be secondary to alcohol abuse, especially in elderly persons living alone in poorly heated homes. Pancreatitis may sometimes be the primary disease, with hypothermia a result of the social circumstances.[94]

Drug-Induced Acute Pancreatitis

Drugs associated with pancreatitis are listed in Table 5–4. Many drugs have been implicated anecdotally, but a definite causal relationship has been demonstrated with thiazides, azathioprine, asparaginase, furosemide, tetracyclines, estrogens, cimetidine, interferon-α, methyldopa, metronidazole, olsalazine, and oxyphenbutazone.[95–99] Other anecdotal cases frequently reported to the World Health Organization involve angiotensin-converting enzyme inhibitors, H_2-receptor blockers, valproate, sulindac, gemfibrozil, lovastatin, pentamidine, and didanosine.[98] Drugs appear to account for 1.4% of cases of acute pancreatitis.[97] The pancreatitis runs a benign course and pseudocysts do not occur.[97] Rechallenge with the drug can prove causation,[100] but this is not practical in every clinical situation. Clinical circumstances often include several other possible pathogenic factors.[101] Whether drug use can cause chronic pancreatitis is not clear.

Primary Sphincter of Oddi Dysfunction (SOD)

SOD is regarded as a potential cause of acute pancreatitis in its own right and as a contributory factor in pancreatitis of other causes.[102] One definition of SOD is "partial obstruction of the SO biliary segment giving rise to intermittent episodic upper abdominal pain, deranged liver function tests, dilatation or delayed drainage of injected contrast from the bile duct. Likewise, a similar condition of the pancreatic segment can give rise to pancreatitis or episodic pain, suggesting a pancreatic origin."[103] Thus, two syndromes are ascribed to the dysfunction, one biliary and one pancreatic. SOD may predispose to gallstone pancreatitis and may itself cause acute pancreatitis. Circumstantial evidence suggests that some instances of recurrent pancreatitis may be caused by SOD, including both pancreatitis that follows scorpion bites and organophosphate insecticide intoxication.[102] The incidence of post-ERCP pancreatitis is substantially higher (11%–31%) in patients undergoing sphincterotomy for SOD than in patients without dysfunction (5%).[104,105] Indeed, patients with SOD are five times more likely to develop post-ERCP pancreatitis after biliary sphincterotomy than are patients with other indications.[104] SOD may be due to hypertonia or dysmotility; manometry is the gold standard for diagnosis. The condition is considered to be present where there is an abnormally increased basal pressure (>40 mm Hg) with a response to endoscopic sphincterotomy. The term *pancreatic sphincter hypertension* is more accurate than is SOD, although *SOD* is the most widely used term. Manometry reveals that SOD persists after biliary sphincterotomy in two thirds of patients and that these patients have a vastly increased risk of post-ERCP pancreatitis.[105] Pancreatic stenting significantly decreases the risk of pancreatitis from 26% to 7%.[105]

Infections

Infection appears to be a secondary event in the vast majority of cases of severe acute pancreatitis. Primary bacterial acute infectious pancreatitis is not a well-accepted entity, and although there are occasional references to acute phlegmonous pancreatitis characterized by a heavy neutrophil infiltrate and duct destruction at autopsy,[106] a clinical picture of acute suppurative bacterial infection, with rapid onset of fever, abdominal pain, leukocytosis, and positive blood cultures, is rare and reportable. Specific infections that do involve the pancreas are mumps, Coxsackie B,[107] other enteroviruses, cytomegalovirus (CMV), Epstein–Barr virus, rubella, arbovirus, *Toxoplasma gondii,* syphilis, clonorchiasis, ascariasis, tuberculosis, and leptospirosis. The pancreatic involvement is usually not significant in the overall context of the disease, except in mumps, where the pancreatitis can be severe. Little is known of the morphology of the pancreatitis of mumps. In rare instances, chronic pancreatitis has followed mumps, possibly by chance.[108] Viruses may have a direct cytopathic effect or else may have an indirect effect via ductal obstruction. Acute pancreatitis has rarely complicated fulminant hepatitis B.[109] CMV infection is rare, except in the context of neonatal infection, immunosuppression, or acquired immunodeficiency syndrome, and can produce clinical pancreatitis.[110] Fibrosis is the main effect of congenital syphilis.

Clonorchis sinensis migrates into the pancreatic duct in about one third of patients with hepatic clonorchiasis. It induces mucus gland hyperplasia or squamous metaplasia, mild inflammation, and eosinophil infiltration in the duct, similar to the changes in the bile ducts, and it can precipitate acute pancreatitis. *Ascaris lumbricoides* occasionally enters the pancreatic duct, causing acute obstructive pancreatitis. Hydatid cyst occurs rarely in the pancreas and is recognized by the scolices and cyst wall in the active phase. Ancient hydatid cysts can be identified by finding hooklets, which are birefringent in polarized light and Ziehl–Neelsen positive, in the cyst wall. Acute pancreatitis has followed rupture of an hydatid cyst of the liver into the bile ducts, with presumed obstruction of the main pancreatic duct.[111] Primary pancreatic hydatid disease is rare and accounts for only 0.25% of cases of hydatid disease.[112] These patients present with a variety of symptoms and signs. Large cysts produce epigastric pain, abdominal mass, and jaundice if the bile duct is obstructed.[113] Complications comprise infection and pancreatic abscess,[114] atrophy of the pancreas distal to the cyst, diabetes,[115] and spontaneous fistula to the duodenum.[112]

Tuberculosis of the pancreas has been reported to cause biliary obstruction, pancreatic abscess, acute or chronic pancreatitis, or epigastric mass,[116] but even in miliary tuberculosis, involvement of the pancreas is rare.

Rare associations of acute pancreatitis include systemic lupus erythematosus (SLE),[117] Behçet's disease, Ehlers–Danlos syndrome,[118] and hemorrhagic pancreatitis due to potassium permanganate poisoning.

Specific Clinical Situations

Liver disease is often associated with pancreatitis in the context of alcohol abuse. However, the association between acute pancreatitis and liver disease is so strong in autopsy series,[119] that it raises the question of whether liver disease per se may cause acute pancreatitis. Most authorities strongly resist this idea. Acute pancreatitis is recorded in association with liver failure or hepatoma,[120] viral hepatitis,[109,121] HELLP syndrome, and liver transplantation. Alcoholic cirrhosis and pancreatitis do not appear to share the same susceptibility factors but can affect the same patient.[122] In one study, 5 of 32 patients with cirrhosis had ERCP features of chronic pancreatitis and 5 of 40 patients with chronic pancreatitis had cirrhosis.[122] At autopsy, chronic pancreatitis is found in 20% of patients with alcoholism and cirrhosis and acute pancreatitis is found in 8%, whereas only 2.6% of controls without alcoholism have any form of pancreatitis.[109] There is a 50% prevalence of chronic pancreatitis in patients with sclerosing hyaline necrosis, a form of severe alcoholic liver disease.[109] Patients with alcoholic pancreatitis tend to have a more intermittent pattern of alcohol consumption than do patients with alcoholic cirrhosis, and the amount of alcohol required to cause pancreatitis seems to be smaller than what is necessary to produce cirrhosis.[123]

Acute pancreatitis during pregnancy or the postpartum period is rare and is most often due to gallstones; it has little to do with the pregnancy itself. Among 519 patients with pancreatitis, 7 had it during pregnancy, 12 in the postpartum period, and 1 after an abortion.[124] Gallstones were present in 18 of these, type I hyperlipidemia in 1, and chronic alcoholism in 1. The predominance of gallstones has been confirmed in other series,[125] and if gallstones are ruled out, hyperlipidemia should be suspected.[126] Hyperlipidemic patients are at increased risk of gestational pancreatitis, owing to the increase in VLDL and low-density lipoprotein in pregnancy. Dietary treatment is often enough to carry them through the pregnancy, but apheresis has sometimes been used.[126] Primary hyperparathyroidism is a rare cause of pancreatitis in pregnancy.[127]

Pancreatitis in children is due to a range of causes similar to those in adults, excepting alcohol. Table 5–6 lists causes in a large recent series of pediatric pancreatitis.[128] The sex ratio in children is equal. A higher proportion of cases are idiopathic or hereditary; hyperlipidemia is one hereditary cause. It remains to be determined what proportion has mutations of the CF gene. A higher proportion of cases are due to anatomic abnormalities, such as anomalous union of the pancreatic and biliary ducts[60] (see Chapter 2).

Acute pancreatitis in the elderly is most often due to gallstones but is sometimes secondary to pancreatic cancer.[129,130] In as many as 30% to

Table 5–6. Pediatric Acute Pancreatitis: Epidemiology and Causes

	Mild	Severe
Age (y)	9.7	7.1
M:F ratio	79:88	20:21
Weight (kg)	38.9	23.2
Cause		
Trauma	23	10
Unknown	68	9
Drug	18	3
Gallstone	13	2
Familial	11	3
Hemolytic-uremic syndrome	3	7
Pancreas divisum	5	2
Other	26	4
Total	**167**	**41**

Key: M:F, males to females.
Adapted from DeBanto JR, Pedroso MRA, Whitcombe DC, et al.: Epidemiology of pediatric acute pancreatitis. Gastroenterology 116:A1117, 1999.

40% of elderly patients with acute pancreatitis, the condition is idiopathic; these patients have higher Ranson scores and greater morbidity and mortality than do patients with pancreatitis of known cause.[131] The elderly patient has an increased risk of complications, especially organ failure, and is at greater risk of death.[67,106,131] The presentation of acute pancreatitis in the elderly is often atypical; many times, the disease is first diagnosed at autopsy.[106,129]

Pancreatitis in patients with end-stage renal disease (ESRD) is uncommon, occurring in 6.4% of a large series,[132] being significantly more common in those with alcohol abuse, SLE, and polycystic kidney disease. Chronic calcific pancreatitis that precedes ESRD is almost invariably due to alcohol abuse. Acute pancreatitis occurring for the first time on dialysis is generally benign. A significant elevation of the calcium X phosphate product is observed in about half the patients without any other known precipitating factor. Pancreatitis that follows renal transplantation is associated with a higher morbidity and mortality. Chronic calcific pancreatitis that is first diagnosed after ESRD is established is seen only in patients with SLE and may be a manifestation of long-standing disease, chronic corticosteroid therapy, or both.[132]

Acute pancreatitis, often subclinical, was found in 28% of 184 bone marrow transplantation patients at autopsy and multivariate analysis showed that independent risk factors for its development were graft-versus-host disease (GVHD), increased length of survival after transplantation, and major infection. Its development may be associated with a high prevalence of biliary sludge and prolonged treatment of GVHD with cyclosporine and prednisone.[101]

Many factors have been implicated in recurrent acute pancreatitis, including abuse of alcohol, biliary tract disease, gallstones, choledochal cyst, papillary stenosis, duodenal diverticula, metabolic disorders, such as hypercalcemia and hyperlipidemia, SLE, CF, pancreas divisum, periampullary cysts, and enteric duplication cysts.[133–137]

Pathogenesis

Pathologists have believed since Chiari's time that acute pancreatitis is an autodigestion of the pancreas by its own enzymes,[138] a view that has been substantiated by recent research. Pancreatitis results when the many protective barriers to autodigestion are overthrown. These barriers include

- Sequestration of the digestive enzymes in the endoplasmic reticulum, golgi, and zymogen granules
- Secretion of the pancreatic enzymes as proenzymes
- Trypsin-sensitive sites so that trypsin is self-inactivating. This mechanism represents an important brake on autodigestion, as evidenced by the fact that hereditary pancreatitis is caused by mutation of cationic trypsinogen at the trypsin-sensitive site.[139]
- Natural antiproteases, particularly pancreatic secretory trypsin inhibitor and α_1-antitrypsin, which inactivate free enzyme in the interstitial fluid or within cells
- Lymphatic flow, which removes interstitial fluid and any activated enzyme or mediators of inflammation that it contains

Acinar Cell Injury

Acinar cell injury is the crucial event that releases digestive enzymes into the interstitium through exocytosis of secretory granules by fusion with the basolateral cell membrane.[140–142] Animal studies have shown that the lysosomal enzyme cathepsin B activates trypsinogen intracellularly and that it therefore may do so also in humans,[140] but other authors think that no activating enzyme may be necessary, because human cationic trypsinogen may self-activate under certain conditions.[89] Ethanol sensitizes the acinar cell to CCK, so that together the effect is similar to CCK hyperstimulation and results in intracellular zymogen activation.[33]

Evidence is mounting that activation of trypsin is the key precipitating event in pancreatitis and that trypsin, in turn, activates the other digestive enzymes and also initiates inflammation through the kallikrein-kinin system.[141] Among the important data are the following:

- In several animal models, premature intracellular activation of trypsinogen has been shown.[142]
- A mutation of cationic trypsinogen, which makes the active molecule resistant to hydrolysis, is a cause of hereditary pancreatitis.
- The protease inhibitor gabexate prevents or modifies the pancreatitis that follows ERCP.
- Activation of trypsinogen in the interstitial space of the pancreas transforms mild experimental pancreatitis into necrotizing pancreatitis.[143]

A finding common to the earliest phase of injury in different animal models of pancreatitis is the colocalization of lysosomal and secretory enzymes in the same organelles, indicating autophagosome formation and cellular injury. Trypsinogen is activated by the lysosomal hydrolase cathepsin B within subcellular organelles and is closely related to acinar cell injury.[140,144,145] The site and mechanism of trypsinogen activation within the acinar cell has been disputed, whether in the normal secretory pathway or in secondary lysosomes, but recent studies suggest the answer may be neither. Trypsinogen activation peptide was identified by immunoelectromicroscopy within cytoplasmic vacuoles, colocalized with cathepsin B, within 30 minutes of hyperstimulation of the pancreas with caerulein.[144] However, the vacuoles were too small (<1 μm in diameter) to be fusion products of lysosomes with zymogen granules. The immunoreactivity shifted to larger vesicles within an hour of injury and these contained a granule membrane protein characteristic of lysosomes and recycling endosomes.[145] Thus, there may be a second pathway of enzyme secretion other than the path to zymogen granules, and this may be where the first enzyme activation occurs.[145] Cationic trypsinogen is the main form of trypsinogen in the human, whereas anionic trypsinogen is the main molecule in animals. Cationic trypsinogen is the precursor of two thirds of the trypsin activity in normal human pancreatic juice and has a propensity to autoinactivate, especially below pH 6. Two other enzymes, mesotrypsin and enzyme Y, rapidly degrade trypsin in vitro by digesting it at arginine or lysine residues.[89] Cationic trypsinogen autoactivates more readily than does anionic trypsinogen and cationic trypsin is resistant to autolysis in the presence of elevated calcium concentrations.[89] These features, and the known role of cationic trypsinogen in hereditary pancreatitis, point to the likelihood of spontaneous activation of cationic trypsinogen without the need for cathepsin B.[89] In experimental animals, induction of acinar cell apoptosis can reduce the severity of pancreatitis.[146,147] This finding supports the central role of autodigestion in pancreatitis, as apoptosis removes acinar cells and their content of digestive enzymes. The autodigestion that is the main feature of severe acute pancreatitis results from activation of pancreatic enzymes released into the interstitial fluid.[143] In mild pancreatitis, it seems that the enzymes released into the interstitial fluid are rapidly washed away by lymphatic flow without being activated, but in the severe form of disease, activation occurs locally in the interstitium, bringing about autodigestive necrosis and multiplying its effect by releasing more enzyme from necrotic acinar cells.[143] A variety of events could affect enzyme activation in the interstitium—infection, inflammatory cell infiltrates, antiproteases, free radicals, and efficiency of lymphatic flow, among others. It seems that the severity of pancreatitis is determined by the intensity of the initiating process, the balance between protective and injurious influences, and the presence or absence of complications, such as infection, the key event being activation of enzymes in the extracellular space.

Fat Necrosis

Phospholipase is the most potentially noxious of the pancreatic enzymes[148] and is thought to be the main mediator of the fatty tissue injury, though several enzymes act in concert. Digestion of the membranes of fat cells releases lipids, which undergo lipolysis by lipase and phospholipase. Hydrolysis of triglycerides releases free fatty acids, which are cytotoxic. Severe injury is characterized by rupture of blood vessels, hemorrhage, and release of toxic hemoglobin digestion products. Digestive enzymes that are released and activated within the pancreatic interstitium can puncture acinar cell membranes, multiplying the quantity of proenzyme released. Cytokines released by cell damage initiate the acute inflammatory response.

Cytokines

The complement components C3a and C5a are activated by trypsin early in pancreatitis and attract neutrophils and macrophages.[149,150] In turn, activated macrophages amplify the response by releasing tumor necrosis factor-α (TNF-α), interleukin-1 (IL-1), interleukin-10 (IL-10), platelet-activating factor (PAF), and nitric oxide (NO). The pancreatic acinar cells are capable of releasing some of these mediators, too, but in lesser quantities. The serum levels of cytokines rise to a peak at 8 hours after induction of experimental cerulein pancreatitis.[151] In human pancreatitis, interleukin-6 (IL-6) and IL-10 levels peak on admission and interleukin-8 (IL-8) levels peak at 2 to 5 days.[152] IL-10 is a potent anti-inflammatory cytokine that inhibits inflammatory cytokine release from all tissue sites. IL-10 decreases the severity of experimental acute pancreatitis, and neutralization of IL-10 by antibody administration increases the severity both of the pancreatitis and the associated lung injury. It also increases both the serum TNF protein level and TNF messenger expression in pancreas, lung, and liver.[152] IL-8 plays a role in the systemic effects of pancreatitis, particularly the lung injury.[153] Animals that lack receptors for either IL-1 or TNF demonstrate increased survival rates after experimental pancreatitis, but the effect is not additive in animals lacking both receptors.[154,155] Abrogation of the effect of interleukin-1β (IL-1β), by inhibition of IL-1–converting enzyme (ICE) or by homozygous knockout of the ICE gene, causes pancreatitis to be attenuated and dramatically improves survival in animal models.[156]

Nuclear Factors

In experimental acute pancreatitis, the nuclear factor–κB (NF-κB), a member of the Rel family of transcriptional regulatory proteins, is activated. NF-κB may mediate the multiorgan dysfunction of acute pancreatitis. Pretreatment with pyrrolidine dithiocarbamate, an inhibitor of NF-κB, results in increased survival of the animals.[157] Mice deficient in T cells (nude mice) and mice deficient in mast cells are resistant to developing the pulmonary complications of acute pancreatitis, indicating that both of these cell types modify the systemic response to acute pancreatitis.

Nitric Oxide

In experimental pancreatitis, inducible NO synthase and oxidative tissue damage in the pancreas is associated with raised systemic NO and arterial hypotension, and this may be an important factor in the systemic and local hemodynamic disturbances associated with acute pancreatitis.[158] NO donor agents reduce the grade of inflammation, whereas NO inhibitors increase the severity of inflammation and decrease pancreatic tissue oxygenation. It is likely that NO inhibits leukocyte activation and preserves capillary perfusion.[159]

Microcirculatory Changes and Anoxic Injury

Microcirculatory changes and anoxic injury might account for acinar injury around the periphery of lobules, the area most remote from the arteriole supplying the lobule. This mode of injury could be operative in hypotension, cardiovascular or other surgery, and possibly in hypothermia.

Oxidative Stress

Oxidative stress, indicating the release of free radicals, is universally found in animal models of pancreatitis. Oxidative stress has also been shown in humans with pancreatitis, by measurement of oxidatively altered linoleic acid and vitamin C in serum and plasma, and this stress is in excess of that seen in controls with other intra-abdominal crises of similar severity.[160] Reactive oxygen species are determinants of disease severity,[140] along with inflammatory cytokines, altered redox states, ischemia, and apoptosis.

Laboratory Diagnosis

The diagnosis of acute pancreatitis is difficult because there are no pathognomic symptoms and the amylase and lipase tests lack sensitivity and specificity. Serum amylase is considered diagnostic only when the level is greater than three times the upper limit of the normal range. However, patients with pancreatitis often have levels lower than this. Newer serum tests may prove more specific. The time course profiles of trypsinogen-2 (anionic trypsinogen) and the trypsin-2-α-1-antitrypsin complex are favorable for diagnosing acute pancreatitis.[161] The elevation starts within hours of the onset of disease and is very steep. The rise of both markers lasts longer than that of amylase, up to 42 days. The magnitude of the elevation correlates with the severity of the disease.[161] Urine screening with a rapid urine trypsinogen-2 test strip has been found to be reliable in excluding acute pancreatitis with a high degree of probability.[162] Lipase and IL-6 levels have been used together for early diagnosis and prognosis of acute pancreatitis.[163] A variety of tests have been advocated to distinguish between mild and severe cases. These include polymorphonuclear neutrophil leukocyte elastase, C-reactive protein, phospholipase A_2, cytokines, and antiproteases. Trypsinogen-2 can be measured in urine and its level correlates with disease severity.[164] The trypsinogen activation peptide can also be measured in urine and its level correlates with disease severity, but the test for it is not commercially available at the time of writing. The activation peptide of carboxypeptidase B is a large molecule that can be measured reliably in serum and urine and, in early studies, its level has correlated well with the severity of acute pancreatitis, though the test's sensitivity and specificity are not known yet.[165]

Gross Pathology

In mild acute pancreatitis (interstitial pancreatitis), the pancreas is swollen and edematous and the peripancreatic tissue is edematous. Fat necrosis may appear as whitish yellow plaques and nodules on the surface and sometimes patchily in the septa throughout the gland (Fig. 5–1). Occasionally, purulent material exudes from the ducts. With increasing disease severity, there is marked induration of the pancreas and more widespread necrosis. Foci of fat necrosis become large and confluent on the surface. On the cut surface, the fat necrosis is more extensive and outlines the lobules, especially if there is partial fatty infiltration of the pancreas. Fat necrosis can affect extrapancreatic tissue, such as the mesentery, transverse mesocolon, omentum, omental bursa, and retroperitoneum. Occasionally, pleural surfaces or mediastinum may be involved. The pancreas is well preserved in mild pancreatitis, but more extensive necrosis results in regions of soft gray material, or mushy brown and black material, due to pancreatic hemorrhage. The hemorrhagic zones are usually most prominent on the surface and rapidly become dark brown or black by alteration of hemoglobin.[166] In extreme examples, the pancreas is swollen and marbled with blackened hemorrhagic zones, confluent pale yellow areas of fat necrosis, and patchy gray areas of parenchymal necrosis, both on the exterior and on the cut surface. The consistency of the gland is usually firm with foci of softening. The extent of necrosis varies from peripheral foci to almost the entire gland. A fluid collection or abscess may complicate the picture.

Microscopic Pathology

The most common form of acute pancreatitis affects the peripheral lobular zones and the

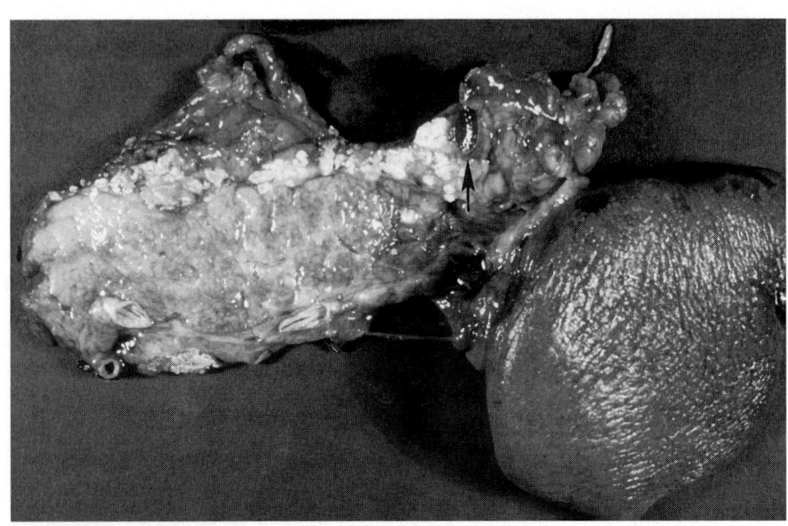

Figure 5–1. Acute pancreatitis with fat necrosis. The pancreas is swollen and has lost the normal lobular definition. The adjacent fat shows patchy pale areas of necrosis. Venous thrombosis is present (*arrow*).

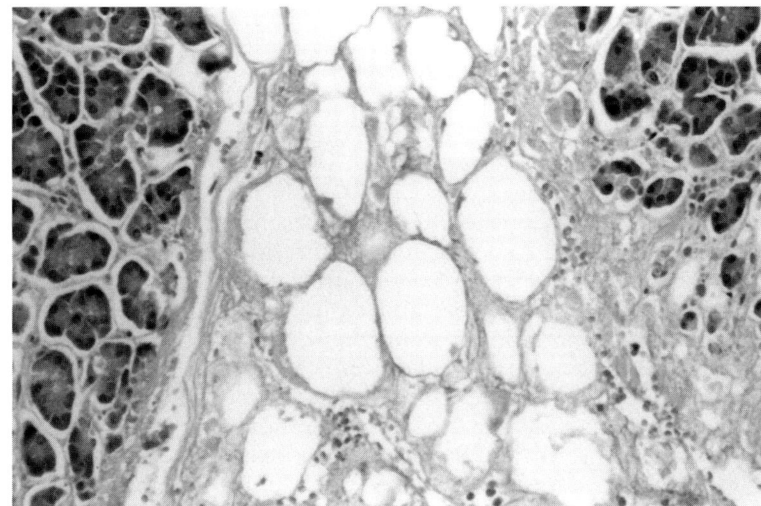

Figure 5–2. Acute pancreatitis with fat necrosis. Note the viable pancreatic acini with intervening ghost outlines of necrotic adipocytes.

surrounding fatty tissue. The earliest change is edema of the interstitial connective tissue, but this phase is rarely seen in a pure form in humans and our knowledge of it derives mostly from experimental animals. "Grossly unmodified" areas in 20 specimens from total pancreatectomy revealed changes believed to be the earliest alterations of acute pancreatitis—namely, homogenization of acinar cells, ductal dilation with epithelial degeneration, diffuse interstitial edema with fibroblastic proliferation, and vascular necrosis.[167] The initial necrosis is in peripancreatic fatty tissue, which seems more susceptible to autodigestion than does the acinar tissue itself. The amount of necrosis increases with the time elapsed from onset of symptoms.[166] Severe pancreatitis shows copious fat necrosis (Fig. 5–2) and the acinar cells adjacent to the fat, at the periphery of lobules, are also necrotic. Adjacent to the necrotic area, acinar lumina contain eosinophilic secretions and show variable cellular necrosis and reduced cytoplasmic granularity.[168] Acinar cells at the periphery of lobules undergo necrosis and centrilobular acini survive (Fig. 5–3). The dying cells lose their cohesion and their cytoplasmic boundaries become fuzzy. The nuclei become pyknotic and either disintegrate into fragments

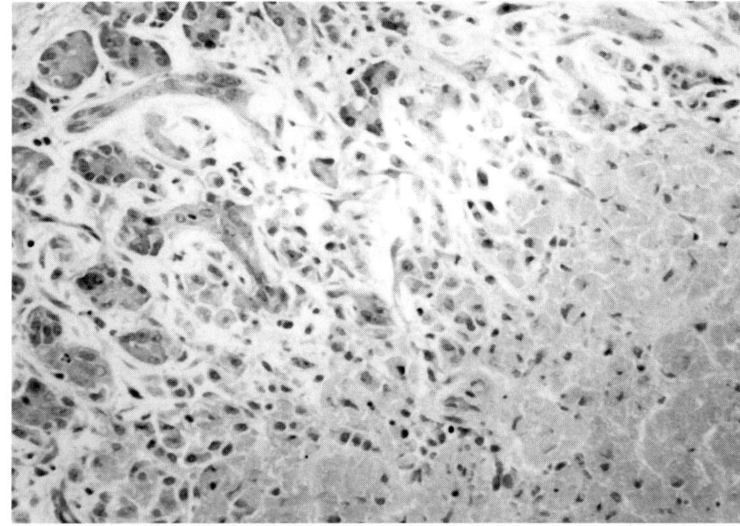

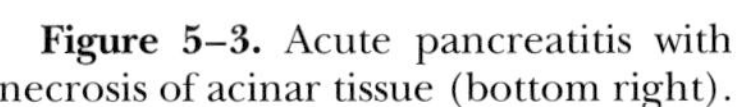

Figure 5–3. Acute pancreatitis with necrosis of acinar tissue (bottom right).

or lose their staining. Finally, the necrotic zone becomes a mass of granular debris and hemorrhage, resulting from autodigestion of blood vessels and rupture. Typically, there is an inflammatory reaction at the junction of necrotic and viable tissue. The necrotic fat cells may coalesce into fat cysts and calcification of the fat necrosis rapidly ensues. The inflammatory reaction, comprising edema, congestion, hemorrhage, and an infiltrate of neutrophils, is located in interlobular spaces and tissue septa, beginning at the periphery of the gland.[166] The scantiness of the neutrophils may reflect injury to venules, inhibition of chemotaxis, or participation of neutrophils in the necrosis. After 3 or 4 days, macrophages accumulate, infiltrate the fat, and become foamy, as they phagocytose lipid.

Small arteries, arterioles, and capillaries undergo thrombosis and segmental necrosis. The veins at the junction of viable and necrotic tissue show thrombosis without phlebitis.[166] Hemorrhage is related to vessel necrosis. Coagulative (ischemic) necrosis has been described in the central parts of the pancreas in some cases.[166,167] Resolution of fat necrosis and pancreatic necrosis is effected by the usual macrophage infiltrate, granulation tissue, and fibrosis over a period of weeks, depending on the size of the necrotic foci. After a single bout of mild or moderate pancreatitis, there is often restitution of the gland without functional deficits, but if the necrosis–fibrosis sequence takes place repeatedly, acute pancreatitis may evolve into chronic disease.[169–171] Ultrastructural changes in the cells at the border of necrotic areas comprise numerous lipid droplets, autophagosomes, residual bodies, aggregates of filaments, degenerated zymogen granules, and dilation and vesiculation of endoplasmic reticulum.[168] Some cells show features of early necrosis, including swelling of mitochondria, folding of nuclear membranes, and clumping of chromatin. Fibrin and fibrillar material are present between the cells, and the eosinophilic deposits in acinar lumina are also fibrillar in fine structure.[168] Immunostaining has shown that the border of fat necrosis in acute pancreatitis contains phospholipase A_2, lipase, and colipase and that these are absent from mammary fat necrosis, suggesting that these enzymes may be instrumental in causing the fat necrosis of pancreatitis.[172] Although the usual pattern of necrosis primarily affects the microcirculatory periphery of the lobules, only a minority of cases actually appear to be due to ischemia or hypotension. The islets of Langerhans are generally spared, unless directly involved in necrosis.

There is a second gross pattern of acute pancreatitis, in which the ductal and periductal areas are primarily affected and the main pancreatic duct and large tributaries undergo necrosis.[106,173] Ductal necrosis starts with precipitation of eosinophilic protein and neutrophil emigration into the lumens of small and medium-size interlobular ducts.[9] The duct epithelium ulcerates and the inflammatory infiltrate pours into the interstitium. Focally, there may be complete ductal necrosis. The acinar tissue is relatively unaffected. This pattern may be seen in patients with alcoholism and cholelithiasis.[173] Impaired secretion and activation of trypsinogen within the ductal system could give rise to this injury, but infection is also plausible, though it is unproven.

A third pattern of acute pancreatitis is a spotty acinar or ductal cell death, without fat necrosis or ductal necrosis, typical of infection by CMV, mumps, Coxsackie B virus, or bacterial infection, such as leptospirosis.[9] It is rarely encountered histologically, as most patients survive the infection.

Autopsy Findings

Despite modern imaging and biochemical testing, 30% to 35% of cases of fatal pancreatitis are first diagnosed at autopsy and are missed during life.[18,174] The cases missed include examples of pancreatitis due to alcoholism, to gallstones, to hypothermia and to upper abdominal surgery. Abdominal pain is absent in virtually all cases that are missed. Autopsies have given us much of our information about the pathology of pancreatitis. The prevalence of acute pancreatitis in adult autopsies is 2.6% to 3.3%.[19,109,119] It is strongly associated with liver diseases, such as subacute hepatitis (16.1%), fulminant hepatitis (13.5%), biliary cirrhosis (10.5%), cholangiocarcinoma (8.6%), and macronodular cirrhosis (7.1%).[119] Death due to acute pancreatitis is ascribed to shock or circulatory failure,[23] or to pulmonary edema in patients dying before 7 days and to infection in patients dying after 7 days.[109] The lung pathology at autopsy comprises edema and diffuse alveolar damage and is sometimes complicated by bronchopneumonia, atelectasis, and pleural effusion.[109] The elderly are at greater risk of death from acute pancreatitis.[67]

Treatment and Prognosis

A full account of treatment is beyond the scope of this chapter, but the pathologist needs to be aware of the general approach. Supportive measures, including fluid replacement and nutritional support, are important and may be the main treatment required for mild or interstitial pancreatitis. Enteral feeding, via a nasoenteric feeding tube placed distal to the ligament of Treitz, is well tolerated in patients who do not have ileus. It costs far less and results in fewer complications than does total parenteral nutrition.[175,176] Endoscopic sphincterotomy is appropriate for severe acute gallstone pancreatitis but not for mild pancreatitis.[57] The effectiveness of sphincterotomy is due in part to reduction of the acute ascending biliary sepsis that accompanies the pancreatitis in about one half of these patients.[177]

Necrosis is the principal determinant of prognosis. Infection develops in 30% to 70% of patients with acute necrotizing pancreatitis and accounts for more than 80% of deaths from acute pancreatitis.[178–180] The distinction between infected and noninfected necrosis is made by percutaneous needle aspiration under CT imaging control, a procedure that is both safe and efficacious. The aspirated material is sent for culture and Gram stain. Infected pancreatic necrosis is a major cause of morbidity and mortality. Antibiotic prophylaxis against infection is efficacious, and imipenim, alone or with cilastatin, is currently the antibiotic of choice.[181,182] A meta-analysis of clinical trials suggests that mortality is significantly reduced in patients with severe pancreatitis who are given broad-spectrum antibiotics to prevent infection of the necrotic tissue.[183] The pancreas has a tissue barrier comparable to the blood–brain barrier,[184] which excludes aminoglycosides, but allows the quinolones and imipenem to achieve a high pancreatic tissue concentration. Metronidazole is added for anaerobic infection. Selective decontamination of the digestive tract has been found to prevent infection in patients with multiple trauma.[185] The anaerobic colonic flora is reduced by giving nonabsorbable antibiotics through a nasogastric tube. A similar approach in pancreatitis resulted in improved survival and possibly reduced pancreatic infection, although intravenous antibiotics are now the standard of care and it is hard to distinguish the effect of selective decontamination of the digestive tract from that of intravenous antibiotics. Débridement of noninfected necrosis is now performed infrequently, as it introduces the risk of infection. The main reason for surgical intervention in necrotizing pancreatitis is to débride infected necrosis, which is uniformly fatal otherwise.[186] The details of which procedure should be done are controversial. As a general principle, optimal conditions for necrosectomy are not present until the second or third week. The surgery involves débriding the necrotic tissue and ensuring postoperative clearance of exudate and debris.[187] Laparotomy or open drainage is the standard method. Endoscopic closed drainage and percutaneous drainage are currently under evaluation.[188–191] Endoscopic drainage consists of insertion of several tubes through the stomach or duodenum into the retroperitoneal space.[191] Percutaneous drainage, via large-bore tubes inserted by an interventional radiologist under CT guidance into infected necrosis through several sites, has been used,[188] and stone retrieval baskets have been used to remove solid debris.[190] However, percutaneous drainage may predispose to secondary infection,[189] and for some of these patients, conversion to open surgery is required.

Central cavitary necrosis is a term applied when the necrosis is almost entirely confined within the pancreatic parenchyma and there is little if any extrapancreatic necrosis. The episodes of pancreatitis are initially severe, with high Ranson scores (see Table 5–1), and need intensive care. However, the rates of infection (20%) and mortality (10%) are low. The condition is diagnosed by CT scan a mean of 19.8 days after onset.[192]

Factors that correlate positively and significantly ($p > 0.05$) with death from *sterile* pancreatic necrosis are: high Ranson score during the first 48 hours, high APACHE II score at admission and at 48 hours, shock, renal insufficiency, multiple systemic complications, and high body mass index.[193] Sixty percent of fatalities occur within 7 days of the patient's admission to hospital, and pulmonary complications are the most significant factor contributing to death.[109] The proinflammatory cytokine PAF is implicated in the pathogenesis of systemic organ failure in severe acute pancreatitis, and an antagonist to it was recently shown to reduce the incidence of organ failure and death if administration of it is started within 48 hours of disease onset.[194]

Obesity is an important prognostic factor; the severity of pancreatitis is directly related to the degree of obesity.[193,195–197] There is a significant increase in respiratory insufficiency in obese patients, necessitating artificial ventilation.[195,197,198] The rate of pancreatic and peripancreatic necrosis is higher in obese than in nonobese subjects.[197] Respiratory insufficiency requiring artificial ventilation is seen in 12.5% of obese patients with pancreatitis; dialysis is required in 7% and the mortality rate is 6.1%.[195]

A study, using stepwise logistic regression analysis, of 270 patients revealed that five other factors are associated with an adverse outcome: advanced age, need for inotropic support, renal failure requiring dialysis, respiratory failure, and previous medication.[199]

Complications

Complications of acute pancreatitis are listed in Table 5–7.

Fluid Collections and Pseudocysts

An acute fluid collection occurs early in the course of acute pancreatitis, has a duration of <4 weeks, is located in or near the pancreas, and always lacks a wall of granulation or fibrous tissue. An acute fluid collection occurs in 30% to 50% of cases of acute pancreatitis. It is detected by imaging. It regresses spontaneously more than 50% of times. The precise composition of a collection is not known. Bacteria are variably present. The critical distinction between an acute fluid collection and a pseudocyst (or a pancreatic abscess) is the lack of a defined wall.[7] The most common site for acute fluid collection is the lesser sac, closely followed by the left anterior pararenal space.[200]

A pseudocyst is a collection of pancreatic juice, enclosed by a wall of fibrous or granulation tissue, that arises as a consequence of acute pancreatitis, pancreatic trauma, or chronic pancreatitis.[7] It arises from a collection of fluid or necrotic material that becomes walled off from adjacent tissues and into which ruptured ductules empty their pancreatic juice. Granulation tissue forms at the margin and gradually matures over 3 to 4 weeks to form a fibrous capsule (Fig. 5–4). There is no epithelial lining. Some pseudocysts spontaneously shrink and resolve. Others continue to expand, owing to inflowing pancreatic juice. A pseudocyst may then compress adjacent organs, such as the stomach, duodenum, or common bile duct, and require surgical drainage.[201] Rarely, one ruptures spontaneously into the stomach.[202] Most are located around the head of the pancreas.[203] Infection of a developing pseudocyst is a particular risk, as the infected necrotic debris may be beyond the reach of antibiotics and may spread to the peritoneal cavity. Pseudocysts are most often detected by imaging but are occasionally palpable. They are usually round or ovoid and have a well-defined wall as demonstrated by CT or ultrasonography. Formation of a pseudocyst requires 4 weeks from the onset of acute pancreatitis. Pseudocysts complicate about 14% of cases of pancreatitis,[13] and about 95% of pseudocysts are due to pancreatitis,[204] the others being due to trauma or carcinoma. In a recent series, one quarter of cases were due to acute pancreatitis and three quarters were due to chronic pancreatitis.[205] The mean age was 44 ± 12 years.[205] Pseudocysts complicate alcohol-induced pancreatitis more often than biliary pancreatitis.[206] Only the small proportion of biliary pancreatitis patients who have a high Ranson score (> 5) (see Table 5–1) and necrotizing pancreatitis need repeat imaging for pseudocyst.[206] Pseudocysts that complicate trauma with laceration of the pancreas and ruptured pancreatic ducts may resolve spontaneously, if the injured duct is peripheral.[207] Distal duct injury can be treated by percutaneous drainage, but proximal duct injury requires surgical treatment.[207] Pseudocysts are rarely due to carcinomas that obstruct the pancreatic duct and induce pancreatitis upstream of the obstruction.[208] Thirty-seven percent of pseudocysts are located in the head of the pancreas, 21.3% in the body, and 37.8% in the tail.[204] Pseudocysts due to acute or biliary pancreatitis are more often located in the tail of the pancreas, whereas those due to chronic pancreatitis are more often located in the head.[204] The mean diameter of pseudocysts in the head is 5.9 cm; in the body, 7.9 cm; and in the tail, 8.6 cm.[204] Pseudocysts that follow biliary pancreatitis are more often complicated by infection (31.3%) than are those that result from alcoholic pancreatitis (8%).[204] Occasionally, hemorrhage into pseudocysts may occur (Fig. 5–5).

Table 5–7. Complications of Acute Pancreatitis

Fluid collections and pseudocysts
Pancreatic necrosis
Infection and abscess
Persistent inflammation
Infarction of the colon
Pancreatic ascites
Systemic complications

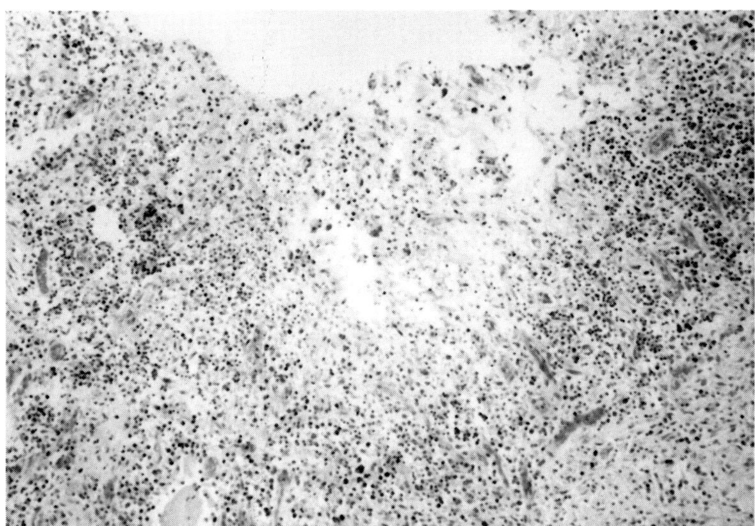

Figure 5–4. Inflamed granulation tissue lining a pseudocyst.

Ultrasonography is the method of choice for detecting pseudocysts in acute pancreatitis. Fine-needle aspiration (FNA) cytology is a reliable way to diagnose pseudocysts and shows acute inflammation, histiocytes, and absence of glandular epithelium.[209] Cyst fluid amylase >5,000 U/L had a 94% sensitivity and a 74% specificity for pseudocyst.[210] Cyst fluid viscosity, carcinoembryonic antigen, CA 125, and cytology can reliably distinguish mucinous cystic tumors (malignant, borderline, and benign) from pseudocysts and microcystic cystadenomas[211] (Fig. 5–6).

Approximately one fifth of pseudocysts undergo spontaneous resolution. Occasionally, pseudocysts undergo spontaneous cyst-enteric fistulization.[212] The spontaneous remission rate is related to the size of the pseudocyst as well as the cause of the pancreatitis.[205] The mean diameter of pseudocysts that remit spontaneously is 5.4 cm, compared with 6.8 cm for cases that do not remit. Two of every three pseudocysts with a diameter >6 cm require an intervention. Postnecrotic pseudocysts remit more often than do pseudocysts due to chronic pancreatitis (32% versus 17.9%; $p < 0.05$).[205] Pseudocysts caused by chronic pancreatitis require significantly more frequent intervention, compared with those induced by acute pancreatitis (55.5% versus 37.5%; $p < 0.05$). The occurrence of complications correlates with the size of the pseudocyst and the type of underlying pancreatitis, being more likely in larger cysts and those occurring after acute pancreatitis.[205] Endoscopic retrograde pancreatography (ERP) can provide important information in the management of pseudocysts, particularly whether there is communication with a hollow viscus such as the stomach.[203]

Pseudocysts are treated by drainage as appropriate to each individual case. Percutaneous catheter drainage has a low mortality rate, does

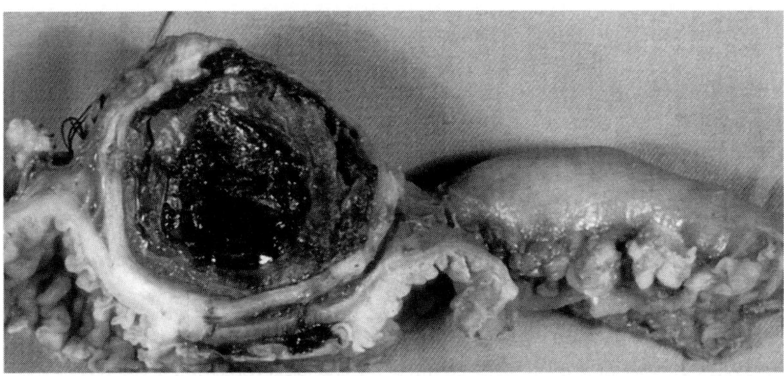

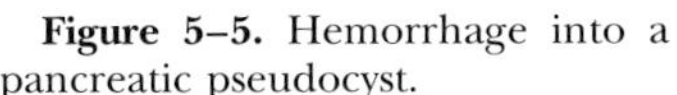

Figure 5–5. Hemorrhage into a pancreatic pseudocyst.

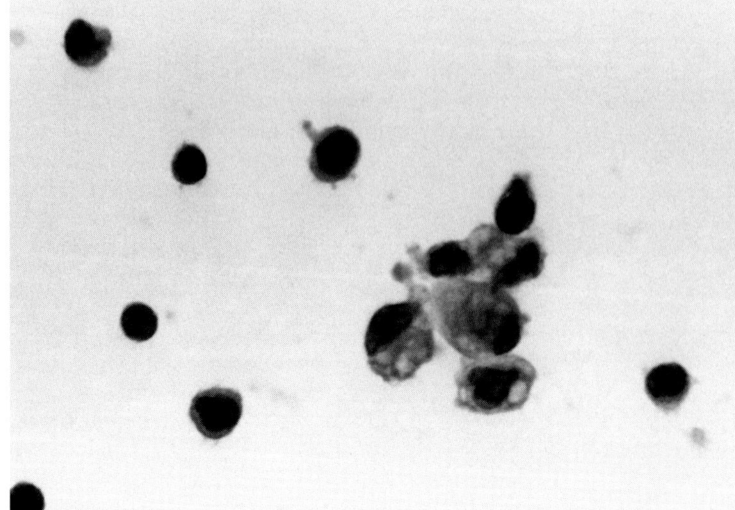

Figure 5–6. Fine-needle aspiration of a pancreatic pseudocyst yielded small numbers of histiocytes and lymphocytes but no epithelial cells.

not require a major operation, and does not violate the surgical field in cases in which subsequent retrograde duct drainage is required,[213] but it is contraindicated when cysts are due to chronic pancreatitis with ductal stricture.[214] When a bulge into the stomach or duodenum is visible endoscopically, endoscopic drainage has been used successfully.[215,216] Surgery provides definitive management and has a low risk of recurrence, but pancreatic resection may be required. Surgical drainage allows biopsy of the cyst wall to exclude a cystic neoplasm.[217] A risk of draining a sterile pancreatic pseudocyst by endoscopic or radiologic approaches is the introduction of infection and conversion to abscess.[218]

A pseudocyst can erode into a blood vessel and cause hemobilia and chronic gastrointestinal blood loss.[219,220] Massive hemorrhage into a pseudocyst can result in a pulsatile mass or false aneurysm. Angiographically, these are saccular, not fusiform. Acute bleeding into a pseudocyst can derive from the splenic artery or vein, the superior or inferior pancreaticoduodenal artery, the gastroduodenal artery, the renal artery, the aorta, or the splenic parenchyma.[221,222] It is treated by surgical hemostasis and/or drainage/resection of the cyst. Vascular necrosis can be found in some cases.[223]

Intrasplenic pseudocysts are a rare complication of acute pancreatitis and may arise by direct extension of a pseudocyst into the splenic hilum or pancreatitis occurring in ectopic intrasplenic pancreatic tissue.[224] They are treated by distal pancreatectomy combined with splenectomy.[225] Intrahepatic pseudocysts in the left lobe of liver, one after a traumatic injury and the other after alcoholic pancreatitis, were described by Okuda et al.[226] Three pseudocysts involving the kidney have been described. The clinical findings and diagnostic imaging favored intrinsic renal disease, but the correct diagnosis was established by amylase determinations from the cyst fluid.[227] The authors concluded that any patient with a fluid collection in the kidney region may have a pancreatic pseudocyst, despite lacking a clear-cut history of pancreatitis or trauma. The wall of a pseudocyst that intrudes on the kidney can become opacified on infusion pyelography, possibly because of parasitizing renal capsular vessels.[228] Rarely, pseudocysts extend into the mediastinum and present with weight loss, chest or abdominal pain, and dyspnea. Chest radiographs frequently demonstrate a posterior mediastinal mass, and esophagograms always shows esophageal displacement. The diagnosis is confirmed by CT of the chest and abdomen. Cyst-gastrostomy is the operation of choice for this condition.[229] Mediastinal pseudocysts arise from posterior leaks of the pancreatic duct that track along the aorta or esophageal hiatus. If the pseudocyst ruptures into a pleural space, it forms a pancreaticopleural fistula and a pancreatic pleural effusion that often reaches massive size.[230] Pancreatic ascites is caused by leakage into the peritoneal cavity from a disrupted pancreatic duct or pseudocyst. Massive pancreatic pleural effusion is the equivalent leak into a pleural cavity. These two conditions are internal pancreatic fistulas. The incidence of pancreatic ascites in patients with pseudocysts is 14.5%.[231] Massive pancreatic pleural effusion is found in 1.3% of patients with pancreatitis.[232] Internal fistulas arise in alcoholic pancreatitis or after trauma but rarely, if ever, follow biliary pancreatitis. These effusions are characterized by high amylase level and protein content above 25 g/L.[231] In about 50% of patients, effusions will respond to conservative treatment, such as somatostatin, parenteral nutrition, and drainage, but this treatment is not employed for longer than 2 to 3 weeks. Pancreatography is used to identify the site of leakage and design a rational approach to treatment. Stenting is sometimes possible, but more often the leaking duct is drained into a defunctionalized Roux-en-Y loop of jejunum.

A presumptive diagnosis of pseudocyst, based upon CT appearance alone, proves to be in error in as many as one third of patients.[180] Lesions that are mistaken for pseudocysts include cystic epithelial or endocrine neoplasms,[233] abdominal lymphoma,[234] cystic teratomas,[235] endometriosis,[236,237] and tumors of the duodenum, including smooth muscle or stromal tumors that undergo cystic change.[238] It is important to correctly diagnose pancreatic cysts, so that neoplasms are not marsupialized to viscera inappropriately.[239] Cysts of uncertain type should be aspirated for cytology and the fluid should be analyzed for markers of neoplasia. Ultimately, biopsy of the cyst wall with frozen section histologic examination may be necessary.

Infected Pancreatitis

Early acute pancreatitis is dominated by the toxic and vasoactive events, and late pancreatitis, by infectious complications.[187] Pancreatic infection develops in 40% to 70% of patients with necrotizing pancreatitis and is a major life-threatening complication with a mortality in the region of 50%. Infection is suspected when fever, elevated white blood cell count, and hypotension develops and is confirmed by FNA under CT guidance for culture and Gram stain.[240] Animal studies have shown that bacteria can reach the pancreas by a variety of routes: via the biliary and pancreatic ducts; via lymphatics; hematogenously; via ascites; and by traversing the colonic wall. The latter route is now considered the route of infection in most human cases. In most instances, the infection is monomicrobial, but polymicrobial flora is reported in 13% to 40% of cases. Gram-negative aerobic bacteria, such as *Escherichia coli, Klebsiella* species, *Pseudomonas* species, and *Proteus,* predominate, but gram-positive organisms, such as *Staphylococcus aureus, Streptococcus faecalis,* and *Enterococcus,* anaerobes (*Bacteroides*), and *Candida* may also be found. The likelihood of infection increases with the duration of pancreatitis, and the frequency of infection overall is in the range of 40% to 60%.[187] The extent of necrosis on CT scans correlates with increasing rates of infection. When necrosis exceeds 50% on CT scanning, the disease is clinically severe and the patient is highly susceptible to secondary infection. Beger et al. reported on 170 patients with severe acute pancreatitis who underwent surgery and found an infection rate of 24% within the first week, 46% in the second, and 71% in the third.[241] Overall, 42% were infected and 58% were sterile. The mortality rate was significantly higher in the infected group (14/71, 20%) than in the uninfected (10/99, 10%).

Pancreatic abscess is a circumscribed collection of pus, in proximity to the pancreas, that arises as a consequence of acute pancreatitis or pancreatic trauma.[7] Pancreatic abscess is almost always a bacterially infected pseudocyst. Most commonly, the clinical picture is that of infection. Pancreatic abscess occurs late in the course of severe acute pancreatitis, often 4 weeks or more after onset.[242]

Persistent inflammation is a rare complication that is characterized by signs of inflammation persisting for months without fluid collections or pseudocysts but never permitting release from the hospital.[243] Eating provokes a flare-up of inflammation. Pancreatography or cholangiography shows stenosis or occlusion of the main pancreatic duct, in most cases. This complication is treated by pancreatoduodenectomy or total pancreatectomy. In addition to acute inflammation and fat necrosis, the resected specimens show main pancreatic duct stenosis or occlusion or pancreatoduodenal fistula.[243]

Rare Complications

Infarction of the colon is a rare complication of acute pancreatitis that can be due to a variety of mechanisms, including thrombosis of mesenteric vessels, direct extension of the pancreatitis, necrosis, and infection.[244–247] In acute pancreatitis, the next most frequent complication is pancreatocolonic fistula.[244]

Vascular complications of acute pancreatitis include occlusion of the splenic vein and erosion of arteries by autodigestion with pseudoaneurysm formation. The splenic artery is most often involved, followed by the gastroduodenal, inferior pancreaticoduodenal, and superior pancreaticoduodenal arteries.[248] They are treated by embolization with a steel coil or Gelfoam or by surgery. Severe hemorrhage can be a life-threatening complication of pseudoaneurysm.

Complement activation occurs in acute pancreatitis in proportion to the severity of the inflammation and has been proposed as a mediator of remote complications.[150] The terminal complement components increase vascular permeability and may contribute to lung injury, which is a major cause of death in patients with acute pancreatitis.[109] Activation of trypsinogen extracellularly may contribute to lung injury.[249] Neutrophils are strongly implicated in causing the lung injury and neutrophil depletion diminishes the severity of experimental acute pancreatitis and the severity of lung injury.[250,251] Intercellular adhesion molecule-1 (ICAM-1) is upregulated in the lung and precedes leukocytic infiltration.[252] TNF-α appears to mediate the increased pulmonary capillary permeability in the lung and the severity of lung injury, and p38 mitogen-activated protein kinase mediates TNF production within the macrophage.[253]

CHRONIC PANCREATITIS

To the clinician, the definition of chronic pancreatitis is "a continuing inflammation of the pancreas with irreversible morphological changes that typically causes pain and permanent functional impairment."[7] To the pathologist, it is a chronic destructive disorder of the exocrine tissue with inflammation, reparative fibrosis, and secondary changes in the islets of Langerhans and pancreatic ducts. Ultimately, it presents with abdominal pain, maldigestion due to exocrine enzymatic deficiency, and diabetes mellitus due to destruction of the islets. In 95% of patients, it ends up as chronic calcifying pancreatitis, a common end stage of multiple causes, including alcoholic, tropical, hereditary, hypercalcemic, hyperlipidemic, drug-induced, and idiopathic pancreatitis. Obstructive pancreatitis does not calcify or cause diabetes but may cause exocrine insufficiency.

The prevalence of chronic pancreatitis is not well documented. The incidence among 107,754 adult autopsies in Japan was 2.1%.[119] The incidence in the population in Denmark is 8 to 10 per 100,000 per year.[254,255] The incidence is increasing, owing to the greater availability of alcohol in affluent societies,[254–256] and there is a close correlation between the per capita alcohol consumption and the incidence.[257] Chronic alcoholic pancreatitis is mainly a disease of men in early to middle adulthood,[258,259] and thus the male-to-female ratio for chronic pancreatitis overall is about 2:1, with the median age at diagnosis being 44 years. The idiopathic cases cluster in two age groups, a younger group between the ages of 15 and 30 years and an older group between the ages of 50 and 70 years. Younger patients present with severe pain, whereas older patients do not.[258] Racial factors play a role and, in the United States, chronic pancreatitis is two to three times more common in blacks than in whites.[259] Tropical chronic pancreatitis is a disease of young people and is more common in men than in women. Occupational exposure to hydrocarbons has been implicated as a contributory cause in one center.[260]

Causes

Chronic alcoholism is the most common cause of chronic pancreatitis in affluent countries and accounts for 60% to 80% of cases.[9,170,256,261–264] Table 5–8 lists causes of chronic pancreatitis. Only 5 of every 100 people with alcoholism develop chronic pancreatitis. Patients with alcoholism who develop severe acute pancreatitis are more likely to develop chronic pancreatitis.[265] Usually, the pancreas returns to normal after an attack of acute pancreatitis, but sometimes acute pancreatitis progresses to chronic disease.[4] Race is a strong predictor for chronic pancreatitis among those who abuse alcohol, and black patients are two to three times more likely to be hospitalized for

Table 5–8. Causes of Chronic Pancreatitis

Relapsing acute alcoholic pancreatitis
Idiopathic
Mutations of the cystic fibrosis gene
Heredity
Hyperparathyroidism
Obstruction by stones, tumor, or ductal anomalies
Pancreas divisum
Autoimmunity (lymphocytic sclerosing pancreatitis)
Tropical pancreatitis

chronic pancreatitis than for alcoholic cirrhosis. This significant difference ($p < 0.001$) is observed in both men and women.[266] Chronic alcoholic pancreatitis occurs in patients with a history of long-standing alcohol abuse. Usually, patients have ingested large amounts of alcohol on a regular basis for an average of 15 years before the first clinical manifestation of chronic pancreatitis,[267,268] and it is estimated that the cumulative intake of alcohol by then is equivalent to ≥ 1,000 L of 100% ethanol.[268] Cigarette smoking independently increases the risk of pancreatitis in patients with alcoholism.[269] The mechanism of disease is likely a necrosis-fibrosis sequence, in which secondary perilobular fibrosis distorts the ducts, leading to precipitation of protein and calcification.[170] Calcification is present in only 2.8% of patients at the onset of the pancreatitis,[264] indicating that it follows the pancreatitis rather than initiates it. The common mutations of the CF transmembrane conductance regulator (CFTR) gene are not found in patients with alcoholic pancreatitis, nor is polymorphism of the variable-length polythymidine tract present (*5T* allele).[270] The *5T* allele in intron 8 is associated with a lower proportion of normal CFTR messenger RNA and functional protein than normal.

Idiopathic chronic pancreatitis is seen in two age groups. The early-onset group begins at a median age of 19 years and the late-onset at a median age of 56 years.[268] Early-onset disease is painful, whereas pain is absent in nearly 50% of late-onset patients.[268] The latter group was first described as having a peak age of 65 years, a predilection for men, a painless clinical course, steatorrhea, weight loss, and pancreatic calcification.[258] Others found an equal incidence in the sexes.[268] Idiopathic chronic pancreatitis was originally said to comprise 20% to 45% of cases of chronic pancreatitis,[256,262–264,271] but this number will shrink because of the discovery in the late 1990s that mutations of the CF gene or of the cationic trypsinogen gene occur with increased frequency in patients with idiopathic chronic pancreatitis.[271–275] The CFTR protein is a cyclic adenosine monophosphate–regulated chloride channel that mediates the secretion of a bicarbonate-rich alkaline fluid, which maintains luminal hydration and keeps the secreted proteins in the pancreatic ducts in solution. Hundreds of putative mutations of the CFTR gene have been identified and, when inherited homozygously or as double heterozygotes, patients develop CF, in which the exocrine secretions become inspissated, leading to obstruction, distal atrophy, and exocrine deficiency. DNA from 134 consecutive patients with any form of chronic pancreatitis (71 alcoholic, 60 idiopathic, 2 hyperparathyroid, and 1 hypertriglyceridemic) was probed for the 22 most common allelic mutations of CFTR.[271] Eighteen (13.4%) patients with mutations were detected, as compared with 5.3% of controls ($p < 0.001$). None of them met the criteria for atypical CF. The most common mutation was ΔF508 (66.6%). Only one third of the patients with mutations had alcoholism. The *5T* allele was found with the expected frequency but sometimes in conjunction with an abnormal allele.[272] A second study probed the DNA from 27 patients (5 male, 22 female) with idiopathic chronic pancreatitis for the 16 most common CF allelic mutations. Ten (37%) had one abnormal CFTR allele.[273] Four patients from the first study and 3 patients from the second had mutations of both alleles but did not fulfill the criteria for diagnosis of CF. A third study employed complete gene sequencing of 16 patients with idiopathic chronic pancreatitis and found that 10 of 16 (62%) carried one or more mutant alleles, indicating that a more thorough search for mutations will yield positive results.[274] In the same study, 4 patients (25%) carried CFTR gene mutations or CF variants on both alleles and 6 (37.5%) were heterozygous. Sweat chloride values were borderline or abnormal in 5 of 13 (38%) patients.[274] The pathogenesis of pancreatitis in these patients presumably relates to the defective CFTR and the mechanism of disease may be similar to that in CF. The incidence of hereditary pancreatitis in a series of 48 cases of presumed idiopathic chronic pancreatitis, reported in 1999, was a surprising 19%.[275]

Hereditary pancreatitis with an autosomal-dominant inheritance pattern is rare and occurs mainly in people of European ancestry.[276–279] The illness usually begins in childhood with episodes of acute pancreatitis and progresses to chronic pancreatitis in adulthood. It is often associated with intraductal stones and complicated by diabetes mellitus. The pathogenesis was recently illuminated by the identification in several kindreds of a mutation in the cationic trypsinogen gene, which is located on chromosome 7*q*35.[279] The mutation is an arginine–histidine substitution at residue 117 of the cationic trypsinogen gene (*R117H*). This is a trypsin-sensitive site and cleavage of trypsin at this site is probably a fail-safe mechanism, by which any trypsin that is activated within the pancreas is promptly inactivated; loss of this cleavage site would permit trypsin to persist and to activate the other proenzymes and begin autodigestion, resulting in pancreatitis.[279] A second mutation, found in two kindreds with hereditary pancreatitis, is an *A* to *T* mutation that results in a transition from asparagine to isoleucine at position 21 (*N21I*) in cationic trypsinogen. An electrostatic bond may form from this altered residue to *R117,* thus inhibiting tryptic autodigestion.[279] One of these families had been reported to show hypertrophy of the sphincter of Oddi and clinical improvement with surgical sphincterotomy, but at follow-up, it was found that the disease had progressed to chronic pancreatitis with insulin dependent diabetes.[280] A third defect, an alanine-to-valine substitution in codon 16 (*A16V*) of the cationic trypsinogen gene, was found both in patients with hereditary pancreatitis and in those with idiopathic pancreatitis.[281] Other genetic defects may yet be found, as some families have unexplained aminoaciduria. In familial pancreatitis, there is an increased risk of carcinoma.[259] Although hereditary pancreatitis is rare, 246 patient records were collected by physicians in 10 countries and eight pancreatic adenocarcinomas were found (as against an expected 0.150, standardized incidence ratio of 53) during a mean follow-up time of 34.6 years. Paternal inheritance was associated with an increased risk of cancer. The estimated cumulative risk of pancreatic cancer to age 70 years approaches 40% and, for patients with a paternal inheritance pattern, 75%.[259]

Obstruction of the main pancreatic ducts by stones, strictures, pseudocysts, or periampullary tumors can result in chronic pancreatitis.[282] Typically, the pancreatic duct is dilated and there are no stones or proteinaceous plugs. The changes may regress, if the obstruction is relieved.[283] Pancreas divisum may also cause obstructive chronic pancreatitis, because of the narrow caliber of the accessory duct and minor papilla.[284]

Pancreas divisum (dominant dorsal duct) is a failure of fusion of the dorsal and ventral pancreatic ducts, so that the dorsal pancreas, including the neck, body, and tail, drains through the minor papilla and the ventral pancreas drains through the papilla of Vater. Pancreas divisum is found by ERCP or by magnetic resonance cholangiopancreatography (MRCP) in between 1% and 9% of patients depending on selection,[285] an average being 3.6% to 5.5% of patients.[286,287] Pancreas divisum is sometimes inherited.[288] Some studies show the expected number of cases of associated pancreatitis and similar behavior to other cases of pancreatitis.[287,289–291] However, among patients with idiopathic recurrent pancreatitis, the incidence of pancreas divisum can be as high as 25%,[286] and the incidence of pancreas divisum is in the range of 12% to 25% in children with pancreatitis.[286,290,292,293] Also, there are several examples of chronic pancreatitis confined to the part drained by the dorsal duct, supporting the idea that the anatomic abnormality predisposes to pancreatitis.[284,285,294] It is proposed that high pressure in the dorsal duct may induce pancreatitis because of the narrowness of the accessory papilla. Sphincterotomy of the minor papilla prevents relapse of acute pancreatitis in cases of pancreas divisum but has no effect in chronic pancreatitis.[295] The results of a variety of therapeutic procedures aimed at widening the minor papilla or the duct of Santorini, including papillotomy, stenting, and sphincteroplasty, are hard to compare with one another because of different diagnostic indications and differences in the procedures employed.[296]

Autoimmune pancreatitis is a rare condition that was initially described as nonalcoholic duct destructive chronic pancreatitis by Ectors et al.[297] in 12 patients who were treated surgically for nonalcoholic chronic pancreatitis. Four of the patients had associated disease with autoimmune features, namely Sjögren's syndrome, primary sclerosing cholangitis, chronic ulcerative colitis, and Crohn's disease, but the other 8 did not. Two identical cases had been described previously as lymphocytic sclerosing pancreatitis in patients with primary sclerosing cholangitis.[298] The distinctive morphologic features are a predominantly T-cell lymphocytic infiltrate around interlobular ducts of medium size, with secondary duct obstruction and occasional duct destruction. There is no calcification, pseudocyst, or fat necrosis. In series reported by Ectors et al., there were 5 women and 7 men with a mean age of 41 years (range 17 to 77 years). In 5 patients, the presenting feature was abdominal pain and in another 5, jaundice. In most cases. there was compression of the duct of Wirsung and of the distal third of the bile duct, sometimes with echographic tumor of the head of pancreas, and the usual operation performed was duodenohemipancreatectomy. These patients may represent the extreme end of a spectrum of disease that sometimes runs a milder course. In 24% of patients with primary sclerosing cholangitis, pancreatic ductal changes were observed at ERCP,[299] and when multiple tests of pancreatic function were performed in patients with Sjögren's syndrome, all patients had abnormalities of exocrine function or ductal morphology. Proposed criteria for autoimmune pancreatitis are listed in Table 5–9.[300] Using these criteria, Horiuchi et al. identified 24 patients with autoimmune pancreatitis, 19 men and 5 women, with a mean age 60.6 years.[301] The main symptoms were jaundice (19 patients), aggravated diabetes mellitus (5 patients), and mild abdominal pain (2 patients). Serum immunoglobulin G (IgG) was elevated in 19 patients and serum immunoglobulin E (IgE) was elevated in 5, but autoimmune diseases were present in only 5 patients. Imaging showed a swollen pancreas with diffuse or irregular narrowing of the pancreatic duct. Twenty-three patients had stricture of the lower end of the common bile duct. Histologically, large interlobular ducts were surrounded by a dense inflammatory infiltrate, composed of lymphocytes, eosinophils, and plasma cells. The majority of the infiltrating lymphocytes in the pancreatic ducts were CD8(+) cells. Functional and morphologic improvements in response to corticosteroid therapy were obtained in all 19 patients so treated.[301]

Hyperparathyroidism is a rare cause of chronic pancreatitis.[256,262,264]

Tropical pancreatitis is a poorly understood entity, but it accounts for most cases of chronic pancreatitis in impoverished parts of tropical Africa and Asia. It begins in childhood and runs a virulent course to premature death from diabetes mellitus, malnutrition, or pancreatic cancer.[302] Tropical pancreatitis is the principal cause of diabetes mellitus in the tropics (so-called fibrocalculous pancreatic diabetes) and the frequency of diabetes is much higher than with alcoholic chronic pancreatitis. Two theories of causation are proposed. The toxin theory posits that it may be caused by dietary toxins, such as the cyanogens in cassava root.[303] The nutritional theory suggests that multiple nutrient deficiencies, especially of the antioxidants ascorbate, β-carotene, and selenium, are associated with the pancreatitis.[262,302] The disease is prevalent where protein and fat malnutrition occur. The *R117H* mutation is not found in these patients.[304]

Rare cases of chronic pancreatitis complicating SLE have been reported that did not appear to be due to drug medication or other causes.[305] There is no obvious mechanism for such an association other than vasculitis.

Acute gallstone pancreatitis rarely, if ever, progresses to chronicity. The mild acute pancreatitis of gallstone disease is generally resolved completely and even repeated attacks do not result in chronic pancreatitis. However, an occasional survivor of necrotizing acute gallstone pancreatitis is left with little residual functional pancreas, exocrine insufficiency, and diabetes mellitus.

Hyperlipidemia has been included as a rare cause of chronic pancreatitis in some series.[262,306]

Chronic pancreatitis in childhood is uncommon and often goes undiagnosed and untreated for years. It may be familial or due to CF, hereditary hyperparathyroidism, hyperlipidemia, or ductal obstruction by choledochal cyst, gastric duplication, or ampullary stenosis.[306,307] Intractable recurrent abdominal pain is a common presenting feature. Puestow procedure (longitudinal pancreatojejunostomy) often relieves the pain and may prevent the progression of exocrine and endocrine insufficiency, if performed early in the course of the disease.[306,307]

Table 5–9. Criteria for Autoimmune Pancreatitis*

Increased serum γ-globulin or immunoglobulin G levels
Presence of antinuclear antibody
Diffuse enlargement of the pancreas
Diffuse irregular narrowing of the main pancreatic duct
An extrinsic stenosis of the common bile duct in the pancreas on endoscopic retrograde pancreatography and cholestatic liver dysfunction
Effectiveness of steroid therapy

* All criteria must be met.

Adapted from Yoshida Y: Chronic pancreatitis caused by an autoimmune abnormality. Proposal of the concept of autoimmune pancreatitis. Dig Dis Sci 40:1561–1568, 1995.

Evolution and Pathogenesis

The most plausible theory of pathogenesis is that chronic pancreatitis is an outcome of repeated attacks of acute pancreatitis, indeed that it arises from relapsing acute pancreatitis as a result of pancreatic injury, inflammation, and reparative fibrosis.[169,170] This point of view is now favored because

- A progression clinically from acute pancreatitis to chronic pancreatitis is well recognized[261]

- Acute exacerbations of chronic pancreatitis are clinically indistinguishable from bouts of acute pancreatitis
- Both acute and chronic pancreatitis are strongly associated with alcohol abuse
- In the hereditary disease, recurrent bouts of acute pancreatitis inevitably lead to chronic pancreatitis
- The histology of the early perilobular fibrosis in resolving acute pancreatitis resembles the established perilobular fibrosis of chronic pancreatitis[169,170]
- Pseudocysts are identical in acute and chronic pancreatitis[169,170]

Whitcomb et al. postulated that a sentinel acute pancreatitis is an essential step in the development of chronic pancreatitis,[279] but patients often present with established chronic pancreatitis without the history of acute episodes. Severe acute alcoholic pancreatitis can lead to intrapancreatic necrosis and reparative fibrosis that can distort the main pancreatic duct and make progression to chronicity likely.[169]

Continuing acinar cell injury and deletion is essential to chronic pancreatitis until the end stage of burned-out disease. There is a significant increase in the number of proliferating cells in the acini in chronic pancreatitis and thus the disease represents not a failure of proliferation but the triumph of acinar cell death over regeneration.[308] Injured cells produce cytokines that elicit inflammation and promote fibrosis. The fibrosis of chronic pancreatitis is likely a product of periacinar stellate cells that store vitamin A, similar to Ito cells in the liver.[309] Fibroblast growth factor 5 is strongly expressed in ductal, acinar, and islet cells of chronic pancreatitis but only faintly in the normal pancreas and may contribute to fibrogenesis in chronic pancreatitis.[310] Transforming growth factor-β is released by resident macrophages and suppresses inflammation but also stimulates fibrogenesis by the stellate cells. Fibrosis itself limits the capacity of the acinar cells to regenerate.

Clinical Manifestations and Course

The main manifestations of chronic pancreatitis are pain, steatorrhea, and diabetes mellitus. Recurrent attacks of upper abdominal pain lasting several days are characteristic. The pain may radiate to the back or scapula and is exacerbated by eating and relieved by leaning forward. In 10% to 20% of cases, there is no pain. Peptic ulcer was found in 17% to 33% of cases in older studies,[256,263,311,312] but whether it is due to *Helicobacter pylori* or self-medication with nonsteroidal anti-inflammatory drugs is unclear. Steatorrhea and diabetes are symptoms of late-stage disease. Enzyme secretion must be reduced to 5% to 10% of normal for steatorrhoea to result.[313] Patients with alcoholic pancreatitis experience lasting pain relief when exocrine secretion declines, after a long duration of disease, and with the onset of diabetes.[1,263] About 50% of patients never require surgery or endoscopic intervention, whereas the others do.[263] The presence of pseudocysts in chronic pancreatitis indicates an early stage of the disease.[169,170]

The 50% survival time in alcoholic chronic pancreatitis (with or without pancreatic surgery) is 20 to 24 years (after onset), markedly shorter than in nonalcoholic pancreatitis. About 20% of deaths are related to pancreatitis and its complications. The extrapancreatic causes of death are trauma, malignancies of the lung or larynx related to smoking, cardiovascular and cerebrovascular diseases, severe infections, and nonpancreatic surgery, some of which relates to use of tobacco.[264] The risk that pancreatic carcinoma will develop within 20 years of the diagnosis of chronic pancreatitis is about 4%.[259,314]

Diagnosis

Many authors consider the diagnosis of chronic pancreatitis established when two of the following three criteria are fulfilled: (1) *clinical:* abdominal pain, acute pancreatitis, or alcohol abuse; (2) *functional:* reduced exocrine pancreatic function; (3) *morphologic:* calcifications, pseudocysts, irregular ducts, histologic evidence.[256] ERCP is indicated to define the ductal anatomy when the diagnosis of chronic relapsing pancreatitis is suspected. One useful outcome of an international meeting held under the auspices of the Pancreatic Society of Great Britain and Ireland in Cambridge, England in 1983 was the agreed-on definition of changes on pancreatography in chronic pancreatitis (Table 5–10).[315] Recent work suggests that MRCP can replace ERCP in the diagnosis of chronic pancreatitis.[316]

Tests of pancreatic exocrine function are divided into (1) those that require a test meal and intubation to sample the duodenal contents and (2) noninvasive tests. The Lundh test meal is the gold standard. The gland is stimu-

Table 5–10. Classification of Pancreatograms in Chronic Pancreatitis*

Terminology	Main Duct	Abnormal Side Branches	Additional Features
Normal	Normal	None	
Equivocal	Normal	< 3	
Mild changes of CP	Normal	≥ 3	
Moderate CP	Abnormal	> 3	
Marked CP	Abnormal	> 3	One or more of: large cavity, obstruction, filling defects, severe dilation, or irregularity

* If pathologic changes are limited to one third or less of the gland, they are said to be local and are designated as being in the head, body, or tail; if more than one third is affected, they are diffuse. Key: CP, chronic pancreatitis.

Adapted from Axon ATR, Classen M, Cotten PB, et al: Pancreatography in chronic pancreatitis. International definitions. Gut 25:1107–1112, 1984.

lated maximally by ingestion of a standard meal and with intravenous secretin and pancreozymin. The duodenum is then aspirated and the volume of secretion and its bicarbonate and protein content is measured. Noninvasive tests involve giving a synthetic molecule that is hydrolyzed by a pancreatic enzyme with the release of a marker molecule that can be measured in blood, stool, or urine. These tests are not used in routine clinical practice because they lack sensitivity and specificity. For example, fluorescein dilaurate (pancreolauryl) is hydrolyzed with the release of fluorescein and *N*-benzoyl-L-tyrosyl-*p*-aminobenzoic acid (bentiromide) with the release of para-aminobenzoic acid. Both of these products are measured in urine. The tests may give false positive results in liver disease, kidney failure, and intestinal malabsorption. Another noninvasive group of tests measures excretion in the breath of radioactive carbon dioxide after ingestion of a labeled substrate that is metabolized to carbon dioxide. Examples are cholesteryl octanoate, triolein, mixed triglyceride, and starch. The amino acid consumption test and the fecal elastase test are also noninvasive. The noninvasive tests are, in general, less sensitive than those that require intubation. The sensitivity of the pancreolauryl test for detecting mild exocrine dysfunction is about 50% and for detecting severe insufficiency about 85%.[317] Where detection of definite pancreatic disease is important, the invasive tests are employed.[317]

Gross Pathology

The pancreas is enlarged early in the course of the disease and shows patchy involvement, especially at the periphery of the gland. The affected areas are indurated and associated with foci of fibrosis or fat necrosis. Fat necrosis is yellowish and firm and becomes calcified and whiter with time. On cut surface, affected areas show septal fibrosis and occasionally necrotic foci or intrapancreatic fat necrosis. Pseudocysts may be found early in the disease. At this stage, the main ducts are not affected, but the branch ducts in the affected areas may be irregular and scarred.[169] In advanced disease, the pancreas is shrunken and firm to hard. The cut surface is fibrotic and whitish. There may be considerable fatty replacement. The ducts have irregular calibers and the degree of ductal irregularity and distortion correlates positively with the extent of pancreatic fibrosis.[169,170] Calculi are often present in the large ducts and may measure up to 1 cm in diameter. The frequency of calculi correlates positively with the extent of parenchymal fibrosis.[169] Ducts that contain calculi display saccular dilations alternating with strictures.[169,170] Pancreatic fibrosis may compress the intrapancreatic portion of the distal common bile duct and cause low-grade biliary obstruction. In the intermediate stages, a variety of pancreatic damage may be found.

Pseudocysts are found in about one quarter of cases that undergo pancreatic resection.[170] Pseudocysts are usually solitary, localized on the pancreatic surface in the body or tail, and 3 to 10 cm in diameter. They may contain fluid or necrotic debris. They are lined by granulation tissue and fibrous tissue, in which there may be hemosiderin-laden macrophages and variable numbers of inflammatory cells (see Fig. 5–4). Intrapancreatic pseudocysts are also found, especially in the head of pancreas.[170] Rarely, pseudocysts are connected to the main pancreatic duct. Pseudocysts are found in 50% of pancreata that show focal fibrosis and in 36% of those with advanced fibrosis.

Segmental chronic pancreatitis, or "groove pancreatitis," can affect that part of the head of pancreas between the duodenum and the common bile duct and leave the remaining pancreas intact.[318] The main finding is often duodenal stenosis. The main scarring is in or beneath the duodenal wall. In some instances, there is pancreatitis of heterotopic pancreas within the duodenal wall, and in 36% of cases, there are true cysts in the duodenal wall. In general, there is only mild fibrosis in the affected part of pancreas. The terminal common bile duct is usually surrounded by fibrosis, and there is a history of biliary disease in one of four patients. Previous peptic ulcer (41.2%) or partial gastrectomy (11.8%) may have contributed. It is important that this condition not be confused with cancer on imaging studies.[318]

Microscopic Pathology

The cardinal features of chronic pancreatitis are three: fibrosis, loss of exocrine tissue, and inflammation. Fibrosis begins focally and progresses to diffuse involvement; it begins as perilobular fibrosis, but intralobular fibrosis then follows, and as the disease advances, the acinar cells are progressively destroyed and replaced by fibrosis.[169,170] Despite this, the basic lobular architecture is still visible under low magnification until the end stage of the disease; in advanced disease, where every section shows perilobular fibrosis, the intralobular fibrosis shows a patchy distribution[169,170] (Fig. 5–7). Periductal fibrosis is sometimes prominent. The exocrine glandular atrophy is patchy in distribution and it is not uncommon to see foci of persisting relatively normal exocrine tissue until late in the disease. The interlobular and intralobular ducts and ductules persist long after the exocrine elements have disappeared, but they may appear to be increased in number, distorted, and tortuous, and the cuboidal epithelial lining may show nuclear and cellular irregularity (Fig. 5–8). Islets of Langerhans are isolated in the fibrous tissue and sometimes clustered together, indicating the extent of the loss of exocrine tissue. New islets, budding from interlobular ducts, are sometimes seen and appear to be a regenerative response to loss of islets.

The larger ducts may contain eosinophilic proteinaceous plugs of precipitated secretion that subsequently calcify (Fig. 5–9). Calculi are found in association with advanced fibrosis.[169] The ductal epithelium is consistently damaged around calculi that fill the lumen.[169] Ductal epithelial alterations are present in 40% of resected specimens of chronic pancreatitis. Eighty percent are classified as dysplasia grade I or benign mucosal changes and 20% as dysplasia grade II or atypical hyperplasia. High-grade dysplasia is uncommon. The grade I changes are simple extra-tall cylindrical epithelium, double rows of cylindrical epithelium, mucoid transformation of the epithelium, pseudopapillary hyperplasia of the epithelium without connective tissue cores, papillary hyperplasia, multilayered epithelial hyperplasia, and tubular accumulations (see Fig. 5–8). Grade II changes, or

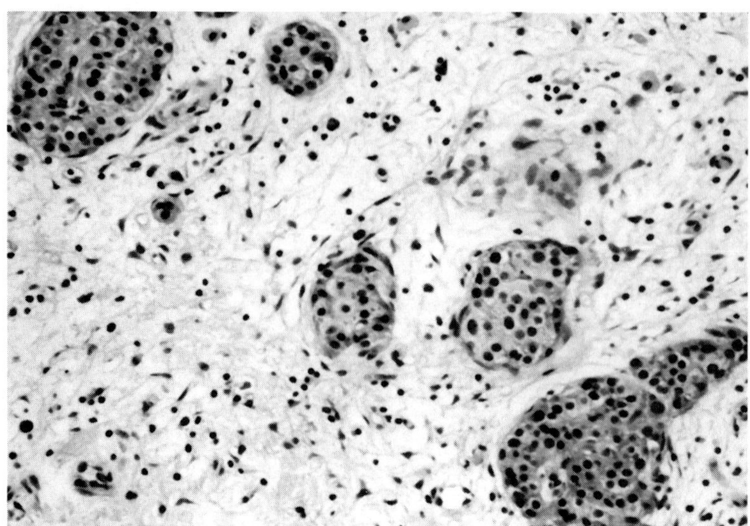

Figure 5–7. Chronic pancreatitis with loss of acinar tissue and preservation of islets.

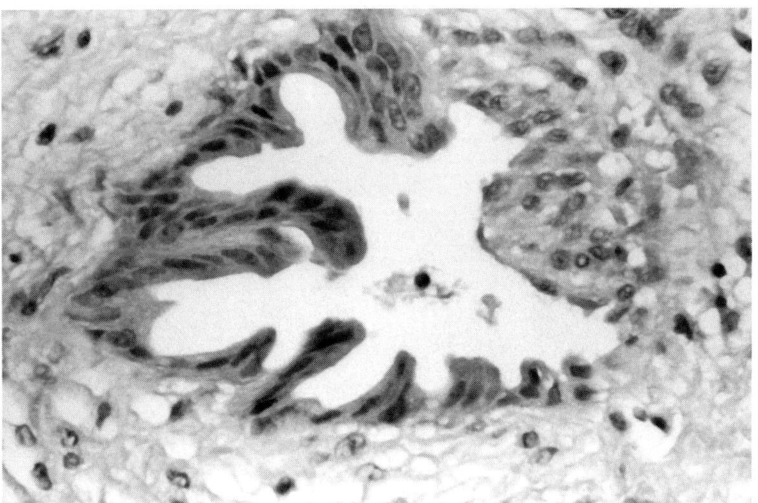

Figure 5–8. Hyperplastic changes in a medium-size duct from a patient with chronic pancreatitis. Note the squamous metaplasia and pseudopapillary hyperplasia.

atypical hyperplasia, has three variants: pseudopapillary hyperplasia with atypia, papillary hyperplasia with atypia, and multilayered epithelial metaplasia with atypia.[319] In addition, the ducts may show regenerative hyperchromatism, focal atrophy or ulceration, pyloric gland metaplasia, or squamous metaplasia (see Fig. 5–8). As in the cervix uteri, immature metaplasia may be capped by a single layer of columnar, mucus-secreting cells. Squamous metaplasia is not associated with pancreatic cancer. Smaller ducts may also become dilated and plugged with protein. The degree of duct distortion and periductal fibrosis correlates closely with the extent of pancreatic fibrosis.[169] Other causes of ductal metaplasia are *Clonorchis sinensis* infection and stenting.

As the exocrine elements atrophy, the islets become more conspicuous, by virtue of being more numerous per unit area, and often show intrainsular or perisinusoidal fibrosis. Islets are lost as the disease advances and diabetes mellitus becomes more common. Hyperplasia of islets can occur to the extent of being pseudoneoplastic and the newly formed islets sprout from the ducts.[320]

Nerves appear prominent in many cases and they are relatively or absolutely increased in number and in size. Apparent perineural invasion by hyperplastic islet cells may be seen (Fig.

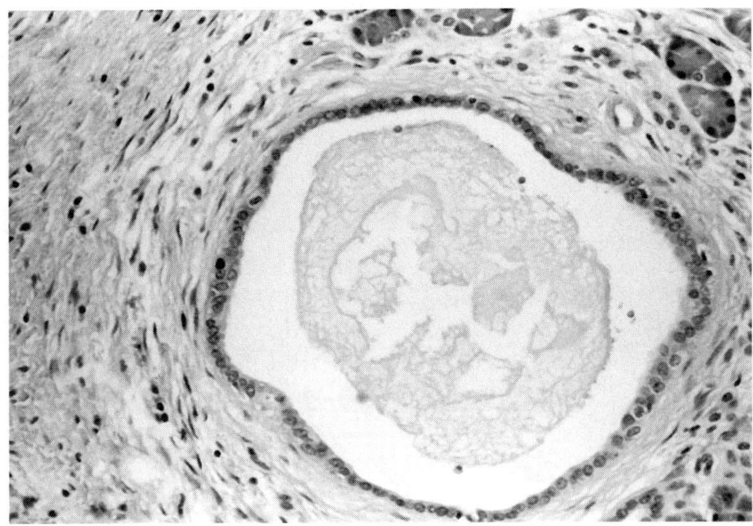

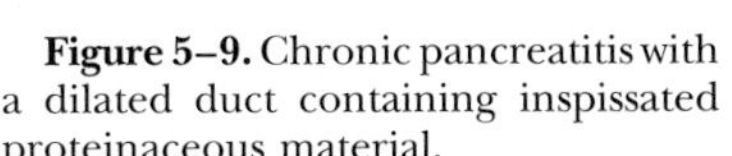

Figure 5–9. Chronic pancreatitis with a dilated duct containing inspissated proteinaceous material.

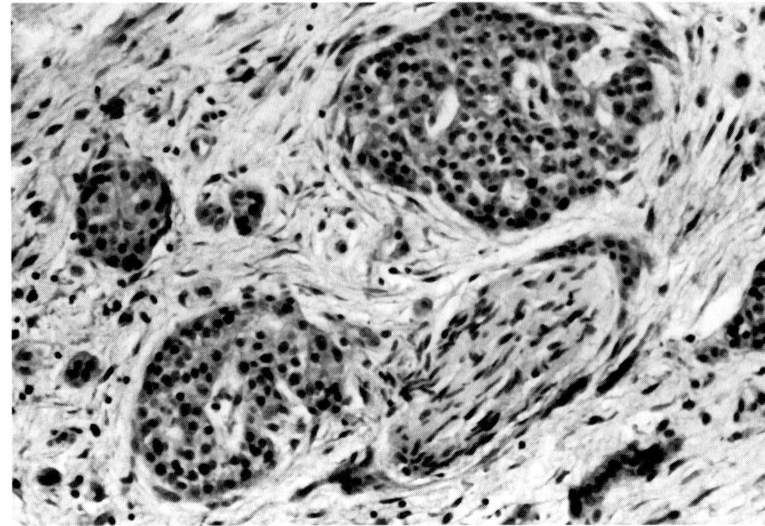

Figure 5–10. Proliferating benign islet cells alongside a small nerve.

5–10). There may be lymphocytic cuffing of the nerves or perineural fibrosis. Both of these changes may be related to the pain of chronic pancreatitis. Both arteries and veins display intimal fibrous thickening and luminal narrowing. Fat necrosis is minimal, but there may be calcified or resolving foci of fat necrosis at the margins of lobules or around the periphery of the gland. Such areas contain foamy macrophages, fat cysts, and hemosiderin.

The inflammation is usually mild to moderate in quantity and comprises lymphocytes, plasma cells, and macrophages, both scattered through the fibrous tissue and in small aggregates (Fig. 5–11). Lymphoid aggregates are found near ducts or beside nerves. Granulocytes are scanty. Activated cytotoxic T cells have been identified in alcoholic chronic pancreatitis.[321] Small arteries display intimal fibrosis.

Fat necrosis may be seen throughout the course of chronic pancreatitis. It consists of fat cells, fat cysts, and foamy macrophages but progresses to macrophage-predominant lesions, sometimes with cystic spaces full of foamy macrophages and surrounded by fibrosis and chronic inflammation. FNA cytology specimens show a mixture of inflammatory cells, acinar cells, and ductal cells. In duodenopancreatectomy specimens for chronic pancreatitis, diffuse hyperplasia of Brunner's glands is seen in 75% of cases.[322]

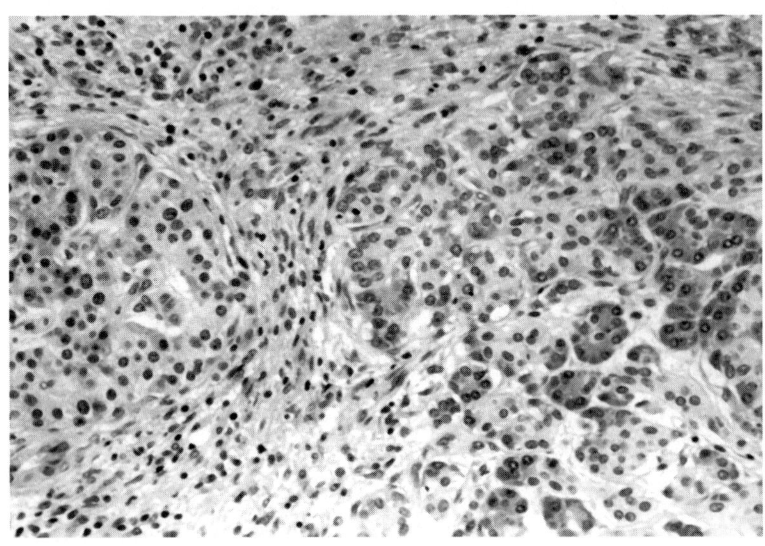

Figure 5–11. Chronic pancreatitis with atrophy, early fibrosis, and parenchymal inflammation.

The features of autoimmune pancreatitis have been described above. Eosinophil leukocytic infiltration of the pancreas has been reported rarely in association with eosinophilic gastroenteritis, idiopathic hypereosinophilic syndrome, and progressive lipodystrophy.[323–326] At frozen section, chronic pancreatitis can be difficult to distinguish from adenocarcinoma. Low-power magnification characteristically shows preservation of a basic lobular pattern in pancreatitis. However, the residual ductules that follow exocrine atrophy and the irregular budding of islets from ductules can be mistaken for cancer. They do not tend to show the cytologic features of malignancy and particularly not the marked variation of nuclear size that is a criterion for cancer. Perineural invasion by tumor cells can be an important distinguishing feature. The pathologist must remember that pancreatitis predisposes to adenocarcinoma and that changes of chronic pancreatitis occur distal to carcinomas. Thus, a frozen-section diagnosis of pancreatitis does not exclude the presence of an adjacent neoplasm.

Treatment

The symptoms of chronic pancreatitis require individual management. Pain is treated with alcohol avoidance, analgesics, and pancreatic enzymes. The role of somatostatin analogues in treatment of pain is under investigation. If pain persists after conservative treatment, ERP is performed to define the caliber of the ducts. It reveals a "chain of lakes" appearance in a large proportion of cases. Ducts larger than 8 mm diameter can be successfully decompressed by longitudinal pancreatojejunostomy (modified Puestow procedure).[327,328] This procedure gives short-term pain relief to a majority of patients but long-term relief to only 50%. Pancreatoduodenectomy has been used for patients with intractable pain whose ducts are of normal size or slightly dilated, especially if an ampullary procedure has failed.[329] Only about one quarter of patients have diabetes or exocrine deficiency before surgery, but most have afterward and require insulin and pancreatic enzymes.[329] Endoscopic treatment is increasingly important and permits postponement or avoidance of surgery, both in adults and in children.[330–332] Endoscopy permits sphincterotomy, extraction of distal stones, insertion of stents or endoprostheses into the pancreatic duct or common bile duct, and drainage of pseudocysts. The indications for endoscopic intervention in chronic pancreatitis include impacted or distal calculi, distal stricture, paraduodenal cyst bulging into the duodenum, and jaundice or cholestasis due to stricture of the intrapancreatic common bile duct. With modern imaging and an experienced surgeon, the complication rate is low and usually consists of mild pancreatitis that is controlled medically. Endoscopic treatment does not compromise later surgery and aids in defining and selecting patients who require palliative surgery. Resolution of subcutaneous panniculitis has been described after insertion of a stent.[333]

Malabsorption is treated with a low-fat diet, to which medium-chain triglycerides may be added. Pancreatic enzyme replacements are used for persisting steatorrhea, sometimes with gastric acid suppression.

Small pseudocysts need no treatment and the majority regress spontaneously. A pseudocyst that persists longer than 6 weeks and continues to enlarge may require intervention, the nature of which depends on the location of the cyst. A pseudocyst in the tail of the pancreas may be treated by resection. For other pseudocysts, internal drainage is performed endoscopically, or else it is marsupialized at open surgery to stomach, duodenum, or jejunum.

Complications

About 70% of patients with chronic pancreatitis develop regional complications (Table 5–11) consisting of biliary, duodenal, or colonic obstruction; pseudocysts; hemorrhage; pancreatic ascites; and gastric varices.[334] Although the

Table 5–11. Complications of Chronic Pancreatitis

Biliary obstruction
Duodenal obstruction
Pseudocyst
Intrapancreatic cyst
Pseudoaneurysm
Portal or splenic vein thrombosis
Colonic complications
Carcinoma of pancreas
Pancreatic and liver abscess
Pancreatic stones
Pancreatic ascites
Giardiasis

majority could be treated conservatively, surgical intervention is needed in 30% of cases.

Stenosis of the common bile duct is a common complication arising from compression of the intrapancreatic portion of the common bile duct by fibrosis of the head of pancreas.[168,335–338] Obstruction is rarely complete and the bile duct is only mildly dilated. Stenosis may present with pain and jaundice or with elevated alkaline phosphatase and bilirubin. Stenosis is identified at ERCP.[338] It behaves benignly in patients who do not have persistent jaundice. Secondary biliary cirrhosis is rare. In the majority of patients, stenosis may be safely managed without biliary bypass.[338]

Duodenal stenosis of a mild degree is common but usually resolves spontaneously as the pancreatitis wanes. Severe stenosis is rare and it may require pancreatoduodenectomy[339] or gastrojejunostomy.[340]

Pseudocysts can give rise to a variety of complications, including rupture of the pseudocyst into adjacent organs. Rupture into the portal vein can present with subcutaneous and generalized fat necrosis.[341,342]

Intrapancreatic true cystic dilations of the pancreatic duct can be identified by ERP in patients with a clinical diagnosis of relapsing pancreatitis.[343] The cysts range in diameter from 0.6 to 5 cm and are frequently associated with a prolonged elevation of the serum amylase level. Intracystic hemorrhage with obstructive jaundice requires early surgical decompression and drainage.[344] Intrapancreatic cysts can be managed nonsurgically, because complications are infrequent and spontaneous resolution may occur.

Pseudoaneurysm is a result of rupture of an artery into a pseudocyst and containment of the periarterial hematoma within a restricted tissue space. It can involve any of the regional arteries that are in contact with pancreatic juice or abscess—the splenic, gastroduodenal, pancreaticoduodenal, gastric, or hepatic arteries. False aneurysms present with massive bleeding or severe anemia.[345] They are diagnosed by angiography, and this permits initial treatment by arterial embolization as well. They range in size from 8 mm to 4.5 cm in one series.[346] Definitive surgery can then follow.

Portal or splenic vein thrombosis, secondary to chronic pancreatitis, is usually due to local inflammation or compression by a pseudocyst. The thrombosis presents as esophagogastric varices with splenomegaly and without cirrhosis. The varices rarely bleed massively.[346,347] If splenic vein thrombosis occurs secondary to left-sided pancreatitis, then distal pancreatectomy and splenectomy is the treatment.

Colonic complications of pancreatitis occur in 6% of cases.[213] Pancreatocolonic fistula is the most common; colonic stenosis that can mimic cancer is rare. Carcinoma is excluded by endoscopic biopsy and ischemic changes may be identified. Spontaneous resolution is the norm, but sometimes segmental resection is required.

Carcinoma of pancreas is a significant risk in chronic pancreatitis,[259,348] and epithelial dysplasia of the ductal epithelium precedes cancer.

Pancreatic and liver abscesses are an uncommon spontaneous late complication of advanced calcific chronic pancreatitis, especially in patients with pancreatojejunostomy.[349]

Pancreatic stones often form within the ductal system in chronic pancreatitis. They consist of protein encrusted with calcium carbonate, a major component of exocrine secretion. The protein contains pancreatic stone protein or lithostathine, an acid phosphoprotein of 14,000 d that is secreted by pancreatic acinar cells, normally serves to prevent calcium carbonate precipitation, and is one of a family of related proteins found in the pancreatic juice.[350] It is postulated that the stones in chronic alcoholic pancreatitis result from decreased secretion of pancreatic stone protein, whereas the radiolucent stones found principally in patients without alcoholism contain degradation products of the protein that are insoluble at the neutral pH of pancreatic juice. In early pancreatitis, eosinophilic proteinaceous material is deposited in the ducts, and this appears to calcify later so that calcific material correlates with severe fibrosis.[168] Calcification diminishes in the last stages of disease and after drainage procedures, indicating that calcification is a dynamic process.[351]

Pancreatic ascites (see under Acute Pancreatitis, earlier) is caused by the leakage of pancreatic juice into the abdominal cavity through a rupture of the pancreatic duct or a pancreatic cyst.[352,353] Surprisingly, ascites can be the presenting feature of chronic pancreatitis, especially in young men with alcoholism.[354]

Giardiasis, occurring in patients with chronic pancreatitis, can lead to increased diarrhea and weight loss.[355–357] In two small series, giardiasis has been reported in 28% of patients with CF and in 27% of patients with chronic pancreatitis.[356,357] It may be that deficiency of trypsin facilitates adherence of *Giardia* to the enterocytes.[357]

REFERENCES

1. Sarles H (Ed): Pancreatitis. Symposium of Marseille 1963. Basel: S Karger, 1965.
2. Sarner M, Cotton PB: 1984 Classification of pancreatitis. Gut 25:756–759, 1984.
3. Sarles H: Revised classification of pancreatitis—Marseilles 1984. Dig Dis Sci 30:573–574, 1985.
4. Seidensticker F, Otto J, Lankisch PG: Recovery of the pancreas after acute pancreatitis in not necessarily complete. Int J Pancreatol 17:225–229, 1995.
5. Sarles H, Adler G, Dani R, et al.: Classification of pancreatitis and definition of pancreatic diseases. Digestion 43:243–246, 1989.
6. Sarner M: Pancreatic inflammatory disease. Gut 37: 455–456, 1995.
7. Bradley EL: A clinically based classification system for acute pancreatitis. Summary of the International Symposium on Acute Pancreatitis, Atlanta, Ga, September 11 through 13, 1992. Arch Surg 128:586–590, 1993.
8. Becker V: Pathological anatomy and pathogenesis of acute pancreatitis. World J Surg 5:303–313, 1981.
9. Kloppel G, Maillet B: Pathology of acute and chronic pancreatitis. Pancreas 8:659–670, 1993.
10. Ranson JH, Rifkind KM, Roses DG, et al.: Prognostic signs and the role of operative management in acute pancreatitis. Surg Gynecol Obstet 139:69–81, 1975.
11. Knaus WA, Draper EA, Wagner DP, et al.: APACHE II: A severity of disease classification system. Crit Care Med 13:818–829, 1985.
12. Larvin M, Mc Mahon MJ: APACHE II score for assessment and monitoring of acute pancreatitis. Lancet ii:201–205, 1989.
13. Lankisch PG, Burchard-Reckert S, Petersen M, et al.: Morbidity and mortality in 602 patients with acute pancreatitis seen between the years 1980–1994. Z Gastroenterol 34:371–377, 1996.
14. Baron TH, Morgan DE: Acute necrotizing pancreatitis. N Engl J Med 340:1412–1417, 1999.
15. Balthazar EJ, Robinson DL, Megibow AJ, et al.: Acute pancreatitis: Value of CT in establishing prognosis. Radiology 174:331–336, 1990.
16. Balthazar EJ, Freeny PC, vanSonnenberg E: Imaging and intervention in acute pancreatitis. Radiology 193:297–306, 1994.
17. Appelros S, Borgstrom A: Incidence, aetiology and mortality rate of acute pancreatitis over 10 years in a defined urban population in Sweden. Br J Surg 86:465–470, 1999.
18. Corfield AP, Cooper MJ, Williamson RCN: Acute pancreatitis. A lethal disease of increasing incidence. Gut 26:724–729, 1985.
19. Renner IG, Savage WT IIIrd, Stace NH, et al.: Pancreatitis associated with alcoholic liver disease. A review of 1022 autopsy cases. Dig Dis Sci 29:593–599, 1984.
20. Akoojee SB: Pancreatitis in Natal. An autopsy study. S Afr Med J 54:667–669, 1978.
21. Trapnell JE, Duncan EHL: Patterns of incidence of acute pancreatitis. Br Med J ii:179–183, 1975.
22. Halvorsen FA, Ritland S: Acute pancreatitis in Buskerud county, Norway. Incidence and etiology. Scand J Gastroenterol 31:411–414, 1996.
23. Storck G, Pettersson G, Edlund Y: A study of autopsies upon 116 patients with acute pancreatitis Surg Gynecol Obstet 143:241–245, 1976.
24. Malagelada JR: The pathophysiology of alcoholic pancreatitis. Pancreas 1:270–278, 1986.
25. Durbec JP, Sarles H: Multicenter survey of the etiology of pancreatic diseases. Relationship between the relative risk of developing chronic pancreatitis and alcohol, protein and lipid consumption. Digestion 18:337–350, 1978.
26. Wilson JS, Pirola RC: The drinker's pancreas: molecular mechanisms emerge. Gastroenterology 113:355–358, 1997.
27. Wilson JS, Gossat D, Tait A, et al.: Evidence for an inherited predisposition to alcoholic pancreatitis. A controlled HLA typing study. Dig Dis Sci 29:727–730, 1984.
28. Norton ID, Apte MV, Haber PS, et al.: Cytochrome P4502E1 is present in rat pancreas and is induced by chronic ethanol administration. Gut 42:426–430, 1998.
29. Nordback IH, MacGowan S, Potter J, et al.: The role of acetaldehyde in the pathogenesis of acute alcoholic pancreatitis. Ann Surg 214:671–678, 1991.
30. Czako L, Takacs T, Varga IS, et al.: Involvement of oxygen-derived free radicals in L-arginine–induced acute pancreatitis. Dig Dis Sci 43:1770–1777, 1998.
31. Furukawa M, Kimura T, Yamaguchi H, et al.: Role of oxygen-derived free radicals in hemorrhagic pancreatitis induced by stress and cerulein in rats. Pancreas 9:67–72, 1994.
32. Steer ML, Rutledge PL, Powers RE, et al.: The role of oxygen-derived free radicals in two models of experimental acute pancreatitis: Effects of catalase, superoxide dismutase, dimethylsulfoxide, and allopurinol. Klin Wochenschr 69:1012–1017, 1991.
33. Katz M, Carangelo R, Miller LJ, et al.: Effect of ethanol on cholecystokinin-stimulated zymogen conversion in pancreatic acinar cells. Am J Physiol 270:G171–G175, 1996.
34. Saluja AK, Lu L, Yamaguchi Y et al.: A cholecystokinin-releasing factor mediates ethanol-induced stimulation of rat pancreatic secretion. J Clin Invest 99:506–512, 1997.
35. Levant JA, Secrist DM, Resin H, et al.: Nasogastric suction in the treatment of alcoholic pancreatitis. A controlled study. JAMA 229:51–52, 1974.
36. Naeije R, Salingret E, Clumeck N, et al.: Is nasogastric suction necessary in acute pancreatitis? Br Med J 2:659–660, 1978.
37. Sarr MG, Sanfey H, Cameron JL: Prospective randomized trial of nasogastric suction in patients with acute pancreatitis. Surgery 100:500–504, 1986.
38. Meshkinpour H, Molinari MD, Gardner L, et al.: Cimetidine in the treatment of acute alcoholic pancreatitis. A randomized, double-blind study. Gastroenterology 77:687–690, 1979.
39. Harvey MH, Cates MC, Reber HA: Possible mechanisms of acute pancreatitis induced by ethanol. Am J Surg 155:49–56, 1988.
40. Acosta JM, Pellegrini CA, Skinner DB: Etiology and pathogenesis of acute biliary pancreatitis. Surgery 88:118–125, 1980.
41. Acosta JM, Ledesma CL: Gallstone migration as a cause of acute pancreatitis. N Engl J Med 290:484–488, 1974.
42. Kelly TR: Gallstone pancreatitis: Pathophysiology. Surgery 80:488–492, 1976.
43. Kelly TR: Gallstone pancreatitis. Local predisposing factors. Ann Surg 200:479–485, 1984.
44. Armstrong CP, Taylor TV, Jeacock J, et al.: The biliary tract in patients with acute gallstone pancreatitis. Br J Surg 72:551–555, 1985.

45. Lee SP, Nicholls JF, Park HZ: Biliary sludge as a cause of acute pancreatitis. N Engl J Med 326:589–593, 1992.
46. Goldstein F, Kucer FT, Thornton JJ IIIrd, et al.: Acute and relapsing pancreatitis caused by bile pigment aggregates and diagnosed by biliary drainage. Am J Gastroenterol 74:225–230, 1980.
47. Negro P, Flati G, Flati D, et al.: Occult gallbladder microlithiasis causing acute recurrent pancreatitis. A report of three cases. Acta Chir Scand 150:503–506, 1984.
48. Neoptolemos JP, Davidson BR, Winder AF, et al.: Role of duodenal bile crystal analysis in the investigation of "idiopathic pancreatitis." Br J Surg 75:450–453, 1988.
49. Ros E, Navarro S, Bru C, et al.: Occult microlithiasis in "idiopathic" acute pancreatitis: Prevention of relapses by cholecystectomy or ursodeoxycholic acid therapy. Gastroenterology 101:1701–1709, 1991.
50. Marotta PJ, Gregor JC, Taves DH: Biliary sludge: A risk factor for "idiopathic" pancreatitis. Can J Gastroenterol 10:385–388, 1996.
51. Csendes A, Kruse A, Funch-Jensen P, et al.: Pressure measurements in the biliary and pancreatic duct systems in controls and in patients with gallstones, previous cholecystectomy, or common bile duct stones. Gastroenterology 77:1203–1210, 1979.
52. Di Magno EP, Shorter RG, Taylor WF, et al.: Relationships between pancreaticobiliary ductal anatomy and pancreatic ductal and parenchymal histology. Cancer 49:361–368, 1982.
53. Armstrong CP, Taylor TV, Torrance HB: Pressure, volume and the pancreas. Gut 26:615–624, 1985.
54. Arendt T: Bile-induced acute pancreatitis in cats: Roles of bile, bacteria, and pancreatic duct pressure. Dig Dis Sci 38:39–44, 1993.
55. Arendt T, Nizze H, Monig H, et al.: Biliary pancreatic reflux–induced acute pancreatitis—myth or possibility? Eur J Gastroenterol Hepatol 11:329–335, 1999.
56. Frey C: Gallstone pancreatitis. Surg Clin N Am 61:923–938, 1981.
57. Folsch UR, Nitsche R, Ludtke R, et al.: Early ERCP and papillotomy compared with conservative treatment for acute biliary pancreatitis. N Engl J Med 336:237–242, 1997.
58. Sugiyama M, Atomi Y: Anomalous pancreaticobiliary junction without congenital choledochal cyst. Br J Surg 85:911–916, 1998.
59. Mori K, Nagakawa T, Ohta T, et al.: Acute pancreatitis associated with anomalous union of the pancreaticobiliary ductal system. J Clin Gastroenterol 13:673–677, 1991.
60. Mori K, Nagakawa T, Ohta T, et al.: Pancreatitis and anomalous union of the pancreaticobiliary ductal system in childhood. J Pediatr Surg. 28:67–71, 1993.
61. Lin A, Feller ER: Pancreatic carcinoma as a cause of unexplained pancreatitis: Report of ten cases. Ann Intern Med 113:166–167, 1990.
62. Wilson C, Imrie CW: Occult pancreatic cancer with recurrent acute pancreatitis. Postgrad Med J 62:765–767, 1986.
63. Guzzardo G, Kleinman MS, Krackov JH, et al.: Recurrent acute pancreatitis caused by ampullary villous adenoma. J Clin Gastroenterol 12:200–202, 1990.
64. Dixon JM, Chapman RW, Berry AR: Carcinoid tumor of the ampulla of Vater presenting as acute pancreatitis. Gut 10:1296–1297, 1987.
65. Mergener K, Gottfried MR, Feldman JM, et al.: Carcinoid of the ampulla of Vater presenting as acute pancreatitis. Am J Gastroenterol 91:2426–2427, 1996.
66. Robertson JF, Imrie CW: Acute pancreatitis associated with carcinoma of the ampulla of Vater. Br J Surg 74:395–397, 1987.
67. De Beaux AC, Palmer KR, Carter DC: Factors influencing morbidity and mortality in acute pancreatitis; an analysis of 279 cases. Gut 37:121–126, 1995.
68. Gutman M, Inbar M, Klausner JM: Metastases-induced acute pancreatitis. Eur J Surg Oncol 19:302–304, 1993.
69. Richter JM, Schapiro RH, Mulley AG, et al.: Association of pancreas divisum and pancreatitis, and its treatment by sphincteroplasty of the accessory ampulla. Gastroenterology 81:1104–1110, 1981.
70. Lavine JE. Harrison M. Heyman MB: Gastrointestinal duplications causing relapsing pancreatitis in children. Gastroenterology 97:1556–1558, 1989.
71. Beckingham IJ, Cullis SNR, Krige JEJ, et al.: Management of hepatobiliary and pancreatic *Ascaris* infestation in adults after failed medical treatment. Br J Surg 85:907–910, 1998.
72. Weiner GR, Geenan E, Hogan WJ, et al.: Use of corticosteroids in the prevention of post-ERCP pancreatitis. Gastrointest Endosc 42:579–583, 1995.
73. Dumot JA, Conwell DL, O'Connor JB, et al.: Pretreatment with methylprednisolone to prevent ERCP-induced pancreatitis: A randomized, multicenter, placebo-controlled clinical trial. Am J Gastroenterol 93:61–65, 1998.
74. Rocca R, Masoero G, Rocca G, et al.: Is post-ERCP acute pancreatitis predictable? A prospective study. Gastroenterology 116:A1159, 1999.
75. Johnson, GK, Geenen JE, Johanson JF, et al.: Evaluation of post-ERCP pancreatitis: Potential causes of differing contrast media. Gastrointest Endosc 46:217–222, 1997.
76. Fung AS, Tsiotos GG, Sarr MG. ERCP-induced acute necrotizing pancreatitis: Is it a more severe disease? Pancreas 15:217–221, 1997.
77. Tarnasky PR, Palesch YY, Cunningham JT, et al.: Pancreatic stenting prevents pancreatitis after biliary sphincterotomy in patients with sphincter of Oddi dysfunction. Gastroenterology 115:1518–1524, 1998.
78. Cavallini G, Tittobello A, Frulloni L, et al.: Gabexate for the prevention of pancreatic damage related to endoscopic retrograde cholangiopancreatography. N Engl J Med 335:919–923, 1996.
79. White TT, Morgan A, Hopton D: Postoperative pancreatitis. A study of seventy cases. Am J Surg 120:132–137, 1970.
80. Fernandez-del Castillo C, Harringer W, Warshaw AL, et al.: Risk factors for pancreatic cellular injury after cardiopulmonary bypass. N Engl J Med 325:382–387, 1991.
81. Lefor AT, Vuocolo P, Parker FB, et al.: Pancreatic complications following cardiopulmonary bypass. Factors influencing mortality. Arch Surg 127:1225–1230, 1992.
82. Gullo L, Cavicchi L, Tomassetti P, et al.: Effects of ischemia on the human pancreas. Gastroenterology 111:1033–1038, 1996.
83. Dominguez-Munoz JE, Malfertheimer P, Ditschuneit HH, et al.: Hyperlipidemia in acute pancreatitis. Relationship with etiology, onset, and severity of the disease. Int J Pancreatol 10:261–267, 1991.
84. Dominguez-Munoz JE, Junemann F, Malfertheimer P: Hyperlipidemia in acute pancreatitis. Cause or epiphenomenon? Int J Pancreatol 18:101–106, 1995.
85. Hofbauer B, Friess H, Weber A, et al.: Hyperlipaemia intensifies the course of acute oedematous and acute

necrotizing pancreatitis in the rat. Gut 38:753–758, 1996.

86. Rollan A, Guzman S, Pimentel F, et al.: Catabolism of chylomicron remnants in patients with previous acute pancreatitis. Gastroenterology 98:1649–1654, 1990.
87. Malagelada JR, Holtermuller KH, Sizemore GW, et al.: The influence of hypercalcemia on basal and cholecystokinin-stimulated pancreatic, gallbladder, and gastric functions in man. Gastroenterology 71:405–408, 1976.
88. Frick T, Fernandez-del Castillo C, Bimmler D, et al.: Elevated calcium and activation of trypsinogen in rat pancreatic acini. Gut 41:339–343, 1997.
89. Whitcomb DC: Hereditary pancreatitis: New insights into acute and chronic pancreatitis. Gut 45:317–322, 1999.
90. Mithofer K, Fernandez-del Castillo C, Frick TW, et al.: Acute hypercalcemia causes acute pancreatitis and ectopic trypsinogen activation in the rat. Gastroenterology 109:239–246, 1995.
91. Frick TW, Mithofer K, Fernandez-del Castillo C, et al.: Hypercalcemia causes acute pancreatitis by pancreatic secretory block, intracellular zymogen accumulation, and acinar cell injury. Am J Surg 169:167–172, 1995.
92. Cates MC, Singh SM, Peick AL, et al.: Acute hypercalcemia, pancreatic duct permeability, and pancreatitis in cats. Surgery 104:137–141, 1988.
93. Savides EP, Hoffbrand BI: Hypothermia, thrombosis, and acute pancreatitis. Br Med J 1:614, 1974.
94. Foulis AK: Morphological study of the relationship between accidental hypothermia and acute pancreatitis. J Clin Pathol 35:1244–1248, 1982.
95. Weaver GA, Bordley J IVth, Guiney WB, et al.: Chronic pancreatitis with cyst formation after prednisone and thiazide treatment. Am J Gastroenterol 77:164–168, 1982.
96. Sturdevant RA, Singleton JW, Deren JL, et al.: Azathioprine-related pancreatitis in patients with Crohn's disease. Gastroenterology 77:883–886, 1979.
97. Lankisch PG, Droge M, Gottesleben F: Drug induced acute pancreatitis: Incidence and severity. Gut 37: 565–567, 1995.
98. Bergholm U, Langman M, Rawlins M, et al.: Drug-induced acute pancreatitis. Pharmacoepidemiol Drug Safety 4:329–334, 1995.
99. Eland IA, van Puijenbroek EP, Sturkenboom MJCM, et al.: Drug-associated acute pancreatitis: Twenty one years of spontaneous reporting in the Netherlands. Am J Gastroenterol 94:2417–2422, 1999.
100. Herrmann R, Shaw RG, Fone DJ: Ranitidine-associated recurrent acute pancreatitis. Aust N Z J Med 20:243–244, 1990.
101. Ko CW, Gooley T, Schoch HG, et al.: Acute pancreatitis in marrow transplant patients: Prevalence at autopsy and risk factor analysis. Bone Marrow Transplant 20:1081–1086, 1997.
102. Chen JWC, Saccone GTP, Toouli J: Sphincter of Oddi dysfunction and acute pancreatitis. Gut 43:305–308, 1998.
103. Hogan WJ, Sherman S, Pasricha P, et al.: Sphincter of Oddi manometry. Gastrointest Endosc 45:342–348, 1997.
104. Freeman ML, Nelson DB, Sherman S, et al.: Complications of endoscopic biliary sphincterotomy. N Engl J Med 335:909–918, 1996.
105. Tarnasky P, Cunningham J, Cotton P: Pancreatic sphincter hypertension increases the risk of post-ERCP pancreatitis. Endoscopy 29:252–257, 1997.
106. Kimura W, Ohtsubo K: Clinical and pathological features of acute interstitial pancreatitis in the aged. Int J Pancreatol 5:1–10, 1989.
107. Imrie CW, Ferguson JC, Sommerville RG: Coxsackie and mumps virus infection in a prospective study of acute pancreatitis. Gut 16:866–870, 1975.
108. Brown M, Smiley RK: Chronic pancreatitis with steatorrhea following mumps with acute pancreatitis. Am J Dig Dis 17:280–282, 1950.
109. Renner IG, Savage WT, Pantoja JL, et al.: Death due to acute pancreatitis. A retrospective analysis of 405 autopsy cases. Dig Dis Sci 30:1005–1018, 1985.
110. Wilcox CM, Forsmark CE, Grendell JH, et al.: Cytomegalovirus-associated acute pancreatic disease in patients with acquired immunodeficiency syndrome. Gastroenterology 99:263–267, 1990.
111. Mentes A, Batur Y, Eldem A, et al.: Pancreatitis as a complication of a hydatic liver cyst—a case report. Jpn J Surg 20:356–358, 1990.
112. Cosme A, Orive V, Ojeda E, et al.: Hydatid cyst of the head of the pancreas with spontaneous fistula to the duodenum. Am J Gastroenterol 82:1311–1313, 1987.
113. Morton PC, Terblanche JT, Bornman PC, et al.: Obstructive jaundice caused by an intrapancreatic hydatid cyst. Br J Surg 68:474–476, 1981.
114. Papadimitriou J: Pancreatic abscess due to infected hydatid disease. Surgery 102:880–882, 1987.
115. Arnaud A, Sarles JC, Sahel J, et al.: Distal pancreatic atrophy and diabetes associated with an intrapancreatic hydatid cyst [letter]. Pancreas 7:394–396, 1992.
116. Dhall JC, Bishnoi PK, Dalal AK, et al.: Tuberculosis of the pancreas: A clinical rarity. Am J Gastroenterol 92:172, 1997.
117. Reynolds JC, Inman RD, Kimberly RP, et al.: Acute pancreatitis in systemic lupus erythematosus: Report of twenty cases and a review of the literature. Medicine 61:25–31, 1982.
118. Sarra-Carbonell S, Jiminez SA: Ehlers–Danlos syndrome associated with acute pancreatitis. J Rheumatol 16:1390–1394, 1989.
119. Ichihara S, Sato M, Kozuka S: Prevalence of pancreatitis in liver diseases of various etiologies: An analysis of 107,754 adult autopsies in Japan. Digestion 51:86–94, 1992.
120. Kuo PC, Plotkin JS, Johnson LB: Acute pancreatitis and fulminant hepatic failure. J Am Coll Surg 187: 522–528, 1998.
121. Mishra A, Saigal S, Gupta R, et al.: Acute pancreatitis associated with viral hepatitis: A report of six cases with review of literature. Am J Gastroenterol 94:2292–2295, 1999.
122. Angelini G, Merigo F, Degani G, et al.: Association of chronic alcoholic liver and pancreatic disease: A prospective study. Am J Gastroenterol 80:998–1003, 1985.
123. Stigendal L, Olsson R: Alcohol consumption pattern and serum lipids in alcoholic cirrhosis and pancreatitis. A comparative study. Scand J Gastroenterol 19:582–587, 1984.
124. McKay AJ, O'Neill J, Imrie CW: Pancreatitis, pregnancy, and gallstones. Br J Obstet Gynaecol 87:47–50, 1980.
125. Jouppila P, Mokka R, Larmi TKI: Acute pancreatitis in pregnancy. Surg Gynecol Obstet 139:879–882, 1974.
126. Roberts IM: Hyperlipidemic gestational pancreatitis. Gastroenterology 104:1560–1561, 1993.
127. Kelly TR: Primary hyperparathyroidism during pregnancy. Surgery 110:1028–1034, 1991.

128. DeBanto JR, Pedroso MRA, Whitcombe DC, et al.: Epidemiology of pediatric acute pancreatitis. Gastroenterology 116:A1117, 1999.
129. Gullo L, Sipahi HM, Pezzilli R: Pancreatitis in the elderly. J Clin Gastroenterol 19:64–68, 1994.
130. Lillemoe KD: Pancreatic disease in the elderly patient. Surg Clin North Am 74:317–344, 1994.
131. Browder W, Patterson MD, Thompson JL, et al.: Acute pancreatitis of unknown etiology in the elderly. Ann Surg 217:469–474, 1993.
132. Padilla B, Pollak VE, Pesce A, et al.: Pancreatitis in patients with end-stage renal disease. Medicine 73:8–21, 1994.
133. Leinkram C, Roberts-Thomson IC, Kune GA: Duodenal diverticula related to gallstones and pancreatitis. Med J Aust 1:209–210, 1980.
134. Kalvaria I, Bornman PC, Girdwood AH, et al.: Periampullary cyst: A surgically remediable cause of pancreatitis. Gut 28:358–362, 1987.
135. Shimada H, Nakagawara G, Nakano A, et al.: A duodenal duplication cyst communicated with an accessory pancreatic duct. Jpn J Surg 14:320–326, 1984.
136. Ng KY, Desmond PV, Collier N: Relapsing pancreatitis due to juxta-pancreatic duodenal duplication cyst with pancreatic ductal communication. Austral N Z J Surg 63:224–229, 1993.
137. Hoffman M, Sugerman HJ, Heuman D, et al.: Gastric duplication cyst communicating with aberrant pancreatic duct: A rare cause of recurrent acute pancreatitis. Surgery 101:369–372, 1987.
138. Chiari H: Über Selbstverdauung des menschlichen Pankreas. Z Heilkunde 17:69–95, 1896.
139. Gorry MC, Gabbaizedeh D, Furey W, et al.: Mutations in the cationic trypsinogen gene are associated with recurrent acute and chronic pancreatitis. Gastroenterology 113:1063–1068, 1997.
140. Steer ML: The early intraacinar cell events which occur during acute pancreatitis. Pancreas 17:31–37, 1998.
141. Kloppel G, Dreyer T, Willemer S, et al.: Human acute pancreatitis: Its pathogenesis in the light of immunocytochemical and ultrastructural findings in acinar cells. Virchows Arch A Pathol Anat Histopathol 409:791–803, 1986.
142. Adler G, Rohr G, Kern HF: Alteration of membrane fusion as a cause of acute pancreatitis in the rat. Dig Dis Sci 27:993–1002, 1982.
143. Hartwig W, Jiminez RE, Werner J, et al.: Interstitial trypsinogen release and its relevance to the transformation of mild into necrotizing pancreatitis in rats. Gastroenterology 117:717–725, 1999.
144. Hofbauer B, Saluja AK, Lerch MM, et al.: Intra-acinar cell activation of trypsinogen during caerulein-induced pancreatitis in rats. Am J Physiol 275:G352–G362, 1998.
145. OtaniT, Chepilko SM, Grendell JH, et al.: Codistribution of TAP and the granule membrane protein, GRAMP-92, in rat caerulein-induced pancreatitis. Am J Physiol 275:G999–G1000, 1998.
146. Bhatia W, Wallig MA, Hofbauer B, et al.: Induction of apoptosis in pancreatic acinar cells reduces the severity of acute pancreatitis. Biochem Biophys Res Commun 246:476–483, 1998.
147. Saluja A, Hofbauer B, Yamaguchi Y, et al.: Induction of apoptosis reduces the severity of caerulein-induced pancreatitis in mice. Biochem Biophys Res Commun 220:875–878, 1996.
148. Keynes M: Heretical thoughts on the pathogenesis of acute pancreatitis. Gut 29:1413–1423, 1988.
149. Roxvall LI, Bengtson LA, Heideman JM: Anaphylatoxins and terminal complement complexes in pancreatitis. Evidence of complement activation in plasma and ascites fluid of patients with acute pancreatitis. Arch Surg 125:918–921, 1990.
150. Roxvall LI, Benjtson A, Sennerby L, et al.: Activation of the complement cascade by trypsin. Biol Chem Hoppe Seyler 372:273–278, 1991.
151. Van Laethem J-L, Eskinazi R, Louis H, et al.: Multisystemic production of interleukin 10 limits the severity of acute pancreatitis in mice. Gut 43:408–413, 1998.
152. Berney T, Gasche Y, Robert J, et al.: Serum profiles of interleukin-6, interleukin-8, and interleukin-10 in patients with severe and mild acute pancreatitis. Pancreas 18:371–377, 1999.
153. Osman MO, Kristensen JU, Jacobsen NO, et al.: A monoclonal anti-interleukin 8 antibody (WS-4) inhibits its cytokine response and acute lung injury in experimental severe acute necrotising pancreatitis in rabbits. Gut 43:232–239, 1998.
154. Denham W, Yang J, Fink G, et al.: Gene targeting demonstrates additive detrimental effects of interleukin-1 and tumor necrosis factor during pancreatitis. Gastroenterology 113:1741–1746, 1997.
155. Gukovskaya AS, Gukovsky I, Zaninovic V, et al.: Pancreatic acinar cells produce, release, and respond to tumor necrosis factor alpha. Role in regulating cell death and pancreatitis. J Clin Invest 100:1853–1862, 1997.
156. Norman J, Yang J, Fink G et al.: Severity and mortality of experimental pancreatitis are dependent on IL-1 converting enzyme (ICE). J Interferon Cytokine Res 17:113–118, 1997.
157. Satoh A, Shimosegawa T, Fujita M, et al.: Inhibition of nuclear factor κB activation improves the survival of rats with taurocholate pancreatitis. Gut 44:253–258, 1999.
158. Al-Mufti RA, Williamson RCN, Mathie RT: Increased nitric oxide activity in a rat model of acute pancreatitis. Gut 43:564–570, 1998.
159. Werner J, Fernandez-del Castillo C, Rivera JA, et al.: On the protective mechanisms of nitric oxide in acute pancreatitis. Gut 43:401–407, 1998.
160. Braganza JM, Scott P, Bilton D, et al.: Evidence for early oxidative stress in acute pancreatitis, Clues for correction. Int J Pancreatol 17:69–81, 1995.
161. Kemppainen E, Puolakkainen P, Hietaranta A, et al.: Time-course profile of serum trypsinogen-2 and trypsin-2-alpha-1-antitrypsin in patients with acute pancreatitis. Gastroenterology 116:A1137, 1999.
162. Kylanpaa-Back L, Kemppainen E, Hedstršm J, et al.: Reliable screening for acute pancreatitis with rapid urine trypsinogen-2 test strip. Gastroenterology 116: A1141, 1999.
163. Pezzilli R, Morselli-Labate AM, Miniero R, et al.: Simultaneous serum assays of lipase and interleukin-6 for early diagnosis and prognosis of acute pancreatitis. Clin Chem 45:1762–1767, 1999.
164. Hedstrom J, Sainio V, Kemppainen E, et al.: Serum complex of trypsin 2 and alpha-1-antitrypsin as diagnostic and prognostic marker of acute pancreatitis: Clinical study in consecutive patients. Br Med J 313:333–337, 1996.
165. Appelros S, Thim L, Borgstrom A: Activation peptide of carboxypeptidase B in serum and urine in acute pancreatitis. Gut 42:97–102, 1998.

166. Nordback I, Lauslahti K: Clinical pathology of acute necrotizing pancreatitis. J Clin Pathol 39:68–74, 1986.
167. Phat VN, Guerrieri MT, Alexandre JH, et al.: Early histological changes in acute necrotizing hemorrhagic pancreatitis. A retrospective pathological study of 20 total pancreatectomy specimens. Pathol Res Pract 178:273–279, 1984.
168. Aho HJ, Nevalainen TJ, Havia VT, et al.: Human acute pancreatitis. A light and electron microscopic study. Acta Path Microbial Immunol Scand Sect A 90:367–373, 1982.
169. Kloppel G, Maillet B: Chronic pancreatitis: evolution of the disease. Hepatogastroenterol 38:408–412, 1991.
170. Kloppel G, Maillet B: Pseudocysts in chronic pancreatitis: a morphological analysis of 57 resection specimens and 9 autopsy pancreata. Pancreas 6:266–274, 1991.
171. Kloppel G, Maillet B: The morphological basis for the evolution of acute pancreatitis into chronic pancreatitis. Virchows Arch A Pathol Anat Histopathol 420:1–4, 1992.
172. Aho HJ, Sternby B, Nevalainen TJ: Fat necrosis in human acute pancreatitis. Acta Pathol Microbiol Scand Sect A 94:101–105, 1986.
173. Foulis AK: Histological evidence of initiating factors in acute necrotizing pancreatitis in man. J Clin Pathol 33:1125–1131, 1980.
174. Lankisch PG, Schirren CA, Kunze E: Undetected fatal acute pancreatitis: Why is the disease so frequently overlooked? Am J Gastroenterol 86:1852–1854, 1991.
175. Kalfarentzos F, Kehagias J, Mead N, et al.: Enteral nutrition is superior to parenteral nutrition in severe acute pancreatitis: Results of a randomized prospective trial. Br J Surg 84:1665–1669, 1997.
176. Windsor AC, Kanwar S, Li AG, et al.: Compared with parenteral nutrition, enteral feeding attenuates the acute phase response and improves disease severity in acute pancreatitis. Gut 42:431–435, 1998.
177. al Karawi MA, el Shiekh Mohamed AR, al Shahri MG, et al.: Endoscopic sphincterotomy in acute gallstone pancreatitis and cholangitis: A Saudi hospital experience. Hepatogastroenterol 40:396–401, 1993.
178. Beger HG, Rau B, Mayer J, et al.: Natural course of acute pancreatitis. World J Surg 21:130–135, 1997.
179. Rau B, Uhl W, Buchler MW, et al.: Surgical treatment of infected necrosis. World J Surg 21:155–161, 1997.
180. Lumsden A, Bradley EL IIIrd: Pseudocyst or cystic neoplasm? Differential diagnosis and initial management of cystic pancreatic lesions. Hepatogastroenterol 36:462–466, 1989.
181. Bassi C, Falcone M, Talamini G, et al.: Controlled trial of perfloxacin versus imipenim in severe acute pancreatitis. Gastroenterology 115:1513–1517, 1998.
182. Powell JJ, Miles R, Siriwardena AK: Antibiotic prophylaxis in the initial management of severe acute pancreatitis. Br J Surg 85:582–587, 1998.
183. Golub R, Siddiqi F, Pohl D: Role of antibiotics in acute pancreatitis: a metaanalysis. J Gastrointest Surg 2:496–503, 1998.
184. Burns GP, Stein TA, Kabnick LS: Blood-pancreatic juice barrier to antibiotic excretion. Am J Surg 151:205–208, 1986.
185. Stoutenbeek CP, van Saene HK, Miranda DR, et al.: The effect of selective decontamination of the digestive tract on colonization and infection rate in multiple trauma patients. Intensive Care Med 10:185–192, 1984.
186. Banks PA: Infected necrosis: Morbidity and therapeutic consequences. Hepatogastroenterol 38:116–119, 1991.
187. Schmid SW, Uhl W, Friess H, et al.: The role of infection in acute pancreatitis. Gut 45:311–316, 1999.
188. Freeny PC, Hauptmann E, Althaus SJ, et al.: Percutaneous CT-guided catheter drainage of infected acute necrotizing pancreatitis: Techniques and results. Am J Roentgenol 170:969–975, 1998.
189. Paye F, Rotman N, Radier C, et al.: Percutaneous aspiration for bacteriological studies in patients with necrotizing pancreatitis. Br J Surg 85:755–759, 1998.
190. Echenique AM, Sleeman D, Yrizarry J, et al.: Percutaneous catheter-directed debridement of infected pancreatic necrosis: Results in 20 patients. J Vasc Interv Radiol 9:565–571, 1998.
191. Baron TH, Thaggard WG, Morgan DE, et al.: Endoscopic therapy for organized pancreatic necrosis Gastroenterology 111:755–764, 1996.
192. Casey JE, Porter KA, Langevin RE, et al.: Clinical features and natural history of central cavitary necrosis. Pancreas 8:141–145, 1993.
193. Karimgami I, Porter KA, Langevin RE, et al.: Prognostic factors in sterile pancreatic necrosis. Gastroenterology 103:1636–1640, 1992.
194. Kingsnorth AN: Early treatment with Lexipafant, a platelet-activating factor antagonist, reduces mortality in acute pancreatitis: A double blind, randomized, placebo-controlled study. Gastroenterology 112(suppl): A453, 1997.
195. Lankisch PG, Schirren CA: Increased body weight as a prognostic parameter for complications in the course of acute pancreatitis. Pancreas 5:626–629, 1990.
196. Funnell IC, Bornman PC, Weakley SP, et al.: Obesity: An important prognostic factor in acute pancreatitis. Br J Surg 80:484–486, 1993.
197. Suazo-Barahona J, Carmona-Sanchez R, Robles-Diaz G, et al.: Obesity: A risk factor for severe acute biliary and alcoholic pancreatitis. Am J Gastroenterol 93: 1324–1328, 1998.
198. Porter KA, Banks PA: Obesity as a predictor of severity in acute pancreatitis. Int J Pancreatol 10:247–252, 1991.
199. Halonen K, Puolakkainen P, LeppSniemi A, et al.: Severe acute pancreatitis—prognostic factors in 270 consecutive patients. Gastroenterology 116:A1130, 1999.
200. Siegelman SS, Copeland BE, Saba GP, et al.: CT of fluid collections associated with pancreatitis. AJR 134:1121–1132, 1980.
201. Hartong WA, Skibba RM, Greenberger NJ: Spontaneous pseudocystogastrostomy associated with pancreatitis. Arch Int Med 136:1287–1289, 1976.
202. Sugawa C: Pancreatic pseudocysts communicating with the stomach: Demonstration by endoscopic retrograde pancreatography. Arch Surg 112:1050–1053, 1977.
203. Skellenger ME, Patterson D, Foley NT, et al.: Cholestasis due to compression of the common bile duct by pancreatic pseudocysts. Am J Surg 145:343–348, 1983.
204. Stoeckmann F, Ahrens G, Klockmann K, et al.: Pancreatic pseudocysts: Natural history and treatment. Gastroenterology 116:A1165, 1999.
205. Plath F, Meyerfeldt R, Emmrich J, et al.: Clinical course of pancreatic pseudocysts. Gastroenterology 116: A1156, 1999.
206. Lankisch PG, Mahlke R, Assmus C, et al.: Which patients with acute pancreatitis are at risk to develop pancreatic pseudocyst? Gastroenterology 116:A1142, 1999.

207. Lewis G, Krige JE, Bornman PC, et al.: Traumatic pancreatic pseudocysts. Br J Surg 80:89–93, 1993.
208. Kimura W, Sata N, Nakayama H, et al.: Pancreatic carcinoma accompanied by pseudocyst: Report of two cases. J Gastroenterol 29:786–791, 1994.
209. Centeno BA, Lewandrowski KB, Warshaw AL, et al.: Cyst fluid cytologic analysis in the differential diagnosis of pancreatic cystic lesions. Am J Clin Pathol 101:483–487, 1994.
210. Hammel P, Levy P, Voitot H, et al.: Preoperative cyst fluid analysis is useful for the differential diagnosis of cystic lesions of the pancreas. Gastroenterology 108:1230–1235, 1995.
211. Lewandrowski KB, Southern JF, Pins MR, et al.: Cyst fluid analysis in the differential diagnosis of pancreatic cysts. A comparison of pseudocysts, serous cystadenomas, mucinous cystic neoplasms, and mucinous cystadenocarcinoma. Ann Surg 217:41–47, 1993.
212. Gonzalez AC, Bradley EL, Clements JL Jr: Pseudocyst formation in acute pancreatitis: Ultrasonographic evaluation of 99 cases. Am J Roentgenol 127:315–317, 1976.
213. Adams DB, Davis BR, Anderson MC: Colonic complications of pancreatitis. Am Surg 60:44–49, 1994.
214. D'Egidio A, Schein M: Percutaneous drainage of pancreatic pseudocysts: A prospective study. World J Surg 16:141–145, 1992.
215. Funnell IC, Bornman PC, Krige JE, et al.: Endoscopic drainage of traumatic pancreatic pseudocyst. Br J Surg 81:879–881, 1994.
216. Sharma SS: Endoscopic gastrocystostomy. Preliminary experience. Ind J Gastroenterol 14:11–12, 1995.
217. Moran B, Rew DA, Johnson CD: Pancreatic pseudocyst should be treated by surgical drainage. Ann Roy Coll Surg Engl 76:54–58, 1994.
218. Hariri M, Slivka A, Carr-Locke DL, et al.: Pseudocyst drainage predisposes to infection when pancreatic necrosis is unrecognized. Am J Gastroenterol 89:1781–1784, 1994.
219. Stewart DL, Torma MJ, Meyer GW: Pancreatic retention cyst secondary to chronic pancreatitis. A cause of hemobilia. Am J Dig Dis 23:663–666, 1978.
220. Belli G, Romano G, D'Alessandro V, et al.: Severe hemorrhage associated with pancreatic pseudocysts: Report of two cases. Int J Pancreatol 4:455–460, 1989.
221. Greenstein A, DeMaio EF, Nabseth DC: Acute hemorrhage associated with pancreatic pseudocysts. Surgery 69:56–62, 1971.
222. Henne-Bruns D, Froschle G, Grimm H, et al.: Acute gastrointestinal bleeding as a complication of pancreatic pseudocysts. Hepatogastroenterol 38:75–77, 1991.
223. Ito Y, Tanegashima A, Nishi K, et al.: Necrotizing arteritis causing fatal massive intraperitoneal hemorrhage from a pancreatic pseudocyst. Int J Legal Med 106:324–327, 1994.
224. Hastings OM, Jain KM, Khademi M, et al.: Intrasplenic pancreatic pseudocyst complicating severe acute pancreatitis. Am J Gastroenterol 69:182–186, 1978.
225. Ueda N, Takahashi N, Yamasaki H, et al.: Intrasplenic pancreatic pseudocyst: A case report. Gastroenterologia Japonica 27:675–682, 1992.
226. Okuda K, Sugita S, Tsukada E, et al.: Pancreatic pseudocyst in the left hepatic lobe: A report of two cases. Hepatology 13:359–363, 1991.
227. Baker MK, Kopecky KK, Wass JL: Perirenal pancreatic pseudocysts: Diagnostic management. Am J Roentgenol 140:729–732, 1983.
228. Lilienfeld RM, Lande A: Pancreatic pseudocysts presenting as thick-walled renal and perinephric cysts. J Urol 115:123–125, 1976.
229. Johnston RH Jr, Owensby LC, Vargas GM, et al.: Pancreatic pseudocyst of the mediastinum. Ann Thor Surg 41:210–212, 1986.
230. Jaffe BM, Ferguson TB, Holtz S, et al.: Mediastinal pancreatic pseudocysts. Am J Surg 124:600–606, 1972.
231. Sankaran S, Walt AJ: Pancreatic ascites: Recognition and management. Arch Surg 111:430–430, 1976.
232. Iacono C, Procacci C, Frigo F, et al.: Thoracic complications of pancreatitis. Pancreas 4:228–436, 1989.
233. Thompson NW, Eckhauser FE, Vinik AI, et al.: Cystic neuroendocrine neoplasms of the pancreas and liver. Ann Surg 199:158–164, 1984.
234. Sariban E, Magrath I, Shawker TH: Abdominal lymphoma mimicking a pancreatic pseudo-cyst. Am J Gastroenterol 77:861–863, 1982.
235. Mester M, Trajber HJ, Compton CC, et al.: Cystic teratomas of the pancreas. Arch Surg 125:1215–1218, 1990.
236. Marchevsky AM, Zimmerman MJ, Aufses AH Jr, et al.: Endometrial cyst of the pancreas. Gastroenterology 86:1589–1591, 1984.
237. Goswami AK, Sharma SK, Tandon SP, et al.: Pancreatic endometriosis presenting as a hypovascular renal mass. J Urol 135:112–113, 1986.
238. Sperti C, Pasquali C, Di Prima F, et al.: Duodenal leiomyosarcoma mimicking a pancreatic pseudocyst. HPB Surgery 8:49–52, 1994.
239. Warshaw AL, Rutledge PL: Cystic tumors mistaken for pancreatic pseudocysts. Ann Surg 205:393–398, 1987.
240. Gerzof SG, Banks PA, Robbins AH, et al.: Early diagnosis of pancreatic infection by computed tomography-guided aspiration. Gastroenterology 93:1315–1320, 1987.
241. Beger HG, Bittner R, Block S, et al.: Bacterial contamination of pancreatic necrosis. A prospective clinical study. Gastroenterology 91:433–438, 1986.
242. Bittner R: Clinical significance and management of pancreatic abscess and infected necrosis complicating acute pancreatitis. Ann Ital Chir 66:217–222, 1995.
243. Rutledge PL, Warshaw AL: Persistent acute pancreatitis. A variant treated by pancreatoduodenectomy. Arch Surg 123:597–600, 1988.
244. Adams DB, Anderson MC: Percutaneous catheter drainage compared with internal drainage in the management of pancreatic pseudocyst. Ann Surg 215:571–576, 1992.
245. Madry S, Fromm D: Infected retroperitoneal fat necrosis associated with acute pancreatitis. J Am Coll Surg 178:277–282, 1994.
246. Dallemand S, Farman J, Stein D, et al.: Colonic necrosis complicating pancreatitis. Gastrointest Radiol 2:27–30, 1977.
247. Kukora JS: Extensive colonic necrosis complicating acute pancreatitis. Surgery 97:290–294, 1985.
248. Burke JW, Erickson SJ, Kellum CD, et al.: Pseudoaneurysms complicating pancreatitis: Detection by CT. Radiology 161:447–450, 1986.
249. Hartwig W, Werner J, Jiminez RE, et al.: Trypsin and activation of circulating trypsinogen contribute to pancreatitis-associated lung injury. Am J Physiol 277:G1008–1016, 1999.
250. Bhatia M, Saluja AK, Hofbauer B, et al.: The effects of neutrophil depletion on a completely noninvasive model of acute pancreatitis-associated lung injury. Int J Pancreatol 24:77–83, 1998.

251. Frossard JL, Saluja A, Bhagat L, et al.: The role of intercellular adhesion molecule 1 and neutrophils in acute pancreatitis and pancreatitis-associated lung injury. Gastroenterology 116:694–701, 1999.
252. Werner J, Z'graggen K, Fernandez-del Castillo C, et al.: Specific therapy for local and systemic complications of acute pancreatitis with monoclonal antibodies against ICAM-1. Ann Surg 229:834–840, 1999.
253. Yang J, Murphy C, Denham W, et al.: Evidence of a central role for p38 map kinase induction of tumor necrosis factor alpha in pancreatitis-associated pulmonary injury. Surgery 126:216–222, 1999.
254. The Copenhagen Pancreatitis Study Group: An interim report from a prospective, epidemiology, multicenter study. Scand J Gastroenterol 16:305–312, 1981.
255. Andersen BN, Pedersen NT, Scheel J, et al.: Incidence of alcoholic chronic pancreatitis in Copenhagen. Scand J Gastroenterol 17:247–252, 1982.
256. Pedersen TN, Worning H: Chronic pancreatitis. Scand J Gastroenterol 31 (suppl) 216:52–58, 1996.
257. Johnson CD, Hosking S: National statistics for diet, alcohol consumption, and chronic pancreatitis in England and Wales, 1960–88. Gut 32:1401–1405, 1991.
258. Ammann RW: Chronic pancreatitis in the elderly. Gastroenterol Clin N Am 19:905–914, 1990.
259. Lowenfels AB, Maissonneuve P, DiMagno EP, et al.: Hereditary pancreatitis and the risk of pancreatic cancer. International hereditary pancreatitis study group. J Natl Cancer Inst 89:442–446, 1997.
260. McNamee R, Braganza JM, Hogg J, et al.: Occupational exposure to hydrocarbons and chronic pancreatitis: A case-referent study. Occup Environ Med 51:631–637, 1994.
261. Ammann RW, Muellhaupt B: Progression of alcoholic acute to chronic pancreatitis. Gut 35:552–556, 1994.
262. Braganza JM, Schofield D, Snehalatha C, et al.: Micronutrient antioxidant status in tropical compared with temperate-zone chronic pancreatitis. Scand J Gastroenterol 28:1098–1104, 1993.
263. James O, Agnew JE, Bouchier IAD: Chronic pancreatitis in England: A changing picture? Br Med J 2(909):34–38, 1974.
264. Ammann RW, Akovbiantz A, Largiader F, et al.: Course and outcome of chronic pancreatitis. Longitudinal study of a mixed medical-surgical series of 245 patients. Gastroenterology 86:820-828, 1984.
265. Rosenblatt ML, Whitcomb DC: Development of chronic pancreatitis in humans after acute pancreatitis is associated with severity of acute pancreatitis. Gastroenterology 116:A1160, 1999.
266. Lowenfels AB, Maisonneuve P, Grover H, et al.: Racial factors and the risk of chronic pancreatitis. Am J Gastroenterol 94:790–794, 1999.
267. Almela P, Aparisi L, Grau F, et al.: Influence of alcohol consumption on the initial development of chronic pancreatitis. Rev Esp Enferm Dig 89:741–752, 1997.
268. Layer P, Yamamoto H, Kalthoff L, et al.: The different courses of early- and late-onset idiopathic and alcoholic chronic pancreatitis. Gastroenterology 107: 1481–1487, 1994.
269. Talamini G, Bassi C, Falconi M, et al.: Cigarette smoking: an independent risk factor in alcoholic pancreatitis. Pancreas 12:131–137, 1996.
270. Haber PS, Norris MD, Apte MV, et al.: Alcoholic pancreatitis and polymorphisms of the variable length polythymidine tract in the cystic fibrosis gene. Alcohol Clin Exp Res 23:509–512, 1999.
271. Sharer N, Schwartz M, Malone G, et al.: Mutations of the cystic fibrosis gene in patients with chronic pancreatitis. N Engl J Med 339:645–652, 1998.
272. Malats N, Real FX, Sharer N, et al.: Correction: Mutations of the cystic fibrosis gene in patients with chronic pancreatitis. N Engl J Med 340:1592–1593, 1999.
273. Cohn JA, Friedman KJ, Noone PG, et al.: Relation between mutations of the cystic fibrosis gene and idiopathic pancreatitis. N Engl J Med 339:653–658, 1998.
274. Bishop MD, Freedman SD, Zielenski J, et al.: Does complete DNA analysis identify a higher percentage of cystic fibrosis gene mutations in patients with idiopathic chronic and recurrent acute pancreatitis. Gastroenterology 116:A1113, 1999.
275. Creighton J, Lyall R, Wilson DI, et al.: Mutations of the cationic trypsinogen gene in patients with chronic pancreatitis. Lancet 354:42–43, 1999.
276. Comfort MW, Steinberg AG: Pedigree of a family with hereditary chronic relapsing pancreatitis. Gastroenterology 21:54–63, 1952.
277. Girard RM, Dube S, Archamboult AP: Hereditary pancreatitis: Report of an affected Canadian kindred and review of the disease. Can Med Assoc J 125:576–580, 1981.
278. Roberts IM: Disorders of the pancreas in children. Gastroenterol Clin N Am 19:963–973, 1990.
279. Whitcomb DC, Gorry MC, Preston RA, et al.: Hereditary pancreatitis is caused by a mutation in the cationic trypsinogen gene. Nature Genetics 14:141–145, 1996.
280. Robechek PJ: Hereditary chronic pancreatitis. A clue to pancreatitis in general? Am J Surg 113:819–824, 1967.
281. Witt H, Luck W, Becker M: A signal peptide cleavage site mutation in the cationic trypsinogen gene is strongly associated with chronic pancreatitis. Gastroenterology 117:7–10, 1999.
282. Stelling T, von Rooij WJ, Tio TL, et al.: Pancreatitis associated with congenital duodenal duplication cyst in an adult. Endoscopy 19:171–173, 1987.
283. Steer ML, Waxman I, Freedman S: Chronic pancreatitis. N Engl J Med 332:1482–1490, 1995.
284. Blair AJ III, Russell CG, Cotton PB: Resection for pancreatitis in patients with pancreas divisum. Ann Surg 200:590–594, 1984.
285. Bret PM, Reinhold C, Taourel P, et al: Pancreas divisum: Evaluation with MR cholangiopancreatography. Radiology 199:99–103, 1966.
286. Cotton PB: Congenital anomaly of pancreas division as cause of obstructive pain and pancreatitis. Gut 21:105–114, 1980.
287. Delhaye M, Engelholm L, Cremer M, Pancreas divisum: Congenital anatomic variant or anomaly? Contribution of endoscopic retrograde dorsal pancreatography. Gastroenterology 89:951–958, 1985.
288. Muzaffar AR, Moyer MS, Dobbins J, et al.: Pancreas divisum in a family with hereditary pancreatitis. J Clin Gastroenterol 22:16–20, 1996.
289. Richter JM, Schapiro RH, Mulley AG, et al.: Association of pancreas divisum and pancreatitis, and its treatment by sphincteroplasty of the accessory ampulla. Gastroenterology 81:1104–1110, 1981.
290. Wagner CW, Golladay ES: Pancreas divisum and pancreatitis in children. Am Surg 54:22–26, 1988.
291. Barthet M, Valantin V, Spinosa S, et al.: Clinical course and morphological features of chronic calcifying pancreatitis associated with pancreas divisum. Eur J Gastroenterol Hepatol 7:993–998, 1995.

292. Lindstrom E, Ihse I: Pancreatic disease caused by pancreas divisum. Eur J Surg 160:385–387, 1994.
293. Mitchell CJ, Lintott DJ, Ruddell WSJ, et al.: Clinical relevance of an unfused pancreatic duct system. Gut 20:1066–1071, 1979.
294. Rusnak CH, Hosie RT, Kuechler PM, et al.: Pancreatitis associated with pancreas divisum: Results of surgical intervention. Am J Surg 155:641–643, 1988.
295. Keith RG, Shapero TF, Saibil FG, et al.: Dorsal duct sphincterotomy is effective long-term treatment of acute pancreatitis associated with pancreas divisum. Surgery 106:660–666, 1989.
296. Lehman GA, Sherman S: Pancreas divisum. Diagnosis, clinical significance and management alternatives. Gastroenterol Clin N Am 5:145–170, 1995.
297. Ectors N, Maillet B, Aerts K, et al.: Non-alcoholic duct-destructive chronic pancreatitis. Gut 41:263–268, 1997.
298. Kawaguchi K, Koike M, Tsuruta K, et al.: Lymphoplasmacytic sclerosing pancreatitis with cholangitis: A variant of primary sclerosing cholangitis extensively involving pancreas. Hum Pathol 22:387–391, 1991.
299. Lindstrom E, Bodemar G, Ryden BO, et al.: Pancreatic ductal morphology and exocrine function in primary sclerosing cholangitis. Acta Chir Scand 156:451–456, 1990.
300. Yoshida Y: Chronic pancreatitis caused by an autoimmune abnormality. Proposal of the concept of autoimmune pancreatitis. Dig Dis Sci 40:1561–1568, 1995.
301. Horiuchi A, Kawa S, Hamano H: A clinicopathological study of autoimmune pancreatitis. Gastroenterology 116:A1134, 1999.
302. Segal I, Gut A, Schofield D, et al.: Micronutrient antioxidant status in black South Africans with chronic pancreatitis: Opportunity for prophylaxis. Clin Chim Acta 239:71–79, 1995.
303. Pitchumoni CS: Special problems of chronic pancreatitis. Clin Gastroenterol 13:941–959, 1984.
304. Rossi L, Whitcomb D, Ehrlich GD, et al.: Lack of *R117H* mutation in the cationic trypsinogen gene in patients with tropical pancreatitis from Bangladesh. Pancreas 17:278–280, 1998.
305. Borum M, Steinberg W, Steer M, et al.: Chronic pancreatitis: A complication of systemic lupus erythematosus. Gastroenterology 104:613–615, 1993.
306. Scott HW, Neblett WW, O'Neill JA, et al.: Longitudinal pancreaticojejunostomy in chronic relapsing pancreatitis with onset in childhood. Ann Surg 199:610–620, 1984.
307. Crombleholme TM, deLorimier AA, Way LW, et al.: The modified Puestow procedure for chronic relapsing pancreatitis in children. J Pediatr Surg 25:749–754, 1990.
308. Slater SD, Williamson RC, Foster CS: Proliferation of parenchymal epithelial cells enhanced in chronic pancreatitis. J Pathol 186:104–108, 1998.
309. Apte MV, Haber PS, Applegate TL, et al.: Periacinar stellate shaped cells in rat pancreas: Identification, isolation, and culture. Gut 43:128–133, 1998.
310. Ishiwata T, Kornmann M, Beger HG, et al.: Enhanced fibroblast growth factor 5 expression in stromal and exocrine elements of the pancreas in chronic pancreatitis. Gut 43:134–139, 1998.
311. Fitzgerald O, Fitzgerald P, Fennelly J, et al.: A clinical study of chronic pancreatitis. Gut 4:193–216, 1963.
312. Dreiling DA, Naqvi MA: Peptic ulcer diathesis in patients with chronic pancreatitis. Am J Gastroenterol 51:503–510, 1969.
313. Di Magno EP, Go VL, Summerskill WH: Relations between pancreatic enzyme outputs and malabsorption in severe pancreatic insufficiency. N Engl J Med 288:813–815, 1973.
314. Lowenfels AB, Maisonneuve P, Cavallini G, et al.: Pancreatitis and the risk of pancreatic cancer. N Engl J Med 328:1433–1437, 1993.
315. Axon ATR, Classen M, Cotton PB, et al.: Pancreatography in chronic pancreatitis. International definitions. Gut 25:1107–1112, 1984.
316. Izumisato Y, Mori T, Sugiyama M, et al.: Value of magnetic resonance cholangiopancreatography in the diagnosis of chronic pancreatitis. Gastroenterology 1999;116:A1136, 1999.
317. DiMagno EP: A perspective on the use of tubeless pancreatic function tests in diagnosis. Gut 43:2–3, 1998.
318. Stolte M, Weiss W, Volkholz H, et al.: A special form of segmental pancreatitis: "groove pancreatitis." Hepatogastroenterol 29:198–208, 1982.
319. Volkholz H, Stolte M, Becker V: Epithelial dysplasias in chronic pancreatitis. Virchows Arch Pathol Anat 396:331–349, 1982.
320. Bartow SA, Mukai K, Rosai J: Pseudoneoplastic proliferation of endocrine cells in pancreatic fibrosis. Cancer 47:2627–2633, 1981.
321. Hunger RE, Mueller C, Z'graggen K, et al.: Cytotoxic cells are activated in cellular infiltrates of alcoholic chronic pancreatitis. Gastroenterology 112:1656–1663, 1997.
322. Stolte M, Schwabe H, Prestele H: Relationship between diseases of the pancreas and hyperplasia of Brunner's glands. Virchows Arch Pathol Anat 394:75–87, 1981.
323. Bastid C, Sahel J, Choux R, et al.: Eosinophilic pancreatitis: report of a case. Pancreas 5:104–107, 1990.
324. Flejou JF, Potet F, Bernades P: La pancréatite à éosinophiles: Une manifestation rare de l'allergie digestive? Gastroenterol Clin Biol 13:731–733, 1989.
325. Eugene C, Gury B, Bergue A, et al.: Ictère révélant une atteinte pancréatique au cours d'un syndrome hyperéosinophilique idiopathique. Gastroenterol Clin Biol 8:966–969, 1984.
326. Smith PM, Morgan ME, Clark CG, et al.: Lipodystrophy, pancreatitis and eosinophilia. Gut 16:230–234, 1975.
327. Puestow CB, Gillesby WJ: Retrograde surgical drainage of pancreas for chronic relapsing pancreatitis. Arch Surg 76:898–907, 1958.
328. Partington PF, Rochelle REL: Modified Puestow procedure for retrograde drainage of the pancreatic duct. Ann Surg 152:1037–1043, 1960.
329. Rossi RJ, Rothschild J, Braasch JW, et al.: Pancreatoduodenectomy in the management of chronic pancreatitis. Arch Surg 122:416–420, 1987.
330. Huibregtse K, Schneider B, Vrij AA, et al.: Endoscopic pancreatic drainage in chronic pancreatitis. Gastrointestinal Endoscopy 34:9–15, 1988.
331. Cremer M, Deviere J, Delhaye M, et al.: Endoscopic management of chronic pancreatitis. Acta Gastroenterologica Belgica 56:192–200, 1993.
332. Kozarek RA, Christie D, Barclay G: Endoscopic therapy of pancreatitis in the pediatric population. Gastrointestinal Endoscopy 39:665–669, 1993.
333. Lambiase P, Seery JP, Taylor-Robinson SD, et al.: Resolution of panniculitis after placement of pancreatic duct stent in chronic pancreatitis. Am J Gastroenterol 91:1835–1837, 1996.

334. Huizinga WK, Baker LW: Surgical intervention for regional complications of chronic pancreatitis. Internat Surg 78:315–319, 1993.
335. Hollands MJ, Little JM: Obstructive jaundice in chronic pancreatitis. HPB Surgery 1:263–270, 1989.
336. Wilson C, Auld CD, Schlinkert R, et al.: Hepatobiliary complications in chronic pancreatitis. Gut 30:520–527, 1989.
337. Barthet M, Bernard JP, Duval JL, et al.: Biliary stenting in benign biliary stenosis complicating chronic calcifying pancreatitis. Endoscopy 26:569–572, 1994.
338. Kalvaria I, Bornman PC, Marks IN, et al.: The spectrum and natural history of common bile duct stenosis in chronic alcohol-induced pancreatitis. Ann Surg 210:608–613, 1989.
339. Bradley EL III, Clements JI Jr: Idiopathic duodenal obstruction. An unappreciated complication of chronic pancreatitis. Ann Surg 193:638–648, 1981.
340. Uravic M, Stimac D, Rubinic M, et al.: Duodenal obstruction from chronic pancreatitis. Minerva Chir 52:885–889, 1997.
341. Takayama T, Kato K, Sano H, et al.: Spontaneous rupture of a pancreatic pseudocyst into the portal venous system. AJR 147:935–936, 1986.
342. Zeller M, Hetz HH: Rupture of a pancreatic cyst into the portal vein. JAMA 195:869–871, 1966.
343. Roberts-Thompson IC: Intrapancreatic cysts associated with relapsing pancreatitis. Austral N Z J Surg 49:41–44, 1979.
344. Roberts-Thompson IC: Endoscopic retrograde pancreatography: Analysis of the normal pancreatogram, and changes which are associated with chronic pancreatitis and pancreatic cancer. Med J Aust 10:793–796, 1977.
345. Takeuchi H, Konaga E, Tanemoto K, et al.: A case of chronic pancreatitis with pseudoaneurysm rupturing into a pseudocyst. Acta Medica Okayama 47:59–62, 1993.
346. Hofer BO, Ryan JA, Freeny PC: Surgical significance of vascular changes in chronic pancreatitis. Surg Gynecol Obstet 164:499–505, 1987.
347. Nishiyama T, Iwao N, Myose H, et al.: Splenic vein thrombosis as a consequence of chronic pancreatitis: A study of three cases. Am J Gastroenterol 12:1193–1198, 1986.
348. Fernandez E, La Vecchia C, Porta M, et al.: Pancreatitis and the risk of pancreatic cancer. Pancreas 11:185–189, 1995.
349. Ammann R, Munch R, Largiader F, et al.: Pancreatic and hepatic abscesses: A late complication in 10 patients with chronic pancreatitis. Gastroenterology 103:560–565, 1992.
350. Rao KN, Van Thiel DH: Pancreatic stone protein. What is it and what does it do? Dig Dis Sci 36:1505–1508, 1991.
351. Ammann RW, Muench R, Otto R, et al.: Evolution and regression of pancreatic calcification in chronic pancreatitis. A prospective long-term study of 107 patients. Gastroenterology 95:1018–1028, 1988.
352. Stroeken HJ, Koster BL: Ascites in benign disease of the pancreas. Arch Chir Neerland 28:293–297, 1976.
353. Athow AC, Wilkinson ML, Saunders AJ, et al.: Pancreatic ascites presenting-in infancy, with review of the literature. Dig Dis Sci 36:245–250, 1991.
354. Broe PJ, Cameron JL: Pancreatic ascites and pancreatic pleural effusion. *In* Bradley EL III (ed): Complications of pancreatitis. Philadelphia: WB Saunders, 1982, pp 245–264.
355. Sheehy TW, Holley HP: *Giardia*-induced malabsorption in pancreatitis. JAMA 233:1373–1375, 1975.
356. Roberts DM, Craft JC, Mather FJ, et al.: Prevalence of giardiasis in patients with cystic fibrosis. J Pediatr 112:555–559, 1988.
357. Lopez IJ, Wright JA, Hammer RA, et al.: Chronic pancreatitis is associated with a high prevalence of giardiasis. Can J Gastroenterol 6:73–76, 1992.

Chapter

6

CAUSES AND MOLECULAR BIOLOGY OF PANCREATIC CARCINOMA

The main factors implicated as causes of adenocarcinoma of the pancreas are listed in Table 6–1.

HEREDITY

Heredity plays an important role in pancreatic cancer causation and there is a growing list of familial disorders that predispose to this disease. Only 2.2% of patients in the Japanese pancreatic cancer registry gave a family history of pancreatic cancer, but 25.9% had a family history of other cancers.[1] Falk et al. found an odds ratio for developing pancreatic cancer of 5.25 for individuals who reported pancreatic cancer in a close relative and of 1.86 for those who reported any cancer in a close relative.[2] The relative risk for pancreatic cancer in those with a positive family history is 3.0 in northern Italy.[3–5] Ghadirian et al. interviewed 150 patients with pancreatic cancer and 150 controls and found a positive family history in 10 patients (6.7%) compared with 1 (0.7%) control.[6] Inherited predisposition may contribute to many cases; and Kern has written that "at least 20%, but possibly more than 50% of pancreatic cancers will involve inherited susceptibility."[7]

Pancreatic adenocarcinoma has been reported in family clusters[8–11] and, in their 18 kindreds, Lynch et al. found that the observed sex ratio, age of onset, histologic type, and survival were comparable to published data on unselected patients.[10,11] There are reported instances of pancreaticobiliary cancer in several hereditary conditions (Table 6–2), including familial adenomatous polyposis,[12] hereditary nonpolyposis colonic carcinoma (HNPCC), Lynch syndrome type 2,[9,10] Peutz–Jeghers syndrome,[13] juvenile polyposis coli, hereditary dysplastic nevus syndrome,[14,15] familial melanoma, *BRCA2* mutations,[16] and hereditary pancreatitis.[17,18]

HNPCC is due to germline mutations of genes that encode proteins that conduct DNA mismatch repair (*MSH2, MLH1, PMS1, PMS2, MSH6*). HNPCC is associated with cancers in many organs including the pancreas.[9,10] HNPCC tumors display microsatellite instability, and about 3% to 4% of pancreatic cancers also have this phenotype,[16] although what proportion of pancreatic cancers bear a germline mutation is not determined. The carcinomas of pancreas that show microsatellite instability have a distinctive morphology, characterized by a solid or syncytial growth pattern with pushing borders and a better prognosis than that of average pancreatic cancers. These characteristics are shared by some of the colonic tumors in patients with HNPCC.[18] Two cases of pancreatic carcinoma have been reported as components of the Muir–Torre syndrome,[19] a syndrome now recognized as a variant of HNPCC.[20,21]

A genetic defect that causes some cases of Peutz–Jeghers syndrome is in the *LKB1* gene on chromosome 19p13.[22–24] The encoded protein is serine threonine kinase 11 (*STK11*), a tumor suppressor. The defect in some cases of juvenile polyposis coli is either in the *PTEN* gene on chromosome 10q22-23,[25] in the *APC* gene,[26] or in the *SMAD4* gene.[27,28] The *PTEN*

Table 6–1. Causes and Risk Factors for Pancreatic Cancer

Hereditary factors
- Familial adenomatous polyposis
- Hereditary nonpolyposis colonic carcinoma
- Peutz–Jeghers syndrome and related conditions
- Hereditary dysplastic nevus syndrome
- Familial melanoma
- *BRCA2*
- Hereditary pancreatitis

Cigarette smoking
Diabetes mellitus
Chronic pancreatitis
Partial gastrectomy
Dietary habits
Alcohol use
Autoimmune disease
Work-related carcinogens

gene on 19q is also mutated in Bannayan–Zonana syndrome (Ruvalcaba–Myhre–Smith syndrome), Lhermitte–Duclos disease, and Cowden disease, constituting a link between these hamartomatous conditions.[29,30] Pancreatic cancer has been reported in Cowden disease[31,33] and in juvenile polyposis coli[33] in the kindred in whom the *SMAD4* defect was identified.[26,34] *SMAD4* is somatically mutated in more than 50% of pancreatic carcinomas (see below). It is a component in the signaling pathway of transforming growth factor-β (TGF-β), which suppresses mitosis.

The *BRCA2* mutations are considered to be present in the germline of 6% of pancreatic adenocarcinomas, indicating that the gene may account for a proportion of pancreatic tumors similar to that of breast and ovarian tumors.[35,36] There is a 5- to 10-fold increase in the risk of

Table 6–2. Hereditary Conditions Implicated in Some Cases of Pancreatic Cancer

Condition	Gene	Chromosome
Hereditary nonpolyposis colonic carcinoma	*MSH2*	2p16
	MLH1	3p21
	PMS1	2q31-33
	PMS2	7p22
	MSH6	
Peutz–Jeghers syndrome	*LKB1* (*STK11*)	19p13
Juvenile polyposis coli	*PTEN*	10q22-23
	SMAD4	18q
	FAP	
Bannayan–Zonana syndrome	*PTEN*	10q22-23
Cowden disease		
Familial breast–ovarian cancer	*BRCA2*	
Familial melanoma kindreds	*MTS-1, p16,*[INK4a] *CDKN2A*	9p21
Familial adenomatous polyposis	*FAP*	5p
Hereditary pancreatitis	Cationic trypsinogen	7q35

Genetic Alterations in Pancreatic Cancer

Accumulation of genetic alterations
Chromosomal losses (suppressor genes)
Chromosomal gains (oncogenes)
Point mutations, methylation or hypomethylation
DNA repair genes (caretakers)
Landscaper genes (tissue stroma)
One gene, one pathway; concordance of genetic defects suggests mutual advantage

Effects of Genetic Alterations

Uncontrolled cell proliferation
Abrogation of cell death
Genetic instability and aneuploidy
Altered signal transduction
Reduced cellular adhesion
Digestion of intercellular matrix
Increased cell mobility
Anchorage-independent proliferation

pancreatic cancer in carriers of *BRCA2* mutations.[36]

Melanoma-prone kindreds with *CDKN2* (*p*16, *MTS1, INK4*) mutations are at a 22-fold increased risk of pancreatic cancer[37,38] but still account for very few cases. The kinase inhibitor *p*16 is cyclin dependent and thus is a cell cycle regulator. It appears to be a crucial gatekeeper gene in the pathway to pancreatic cancer. In melanoma kindreds, mutation of *CDKN2* is responsible for about 50% of cases.

Redston has proposed the following criteria for use in clinical research to identify cases of familial pancreatic cancer[39]:

A. Familial pancreatic cancer syndrome (genetic basis not known): Two or more first-, second-, or third-degree relatives with confirmed pancreatic cancer
B. Early onset pancreatic cancer (genetic basis not known): Any individual with pancreatic cancer diagnosed before the age of 50 years, irrespective of family history
C. HNPCC (mismatch repair genes): Mount Sinai Hospital, Toronto, modifications of the Amsterdam criteria:
   i. Three or more relatives with cancer, at least one colorectal, and any gastrointestinal, endometrial, ovarian, or genitourinary cancer in the other two
   ii. Two of the three relatives with cancer are first-degree relatives
D. Familial melanoma (*CDKN2* gene): Two or more melanomas among first-, second-, or third-degree relatives
E. Multiple primary melanoma/pancreatic cancer (*CDKN2* gene): Any individual with both pancreatic cancer and melanoma
F. Breast ovarian syndrome (*BRCA2* gene, possibly *BRCA1* gene): Two or more first-, second-, or third-degree relatives with ovarian cancer at any age; or breast cancer at age 60 years or younger; or one or more male breast cancers

CIGARETTE SMOKING

Cigarette smoking is the main established environmental risk factor for pancreatic cancer, but the strength of the association is much less than for lung cancer. Eight prospective studies have shown a positive association of smoking with pancreatic cancer.[40] The mortality ratios for pancreatic cancer of smokers to nonsmokers in these studies ranged from 1.2 to 3.1.[40] Case-control studies have generally bolstered these findings, showing increased relative risk for current smokers ranging from 1.9 to 5.52, with the average being about 2.5 times the risk of a nonsmoker.[40–45] Most studies have shown a dose–response relationship.[40,41] Cancer of the pancreas also occurs as a second primary in patients who smoke, especially women.[46] One study strengthened the case for a causal link by showing both a dose–response relationship to smoking 15 years before diagnosis and a diminished risk in people who quit smoking.[47] The rapid reduction of risk associated with quitting smoking was confirmed by Fuchs et al.[44] The risk attributable to smoking in northern Italy is 14%.[5] In the United States, the proportion of pancreatic cancer attributable to smoking is about 25%.[43,44] Chewing tobacco is associated with a higher odds ratio (3.6) for pancreatic cancer than is smoking (2.1).[45] The risk to female smokers is comparable to that of male smokers.[45] A potential mechanism for carcinogenesis in the pancreas is mutation at codon 12 in K-*ras* induced by nitrosamines derived from smoke,[48] and activating mutations are more common in the cancers of smokers than in those of nonsmokers.[49] There is also an association between cigarette smoking and the presence of codon 12 K-*ras* mutations in nonneoplastic pancreas.[50]

DIABETES MELLITUS

Controversy persists as to whether there is any true causative association between carcinoma of the pancreas and diabetes mellitus. Several studies have shown an increased risk for pancreatic cancer only in patients with recent onset of diabetes in whom the diabetes could be a symptom of the developing cancer.[40] However, a study of Seventh Day Adventists found a relative risk (RR) of 3.4 for diabetes[51] and a follow-up study of 50,000 college students showed a RR of 6.0 for diabetes.[52,53] Another study found a twofold increase in risk among women with diabetes but not among men with diabetes.[54] Diabetes is present in 16.2% of Japanese patients with pancreatic cancer.[1]

CHRONIC PANCREATITIS

Chronic pancreatitis increases the risk of carcinoma by 5.7 to 15 times, according to several epidemiologic studies.[52,55,56] The risk of pancreatic cancer is appreciably higher 5 or more years after the diagnosis of pancreatitis than in the first 4 years.[3] Evidence of preexisting chronic pancreatitis was found in 5% of patients with pancreatic carcinoma at autopsy,[57] and 5% is the estimated risk attributable to pancreatitis.[3] In the Japanese pancreatic cancer registry, the incidence of chronic pancreatitis is 3%. Like diabetes, pancreatitis can result from cancer of the pancreas, and this confuses the issue. The likelihood that pancreatitis is a premalignant condition is supported by the occurrence of K-*ras* mutations in mucous hyperplasia of ductal epithelium in pancreatitis[58] and by microsatellite instability in pancreatic juice from 100% of patients with pancreatitis.[59] Hereditary pancreatitis predisposes to pancreatic carcinoma several decades after the onset of the pancreatitis.[56] The estimated cumulative risk of pancreatic cancer to age 70 in patients with hereditary pancreatitis is 40%; for patients with a paternal inheritance pattern, it is 75%.[56] However, hereditary pancreatitis accounts for only a small proportion of pancreatic carcinomas. In light of the recent implication of mutant cystic fibrosis transmembrane conductance regulator genes in the causation of chronic pancreatitis, it will be interesting to see whether an association is ultimately found between such genes and pancreatic carcinoma.

OTHER NUTRITIONAL FACTORS

Partial gastrectomy has been found to confer a threefold increase in risk of carcinoma of the pancreas in a study of autopsies.[60] The reasons for this finding are unclear.

Studies of the food habits of patients with pancreatic cancer suggest a role for diet both in causing the cancer and in protecting against it. A population-based case-control study found an increased risk of pancreatic cancer with a high consumption of salt (RR, 4.28), smoked meat (RR, 4.68), dehydrated food (RR, 3.1), fried food (RR, 3.84), and refined sugar (RR, 2.81).[6] Daily consumption of meat has been associated with a 2.5-fold increase in risk.[40] Several case-control studies show a protective effect of diets rich in fiber, raw fruits, and vegetables.[40,51] A number of studies have linked pancreatic cancer to fat consumption, particularly deep-fried foods, saturated fat, and cholesterol,[40] and diets rich in these agents tend to lack raw fruits and vegetables.[61] The attributable risk for high consumption of meat was 14%, and for low consumption of fruit, 12%.[5] Coffee consumption was briefly blamed when it emerged as a significant variable from the control wing of a study,[54] but after several other studies, the initial finding has been rejected, and coffee is generally accepted as not predisposing to pancreatic cancer.[62]

Alcohol is the main risk factor for chronic pancreatitis, and alcohol has also been suggested as an independent risk factor for pancreatic cancer. Alcohol consumption often goes along with smoking and studies that have controlled for the effect of tobacco have largely found no increased risk from alcohol per se.[40] Conversely, moderate wine consumption may have a protective effect against pancreatic cancer.[40]

A Chinese study of host immune function in patients with pancreatic cancer found a twofold increase in risk for prior autoimmune disease. By contrast, a history of allergy diminished the risk to an odds ratio of 0.6.[63] Several other studies have shown diminished risk with allergic disorders and asthma.[40]

ENVIRONMENTAL CARCINOGENS

There is no clear picture of work-related carcinogenesis in pancreatic cancer. A cluster of pancreatic cancer cases has been tentatively linked to oil refining and paper manufacture.[64] A Finnish study found increased risk for a small number of occupations and job titles, but no relationship to specific exposures was found.[65-] Another Finnish study found an elevated odds ratio for exposure to ionizing radiation (4.3), nonchlorinated solvents (1.6 to 1.8), and pesticides (1.7) but not to asbestos, chromates, cleaning agents, waxes, polishes, or other items.[66]

GENETIC ALTERATIONS AND MOLECULAR BIOLOGY

The main cellular disorder in carcinogenesis is the progressive accumulation of genetic alterations.[67,68] In addition to chromosomal losses and gains, the molecular changes in pancreatic carcinoma include mutations of genes in multiple pathways that lead to uncontrolled cell proliferation, abrogation of cell death, genetic instability, altered signal transduction, and reduced cellular adhesion. Potentially self-stimulating autocrine loops, whereby the tumor produces both growth factors and their receptors, may be important. Also, alterations to extracellular substances, such as matrix metalloproteases, may play a role in invasion and metastasis. Traditionally, the genes that feature in cancer causation are classified as oncogenes, or suppressor genes. Oncogenes are cancer-driving genes that may be activated after mutation of a single allele, in contrast to suppressor genes, which require loss of both copies to remove an obstacle to cell growth. When part of a chromosome that contains one allele of a suppressor gene is lost, a mere point mutation or methylation of the second allele can eliminate the function of the gene. DNA hypomethylation may also lead to enhanced rates of mutation, because methylation plays an important role in maintaining genome stability and the mutator phenotype can be produced by inactivation of methylating enzymes.[69]

Some of the genes involved in hereditary predisposition to cancer have been classified as *gatekeeper* genes, *caretaker* genes, *landscaper* genes, and *modifier* genes.[70–72] Gatekeeper genes directly control cell division in specific tissues, and loss of function of these genes leads to runaway growth. Examples are the retinoblastoma gene (p53), *VHL,* and the adenomatous polyposis coli gene. One defective copy is inherited or lost through chromosomal deletion and the second allele is lost through a random "second hit" resulting in deletion of function. In the pancreas, the multitumor suppressor gene (MTS, p16, *CDKN2*) is probably a gatekeeper, because it is inactivated in virtually all carcinomas.

Caretaker genes maintain the integrity of the genetic code by repairing DNA, and when one of these genes is inactivated, there is an increase in mutation rates, predisposing to cancer.[71] Thus, they are indirect tumor suppressor genes. Many of these defects are in so-called cancer families, some of which are now identified as HNPCC or breast cancer predisposing genes, such as *BRCA1* and *BRCA2.* Both HNPCC and *BRCA2* have been implicated in cases of pancreatic cancer.

Landscaper genes are thought to affect the stroma of epithelial cells, thus predisposing the epithelium to cancer. The stromal cells, but not the epithelial cells, contain clonal genetic alterations.[72] Landscaper genes include the genes for juvenile polyposis coli and Peutz–Jeghers syndrome. One gene that causes juvenile polyposis, *SMAD4,* is an important gene in pancreatic cancer.

Modifier genes—for example, those involved in metabolism of carcinogens—are the least understood and may be of considerable importance in cancer causation. They are not a defined "family" of genes; the best-defined members are those responsible for metabolism of xenobiotics, such as variants of cytochrome *P450,* or glutathione-*S*-transferase, both of which increase the risk of lung cancer in smokers.[73]

Chromosomal Abnormalities

Although a small proportion of cancers generate mutations through defective DNA repair (detected by microsatellite instability) and are usually euploid, most cancers are aneuploid and generation of aneuploidy seems to be an alternative more common mechanism driving carcinogenesis. The fractional allelic loss (FAL), or the proportion of chromosomal arms lost, is a predictor of tumor outcome in breast and colorectal carcinomas and there is evidence from one series that this is also the case with pancreatic carcinomas, where long survivals correlate with low FAL.[74] It is estimated that "chromosomal structural anomalies can account for two-thirds of the LOH [loss of heterozygosity] in pancreatic adenocarcinomas and that most homozygous deletions are likely to be interstitial chromosomal deletions, that are below the detection limits of conventional karyotypic analyses."[75] The first mutations of genes that control the mitotic checkpoint, which normally ensures even division of the chromatids at mitosis, have been described in colorectal cancer cell lines[76] and suggest that specific mutations in these genes may drive the acquisition of aneuploidy by tumors, increasing their malignancy through loss of tumor suppressor genes.

Karyotyping studies disclose frequent loss of chromosomes 18, 13, 12, 17, and 6; a gain of chromosomes 20 and 7; and frequent chromosome breakpoints, or other abnormalities of 1p, 3p, 11p, 17p, 1q, 6q, and 19q.[77–81] Comparative genomic hybridization on tumor biopsies reveals frequent gains of 7p, 8q, 5p, 5q, 11p, 11q, 12p, and 18q and losses of 18q, 18p, 6q, and 17p.[81] Additional changes are found in pancreatic cancer cell lines, but their relevance is questionable if not found in native tumors. There is a high frequency of structural rearrangements in chromosome 19, comprising a high frequency of 19p losses and 19q gains.[82] Ten percent of tumors display double-minute chromatin bodies, a cytogenetic manifestation of gene amplification.[79] Allelic losses (and the chromosomal losses cited above) often point to the location of suppressor genes that, if inactivated, release the cell from restraints on propagation. Such losses have been demonstrated at chromosomes 17p (90%), 18q (90%), 1p (67%), and 9p (80%). Alleles at 3p, 6p, 8p, 10q, 12q, 13q, 18p, 21q, and 22q are lost in 40% to 60% of tumors.[83] In a Japanese series, another common site for LOH was 6q.[84] Gene p53 is located on 17p and the MTS gene (MTS-1, p16) is on 9p. The number of other allelic losses suggests that several unrecognized pancreatic tumor suppressor genes are still awaiting discovery.

During carcinogenesis, the cells that acquire alterations of rate-limiting genes in regulatory pathways are positively selected. Mutation of one gene in a specific regulatory sequence obviates the need for a second gene mutation in that pathway. Looked at in another way, the coexistence of mutations in any two genes in a single tumor suggests that these genes are involved in different growth-regulatory pathways.[85] The concordance of specific genetic alterations may indicate that one confers a selective advantage on the other. For example, the concordance of *DPC4* (*SMAD4*) and *p16* (*MTS1*) inactivations ($p = 0.007$) suggests that the inactivation of *p16* increases the selective advantage of later mutation of *DPC4*.[85]

Among the techniques used to find genes that are overexpressed in cancer is cDNA representational difference analysis, which identified 16 cancer-specific genes, 5 recognized and 11 novel, in work from the University of Ulm.[86] One of these genes encoded a novel protein with four K-homologous (KH) domains. By fluorescent in situ hybridization, it was assigned to chromosome 7p11.5. The protein transcript has 580 aminoacids and a mass of 65 kd. The precise function of the protein is unknown, although other KH proteins are RNA-binding proteins and may play a role in transcription or translation of proteins.[87]

Oncogenes

Oncogenes encode proteins that positively promote cell proliferation. Chromosomal and allelic gains suggest the presence of oncogene(s) in the relevant portion of chromosome gained. Oncogenes can be activated by overexpression or by mutation of a single allele that results in a constitutionally activated protein. The picture is not as clearcut as this, however, because, under certain circumstances, they act as tumor suppressors. C-*myc,* in addition to its oncogenic function, also has proapoptotic activity.

Some specific carcinogens cause specific mutations in oncogenes, mutations that act as molecular fingerprints (e.g., K-*ras*). In addition to K-*ras,* the other oncogenes studied in pancreatic cancer include c-*erb*-B1, c-*erb*-B2, c-*erb*-B3, c-*met,* c-*myb,* and *AKT2.*

K-ras Oncogene

The oncogene most thoroughly studied in pancreatic carcinoma is K-*ras,* a member of a family of three *ras* oncogenes, Harvey (H), Kirsten (K), and N-*ras,* that are encoded on chromosome 12p12. K-*ras,* a 2kD guanine-nucleotide-binding protein that has guanosine triphosphatase (GTP-ase) activity, resides on the inner surface of the cell membrane and is involved in signal transduction, binding guanosine triphosphate (GTP) in its active state. It responds to growth factor receptors, such as insulin-like growth factor receptor-1, and it passes the signal to molecules, such as *ras* p21 protein, growth factor receptors, and the c-*raf* oncogene product. Paradoxically, normal expression of *ras* also tends to cause cell-cycle arrest mediated by $p14^{ARF}$, which activates p53 and by $p16^{INK4a}$, which activates RB.[88]

Activating mutations at codons 12, 13, or 61 occur in approximately 80% of pancreatic adenocarcinomas.[89–92] These mutations are more common in patients who smoked cigarettes (88%), than in those who never smoked (68%).[90] The codon 12 mutation, most often a G-to-A conversion at the second nucleotide of a GG pair, can be produced by nitrosamines,[93] which are present in cigarette smoke. This suggests that nitrosamines from cigarette smoke may account for some of the K-*ras* mutations in patients with pancreatic cancer who smoke and may explain the causative link between smoking and pancreatic cancer. Point mutations cause *ras* to remain in its active GTP-bound state, sending signals downstream continuously. Transfection of pancreatic cancer cell lines with a plasmid expressing an antisense K-*ras* gene caused growth suppression of those cell lines that had K-*ras* point mutations but not of those that retained the wild-type K-*ras*.[94] This suggests that cancer cells are dependent on a few crucial regulatory molecules, a weakness that could be exploited by innovative therapies. A novel group of pharmaceuticals, the farnesyltransferase inhibitors, prevent wild-type K-*ras* from binding to cell membrane and may prove useful as cancer chemotherapeutic agents or as prophylactic treatments if the mutant form retains the binding activity.[95]

As with colorectal adenomas, K-*ras* mutations occur early in the course of carcinogenesis in intraductal epithelial proliferations, both in humans and in the Syrian golden hamster model of pancreatic carcinoma.[89,96–100] Also, the rate of K-*ras* mutations is the same in early cancers as in advanced.[101] Mutations of K-*ras* were also found in 10 of 16 (62.5%) mucous cell hyperplasias collected from 10 pancreata resected for chronic pancreatitis.[102] Normal flat mucosa does not show mutations.[102] Immunohistochemical expression of K-*ras* was found in 3% of normal ducts, 30% of ductal papillary hyperplasias, 73% of ductal dysplasias, and 53% of cancers.[103] Initial studies suggested that the rate of mutations in K-*ras* was low in cases of intraductal papillary mucinous tumor, but later studies found a frequency ranging from 55% to 100%.[92]

In patients with pancreatic cancer, K-*ras* mutations have been demonstrated in pancreatic secretions, in fine-needle biopsy specimens,[104,105] in pancreatic juice,[106,107] in peripheral blood,[106] in stools,[108] and in duodenal fluid.[109] Studies on stool specimens show mutations not only in patients with invasive pancreatic cancer but also in patients with intraductal lesions. However, analysis of K-*ras* in stool as a potential screening test for early pancreatic cancer, or its precursor lesions, is unlikely to be useful because K-*ras* mutations were found in pancreatic juice in 2 of 5 cases of pancreatitis[110] and in 3 of 10 pancreata with benign conditions.[109]

Rho *Genes*

The *rho* genes are a *ras*-related small GTP-ase protein family that regulates cytoskeletal structures and has the potential to transform cultured cells. The expression levels of the *rho*C gene were significantly higher in pancreatic cancers than in nonmalignant tissue. There was no increase of *rho*A or B expression and no mutations of the genes.[111]

*c-*fos *and c-*jun *Oncogenes*

The product of c-*fos,* in combination with the related protein c-*jun,* forms a transcription factor called AP1 and has been reported to be overexpressed in a low proportion of pancreatic carcinomas.[112] Another report found c-*jun* expression to be increased in tumor cells in most carcinomas.[113]

*c-*erb*-B1, -2, and -3 Proto-oncogenes*

The c-*erb*-B1 proto-oncogene encodes epidermal growth factor receptor (EGFR), a 170-kd phosphoprotein, on the short arm of chromosome 7. EGFR can be activated not only by epidermal growth factor (EGF) but also by transforming growth factor-α (TGF-α), cripto, and amphiregulin. EGF is a polypeptide that stimulates epithelial growth and differentiation. Cripto is a protein that includes a region of homology to EGF and TGF-α.[114–116] When one of these ligands binds to EGFR, its tyrosine kinase activity is turned on and generates a signal that promotes cell division. EGFR is expressed in the normal endocrine pancreas but not in the normal exocrine pancreas. However, it is frequently overexpressed in well-differentiated adenocarcinomas by an increase in gene transcription.[117–119] TGF-α is also greatly overexpressed in 95% of pancreatic carcinomas; thus, pancreatic carcinoma cells generate both a growth factor and its receptor, making a potential autocrine loop that promotes cell division.[120,121] Furthermore, EGF is itself expressed in 12% of pancreatic cancers and may also stimulate that loop. Bockman et al. showed that TGF-α is abundant in nerves in the pancreas, whereas the adenocarcinoma expresses EGFR, suggesting that interaction of TGF-α in nerves with EGFR on cancer cells constitutes a possible paracrine mechanism that provides a growth advantage for pancreatic adenocarcinoma and may explain its propensity for perineural growth.[122]

The c-*erb*B2 (HER-2/*neu*) oncogene encodes a protein related to EGFR that is not expressed in normal ducts[103] but is overexpressed in between 20% and 80% of pancreatic adenocarcinomas by immunohistochemistry. Expression does not correlate with histologic grade.[123,124] It is also overexpressed in intraductal mucin-hypersecreting neoplasm of the pancreas in 76% of cases.[124] and in most premalignant duct lesions, including 55% of duct hyperplasias,[103] 82% of flat mucinous hyperplasias,[125] 67% of dysplasias, and 100% of carcinomas in situ.[125]

These data suggest that intraductal lesions, formerly designated hyperplasias, may in fact be dysplasias. Immunostaining showed the protein product of HER-2/*neu* in most well-differentiated or moderately differentiated areas of pancreatic carcinoma but in only 19% of poorly differentiated areas. Overall, 58% of cases showed moderate or strong HER-2/*neu* expression inclusive of all histologic grades, and 63 of 79 (80%) cases were positive if weak or focal staining was included.[126]

The *erb*-B3 protein was found on the cell membranes of 90% of pancreatic carcinomas by immunostaining. In 17 of 27 pancreatic cancers, there was a 6.7-fold increase ($p < 0.001$) in *erb*-B3 mRNA levels, but Southern blot analysis did not reveal *erb*-B3 gene amplification. Using a highly specific antibody, faint to moderate immunoreactivity was present in the ductal cells of normal pancreas. In 47% (27 of 58) of the pancreatic cancers, there were many cancer cells with intense *erb*-B3 immunostaining. The presence of *erb*-B3 in the cancer cells was associated with advanced tumor stage and shorter survival postoperatively.[114]

c-met *Proto-oncogene (Hepatocyte Growth Factor Receptor)*

The c-*met* proto-oncogene encodes a transmembrane tyrosine kinase, which is the receptor for hepatocyte growth factor (HGF) and has the ability to modulate cell proliferation and differentiation. It is activated by the HGF. In contrast to weak immunoreactivity in normal acinar and ductal cells, 14 of 16 ductal carcinomas showed intense immunoreactivity. Pancreatic cancers show a seven-fold increase in c-*met* mRNA levels and a 10-fold increase in hepatocyte growth factor mRNA.[127] This concomitant expression of a growth factor and its receptor suggests an autostimulatory loop that may contribute to pancreatic cancer cell growth.

c-myb *Proto-oncogene*

A high copy number amplification on 6q has been found in pancreatic cancer tissue, and two candidates, c-*myb* and a novel gene called eukaryotic release factor 3b (eRF3b), were shown to be amplified. The c-*myb* proto-oncogene was amplified in 10% of the pancreatic carcinoma tissues. The c-*myb* oncogene was overexpressed in the majority of pancreatic cancer tissues, however, indicating that other mechanisms of overexpression are active. The novel gene seems to be coamplified with c-*myb*.[128]

AKT2 *Oncogene*

An oncogene that encodes a protein serine-threonine kinase, *AKT2*, is amplified in some pancreatic ductal carcinoma cell lines, and 20% of ductal carcinomas display positive immunostaining for*AKT2*. This gene amplification on chromosome 19q tallies with the earlier finding of gene amplification involving the 16S gene on this same chromosomal arm.[129,130]

src

The *src* family of tyrosine kinases participate in the regulation of cell adhesion, cell growth, and differentiation. In all 13 pancreatic carcinomas examined by immunohistochemistry, *src* was overexpressed, and *src* protein expression was elevated in 14 of 17 carcinoma cell lines.[131]

Tumor Suppressor Genes

Tumor suppressor genes are genes from pathways that normally suppress tissue growth (mitosis) and that, when inactivated, permit excessive growth. Both copies must be inactivated to permit tumorigenesis. Chromosomal loss can abrogate one allele and the second may then be subject to random mutation or inactivation by methylation. The suppressor genes that have been studied in pancreatic cancer include p53, *SMAD4, MTS-1* (p16), *APC, Rb, FHIT,* and *MKK4.*

p53

The p53 protein, so called for its molecular weight, 53 kd, is encoded on chromosome 17p13 and is the gene that is most commonly mutated in cancer. It is a centrally important negative regulator of the cell cycle at stages G_1 and G_2 and an inducer of apoptosis. It controls entry to the G1/S boundary and, as such, is a tumor suppressor that is implicated in at least half of all human malignancies, including many cancers of the colorectum, breast, lung, liver, and pancreas.[132] The p53 protein also senses DNA damage and then redistributes cytoplasmic Fas to the cell surface to initiate apoptosis. Normally, p53 is maintained at low levels through interaction with Mdm-2, a protein that marks it for degradation. Mdm-2 is a target for DNA-dependent protein kinase, which mediates responses to DNA damage, and phosphorylation of either p53 or Mdm-2 prevents the two proteins from interacting, thus stabilizing and activating p53.[133] Mdm-2 can also be elevated in tumors leading to p53 inactivation. Mdm-2 is also a target for p19,[ARF] the protein encoded by the alternative reading frame in the *Ink4a* locus, which is often deleted in pancreatic cancer.

The loss of 17p in virtually all pancreatic cancers implies loss of one p53 allele. Gene sequencing reveals that 70% of all pancreatic cancers also have p53 gene mutations.[134] Most are missense point mutations within the evolutionarily conserved domains, but intragenic deletions account for 32% of mutations.[134] Mutated p53 is usually more stable than the wild-type molecule, accumulates in the cell, and is demonstrable by immunostaining,[135,136] but staining reveals nothing about function. Approximately half of all human pancreatic carcinomas overexpress p53 on immunostaining, and there is a positive correlation with tumor grade.[89,137,138] Levels of p53 mRNA may be increased without evidence for gene amplification,[138] and wild-type p53 can also be overexpressed.[139] There is some evidence that patients whose pancreatic cancers have p53 mutations may have shorter survival and that their tumors may have a higher histologic grade.[89,134,137]

The p53 protein is overexpressed in the nuclei of about 20% of intraductal epithelial dysplasias[89,103,140] but in 80% of carcinomas,[103] indicating that it is a late phenomenon in tumor progression. Restoration of wild-type p53 to a pancreatic carcinoma cell line (Panc 1) resulted in the induction of apoptosis and differentiation along neuroendocrine lines.[141] The antiproliferative activity of p53 is mediated by transcriptional regulation of p21,[WAF1] a cyclin-dependent kinase (CDK). Immunoreactivity of p21 is found in about 40% of pancreatic cancers.[142]

Another function of p53 is to guard the genome by inspecting DNA before it is copied; if the DNA is in disrepair, the cell is targeted for apoptosis. Loss of this function would promote tumor growth, too.

SMAD4 (DPC4) and Transforming Growth Factor-β

Ninety percent of pancreatic cancers display allelic loss at chromosome 18q, and a tumor suppressor gene was located in this region and called *DPC4* (***d****eleted in* ***p****ancreatic* ***c****arcinoma, locus 4*) or, more recently, *SMAD4.* The *SMAD4* gene is lost or mutated in 50% of pancreatic carcinomas. The *SMAD4* protein has homology to the fruit fly protein MAD, part of the TGF-β signaling pathway, and plays a role in inhibiting cell growth by interacting with p21waf1, which is a downstream target of *SMAD4.*[143–145] This pathway of inhibition of cell proliferation is an important negative control that is eliminated in pancreatic cancer. *SMAD* genes encode proteins that transduce signals from the TGF-β family of cytokines, which inhibit epithelial cell proliferation in vitro. Wild-type *SMAD4* mediates TGF-β–stimulated gene transcription at specific DNA sequences bound by *SMAD4* (*SMAD* binding element). Mutations within the NH2-terminal third of *SMAD4* weakened or ablated DNA binding and cells harboring *SMAD4* alterations had a universal impairment of the TGF-β–stimulated *SMAD* binding element transcriptional response.[145,146] This would tend to diminish apoptosis and promote cell survival. Two *SMAD* genes, *SMAD4* and *SMAD2,* are mutated in human tumors, but not the other four *SMAD* proteins recognized at the time of writing.[147] *SMAD2* and *SMAD4* are vital in early embryonic development, in the phase of gastrulation. *SMAD4* is not mutated in familial pancreatic carcinomas.

The discrepancy between the 90% frequency of chromosome 18 deletions and the 50% loss of *SMAD4* suggests that another pancreatic tumor suppressor may be concealed in this region. The *DCC* gene does reside in this area (18q21.3), but because of the length and complexity of the gene (29 exons spanning 1.4 megabases), its mutational status in pancreatic carcinomas is unknown, although absent or reduced expression of the gene was found in 8 of 11 pancreatic cell lines and 4 of 8 primary tumors.[148] TGF-βs inhibit cell proliferation by regulating the levels and activities of G_1 cyclins and CDKs. Positive immunohistochemistry for transforming growth factor-β_1 (TGF-β_1) is found in one third of pancreatic cancers and identifies low-grade tumors and patients with better survival, according to some authors,[142] but the opposite is true, according to others.[149,150] *SMAD2* was found by immunohistochemistry in the cancer cells of 67% of pancreatic cancers and was coexpressed with TGF-β_1 in those cells.[151] Positive immunostaining for TGF-β receptor types I and II was found in 73% and 56% of tumors, both being present concomitantly in 54%. Positivity for either or both was associated with advanced tumor stage.[152]

Multiple Tumor Suppressor-1 (*MTS-1*, *p16^{INK4a}*, *CDKN2A*) and Retinoblastoma

The multiple tumor suppressor-1 gene (*MTS-1, p16*^{INK4a}, *CDKN2A*), which is encoded on chromosome 9p21, is inactivated in virtually all pancreatic cancers.[153,154] The product of this gene inhibits cdk4 and cdk6, two protein kinases that drive G_1 progression and phosphorylate and inactivate the retinoblastoma protein. Unphosphorylated retinoblastoma protein blocks the G_1–S transition at the G_1 checkpoint, the point at which the commitment to complete the cell cycle is made. Thus, dysfunctional *MTS-1* promotes cell division. Allelic deletions of 9p21-22 occur in 85% of pancreatic carcinomas. Many tumor types inactivate *p16* through homozygous deletions, and this is one of the most common tumor mutations. Homozygous deletions of this gene are found in approximately 40% of pancreatic cancers, sequence changes in 38%, and gene silencing by methylation in virtually all of the remaining cases.[153–155] Of great interest is that this gene is lost in early pancreatic intraductal lesions, often due to hypermethylation of the promotor region,[155] a genetic change that occurs early in many gastrointestinal cancers. The *p15*^{INK4b}/*MTS-2* gene is tandemly linked to *p16/MTS-1* and is usually codeleted with it but is not subject to mutations.[157] Other members of the family of CDK inhibitors are p18^{INK4c} and p19^{INK4d}. By immunostaining, 42% of pancreatic carcinomas have lost p16 expression, and this loss is associated with higher tumor grade.[157]

Within the *Ink4a* gene is an alternative reading frame that encodes a protein p14^{ARF} (the mouse homologue is called p19^{ARF}), which binds to the p53-MDM2 complex and prevents p53 degradation. The p14^{ARF} protein is expressed in response to the transcription factor E2F-1, which is itself activated when Rb is lost. This pathway links the tumor suppressors Rb and p53.[159] In addition, p14^{ARF} is essential for the activation of p53 in response to *ras*.[88]

As alluded to above, families with the atypical mole/melanoma hereditary trait carry a germline mutation of the *p16* gene and are also susceptible to pancreatic cancer.[38] This syndrome should be suspected when pancreatic cancer and melanoma coexist in a pedigree but probably accounts for less than 5% of familial pancreatic cancers and a very small proportion of all pancreatic cancers.[160]

Retinoblastoma Gene

The retinoblastoma (Rb) gene is encoded on 13q14, an area where there is LOH in 50% of pancreatic cancers,[143] and the Rb–p16^{INK4a} tumor suppressive pathway plays a central role in the development of pancreatic carcinomas. The Rb–p16^{INK4a} pathway is abrogated in 49 of 50 carcinomas, all through inactivation of the p16^{INK4a} gene.[161] The mechanisms include intragenic mutations, in nearly half the cases, and homozygous deletion of the gene or methylation of the 5′-CpG island of the wild-type gene in the remainder. Immunostaining reveals normal expression levels of the Rb protein in all carcinomas studied.[143,161–163] Mutations of the p16^{INK4a} gene are found in the intraductal lesions of pancreatic carcinomas in three of four cases where mutations are also present in the invasive tumor but are not demonstrated in intraductal lesions of pancreata having wild-type p16^{INK4a}.[164]

Most human cancers display abrogation of both the p53 and the Rb pathways of cell cycle inhibition. Loss of Rb function leads to overactivity of the E2F transcription factors and abnormal growth but also to activation of p53, which tends to suppress growth. E2F-1 directly activates expression of the human tumor suppressor protein p14,^{ARF} which binds to the MDM2-p53 complex and prevents p53 degradation.[159] This linkage of the p53 and Rb pathways appears to be a fail-safe mechanism to arrest the cell cycle or induce apoptosis. Oncogenic *ras* elicits an antiproliferative response mediated by upregulation of p14^{ARF} and p16,^{INK4a} which in turn activate the tumor suppressors p53 and Rb, respectively.[88] Thus, inactivation of both p53 and Rb pathways leaves the way open for unopposed oncogenic stimulation of growth.

p27Kip1

Like p16, p27-Kip1 is a universal inhibitor of CDKs in mammalian cells. Immunohistochemical staining showed that about half of all cases lose p27Kip1 staining, and this loss correlates strongly with poor survival.[165]

APC

It is controversial whether the adenomatous polyposis coli (*APC*) gene plays any appreciable role in pancreatic carcinogenesis. *APC,* encoded on chromosome 5p, is mutated in the germline of individuals with familial adenomatosis polyposis, and these individuals sometimes develop pancreatic carcinoma. Cytogenetic studies of cases of pancreatic cancer reveal no abnormality of chromosome 5 and neither allelic loss of 5q nor truncated *APC* protein.[166] However, other studies have been at variance with each of these results and have described point mutations in 40% of pancreatic cancers in Japanese patients.[167,168]

FHIT

The *FHIT* gene may be a target tumor suppressor gene in pancreatic cancer. *FHIT* is localized on chromosome 3p14. *FHIT* transcript is lost in 70% of pancreatic carcinoma cell lines, whereas 66% also revealed intragenic homozygous deletions of exons 3, 4, and 5.[169]

MAPKK4

Mitogen-activated protein kinase kinase 4 (*MAPKK4*) is one of a family of kinases that act in signal transduction pathways. Homozygous deletions have been found in two carcinoma cell lines, one pancreatic cancer and one lung cancer, that eliminate coding portions of the *MAPKK4* locus at 17p. In addition, in 88 cancer cell lines prescreened for LOH, two nonsense and three missense mutations were found. These findings suggest that *MAPKK4* may be a tumor suppressor gene.[170]

PTEN/MAC1

The *PTEN/MAC1* candidate tumor suppressor gene, which is encoded at chromosome 10q23, is mutated in the germ line of patients with Cowden disease, Ruvalcaba–Myhre–Smith syndrome, and some families with hereditary juvenile polyposis. It may be involved in pancreatic cancer, as microsatellite analysis showed LOH at markers near the gene in 39% of pancreatic cancers.[171] However, a search of the entire coding region in 8 pancreatic and (170 other) cancers proved negative.[172] *PTEN* is a dual-specificity phosphatase that is essential for embryonic development, and knockout mice studies show that homozygous deficiency is lethal to the early embryo, whereas heterozygosity is associated with hyperplastic/dysplastic changes in several organs.[173] *PTEN* inactivation enhanced the ability of embryonic stem cells to generate tumors in nude and syngeneic mice, owing to increased anchorage-independent growth and aberrant differentiation, supporting the notion that *PTEN* is a tumor suppressor.[173]

p27

The CDK inhibitor p27 has been shown to be upregulated by 24 hours of treatment with 1,25-dihydroxyvitamin D3 and 22-oxa-1,25-dihydroxyvitamin D3. The opposite effect was seen after 7 days. The early effect could block the G_1–S transition and produce growth inhibition.[174]

Other Genetic Results

Microsatellite instability, the manifestation of the replication error phenotype of HNPCC, has been found in pancreatic juice from pancreatitis patients more often than from carcinoma patients, a finding that may be interpreted as saturation of an intact mismatch repair system in pancreatitis.[110] Han et al.[175] found genetic instability in six of nine pancreatic cancers, by looking at four microsatellite loci, but Seymour et al.[166] did not confirm this, and Hahn et al.[143] found widespread microsatellite instability of the type seen with the mutator phenotype of HNPCC in only 1 of 18 patients. Thus, the role of the replication error phenotype in pancreatic cancer is not fully elucidated but does not appear to be a major one.

The arginine-rich protein gene on 3p21.1 shows mutations of codon 50 in 11 of 37 pancreatic carcinomas.[176] Urokinase plasminogen activator, a serine protease that may play a role in cancer invasion and metastasis, is increased in pancreatic cancer, both by immunocytochemistry and Northern blot analysis.[177] It binds to a specific membrane receptor, which activates plasminogen to plasmin. When both urokinase plasminogen activator and its receptor were overexpressed, the patients had a shorter survival than did those patients in whom one or neither was overexpressed.[177]

A new tumor-associated antigen, M4SF5, which has the structure of a transmembrane protein, is overexpressed in pancreatic cancers, as compared with normal pancreas and pancreatitis tissue. It is encoded on chromosome 19p13.3 and bears strong homology with the L6 antigen; its function is unknown.[178,179]

The guanine-nucleoside exchange factor, Mss4, is overexpressed in pancreatic cancer tissue, compared with both normal pancreas and pancreatitis. Mss4 is required in the regulation of intracellular transport, but its precise role in the function and growth of human tumor cells is unknown.[180]

Increased telomerase activity may be demonstrated in 32 (84%) of 38 pancreatic carcinomas and may prove to be a genetic diagnostic marker or a target for future therapy.[181]

A pancreatic cancer cell line has been developed and shown to be dependent on autocrine stimulation by interleukin-1α (IL-1α). Its growth was inhibited by antibody to IL-1α.[182] This cell line secreted large amounts of IL-1α, interleukin-6 and interleukin-8 into the culture medium.

The cyclin D1 gene is amplified in 25% of adenocarcinomas of the pancreas and overexpression of mRNA is observed in 82% of cases. Immunostaining shows nuclear protein expression in 68%, and this protein accumulation correlates significantly with a poor prognosis.[183]

By comparison with normal pancreas and chronic pancreatitis, heat shock protein 89-α (HSP 89-α) is found to be selectively overexpressed in pancreatic carcinoma.[184] HSP 89-β and ubiquitin are constitutively expressed at all levels in all three tissues. Steady-state levels of HSP 70 mRNA are increased in pancreatic carcinoma and in chronic pancreatitis. Thus, these proteins are differentially expressed in cancer and HSP 89-α has some cancer specificity.[184]

APOPTOSIS

Progression of the cell cycle, control of apoptosis, and maintenance of euploidy are intimately linked processes with common controlling proteins. An inhibitor of apoptosis, survivin, is expressed in the G_2–M phase of the cell cycle in a cycle-regulated manner.[185] At the beginning of mitosis, survivin binds to the microtubules of the mitotic spindle, and if this interaction is disrupted, the antiapoptotic function of survivin is lost and caspase-3 is activated.[185] Survivin is overexpressed in pancreatic and many other cancers.[186] The *bcl-2* oncogene acts as an antiapoptotic influence and prolongs cell survival, but the *bax* gene promotes apoptosis. Both show overexpression of mRNA in pancreatic cancers and immunostaining is positive in 28% and 83% of cancers, respectively. Positive immunostaining for *bax* is associated with longer survival.[187]

Pancreatic cancers may evade apoptosis by making nonfunctional Fas receptors, or the aberrant expression of functional Fas ligands may allow them to counterattack T cells.[188]

MATRIX METALLOPROTEASES AND THEIR INHIBITORS

Invasion of carcinomas is believed to depend on their ability to digest the extracellular matrix and to produce a desmoplastic reaction. Therefore, there is great interest in the balance between these proteases and their inhibitors in pancreatic cancers. Matrix metalloprotease 2 (MMP2) is overexpressed, whereas tissue inhibitor of metalloprotease 2 (TIMP2) is underexpressed, changes that may contribute to invasion and metastasis.[189] MMP2 and its activator, membrane-type matrix metalloprotease (MT1-MMP), are highly overexpressed in pancreatic cancer and seem to be related to the desmoplastic reaction.[190] Serum levels of TIMP1 are elevated in pancreatic carcinoma.[191] Another gene overexpressed in pancreatic cancers encodes a novel putative transmembrane protein with two Kunitz-type serine protease inhibitor domains and has been named *kop* (***K***unitz domain containing protein ***o***verexpressed in ***p***ancreatic cancer).[179] It is assigned to chromosome 19q13.1. It is postulated that this protein may play a role in invasion and metastasis and possibly in creation of a desmoplastic reaction. Stromelysin 3 is overexpressed in the stromal cells of 80% of pancreatic adenocarcinomas and in the carcinoma cells of 30% and is inhibited by retinoids.[192]

Expression of plasminogen activators and their inhibitors have been examined immunohistochemically in 97 pancreatic carcinomas. Urokinase-type plasminogen activator was expressed in 76 specimens (78.4) and tissue-type plasminogen activator in 8 specimens (8.2%). Plasminogen activator inhibitor type 1 (PAI-1) expression was detected in 80 carcinoma specimens (82.5%) and plasminogen activator inhibitor type 2 (PAI-2) in 79 carcinoma specimens (81.4%). PAI-2 expression was significantly lower in carcinomas with peritoneal metastasis ($p < 0.02$). Strong PAI-2 expression was associated with significantly higher survival than negative or weak PAI-2 expression ($p < 0.05$).[193]

ANGIOGENESIS AND TUMOR STROMA

Vascular endothelial growth factor, an angiogenic polypeptide, is expressed in the tissue of 64% of pancreatic cancers and was correlated with increased blood vessel number, larger tumor size, and local progression.[194]

MECHANISMS OF CARCINOGENESIS

Little is known about the interaction of environmental carcinogens with pancreatic ductal cells. It has been proposed that the exocrine pancreas might concentrate carcinogens from the blood and thus expose the ductal cells to high concentrations or, alternately, that the ductal cells themselves might convert precursor molecules to carcinogens.[195] The suggestion that bile reflux might play a role is supported only by weak evidence at this time. Cyclooxygenase-2 is overexpressed in between one half and two thirds of pancreatic cancers and this suggests that nonsteroidal anti-inflammatory drugs may be useful in chemoprevention or therapy for this cancer.[196,197] Aberrant E-cadherin expression was found in 42% of pancreatic cancers and it was positively correlated with poor differentiation, lymph node involvement, distant metastases, and advanced tumor stage.[198]

REFERENCES

1. Yamamoto M, Ohashi O, Saitoh Y: Japan pancreatic cancer registry: Current status. Pancreas 16:238–242, 1998.
2. Falk RT, Pickle LW, Fontham ET, et al.: Life-style risk factors for pancreatic cancer in Louisiana: A case-control study. Am J Epidemiol 128:324–336, 1988.
3. Fernandez E, La Vecchia C, Porta M, et al.: Pancreatitis and the risk of pancreatic cancer. Pancreas 11:185–189, 1995.
4. Fernandez E, La Vecchia C, D'Avanzo B, et al.: Family history and the risk of liver, gallbladder, and pancreatic cancer. Cancer Epidemiol Biomarkers Prev 3:209–212, 1994.
5. Fernandez E, La Vecchia C, Dicarli A: Attributable risks for pancreatic cancer in northern Italy. Cancer Epidemiol Biomarkers Prev 5:23–27, 1996.
6. Ghadirian P, Baillargeon J, Simard A, et al.: Food habits and pancreatic cancer: A case-control study of the Francophone community in Montreal, Canada. Cancer Epidemiol Biomarkers Prev 4:895–899, 1995.
7. Kern SE: Advances from genetic clues in pancreatic cancer. Curr Opinion Oncol 10:74–80, 1998.
8. Ehrenthal D, Haeger L, Griffin T, et al.: Familial pancreatic adenocarcinoma in three generations. A case report and a review of the literature. Cancer 59:1661–1664, 1987.
9. Lynch HT, Voorhees GJ, Lanspa SJ, et al.: Pancreatic carcinoma and hereditary nonpolyposis colorectal cancer: A family study. Br J Cancer 52:271–273, 1985.
10. Lynch HT, Smyrk T, Kern SE, et al.: Familial pancreatic cancer: A review. Semin Oncol 23:251–275, 1996.
11. Lynch HT, Fitzsimmons ML, Smyrk TC, et al.: Familial pancreatic cancer: Clinicopathologic study of 18 nuclear families. Am J Gastroenterol 85:54–60, 1990.
12. Jagelman DG: Extracolonic manifestations of familial polyposis coli. Cancer Genet Cytogenet 27:319–325, 1987.
13. Bowlby LS: Pancreatic adenocarcinoma in an adolescent male with Peutz–Jeghers syndrome. Hum Pathol 17:97–99, 1986.
14. Lynch HT, Fusaro L, Lynch JF: Familial pancreatic cancer: A family study. Pancreas 7:511–515, 1992.
15. Lynch HT, Fusaro RM: Pancreatic cancer and the familial atypical multiple mole melanoma (FAMMM) syndrome. Pancreas 6:127–131, 1991.
16. Goggins M, Offerhaus GJ, Hilgers W, et al.: Pancreatic adenocarcinomas with DNA replication errors (RER+) are associated with wild-type K-*ras* and characteristic histopathology. Am J Pathol 152:1501–1507, 1998.
17. Davidson P, Costanza D, Sweiconer JA, et al.: Hereditary pancreatitis: A kindred without gross aminoaciduria. Ann Intern Med 68:88–96, 1983.
18. Bartholomew LG, Gross JB, Comfort MW: Carcinoma of the pancreas associated with chronic relapsing pancreatitis. Gastroenterology 35:473–477, 1958.
19. Cohen PR, Kohn SR, Kurzrock R: Association of sebaceous gland tumors and internal malignancy: The Muir–Torre syndrome. Am J Med 90:606–613, 1991.
20. Kruse R, Lamberti C, Wang Y, et al.: Is the mismatch repair deficient type of Muir–Torre syndrome confined to mutations in the h*MSH2* gene? Hum Genet 98:747–750, 1996.
21. Suspiro A, Fidalgo P, Cravo M, et al.: The Muir–Torre syndrome: A rare variant of hereditary nonpolyposis colorectal cancer associated with h*MSH2* mutation. Am J Gastroenterol 93:1572–1574, 1998.
22. Hemminki A, Markle D, Tomlinson I, et al.: A serine/threonine kinase gene defective in Peutz-Jeghers syndrome. Nature 391:184–187, 1998.
23. Ylikorkala A, Avizienyte E, Tomlinson IPM, et al.: Mutations and impaired function of *LKB1* in familial and non-familial Peutz–Jeghers syndrome and a sporadic testicular cancer. Hum Mol Genet 8:45–51, 1999.
24. Nagakawa H, Koyama K, Miyoshi Y, et al.: Nine novel germline mutations of *STK11* in ten families with Peutz–Jeghers syndrome. Hum Genet 103:168–172, 1998.
25. Olschwang S, Serov-Sinilnikova OM, Lenoir GM, et al.: *PTEN* germ-line mutations in juvenile polyposis coli. Nature Genetics 18:12–14, 1998.
26. Kim JC, Roh SA, Kim HC, et al.: Somatic mutations of the first 14 exons of APC in hamartomatous polyps of the colon. Hum Mutat 14:351–352, 1999.
27. Howe JR, Roth S, Ringold JC, et al.: Mutations in the *SMAD4/DPC4* gene in juvenile polyposis. Science 280:1086–1088, 1998.

28. Houlston R, Bevan S, Williams A, et al.: Mutations in *DPC4* (*SMAD4*) cause juvenile polyposis syndrome, but only account for a minority of cases. Hum Mol Genet 7:1907–1912, 1998.
29. Marsh DJ, Dahia PLM, Zheng Z, et al.: Germline mutations in *PTEN* are present in Bannayan–Zonana syndrome. Nature Genetics 16:333–334, 1997.
30. Zigman AF, Lavine JE, Jones MC, et al.: Localization of the Bannayan–Riley–Ruvalcaba syndrome gene to chromosome 10q23. Gastroenterology 113:1433–1437, 1997.
31. Desai DC, Neale KF, Talbot IC, et al.: Juvenile polyposis. Br J Surg 82:14–17, 1995.
32. Walpole IR, Cullity G: Juvenile polyposis: A case with early presentation and death attributable to adenocarcinoma of the pancreas. Am J Med Genet 32:1–8, 1989.
33. Stemper TJ, Kent TH, Summers RW: Juvenile polyposis and gastrointestinal carcinoma. A study of a kindred. Ann Intern Med 83:639–646, 1975.
34. Howe JR, Ringold JC, Hughes JH, et al.: Direct genetic testing for *SMAD4* mutations in patients at risk for juvenile polyposis. Surgery 126:162–170, 1999.
35. Goggins M, Schutte M, Lu J, et al.: Germline *BRCA2* gene mutations in patients with apparently sporadic pancreatic carcinomas. Cancer Res 56:5360–5364, 1996.
36. Ozcelik H, Schmockler B, Di Nicola N, et al.: Germline *BRCA2* 6174delT mutations in Ashkenazi Jewish pancreatic cancer patients. Nat Genet 16:17–18, 1997.
37. Whelan AJ, Bartsch D, Goodfellow J: A familial syndrome of pancreatic cancer and melanoma with a mutation in the *CDKN2* tumor suppressor gene. N Engl J Med 333:975–977, 1995.
38. Goldstein AM, Fraser MC, Struewing JP, et al.: Increased risk of pancreatic cancer in melanoma-prone kindreds with *p16* mutations. N Engl J Med 333:970–974, 1995.
39. Redston M: Inherited predisposition to pancreatic cancer. Current Oncology 5:S12–S16, 1998.
40. Gold EB: Epidemiology of and risk factors for pancreatic cancer. Surg Clin North Am 75:819–843, 1995.
41. Wynder EL: An epidemiological evaluation of the causes of cancer of the pancreas. Cancer Res 35:2228–2233, 1975.
42. Wynder EL, Hall NE, Polansky M: Epidemiology of coffee and pancreatic cancer. Cancer Res 43:3900–3906, 1983.
43. Silverman DT, Dunn JA, Hoover RN, et al.: Cigarette smoking and pancreas cancer: A case-control study based on direct interviews. J Nat Cancer Inst 86:1510–1516, 1994.
44. Fuchs CS, Colditz GA, Stampfer MJ, et al.: A prospective study of cigarette smoking and the risk of pancreatic cancer. Arch Intern Med 156:2255–2260, 1996.
45. Muscat JE, Stellman SD, Hoffman D, et al.: Smoking and pancreatic cancer in men and women. Cancer Epidemiol Biomarkers Prev 6:15–19, 1997.
46. Neugut AI, Ahsan H, Robinson E: Pancreas cancer as a second primary malignancy. A population-based study. Cancer 76:589–592, 1995.
47. Howe GR, Jain M, Burch JD, et al.: Cigarette smoking and cancer of the pancreas: Evidence from a population-based case-control study in Toronto, Canada. Int J Cancer 47:323–328, 1991.
48. Topal MD: DNA repair, oncogenes and carcinogenesis. Carcinogenesis 9:691–696, 1988.
49. Hruban RH, Van Mansfeld ADM, Offerhaus JGA, et al.: K-*ras* oncogene activation in adenocarcinoma of the human pancreas: A study of 82 carcinomas using a combination of mutant-enriched polymerase chain reaction analysis and allele-specific oligonucleotide hybridization. Am J Pathol 143:545–554, 1993.
50. Berger DH, Chang H, Wood M, et al.: Mutational activation of K-*ras* in nonneoplastic exocrine pancreatic lesions in relation to cigarette smoking status. Cancer 85:326–332, 1999.
51. Mills PK, Beeson WL, Abbey DE, et al.: Dietary habits and past medical history as related to past fatal pancreas cancer risk among Adventists. Cancer 61:2578–2585, 1988.
52. Whittemore AS, Paffenbarger RS, Anderson K, et al.: Early precursors of site-specific cancers in college men and women. J Natl Cancer Inst 74:43–51, 1985.
53. Whittemore AS, Paffenbarger RS, Anderson K, et al.: Early precursors of pancreatic cancer in college men. J Chronic Dis 36:251–256, 1983.
54. MacMahon B, Yen S, Trichopoulos D, et al.: Coffee and cancer of the pancreas. N Engl J Med 304:630–633, 1981.
55. Lowenfels AB, Maisonneuve P, Cavallini G, et al.: Pancreatitis and the risk of pancreatic cancer. N Engl J Med 328:1433–1437, 1993.
56. Lowenfels AB, Maisonneuve P, DiMagno EP, et al.: Hereditary pancreatitis and the risk of pancreatic cancer. J Natl Cancer Inst 89:442–446, 1997.
57. Mao C, Domenico DR, Kim K, et al.: Observations on the developmental patterns and the consequences of pancreatic exocrine adenocarcinoma. Findings of 154 autopsies. Arch Surg 130:125–134, 1995.
58. Yanagisawa A, Ohtake K, Ohashi K, et al.: Frequent c-Ki-*ras* oncogene activation in mucous cell hyperplasias of pancreas suffering from chronic inflammation. Cancer Res 53:953–956, 1993.
59. Brentnall TA, Chen R, Lee JG, et al.: Microsatellite instability and K-*ras* mutations associated with pancreatic adenocarcinoma and pancreatitis. Cancer Res 55:4264–4267, 1995.
60. Offerhaus GJ, Giardiello FM, Moore GW, et al.: Partial gastrectomy: A risk factor for carcinoma of the pancreas? Hum Pathol 18:285–288, 1987.
61. Howe GR, Ghadirian P, Bueno de Mesquita HB, et al.: A collaborative case-control study of nutrient intake and pancreatic cancer within the search program. Int J Cancer 51:365–372, 1992.
62. Fontham ET, Correa P: Epidemiology of pancreatic cancer. Surg Clin North Am 69:551–567, 1989.
63. Dai Q, Zheng W, Ji BT, et al.: Prior immunity-related medical conditions and pancreatic cancer risk in Shanghai. Int J Cancer 63:337–340, 1995.
64. Pickle LW, Gottleib MS: Pancreatic cancer mortality in Louisiana. Am J Public Health 70:256–259, 1980.
65. Partanen T, Kauppinen T, Degerth R, et al.: Pancreatic cancer in industrial branches and occupations in Finland. Am J Ind Med 25:851–866, 1994.
66. Kauppinen T, Partanen T, Degerth R, et al.: Pancreatic cancer and occupational exposures. Epidemiology 6:498–502, 1995.
67. Fearon ER, Vogelstein B: A genetic model for colorectal tumorigenesis. Cell 61:759–767, 1990.
68. DiGiuseppe JA, Yeo CJ, Hruban RH: Review article. Molecular biology and the diagnosis and treatment of adenocarcinoma of the pancreas. Adv Anat Pathol 3:139–155, 1996.
69. Chen RZ, Petterson U, Beard C, et al.: DNA hypomethylation leads to elevated mutation rates. Nature 395:89–93, 1998.

70. Kinzler KW, Vogelstein B: Lessons from hereditary colorectal cancer. Cell 87:159–170, 1996.
71. Kinzler KW, Vogelstein B: Gatekeepers and caretakers. Nature 386:762–763, 1997.
72. Kinzler KW, Vogelstein B: Landscaping the cancer terrain. Science 280:1036–1037, 1998.
73. Hirvonen A: Genetic factors in individual responses to environmental exposures. J Occup Environ Med 1:37–43, 1995.
74. Seymour AB, Hruban RH, Redston M, et al.: Allelotype of pancreatic adenocarcinoma. Cancer Res 54:2761–2764, 1994.
75. Brat DJ, Hahn SA, Griffin CA, et al.: The structural basis of molecular genetic deletions. An integration of classical cytogenetic and molecular analyses in pancreatic adenocarcinoma. Am J Pathol 150:383–391, 1997.
76. Cahill DP, Lengauer C, Yu J, et al.: Mutations of mitotic checkpoint genes in human cancers. Nature 392:300–303, 1998.
77. Johansson B, Bardi G, Heim S, et al.: Non-random chromosomal re-arrangements in pancreatic carcinomas. Cancer 69:1674–1681, 1992.
78. Griffin CA, Hruban RH, Long PP, et al.: Chromosome abnormalities in pancreatic adenocarcinoma. Genes Chromosomes Cancer 9:93–100, 1994.
79. Griffin CA, Hruban RH, Morsberger LA, et al.: Consistent chromosome abnormalities in adenocarcinoma of the pancreas. Cancer Res 55:2394–2399, 1995.
80. Fukushige S, Waldman FM, Kimura M, et al.: Frequent gain of copy number on the long arm of chromosome 20 in human pancreatic adenocarcinoma. Genes Chromosomes Cancer 19:161–169, 1997.
81. Mahlamaki EH, Hoglund M, Gorunova L, et al.: Comparative genomic hybridization reveals frequent gains of 20q, 8q, 11q, 12p, and 17q, and losses of 18q, 9p, and 15q in pancreatic cancer. Genes Chromosomes Cancer 20:383–391, 1997.
82. Hoglund M, Gorunova L, Andren-Sandberg A, et al.: Cytogenetic and fluorescence in situ hybridization analyses of chromosome 19 aberrations in pancreatic carcinomas: Frequent loss of 19p13.3 and gain of 19q13.1-13.2. Genes Chromosomes Cancer 1998;21:8–16, 1998.
83. Hahn SA, Seymour AB, Hoque ATMS, et al.: Allelotype of pancreatic cancer using a xenograft model. Cancer Res 55:4670–4675, 1995.
84. Kimura M, Abe T, Sunamura M, et al.: Detailed deletion mapping on chromosome arm 12q in human pancreatic adenocarcinoma: Identification of a I-cM region of common allelic loss. Genes Chromosomes Cancer 17:88–93, 1996.
85. Rozenblum E, Schutte M, Goggins M, et al.: Tumor-suppressive pathways in pancreatic cancer. Cancer Res 57:1731–1734, 1997.
86. Gress TM, Wallrapp C, Frohme M, et al.: Identification of genes with specific expression in pancreatic cancer by cDNA representational difference analysis. Genes Chromosomes Cancer 19:97–103, 1997.
87. Mueller-Pillasch F, Lacher U, Wallrapp C, et al.: Cloning of a gene highly overexpressed in cancer coding for a novel KH-domain containing protein. Oncogene 14:2729–2733, 1997.
88. Palmero I, Pantoja C, Serrano M: p19^{ARF} links the tumour suppressor p53 to *ras*. Nature 395:125–126, 1998.
89. DiGiuseppe JA, Hruban RH, Goodman SN, et al.: Overexpression of p53 protein in adenocarcinoma of the pancreas. Am J Clin Pathol 101:684–688, 1994.
90. Hruban RH, von Mansfield AD, Offerhaus GJ, et al.: K-*ras* oncogene activation in adenocarcinoma of the human pancreas. A study of 82 carcinomas using a combination of mutant-enriched polymerase chain reaction analysis and allele specific oligonucleotide hybridization. Am J Pathol 143:545–554, 1993.
91. Motojima K, Tsunoda T, Kanematsu T, et al.: Distinguishing pancreatic carcinoma from other periampullary carcinomas by analysis of mutations in the Kirsten-*ras* oncogene. Ann Surg 214:657–662, 1991.
92. Mulligan NJ, Yang S, Andry C, et al.: The role of p21^{ras} in pancreatic neoplasia and chronic pancreatitis. Hum Pathol 30:602–610, 1999.
93. Topal MD: DNA repair oncogenes and carcinogenesis. Carcinogenesis 9:691–696, 1988.
94. Aoki K, Yoshida T, Matsumoto N, et al.: Suppression of Ki-*ras* p21 levels leading to growth inhibition of pancreatic cancer cell lines with Ki-*ras* mutation but not those without Ki-*ras* mutation. Mol Carcinogen 20:251–258, 1997.
95. Kainuma O, Asano T, Hasegawa M, et al.: Inhibition of growth and invasive activity of human pancreatic cancer cells by a farnesyltransferase inhibitor, manumycin. Pancreas 15:379–383, 1997.
96. Tada M, Yokosuka O, Omata M, et al.: Analysis of *ras* gene mutations in biliary and pancreatic tumors by polymerase chain reaction and direct sequencing. Cancer 66:930–935, 1990.
97. Tada M, Omata M, Ohto M: *Ras* gene mutations in intraductal papillary neoplasms of the pancreas. Cancer 67:634–637, 1991.
98. Sugio K, Molberg K, Albores-Saavedra J, et al.: K-*ras* mutations and allelic loss at 5q and 18q in the development of human pancreatic cancers. Int J Pancreatol 21:205–217, 1997.
99. Lemoine NR, Jain S, Hughes CM, et al.: Ki-*ras* oncogene activation in preinvasive pancreatic cancer. Gastroenterology 102:230–236, 1992.
100. Cerny WL, Mangold KA, Scarpelli DG: K-*ras* mutation is an early event in pancreatic duct carcinogenesis in the Syrian golden hamster. Cancer Res 52:4507–4513, 1992.
101. Schaeffer BK, Glasner S, Kuhlmann E, et al.: Mutated c-K-*ras* in small pancreatic adenocarcinomas. Pancreas 9:161–165, 1994.
102. Yanagisawa A: Progress in the study of pancreatic cancer and its pathology. Semin Surg Oncol 15:8–14, 1998.
103. Apple SK, Hecht JR, Lewin DN, et al.: Immunohistochemical evaluation of K-*ras*, p53, and HER-2/*neu* expression in hyperplastic, dysplastic, and carcinomatous lesions of the pancreas: Evidence of multistep carcinogenesis. Hum Pathol 30:123–129, 1999.
104. Trumper LH, Burger R, vonBonin F, et al.: Diagnosis of pancreatic adenocarcinoma by polymerase chain reaction from pancreatic secretions. Br J Cancer 70:278–284, 1994.
105. Kondo H, Suganno K, Fukayama N, et al.: Detection of point mutations in the K-*ras* oncogene at codon 12 in pure pancreatic juice for diagnosis of pancreatic carcinoma. Cancer 73:1589–1594, 1994.
106. Tada M, Omata M, Kawai S, et al.: Detection of *ras* gene mutations in pancreatic juice and peripheral blood of patients with pancreatic adenocarcinoma. Cancer Res 53:2472–2474, 1993.
107. Watanabe H, Sawabu N, Ohta H, et al.: Identification of K-*ras* mutations in the pure pancreatic juice of

patients with ductal pancreatic cancers. Jpn J Cancer Res 84:961–965, 1993.

108. Caldas C, Hahn SA, Hruban RH, et al.: Detection of K-*ras* mutations in the stool of patients with pancreatic adenocarcinoma and pancreatic ductal hyperplasia. Cancer Res 54:3568–3573, 1994.
109. Wilentz RE, Chung CH, Sturm PD, et al.: K-*ras* mutations in the duodenal fluid of patients with pancreatic carcinoma. Cancer 82:96–103, 1998.
110. Brentnall TA, Bronner MP, Byrd DR, et al.: Early diagnosis and treatment of pancreatic dysplasia in patients with a family history of pancreatic cancer. Ann Intern Med 131:247–255, 1999.
111. Suwa H, Ohshio G, Imamura T, et al.: Overexpression of the *rho*C gene correlates with progression of ductal adenocarcinoma of the pancreas. Br J Cancer 77:147–152, 1998.
112. Wakita K, Ohyanagi H, Yamamoto K, et al.: Overexpression of c-Ki-*ras* and c-*fos* in human pancreatic carcinomas. Int J Pancreatol 11:43–47, 1992.
113. Tessari G, Ferrara C, Poletti A, et al.: The expression of proto-oncogene c-*jun* in human pancreatic cancer. Anticancer Res 19:863–867, 1999.
114. Friess H, Yamanaka Y, Kobrin MS, et al.: Enhanced *erb*B-3 expression in human pancreatic cancer correlates with tumor progression. Clin Cancer Res 1:1413–1420, 1995.
115. Friess H, Yamanaka Y, Büchler M, et al.: Cripto, a member of the epidermal growth factor family, is overexpressed in human pancreatic cancer and chronic pancreatitis. Int J Cancer 56:668–674, 1994.
116. Tsutsumi M, Yasui W, Naito A, et al.: Expression of cripto in human pancreatic tumors. Jpn J Cancer Res 85:118–121, 1994.
117. Lemoine NR, Hughes CM, Barton CM, et al.: The epidermal growth factor receptor in human pancreatic cancer. J Pathol 166:7–12, 1992.
118. Yamanaka Y, Freiss H, Kobrin MS, et al.: Overexpression of HER2/*neu* oncogene in human pancreatic carcinoma. Hum Pathol 24:1127–1134, 1993.
119. Lemoine NR, Lobresco M, Leung H, et al.: The erbB-3 gene in human pancreatic cancer. J Pathol 168:269–273, 1992.
120. Barton CM, Hall PA, Hughes CM, et al.: Transforming growth factor alpha and epidermal growth factor in human pancreatic cancer. J Pathol 163:111–116, 1991.
121. Korc M, Chandreskar B, Yamanaka Y, et al.: Overexpression of the epidermal growth factor receptor in human pancreatic cancer is associated with concomitant increases in the levels of epidermal growth factor and transforming growth factor α. J Clin Invest 90:1352–1360, 1992.
122. Bockman DE, Buchler M, Beger HG: Interaction of pancreatic cancer with nerves leads to nerve damage. Gastroenterology 107:219–230, 1994.
123. Hall PA, Hughes CM, Staddon SL, et al.: The c-*erb* B-2 proto-oncogene in human pancreatic cancer. J Pathol 161:195–200, 1990.
124. Satoh K, Shimosegawa T, Moriizumi S, et al.: K-*ras* mutations and p53 protein accumulation in intraductal mucin-hypersecreting neoplasms of the pancreas. Pancreas 12:362–368, 1996.
125. Day JD, DiGiuseppe JA, Yeo CJ, et al.: Immunohistochemical evaluation of HER-2/*neu* oncogene expression in pancreatic adenocarcinoma and pancreatic intraepithelial neoplasms. Hum Pathol 27:119–124, 1996.
126. Dugan MC, Dergham ST, Kucway R, et al.: HER-2/*neu* expression in pancreatic adenocarcinoma: Relation to tumor differentiation and survival. Pancreas 14:229–236, 1997.
127. Ebert M, Yokoyama M, Freiss H, et al.: Coexpression of the c-*met* protooncogene and hepatocyte growth factor in human pancreatic cancer. Cancer Res 54:5775–5778, 1994.
128. Wallrapp C, Muller-Pillasch F, Solinas-Toldo S, et al.: Characterisation of a high copy number amplification at 6q24 in pancreatic cancer identifies c-*myb* as a candidate oncogene. Cancer Res 57:3135–3139, 1997.
129. Miwa W, Yasuda J, Murakami Y, et al.: Isolation of DNA sequences amplified at chromosome 19q13.1-19q13.2, including the *AKT* locus in human pancreatic cancer. Biochem Biophys Res Commun 225:968–974, 1996.
130. Cheng JQ, Ruggeri B, Klein WM, et al.: Amplification of *AKT2* in human pancreatic cancer cells and inhibition of *AKT2* expression and tumorigenicity by antisense RNA. Proc Natl Acad USA 93:3636–3641, 1996.
131. Lutz MP, Esser IB, Flossmann-Kast BB, et al.: Overexpression and activation of the tyrosine kinase Src in human pancreatic carcinoma. Biochem Biophys Res Commun 243:503–508, 1998.
132. Vogelstein B, Kinzler K: Tumor-suppressor genes. X-rays strike at p53 again. Nature 370:174–175, 1994.
133. Evan G, Littlewood T: A matter of life and cell death. Science 281:1317–1322, 1998.
134. Redston MS, Caldas C, Seymour AB, et al.: p53 mutations in pancreatic carcinoma and evidence of common involvement of homocopolymer tracts in DNA microdeletions. Cancer Res 54:3025–3033, 1994.
135. Levine AJ: p53, the cellular gatekeeper for growth and division. Cell 88:323–331, 1997.
136. Hall PA: p53: The challenge of linking basic science and patient management. Oncologist 3:218–224, 1998.
137. Yokoyama M, Yamanaka Y, Freiss H, et al.: p53 expression in human pancreatic cancer correlates with enhanced biological aggressiveness. Anticancer Res 14:2477–2483, 1994.
138. Sessa F, Bonato M, Bisoni D, et al.: Ki-*ras* and p53 gene mutations in pancreatic ductal carcinoma: A relationship with tumor phenotype and survival. Eur J Histochem 42(Spec No):67–76, 1998.
139. Scarpa A, Capelli P, Mukai K, et al.: Pancreatic adenocarcinomas frequently show p53 gene mutations. Am J Pathol 142:1534–1543, 1993.
140. Boschman CR, Stryker S, Reddy JK, et al.: Expression of p53 protein in precursor lesions and adenocarcinoma of human pancreas. Am J Pathol 145:1291–1295, 1994.
141. Lang D, Miknyoczki SJ, Huang L, et al.: Stable reintroduction of wild-type p53 (MTmp53ts) causes the induction of apoptosis and neuroendocrine-like differentiation in human ductal pancreatic carcinoma cells. Oncogene 16:1593–1602, 1998.
142. Coppola D, Lu L, Fruehauf JP, et al.: Analysis of p53, $p21^{WAF1}$, and TGF-β1 in human ductal adenocarcinoma of the pancreas. TGF-β1 protein expression predicts longer survival. Am J Clin Pathol 110:16–23, 1998.
143. Hahn SA, Schutte M, Hoque AT, et al.: *DPC 4,* a candidate tumor suppressor gene at human chromosome 18q21.1. Science 271:350–353, 1996.
144. O'Brien C: New tumor suppressor gene found in pancreatic cancer. Science 271:294, 1996.

145. Grau AM, Zhang L, Wang W, et al.: Induction of p21waf1 expression and growth inhibition by transforming growth factor beta involve the tumor suppressor gene *DPC4* in human pancreatic adenocarcinoma cells. Cancer Res 57:3929–3934, 1997.
146. Dai JL, Turnacioglu KK, Schutte M, et al.: *DPC4* transcriptional activation and dysfunction in cancer cells. Cancer Res 58:4592–4597, 1998.
147. Riggins GJ, Kinzler KW, Vogelstein B, et al.: Frequency of *SMAD* gene mutations in human cancers. Cancer Res 57:2578–2580, 1997.
148. Höhne MW, Halatsch ME, Kahl GF, et al.: Frequent loss of expression of the potential tumor suppressor gene *DCC* in ductal pancreatic adenocarcinoma. Cancer Res 52:2616–2619, 1992.
149. Friess H, Yamanaka Y, Büchler M, et al.: Enhanced expression of the type II transforming growth factor β receptor in human pancreatic cancer cells without alteration of type III receptor expression. Cancer Res 53:2704–2707, 1993.
150. Friess H, Yamanaka Y, Büchler M, et al.: Enhanced expression of transforming growth factor β isoforms in pancreatic cancer correlates with decreased survival. Gastroenterology 105:1846–1856, 1993.
151. Kleeff J, Friess H, Simon P, et al.: Overexpression of *SMAD2* and colocalization with F-beta1 in human pancreatic cancer Dig Dis Sci 44:1793–1802, 1999.
152. Lu Z, Friess H, Graber HU, et al.: Presence of two signalling TGF-beta receptors in human pancreatic cancer correlates with advanced tumor stage. Dig Dis Sci 42:2054–2063, 1997.
153. Caldas C, Hahn SA, da Costa LT, et al.: Frequent somatic mutations and homozygous deletions of the *p16* (*MTS1*) gene in pancreatic adenocarcinoma. Nat Genet 8:27–32, 1994.
154. Schutte M, Hruban RH, Geradts J, et al.: Abrogation of the *RB/p16* tumor-suppressive pathway in virtually all pancreatic carcinomas. Cancer Res 57:3126–3130, 1997.
155. Rozenblum E, Schutte M, Goggins M, et al.: Natural relationships among tumor-suppressive pathways: Application of pancreatic cancer model. Cancer Res 57:1731–1734, 1997.
156. Wilentz RE, Geradts J, Maynard R, et al.: Inactivation of the *p16*(*INK4A*) tumor suppressor gene in pancreatic duct lesions: Loss of intranuclear expression. Cancer Res 58:3942–3945, 1998.
157. Naumann M, Savitskaia N, Eilert C, et al.: Frequent codeletion of *p16/MTS1* and p15.MTS2 and genetic alterations in *p16/MTS1* in pancreatic tumors. Gastroenterology 10:1215–1224, 1996.
158. Hu YX, Watanabe H, Ohtsubo K, et al.: Frequent loss of *p16* expression and its correlation with clinicopathological parameters in pancreatic cancer. Clin Cancer Res 3:1473–1477, 1997.
159. Bates S, Phillips AC, Clark PA, et al.: $p14^{ARF}$ links the tumour suppressors RB and p53. Nature 395:124–125, 1998.
160. Moskaluk CA, Hruban RH, Lietman AS, et al.: Novel germline *p16*(*INK4a*) allele (Asp 145 Cys) in a family with multiple pancreatic carcinomas. Hum Mutat 12:70, 1998.
161. Schutte M, da Costa LT, Hahn SA, et al.: Identification by representational analysis of a homozygous deletion in pancreatic carcinoma that lies within the *BRCA2* region. Proc Nat Acad Sci USA 90:2846–2850, 1993.
162. Ruggeri BA, Huang L, Wood M, et al.: Amplification and overexpression of the *AKT2* oncogene in a subset of human pancreatic ductal adenocarcinomas. Mol Carcinogen 21:81–86, 1998.
163. Huang L, Lang D, Geradts J, et al.: Molecular and immunochemical analyses of RB1 and cyclin D1 in human ductal pancreatic carcinomas and cell lines. Mol Carcinogen 15:85–95, 1996.
164. Moskaluk CA, Hruban RH, Kern SE: p16 and dK-*ras* gene mutations in the intraductal precursors of human pancreatic carcinoma. Cancer Res 57:2140–2143, 1997.
165. Lu CD, Morita S, Ishibashi T, et al.: Loss of p27Kip1 expression independently predicts poor prognosis for patients with resectable pancreatic adenocarcinoma. Cancer 85:1250–1260, 1999.
166. Seymour AB, Hruban RH, Redston M, et al.: Allelotype of pancreatic carcinoma. Cancer Res 54:2761–2764, 1994.
167. Horii A, Nakatsuru S, Miyoshi Y, et al.: Frequent somatic mutations of the *APC* gene in human pancreatic cancer. Cancer Res 52:6696–6698, 1992.
168. Neuman WL, Wasylyshyn ML, Jacoby R, et al.: Evidence for a common molecular pathogenesis in colorectal, gastric, and pancreatic cancer. Genes Chromo Cancer 3:4674–4673, 1991.
169. Simon B, Bartsch D, Barth P, et al.: Frequent abnormalities of the putative tumor suppressor gene *FHIT* at 3p14.2 in pancreatic carcinoma cell lines. Cancer Res 58:1583–1587, 1998.
170. Teng DH, Perry WL, Hogan JK, et al.: Human kitogen-activated protein kinase kinase 4 as a candidate tumor suppressor. Cancer Res 57:4177–4182, 1997.
171. Okami K, Wu L, Riggins G, et al.: Analysis of *PTEN/MMAC1* alterations in aerodigestive tract tumors. Cancer Res 58:509–511, 1998.
172. Sakurada A, Suzuki A, Sato M, et al.: Infrequent genetic alterations of the *PTEN/MMAC* gene in Japanese patients with primary cancers of the breast, lung, pancreas, kidney, and ovary. Jpn J Cancer Res 88:1025–1029, 1997.
173. Di Christofano A, Pesce B, Cordon-Cardo C, et al.: *PTEN* is essential for embryonic development and tumour suppression. Nat Genet 19:348–355, 1998.
174. Kawa S, Nikaido T, Aoki Y, et al.: Vitamin D analogues up-regulate p21 and p27 during growth inhibition of pancreatic cancer cell lines. Br J Cancer 76:884–889, 1997.
175. Han HJ, Yanagisawa A, Kato Y, et al.: Genetic instability in pancreatic cancer and poorly differentiated type of gastric cancer. Cancer Res 53:5087–5089, 1993.
176. Shridhar V, Rivard S, Wang X, et al.: Mutations in the arginine-rich protein gene (ARP) in pancreatic cancer. Oncogene 14:2213–2216, 1997.
177. Cantero D, Friess H, Deflorin J, et al.: Enhanced expression of urokinase plasminogen activator and its receptor in pancreatic carcinoma. Br J Cancer 75:388–395, 1997.
178. Muller-Pillasch F, Wallrapp C, Lacher U, et al.: Identification of a new tumor-associated antigen TM4SF5 and its expression in human cancer. Gene 208:25–30, 1998.
179. Muller-Pillasch F, Wallrapp C, Bartels K, et al.: Cloning of a new Kunitz-type protease inhibitor with a putative transmembrane domain overexpressed in pancreatic cancer. Biochim Biophys Acta 1395:88–95, 1998.
180. Muller-Pillasch F, Zimmerhackl F, Lacher U, et al.: Cloning of novel transcripts of the human guanine-nucleotide-exchange factor Mss4: In situ chromo-

somal mapping and expression in pancreatic cancer. Genomics 46:389–396, 1997.

181. Tsutsumi M, Tsujiuchi T, Ishikawa O, et al.: Increased telomerase activities in human pancreatic duct adenocarcinomas Jpn J Cancer Res 88:971–976, 1997.
182. Yamada T, Okajima F, Adachi M, et al.: Growth dependency of a new human pancreatic cancer cell line, YAPC, on autocrine interleukin-1α stimulation. Int J Cancer 76:141–147, 1998.
183. Gansuage S, Gansauge F, Ramadani M, et al.: Overexpression of cyclin D1 in human pancreatic carcinoma is associated with poor prognosis. Cancer Res 57:1634–1637, 1997.
184. Gress TM, Muller-Pillasch F, Weber C, et al.: Differential expression of heat shock proteins in pancreatic carcinoma. Cancer Res 54:547–551, 1994.
185. Li F, Ambrosini G, Chu EY, et al.: Control of apoptosis and mitotic spindle checkpoint by survivin. Nature 396:580–583, 1998.
186. Ambrosini G, Adida C, Altieri DC: A novel antiapoptosis gene, survivin, expressed in cancer and lymphoma. Nature Medicine 3:917–921, 1997.
187. Friess H, Lu Z, Graber HU, et al.: *bax,* but not *bcl-*2, influences the prognosis of human pancreatic cancer. Gut 43:414–421, 1998.
188. Von Bernstorff W, Spanjaard RA, Chan AK, et al.: Pancreatic cancer cells can evade immune surveillance via nonfunctional Fas (APO-1/CD95) receptors and aberrant expression of functional Fas ligand. Surgery 125:73–84, 1999.
189. Bramhall SR, Neoptolomos JP, Stamp GW, et al.: Imbalance of expression of matrix metalloproteases (MMPs) and tissue inhibitors of the matrix metalloproteases (TIMPs) in human pancreatic carcinoma. J Pathol 182:347–355, 1997.
190. Ellenreider V, Alber B, Lacher U, et al.: Expression of MT-MMP's in pancreatic cancer and chronic pancreatitis. Gastroenterology 114:A590, 1998.
191. Zhou W, Sokoll LJ, Bruzek DJ, et al.: Identifying markers for pancreatic cancer by gene expression analysis. Cancer Epidemiol Biomarkers Prev 7:109–112, 1998.
192. von Marschall Z, Rieken EO, Rosewicz S: Stromelysin 3 is overexpressed in human pancreatic carcinoma and regulated by retinoic acid in pancreatic carcinoma cell lines. Gut 43:692–698, 1998.
193. Takeuchi Y, Nakao A, Harada A, et al.: Expression of plasminogen activators and their inhibitors in human pancreatic carcinoma: Immunohistochemical study. Am J Gastroenterol 88:1928–1933, 1993.
194. Itakura J, Ishiwata T, Friess H, et al.: Enhanced expression of vascular endothelial growth factor in human pancreatic cancer correlates with local disease progression. Clin Cancer Res 3:1309–1316, 1997.
195. Morgan RGH, Wormsley KG: Progress report. Cancer of the pancreas. Gut 18:580–596, 1977.
196. Molina MA, Sitja-Arnau M, Lemoine MG, et al.: Increased cyclooxygenase-2 expression in human pancreatic carcinomas and cell lines: Growth inhibition by nonsteroidal anti-inflammatory drugs. Cancer Res 59:4356–4362, 1999.
197. Okami J, Yamamoto H, Fujiwara Y, et al.: Overexpression of cyclooxygenase-2 in carcinoma of the pancreas. Clin Cancer Res 5:2018–2024, 1999.
198. Karayiannakis AJ, Syrigos KN, Chatzigianni E, et al.: Aberrant E-cadherin expression associated with loss of differentiation and advanced stage in human pancreatic cancer. Anticancer Res 18:4177–4180, 1998.

Chapter

7
DUCTAL ADENOCARCINOMA

Over 80% of exocrine pancreatic tumors are ductal adenocarcinomas; another 10% are variants of ductal carcinoma, either giant cell carcinomas, adenosquamous carcinomas, or mucinous carcinomas[1] (Table 7–1). Ductal adenocarcinomas arise from foci of epithelial dysplasia and replicate to some degree the morphology of the major pancreatic ducts. Ductal adenocarcinomas are rarely curable, even by major surgery. Most patients are dead within 18 months of the onset of symptoms. These tumors are often silent until disease is advanced. There are no natural barriers to local spread; there is a high incidence of metastasis at the time of diagnosis, and current adjuvant therapies are ineffective.

INCIDENCE

Incidence statistics for pancreatic cancer do not distinguish among the different histologic types and include all malignancies of the pancreas, but because the ductal adenocarcinoma is the dominant neoplasm, the numbers mainly represent that tumor type. Carcinoma of the pancreas is the fourth most common cause of cancer death, both in men (after lung, prostate, and colorectum) and in women (after lung, breast, and colorectum).[2–4] Annually, pancreatic cancer is now responsible for 27,800 deaths in the United States, 14,000 deaths in Japan,[5] and 168,000 deaths worldwide.[4] The incidence rate and the mortality rate are approximately equal because the cancer is almost invariably fatal. The incidence of this tumor recently stabilized, both in Great Britain and in the United States, after steadily increasing for several decades.[6,7] Men are affected slightly more often than women are, in a proportion that varies from country to country. In Japan in 1990, the mortality rate per 100,000 was 12.1 in men and 9.6 in women. The age-standardized incidence is 9 per 100,000 men and 8 per 100,000 women, but because of the excess of women in older age groups, the total number of cases in women exceeds that in men.[2] This cancer is rare before the age of 40 years, and the incidence rises progressively after the age of 50, to peak in the ninth decade of life.[8] In the United States, 68.5% of cases are diagnosed in patients over the age of 65.[9]

EPIDEMIOLOGIC ASSOCIATIONS

Pancreatic cancer is associated positively with geographic latitude and negatively with average ambient temperature; thus, it is a disease of the industrialized world[10,11] (Table 7–2). The positive relationship with latitude suggests that diminished exposure to sunlight, diminished vitamin D formation in skin, and consequent diminished calcium absorption might promote pancreatic cancer.[10] Increased food consumption at temperate latitudes and the nature of the diet may also be relevant to pancreatic cancer.[11–13] Race does not appear to account for this effect.

Urban dwellers have higher rates of pancreatic carcinoma than do rural dwellers. The incidence in blacks is 1.5 to 2.0 times that in whites.[4,14] The highest rates of pancreatic cancer are found in Polynesians, particularly native Hawaiians and Maoris, and in these populations, the relative risk for males is about three times that for females.[15]

Table 7–1. Morphologic Variants of Ductal Adenocarcinoma

Mucinous (colloid) carcinoma
Signet ring cell carcinoma
Adenosquamous carcinoma
Squamous cell carcinoma
Composite ductal-endocrine carcinoma
Small cell carcinoma
Pleomorphic, sarcomatoid, and anaplastic carcinoma
Undifferentiated carcinoma with osteoclast-like giant cells
Microadenocarcinoma
Clear cell carcinoma

CLINICAL MANIFESTATIONS

The symptoms and signs of pancreatic carcinoma depend on the location of the tumor. Roughly two thirds of cases involve the head of pancreas and one third the body and tail. The onset is insidious, with dull epigastric pain that sometimes penetrates through to the back, weight loss, anorexia, weakness, and vomiting. Jaundice, due to obstruction of the distal common bile duct, occurs in over 50% of patients at some time, but < 20% of patients present with the classic painless progressive jaundice. Cancers of the body and tail of the pancreas present at a more advanced stage than do cancers of the head and are, on average, larger. About one quarter of patients have a palpable abdominal mass at presentation and some have hepatomegaly. Other manifestations include acute pancreatitis,[16] psychiatric depression, migratory thrombophlebitis,[17] nonbacterial thrombotic endocarditis,[18] recent-onset diabetes mellitus[19] and (rarely) duodenal obstruction, duodenal or gastric hemorrhage, steatorrhea, acanthosis nigricans, disseminated fat necrosis, hypoglycemia,[20] and hypercalcemia.[21] The cause of the pain of pancreatic carcinoma may be ductal obstruction, neural invasion, or secondary pancreatitis, although the mechanisms are not fully elucidated. The afferent pain fibers from the pancreas form part of the sympathetic system. Weight loss appears to be mainly due to the cachexia of cancer, rather than to pancreatic enzyme deficiency and maldigestion. Thromboembolic disease occurs at some time in about 20% of patients, more frequently in those with mucin-producing tumors of the body and tail of the pancreas. The variants of thromboembolic disease include venous thrombosis (superficial or deep), marantic endocarditis, and, rarely, arterial thrombosis or disseminated intravascular coagulation. Ascites is an occasional presenting feature. Skin metastases are a rare feature.[22] Pancreatitis shares symptoms with carcinoma of the pancreas, making diagnosis of cancer difficult in patients with preexisting pancreatitis.

The liver enzymes alkaline phosphatase and 5^1-nucleotidase are elevated in 66% of patients, transaminases in 60%, bilirubin in 44%, and blood glucose in 53%.[23]

DIAGNOSTIC MODALITIES

Ultrasonography detects about 60% of tumors and is usually the first imaging study performed. Computed tomography (CT) is the most accurate diagnostic modality, superseding celiac angiography and selenomethionine scans. Helical CT scan provides the best overall assessment of patients with periampullary malignancies, and it is often the only investigation required before proceeding to surgery.[24] The arterial dominant phase of dynamic CT scan yields the best correlation between CT-measured tumor size and that of the resected specimens ($p < 0.01$), but the correlation coefficient is not high ($r = 0.67$).[25] If no mass is apparent on the helical CT scan, diagnostic endoscopic retrograde cholangiopancreatography (ERCP) is indicated. ERCP detects about 75% of tumors and gives very few false positive results. The value of magnetic resonance cholangiopancreatography in diagnosis of pancreatic carcinoma is being assessed.[26,27]

Ultrasonography has been combined with endoscopy, laparoscopy, and portal venous catheterization in an attempt to determine the extent of tumor infiltration of the portal vein and the resectability of pancreatic cancers. If microscopic proof of the diagnosis will allow avoidance of surgery, then fine-needle aspiration cytology (FNAC) should be performed.[24] Intraportal endovascular ultrasonography may prove useful but is not yet fully assessed.[28] Endoscopic ultrasonography with fine-needle aspiration (FNA) is a highly successful combination that

Table 7–2. Epidemiologic Associations

Latitude and temperature
Urban living
Race and ethnicity

allows staging and confirmation of diagnosis in periampullary tumors. On endoscopic ultrasonography, three signs reliably identify tumor invasion of major veins forming the portal confluence: (1) peripancreatic venous collaterals in the area of a mass that obliterates the normal anatomic location of a major portal confluence vessel, (2) tumor within the vessel lumen, and (3) abnormal vessel contour with loss of the vessel–parenchymal sonographic interface.[29] Fluorodeoxyglucose positron emission tomography (FDGPET) has similar sensitivity to CT in identifying malignant disease of the pancreas, but FDGPET was found to be more specific for malignant versus benign disease than was CT.[30]

Serum markers such as CA19-9, DUPAN-2, carcinoembryonic antigen (CEA), and Span 1 are individually of limited value but can be quite accurate in combination,[31] although they are only ancillary to direct imaging for diagnosis. We may be on the threshold of an exciting advance in diagnosis based on gene expression analysis in specific cancers.[32] Of the 45,000 genes identified, 183 were found to be expressed at significantly elevated levels in pancreatic cancer. A combination of individually suboptimal markers (tissue inhibitor of metalloprotease 1 [TIMP1], CA19-9, and CEA) detected 60% of pancreatic cancers in 85 patients in a highly specific manner.[32] CA 19-9 is elevated in the serum of 80% of patients with pancreatic carcinoma and is superior to CEA alone. A sustained decrease of CA19-9 during the first weeks of chemotherapy with gemcitabine is associated with a better survival of patients with locally advanced or metastatic cancer. Another test that needs further evaluation is the finding of K-*ras* mutations in the plasma DNA from 80% of patients with pancreatic cancer.[33]

Immunostaining for CA 19-9 does not distinguish normal or hyperplastic ducts from malignant, but monoclonal antibodies against epitopes of CEA, the CEA-related antigen, and nonspecific cross-reacting antigen 95 are capable of discriminating among adenocarcinoma, reactive duct changes, and acinar or endocrine cell neoplasms.[34] Other markers, such as Le^x or DUPAN 2, also recognize pancreatic carcinoma but are not specific for it.

PREMALIGNANT LESIONS

The premalignant lesion of pancreatic ductal carcinoma is ductal epithelial dysplasia (or intraepithelial neoplasia), which progresses in a stepwise fashion from low-grade to high-grade epithelial abnormality.[34,35] This sequence is supported by immunostaining for K-*ras,* p53, and HER-2/*neu*.[36] Ductal papillary hyperplasia is defined as "a focal lesion in which the normal duct epithelium is replaced by papillary folds lined by columnar cells displaying mucinous hypertrophy."[37] It may arise in normal pancreas and occurs with increased frequency in chronic pancreatitis and in association with carcinomas. Ductal papillary hyperplasia shows nuclear enlargement but few mitoses, and it is unclear whether it represents low-grade dysplasia.[38] The term *atypical ductal hyperplasia* is a synonym for *dysplasia.* Ductal epithelial dysplasia may be either a flat or a papillary proliferation, with cytologic atypia, increased nucleocytoplasmic ratio, nuclear enlargement, pleomorphism, crowding, and loss of polarity (Fig. 7–1). Dysplasia occurs more frequently in pancreata with ductal adenocarcinoma than in those without[38–41] and is usually found only in close proximity to the carcinomas. High-grade dysplasia is defined as "a change of the ductal epithelium characterised by irregular epithelial budding and bridging, and severe nuclear abnormalities such as loss of polarity, pleomorphism, coarse chromatin, dense nucleoli and mitotic figures. The lesion can be considered as noninvasive ductal adenocarcinoma"[38] (Fig. 7–2). It typically affects medium-size and large ducts. Three cases have been described in which this lesion was found in the ductal resection margin of a partial pancreatectomy specimen, and in all three, a carcinoma subsequently arose in the residual gland.[35] Multicentric intraductal carcinomas can arise from atypical papillary hyperplasia.[42] Activating point mutations of K-*ras* are found in papillary dysplasia and papillary hyperplasia.[43–47] Mutations of *p16*[48] and overexpression of p53 and HER-2/*neu* also occur in the dysplasia, confirming its progress along the neoplastic pathway.[36,49–51] Most carcinomas are positive for p53.

Carcinoma in situ may extend along the main pancreatic ducts for a considerable distance beyond the main tumor and often has a micropapillary growth pattern. This lesion can be distinguished from papillary hyperplasia in which there is minimal cytologic atypia.[38,40,52] The distinction between reactive ductal epithelial changes and premalignant changes is not always easy in cases of ductal obstruction or chronic pancreatitis.

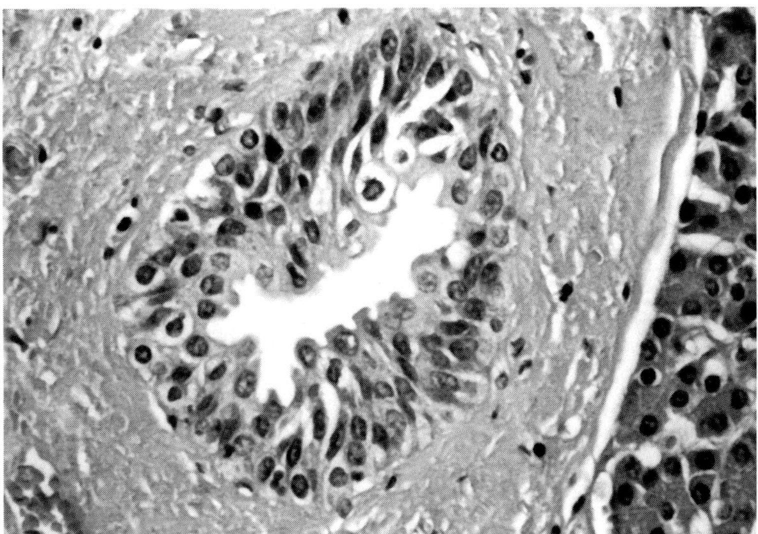

Figure 7–1. Low-grade dysplastic changes within a pancreatic duct.

FINE-NEEDLE ASPIRATION CYTOLOGY

FNAC performed under ultrasonographic guidance is the method of choice for pathologic sampling of pancreatic masses and is capable of definitively establishing the diagnosis. It is especially useful for confirming a diagnosis in those who are too old or too ill to withstand surgery or in those in whom metastases are evident on imaging. If palliative surgery is to be undertaken, it is best to obtain an open biopsy at surgery. If curative surgery is contemplated, FNAC is not usually performed unless the patient will not accept surgery without an established diagnosis.[53] This is because of the risk of seeding along the needle track. FNAC is also used for masses of the body and tail of the pancreas that are unresectable.[54]

The mean sensitivity of FNAC in the diagnosis of malignancy using figures from seven studies is about 72%.[55–61] However, the reliability of a negative FNAC to exclude pancreatic cancer is argued to be too low to warrant its routine preoperative use.[53] The reported false positive rate is very low (about 1%) and is due to pancreatitis.[55,58] Substantial numbers of cases are, however, reported as borderline or suspicious for

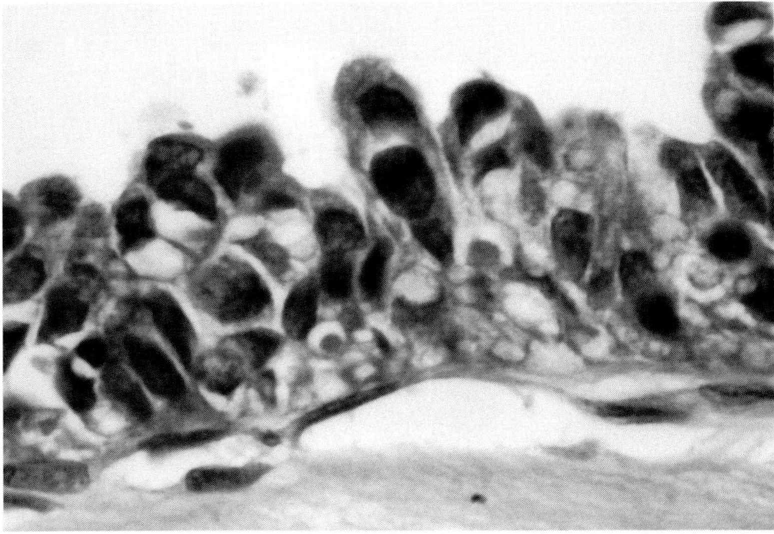

Figure 7–2. High-grade dysplastic changes within a pancreatic duct. Note the severe pleomorphism and loss of polarity.

malignancy. FNAC has been performed under the guidance of endoscopic ultrasound and yielded good results.[59] FNAC has been used in patients with resectable cancer and in cancers treated by neoadjuvant chemoradiation alone and there was no statistical difference in the incidence of peritoneal metastases between patients who had FNAC and those who did not.[60] Intraoperative FNAC is sometimes performed in preference to biopsy and frozen section and, pooling the results of two studies, 76% of carcinomas of pancreas were correctly diagnosed.[62,63] Thus, its value is limited by a false negative rate of 24%. Part of the reason for this is suboptimal needle placement. Endosonography-guided or intraoperative transduodenal FNAC is being used increasingly, as the needle track can be included in the excision specimen, if surgery is subsequently performed. The early results have been excellent, with 100% specificity and 82% sensitivity.[64] FNAC is a safe procedure that has very low morbidity and mortality, although rare instances of death, pancreatitis, abscess, or hematoma may occur.[65] Needle track implants are rare. By contrast, after open biopsy, there may be rapid transperitoneal spread.[66] The addition of either the CEA immunoassay, K-*ras* mutation analysis, or both, enhances the sensitivity of cytologic diagnosis.[67]

The normal ductal epithelium represented in FNAC specimens forms flat sheets with evenly spaced nuclei and distinct cytoplasmic borders, whereas the normal acinar cells form cohesive clusters of smaller cells that have basal nuclei and granular cytoplasm. Most adenocarcinomas display high cellularity with dyscohesion, showing a range from small or large clusters to single cells (Fig. 7–3). Nuclear enlargement, pleomorphism, crowding, overlapping, and loss of polarity are features that favor malignancy. Large angular or irregular nucleoli and thick nuclear membranes may be found (Fig. 7–4). Pleomorphic and giant cell carcinomas may show bizarre malignant cells. In some instances, the distinction of well-differentiated carcinoma from reactive ductal change is a problem. The most helpful criteria for a diagnosis of malignancy are loss of polarity within three-dimensional clusters, threefold variation in nuclear size, and irregular nuclear membranes. Other features, such as necrosis, mitoses, and the absence of inflammation, may help (Table 7–3). Adenosquamous carcinomas show extensive necrosis and sometimes ghosted squamous cells or anucleate squames. The malignant cells may be squamous or may demonstrate a mixture of squamous and glandular features.

Endoscopic pancreatic duct brushings yield specimens suitable for assessment by conventional cytology alone or with the addition of p53 immunostaining.[68]

Laparoscopy detects small liver and peritoneal metastases that are undetectable by other techniques.[69] Pancreatic cancer often sheds malignant cells into the peritoneal cavity that can be picked up on lavage at laparoscopy. Warshaw[68] reported the results of cytologic examination of peritoneal washings from 40 patients with pancreatic ductal adenocarcinoma whose tumors were deemed potentially resect-

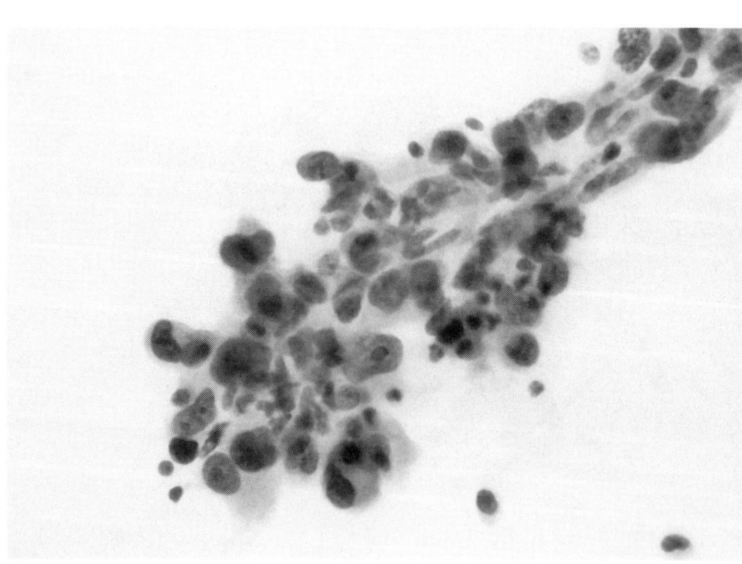

Figure 7–3. Fine-needle aspiration of pancreatic ductal adenocarcinoma. This clump of tumor shows high cellularity with crowding and overlapping nuclei.

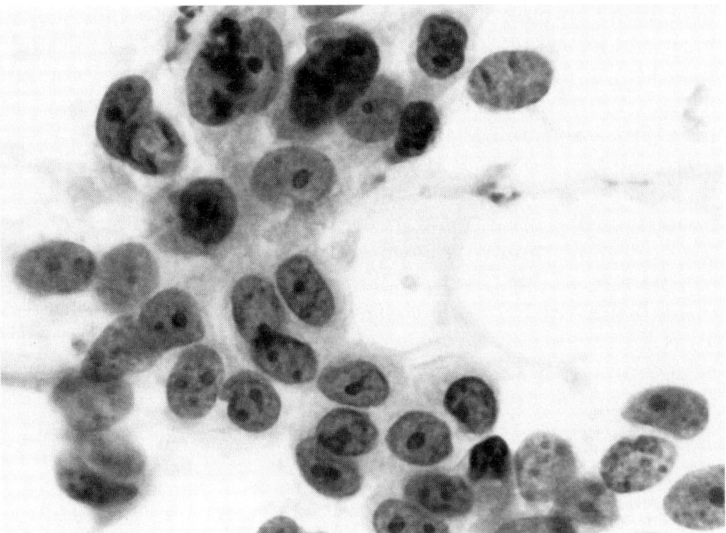

Figure 7–4. Fine-needle aspiration of pancreatic ductal adenocarcinoma showing pleomorphic cells with prominent nucleoli.

able by computed tomography; 100 mL of saline was instilled and aspirated at laparoscopy in 27 patients and at laparotomy in 13. Malignant cells were found in the washings in 30%. These included 4 of 8 patients cases with ascites (50%) and 4 of 32 patients without (12.5%), indicating that the presence of ascites does not necessarily imply peritoneal carcinomatosis. Peritoneal fluid cytology was positive in 6 of 8 patients (75%) who had undergone previous percutaneous needle biopsy, versus 6 of 32 (19%) of those patients who had not ($p < 0.01$), which suggests that intraperitoneal spread of cancer cells may be promoted by tumor biopsy. Only 1 of the 12 patients whose findings on peritoneal cytology were positive had a visible surface implant, but none of the 6 patients found to have liver metastases had positive findings on peritoneal cytology. A judgment on resectability was made independently of cytologic status, and only the tumor of 1 of 10 with positive findings on cytology was resectable (and that with positive margins), whereas tumors in 13 of 25 of those with negative findings on cytology were resectable. The survival of those with positive findings on peritoneal cytology was significantly worse than of those with negative findings.[69] This last finding was confirmed in a follow-up study of 32 patients with positive findings on peritoneal cytology and 30 with negative findings. Visible, biopsy-proven peritoneal metastases were present in 17 of the 32 patients with positive findings and absent in 15. The median survival was 7.8 months in the group with positive findings and visible metastases, 8.6 months in the group with positive findings without visible metastases, and 13.5 months in the group with negative findings.[70] Peritoneal cytology may thus add another unique element to preoperative staging of pancreatic cancer and may possibly also become a method for monitoring the success of treatment. Others authors have made similar observations.[71]

Biopsy should be part of the diagnostic workup for patients with suspected inoperable pancreatic carcinoma, because histologic con-

Table 7–3. Cytologic Comparison of Pancreatitis and Adenocarcinoma

	Pancreatitis	Adenocarcinoma
Cellularity	Low or moderate	High
Cohesiveness	Flat sheets and clumps with retained polarity	Three-dimensional sheets and single cells; loss of polarity
Nucleocytoplasmic ratio	Normal or mildly increased	Mildly to markedly increased
Nuclear enlargement	Mild	Marked
Nuclear contours	Smooth or slightly irregular	Smooth to very irregular
Macronucleoli	Rare	Frequent

firmation aids clinical management. Pancreatic biopsy does not adversely influence survival time for patients with inoperable pancreatic tumors,[72] but it may sometimes be followed by rapid intra-abdominal spread.[66] It is likely that open biopsy may aid spread of adenocarcinoma, and many surgeons still believe in performing a diagnostic pancreatoduodenectomy for tumors or tumorlike lesions of the head of the pancreas and periampullary region, even though that means some patients with pancreatitis are treated in this way.[73,74] This approach is acceptable because of the current low-risk surgical procedures used.

GROSS PATHOLOGY

About 60% of pancreatic carcinomas occur in the head, 15% in the body, 5% in the tail, and 20% in a combination of sites.[9,75,76] Tumors in the head of pancreas often present with obstruction of the common bile duct, as about half of them are located close to the intrapancreatic portion of the duct as it passes through the dorsal part of the pancreatic head. The stenotic segment is usually short, 1 cm or less in length, and the proximal duct is dilated. Tumors also frequently obstruct the pancreatic duct, causing distal dilation and beading of the pancreatic duct, exocrine atrophy, clinical exocrine insufficiency, and secondary pancreatitis with thickening and fibrosis of the body and tail.

Pancreatic carcinomas are usually ill-defined firm or scirrhous masses that are somewhat paler than the normal pancreas, grayish white, and homogeneous, without a lobular pattern (Fig. 7–5). They may contain small cysts that, in a minority of cases, are due to a mucinous component of the tumor but more often are a component of secondary pancreatitis or a remnant of preexisting pancreatitis. Foci of necrosis or hemorrhage are uncommon. The diameter of carcinomas in resected pancreata usually ranges from 1.5 to 5 cm, whereas in autopsy series the averages are larger. Tumors of the body and tail average between 5 and 7 cm in diameter.[41,77] The gross dimensions of pancreatic cancers may be an unreliable measure of their actual size because the tumor infiltration and the associated pancreatitis make the boundaries indistinct. The final estimate of tumor size should be based on the microscopic findings, as tumors may extend well beyond their visible boundaries. Because the pancreas is only ≤ 2.5 cm in thickness and the carcinomas are invasive, not expansile, most larger tumors extend into the peripancreatic fat, where they can spread without hindrance.

At autopsy, carcinoma may have invaded the duodenum, stomach, transverse colon, spleen, left adrenal, kidney, portal vein, splenic vein, or splenic artery. Lymph node and liver metastases

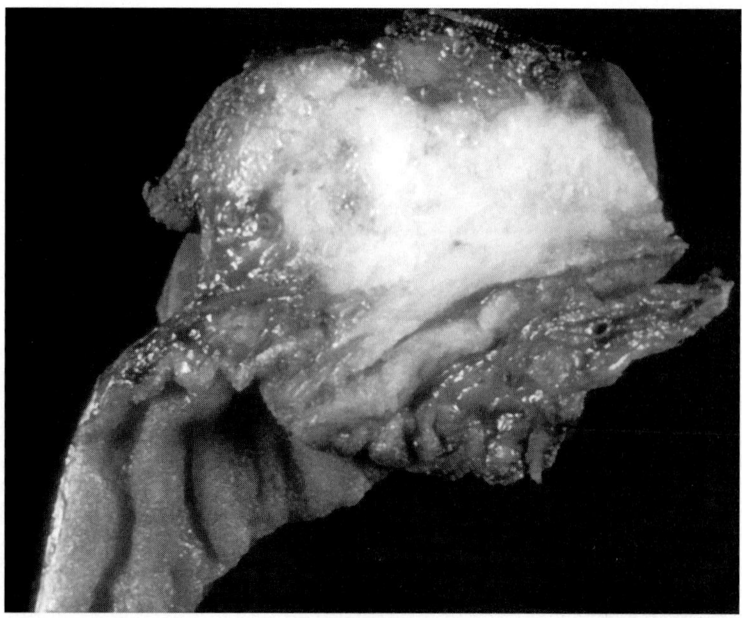

Figure 7–5. Duct carcinoma of the head of the pancreas presenting as an ill-circumscribed homogeneous gray-white mass.

are commonly present. Secondary biliary cirrhosis is rare nowadays because stenting is effective for draining obstructed bile ducts.

GROSS DISSECTION

Orient the specimen and find the cut ends of the common bile duct and pancreatic duct. Ink the soft-tissue margins so that the relationship of tumor to margins of excision can be assessed under the microscope. Open the common bile duct from the back and identify stricture or dilation. Open the main pancreatic duct. Ductal dilation is often present upstream of the tumor. The posterosuperior location of the splenic vessels helps to orient distal pancreatectomy specimens. Identify lymph nodes by palpation and submit them for microscopic examination, one per cassette. Slice the specimen serially to demonstrate the relationship of tumor to ampulla, bile duct, main pancreatic duct, and resection margins. The tumor can usually be identified grossly and classified as to site of origin. Divide whole slices into blocks for histology. Err on the side of submitting too many blocks. Wrap the remaining tissue slices in sequence in anticipation of revisiting them if necessary.

MICROSCOPIC FEATURES OF DUCTAL ADENOCARCINOMA

The center of the tumor usually shows neoplastic glands of variable size in a desmoplastic stroma, with few remnants of normal tissue. Blocks from the tumor margin display invasion of normal structures and secondary changes, such as atrophy or pancreatitis. Cancer may infiltrate widely through the parenchyma and alongside the ducts. Individual tumors often show a range of differentiation. Pancreatic carcinomas have traditionally been graded using subjective criteria. The less differentiated the tumor, the less the resemblance to normal pancreatic ducts. Moderately and poorly differentiated carcinomas predominate over well-differentiated by a ratio 12:1.[41,77] A more satisfactory system would be to grade tumors according to the percentage of the neoplasm that has gland formation, as is done with colorectal carcinomas. The traditional approach is as follows:

- *Well-differentiated tumors* show well-formed glands or tubules in a desmoplastic stroma. The epithelium is typically composed of tall columnar mucin-producing cells with basal nuclei and pale cytoplasm, but it may be focally cuboidal or flattened (Fig. 7–6). Goblet cells are not present. The cytoplasm is eosinophilic or pale. Nuclei are basal, regular, and generally well polarized. The nuclear membranes are thickened and the nuclei are enlarged and often contain nucleoli. The glands may be quite large and duct-like and may form papillary infoldings or cribriform patterns.
- *Moderately differentiated tumors* display more variable gland size and shape, more glandular complexity, and more pronounced cytologic atypia than do well-differentiated tumors

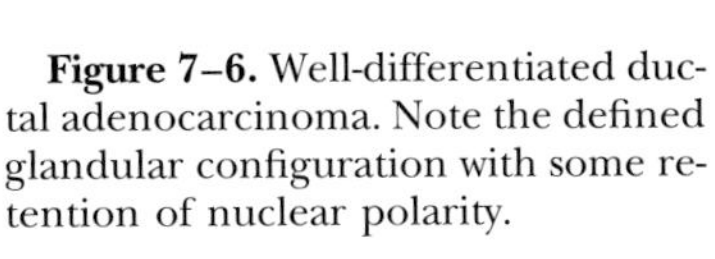

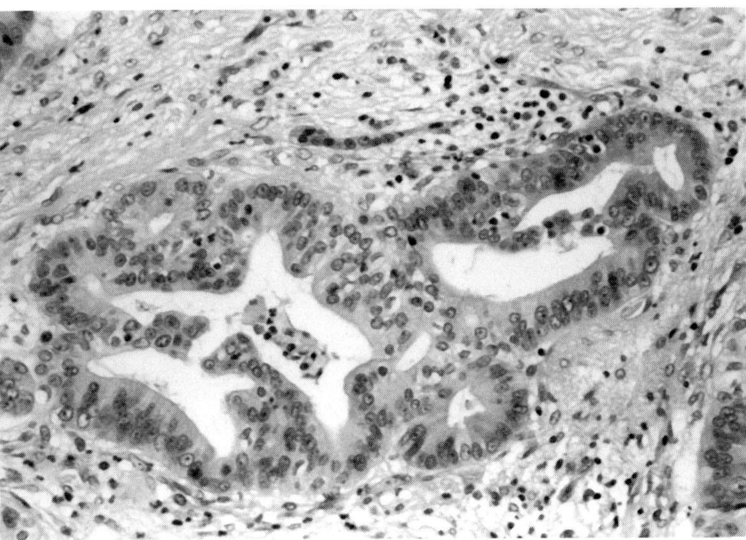

Figure 7–6. Well-differentiated ductal adenocarcinoma. Note the defined glandular configuration with some retention of nuclear polarity.

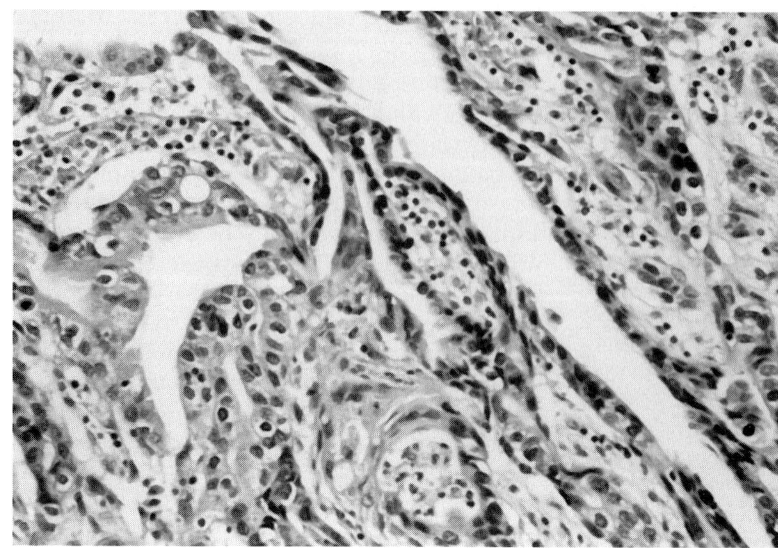

Figure 7–7. Moderately differentiated ductal carcinoma with poorly formed glands and a marked cellular pleomorphism.

(Fig. 7–7). There is more nuclear irregularity, pleomorphism, hyperchromatism, and chromatin clumping and the mitotic index is higher than in well-differentiated tumors. The cytoplasm may be clear or eosinophilic. There may be partial atrophy of the epithelial lining and mucin and cellular debris in the lumina. The stroma is desmoplastic.

- *Poorly differentiated tumors* display ill-formed glands and cellular anaplasia. The glands are highly irregular, confluent, or poorly defined and may meld into infiltrating cords or sheets of cells (Fig. 7–8). They may be devoid of mucin or may contain large cytoplasmic mucin vacuoles. There is considerable nuclear pleomorphism, large irregular nucleoli, and loss of polarity, sometimes with bizarre nuclei and many mitoses. Cytoplasm is variable in quantity but often copious, eosinophilic or amphophilic, and glassy or granular. Foci of necrosis and hemorrhage may be present. Desmoplasia is less prominent than in the

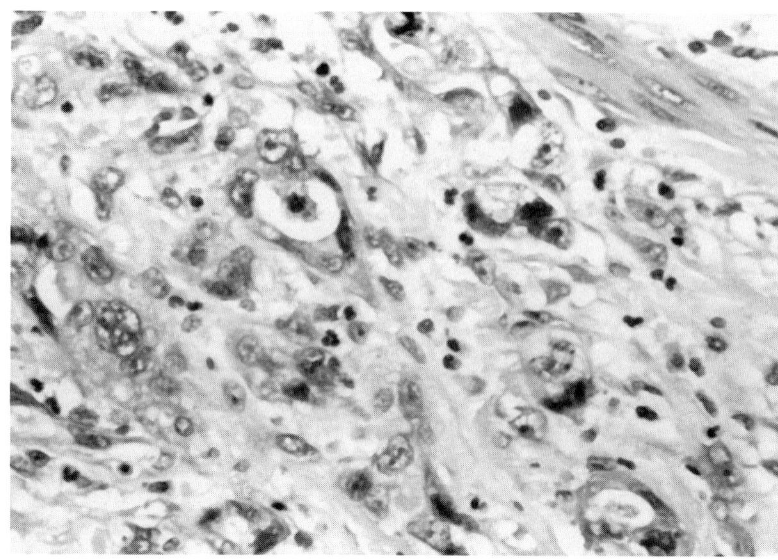

Figure 7–8. Poorly differentiated ductal adenocarcinoma showing ill-formed glands, sheets, and cords of tumor cells.

better-differentiated tumors. There may be a sprinkling of inflammatory cells, either lymphocytes or neutrophils.

Pancreatic carcinomas with the replication error phenotype are often poorly differentiated, have pushing borders and a prominent syncytial growth pattern. These tumors also have wild-type K-*ras*. Patients with this tumor phenotype may have a better-than-average survival rate.[78] A rare example of poorly differentiated pancreatic carcinoma with rhabdoid features has been described.[79]

In small biopsies, the distinction between normal and neoplastic ducts can be difficult. The stroma is desmoplastic and abundant and the glands are distributed irregularly throughout it. Remnants of the normal pancreas are often interspersed with the cancer. Cancerous glands may extend along the ducts or along interlobular septa and can be highlighted by a CEA immunostain. Perineural invasion is commonly present and can be a very useful feature to confirm the neoplastic nature of well-differentiated glandular proliferation (Fig. 7–9).

HISTOCHEMISTRY AND IMMUNOSTAINS

Most pancreatic carcinomas stain positively for mucin with the high iron diamine stain for sulfated acid mucins, alcian blue stain at pH 2.5 for acid mucins, and diastase-PAS (periodic acid–Schiff) for neutral mucins. The staining is cytoplasmic and concentrated at the luminal border. Metastases to liver are usually positive with alcian blue, as are cholangiocarcinomas. Immunostains are not of much practical value in the diagnosis of pancreatic carcinoma or in distinguishing its metastases from those of other primary sites. Positive results are commonly obtained for CEA (near 100%); CA 19-9 (80%); CA125 (50%); TAG 72 (80%); DUPAN 2 (90%); Span 1 (90%); mucinlike antigens; villin; keratins 7, 8, 18, 19, and 20 (near 100%).[80–83] CEA stains the luminal borders of the cells and sometimes the cytoplasm. Staining is strongest in well-differentiated carcinomas and may be only focal or patchy in poorly differentiated tumors. Stains for vimentin, amylase, lipase, trypsin, and chymotrypsin and for general neuroendocrine markers, such as neuron-specific enolase, are negative.[84] Most pancreatic adenocarcinomas contain small numbers of cells that are immunoreactive with antibodies against chromogranin A and pancreatic peptide hormones.[85,86] Abnormal colocation of hormones in the same cell may be found.[86] This finding implies not that all adenocarcinomas are of mixed exocrine-endocrine phenotype but rather that a minor component of endocrine cells can differentiate out of the malignant clone. A similar minor population of endocrine cells is common in many gastrointestinal adenocarcinomas, particularly colonic neoplasms. True mixed exocrine-endocrine tumors are rare. Cytokeratins 20 and 7 give positive

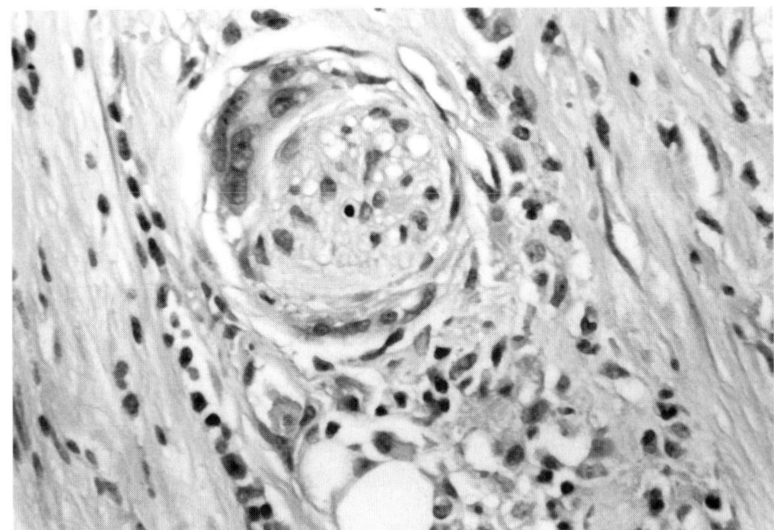

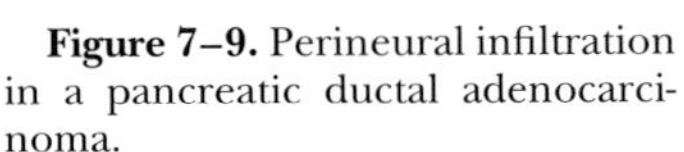

Figure 7–9. Perineural infiltration in a pancreatic ductal adenocarcinoma.

immunoreactivity with ductal adenocarcinomas, and this dual immunopositivity is found in 80% of liver metastases from the pancreas or biliary tract, whereas colorectal carcinoma is positive for cytokeratin 20 and negative for cytokeratin 7.[87]

FROZEN-SECTION DIAGNOSIS

The distinction of carcinoma from chronic pancreatitis is a recognized pitfall for the unwary. Biopsies taken from the surface of the pancreas may show tumor infiltrating normal or altered pancreas, so the diagnosis may be easy. However, in other cases, it may be difficult to distinguish well-differentiated carcinomas from chronic pancreatitis. In advanced foci of chronic pancreatitis, there is extensive fibrosis, loss of exocrine tissue, distortion of ducts, and proliferation of islet tissue from ducts or ductules. The distorted interlobular ducts or islets of Langerhans, combined with fibrosis and loss of exocrine acini, may challenge the diagnostic skills of experienced pathologists, even on permanent sections.[88] About 5% of carcinomas arise in chronic pancreatitis. Typically, infiltrating carcinomas disregard the normal lobular architecture, although focally the tumor may respect lobular architectural outlines. Cytologic features are therefore always important. The criterion of fourfold variation in nuclear size is a useful aid in the diagnosis of cancer at frozen section.[89] Other useful features for a diagnosis of cancer include absent ductal lumina, disorganized duct distribution, irregular large eosinophilic nucleoli, vascular and perineural invasion, and infiltration of the duodenal wall.[89] It must be remembered that normally there are accessory mucus glands around the ampulla that extend into the muscle coat of the duodenum and should not be mistaken for infiltrating carcinoma.[90] Individual cancer cells may show nuclear dyspolarity (irregular placement in the cell), nuclear enlargement, clearing of the nucleoplasm, thickening of the nuclear membranes, and irregular nucleoli. Mitoses may not be plentiful. Perineural or intraneural invasion is a useful diagnostic feature, but be aware that benign pancreatic acini, ducts, or islet cells can, on rare occasions, be found intraneurally.[91]

DIFFERENTIAL DIAGNOSIS

The main differential diagnostic considerations are periampullary carcinomas and pancreatitis. Tumors of special types should also be kept in mind. Chronic pancreatitis is often seen in people younger than 40 years of age, whereas most pancreatic cancer patients are older than 50. Grossly, pancreatic carcinomas are ill-defined solid masses and focal pancreatitis may on occasion assume that appearance. Microscopically, there is a superficial resemblance between chronic pancreatitis and cancer, insofar as both display glands in fibrous stroma, but in the case of cancer, the stroma is desmoplastic and the glands are cytologically atypical and infiltrative. In contrast, in pancreatitis, lobular outlines are preserved, the fibrosis is scarring, the ducts are benign, and remnants of normal pancreas show regenerative proliferation with no cytologic atypia. Islets of Langerhans are present and are sometimes distorted and enlarged by pseudoneoplastic proliferation from ducts. Also, islet cell clusters may be associated with nerves[92] and can be mistaken for perineural invasion. Ampullary carcinoma and carcinoma of the lower end of the common bile duct have similar histomorphology to that of pancreatic adenocarcinoma, and the main method of distinction is careful gross and microscopic examination. Even then, a distinction is not always possible. Only a minority of ampullary and bile duct carcinomas carry the codon 12 mutation in K-*ras*. Carcinomas of the duodenal mucosa usually have goblet cells or a resemblance to colonic carcinoma, and residual adenoma is commonly present. Special types of neoplasm, such as intraductal papillary-mucinous tumor, mucinous cystic tumor, serous cystadenoma, acinar cell carcinoma, solid and cystic pseudopapillary tumor, pancreatoblastoma, and islet cell tumor, each have individual peculiar patterns that make misdiagnosis unlikely. Pancreatoblastomas arise in children and show squamoid nests and acinar cell differentiation. Endocrine cell tumors may include glandular or microglandular foci, but they are mucin negative and associated with trabecular, nested, or solid areas, with a rich capillary vasculature. Acinar cell carcinomas are more likely to be confused with endocrine cell tumors than with adenocarcinomas and they give positive immunostaining for pancreatic enzymes.[1]

PROGNOSTIC FACTORS AND STAGING

Pancreatic cancer has the worst prognosis of all gastrointestinal malignancies. Forty percent of patients are dead within 3 months of diagnosis, 65% within 6 months, and close to 90% within 1 year.[23] Only 0.5% to 3% survive 5 years.[23,93] Radical surgical excision gives the only chance of long-term survival, but even in specialist referral centers, only 15% of patients have resectable tumors at diagnosis; 40% have localized but unresectable tumors and 45% have distant metastases.[9,94] Population studies reveal a much lower resectability rate—4.2% in Sweden and 2.6% in Great Britain,[93,95] although it has increased in Sweden to about 7% overall in recent years.[93] Less than 10% of French patients with left-sided pancreatic cancer are candidates for surgery.[96] The main reasons for irresectability are the presence of distant metastases and retropancreatic spread encasing the great vessels.

The marginal benefit from surgical resection is not great. The National Cancer Data Base report shows a modest survival advantage for resectable versus nonresectable tumors: 1 year—48% versus 23%, 2 years—24% versus 9%, 3 years—17% versus 6%, respectively,[9] and these groups (resectable and nonresectable) are not comparable to begin with. Five-year survival for all resected pancreatic carcinomas is between 15% and 20% in specialized units, but even 5-year survival is not tantamount to cure, because deaths continue to occur past 5 years.[94,97–99] In cases registered at the Japanese pancreatic cancer registry, the resection rate is now 36% and the 5-year survival rate of patients who underwent resection is 18.2% (overall 6.5%).[5] We do not know the natural history of resectable tumors that remain unresected and no trials of surgery versus other therapies have been conducted in patients with operable tumors. The survival picture of patients with carcinoma of the head of pancreas is more gloomy: Only 3 of 81 (3.7%) patients in a recent study survived 4 years.[100] It is likely, too, that we are diagnosing the disease earlier through improved imaging, and these patients would naturally have a somewhat longer survival.

The prognosis for patients whose tumors are unresectable is so poor that individual prognostic factors have not been studied extensively in this context. A French study found that for patients treated surgically but without excision, median survival times were shortest with biliary stenting and cholecystoenteric bypass (2.6 and 3.2 months, respectively) and longest with choledochoenteric bypass with or without gastrojejunostomy (5.0 or 5.5 months, respectively).[101] Jaundice at presentation was the only independent favorable feature identified in one Norwegian study of patient-related factors.[102] This may be because patients with carcinomas of the head of pancreas who present with jaundice have relatively smaller neoplasms than nonicteric patients. Nonicteric carcinomas of the pancreatic head normally arise in an area far from the biliary tree and have grown to be large tumors by the time they present.[103,104]

In the Memorial Sloan-Kettering Cancer Center series of 684 patients with pancreatic cancer, only 17% were treated by resection with curative intent. Median survival after resection was 14.3 months, compared with 4.9 months without resection. The 5-year survival rate for patients who underwent resection was 10.2%, but there were several deaths from the tumor in the sixth postoperative year, so 5-year survival cannot be equated to cure.[94] For patients whose tumors are resected, the influence of individual prognostic factors is not conclusively established, because most series are small. Tumor-related pathologic prognostic factors are listed in Table 7–4.

Histologic Type

Special types of tumor are not comparable to ductal adenocarcinoma. Mucinous cystadenocarcinoma, the malignant form of the mucinous cystic neoplasm, should not be considered alongside ordinary pancreatic adenocarcinoma, as it has a much better prognosis and is morphologically and genetically distinct.[105] Similarly, intraductal papillary carcinoma (papillary mucinous tumor) has a far better prognosis than does ordinary ductal carcinoma, because most cases are noninvasive at the time of presentation.[106,107]

Table 7–4. Pathologic Prognostic Factors for Adenocarcinoma of the Pancreas

Mitotic index
Tumor size
Extrapancreatic extension
Peritoneal involvement
Lymph node involvement
Venous invasion
Involvement of margins of resection
Distant metastases
Histologic type and grade

Histologic Grade

Most studies agree that moderately to poorly differentiated tumors have a worse prognosis than well-differentiated tumors.[77,98,104,108–111] The 5-year survival for poorly differentiated adenocarcinomas was 10% versus almost 50% for well-differentiated carcinomas in the multivariate analysis from Memorial Hospital.[98] There have, however, been dissenting studies,[112] the most important being the Japanese registry figures quoted by Yamamoto et al., which showed no survival difference for the three grades (11.1%, 9.1%, and 9.1%).[113]

Tumor Size

Although it has not been confirmed in some reports,[112–114] most studies have found that small tumors (variously defined as < 4.4 cm, < 4.0 cm, < 2.5 cm, < 2.0 cm) are associated with the greatest chance of cure by surgery and, on average, have the longest survival.[98,113,115,116] Indeed, tumor size was the strongest predictor of prognosis following regional pancreatectomy in one series.[117] In multivariate analysis, tumor size has proved significant, with tumors < 2.5 cm in diameter having a better prognosis.[98] Japanese studies show that tumors < 2.0 cm in diameter are more often (90%) resectable and have longer postoperative survival times.[113] This relatively favorable prognosis of small tumors has also been confirmed by a study from the Netherlands.[115] However, small tumors with distant metastasis seem to carry a worse prognosis than do large tumors with distant metastasis.[115] If tumors are not resectable at the time of operation, the size of the tumor does not appear to affect survival. Many small tumors are not curable: 40% have lymph node metastases, 30% have portal system involvement, and 24% have retroperitoneal involvement at the time of diagnosis.[118] Small pancreatic cancers (< 4 cm), which are macroscopically confined to the pancreas, often show microscopic extrapancreatic tumor extension, especially invasion to the retroperitoneal tissues and to the periaortic lymph nodes. This suggested to Ohta and colleagues that an aggressive surgical approach, including complete resection of surrounding connective tissues in the retroperitoneum and extensive lymph node dissection, is necessary to improve the surgical therapeutic results, even for small pancreatic cancers.[119] Only 12% of resected tumors are T1 (confined to the pancreas), and they tend not to have neural plexus invasion and to have a low rate of lymph node metastasis.[120] Sellner and Machacek found a highly significant negative correlation ($p < 0.0001$) between tumor mass and survival for radically treated periampullary carcinomas.[121] Brower et al. found that tumor size was itself a predictor of nodal status.[108]

Extrapancreatic Extension and Resection Margin Involvement

Extrapancreatic extension is inextricably related to perineural infiltration on the posterior surface of the pancreas and is a significant adverse prognostic indicator.[112,114,122–124] The frequency of extrapancreatic extension is directly related to tumor size. There is extrapancreatic extension in approximately 20% of tumors ≤ 2 cm in size, in 50% of those 2.1 to 4.0 cm in size, in 77% of tumors 4.1 to 6.0 cm in size, and in 90% of tumors > 6.0 cm.[113] Invasion of the anterior pancreatic capsule is also an adverse prognostic indicator.[122,123] Invasion of adjacent organs significantly diminishes survival.[112]

Resection margins are involved in 50% of resections for carcinoma of the head of pancreas.[125] The peripancreatic soft tissue margin is the margin most commonly involved. It should be inked before further specimen dissection.[125] Microscopic involvement of the margins of excision by cancer is an independent predictor of poor survival.[103,122,123] Nagakawa et al. found that all patients with microscopic involvement of margins were dead within 3 years, whereas 68.8% of those with a negative margin survived 5 years or more.[122] The involvement of the margin was invariably a result of perineural spread.[122] Over 70% of failures after curative resection involve a component of local failure, and 20% are local failures only.[126] These findings are the basis for protocols evaluating preoperative or intraoperative radiotherapy. Pancreatic tumor extension into peripancreatic fat or nerves, and invasion of ampullary carcinomas into duodenal wall, unfavorably influenced the N1 category (tumors with local lymph node metastasis).[103] Residual tumor is classified as microscopic (R1) or macroscopic (R2). In the Japanese Cancer Registry, the prognosis for patients with R2 disease was no better than for patients who were treated without resection.[113]

Perineural Invasion

Perineural invasion is extratumoral invasion of perineural spaces and of nerves. It is an important route for the spread of pancreatic carcinoma[103,122,127–129] (see Fig. 7–9). Perineural invasion by adenocarcinoma is not confined to the periphery of nerves but penetrates the perineurium and becomes intimately associated with Schwann cells and axons in the endoneurium, resulting in nerve damage that may provoke pain.[128] If the perineural spread involves the retropancreatic tissue and the pancreatic neural plexus, the tumor is hard to ablate surgically. Perineural spread was present in 95% of carcinomas of head of pancreas in the series of Yamaguchi et al., and it proved a significant adverse prognostic factor.[103,104] Combination of two series of carefully documented resected cancers of the pancreas showed 32 of 38 (84%) had invasion of the pancreatic nerve plexus and retropancreatic tissue.[123] However, the proportion was much lower (43% of 65 patients) in a third study.[127] The degree of extrapancreatic neural invasion tends to increase with the degree of intrapancreatic neural invasion.[123,127] Nerve plexus invasion is also significantly associated with retroperitoneal extension but is not significantly associated with tumor location, tumor size, histologic type, or lymph vessel invasion.[127] Invasion of the nerve plexus is also associated with involvement of the surgical resection margin.[123] These studies make it clear that en bloc resection of the retropancreatic tissue to include the nerve plexus and fat tissue is necessary for the adequate surgical treatment of cancer of the pancreatic head. Transforming growth factor-α (TGF-α) is abundant in nerves in the pancreas, whereas epidermal growth factor receptor (EGFR) is displayed on the cells of the adenocarcinoma, suggesting that interaction of TGF-α in nerves with EGFR on cancer cells may constitute a paracrine mechanism that provides a growth advantage for pancreatic adenocarcinoma.[128]

Peritoneal Involvement

As disseminated peritoneal metastasis renders the cancer incurable and contraindicates excisional surgery, few studies have looked at it objectively. A distinction may need to be drawn between disseminated metastases and a focal peritoneal surface tumor. Tsunoda et al. found a significant difference in the 1-year survival rates between patients whose test findings were positive and those who were negative for serosal involvement and had undergone surgery, but they found no difference in the postoperative cumulative survival curves.[124]

Venous Invasion

Venous invasion is believed to be a function of tumor location, rather than an indicator of aggressive tumor biology.[130] Venous invasion did not seem to affect survival in one study[110] but was a significant adverse finding in another.[124]

Lymph Node Involvement

The presence of lymph node involvement is an independent prognostic factor in most studies.[100,109,112,113,123] Survival diminishes with the involvement of any nodes and again with involvement of secondary or tertiary nodes (n_2 and n_3 in the Japanese staging system).[131–134] Japanese registry figures for cumulative survival are 30.2% at 5 years when no nodes are involved, 7.2% when group 1 nodes are involved, 3.2% when group 2 nodes are involved, and no 3-year survival when group 3 lymph nodes are involved.[113] The surgical pathology report should document the total number of lymph nodes present and the number involved by tumor.

Lymphatic invasion was present in 85% of carcinomas of head of pancreas in one series[113] but was not independently significant, whereas the rate was 73% in another study and was significant.[112]

Distant Metastasis

Distant metastasis, like peritoneal involvement, has the dire clinical connotation of incurability and significantly worsens prognosis.[114] However, in the study of Tsunoda et al., there was no significant difference in postoperative cumulative survival curves between patients who had distant metastases and those who did not. This surprising lack of difference may have been due to the small number of patients in the group who were operated upon despite having metastases.[124]

Tumor Site

Some studies suggest that location in the head of pancreas predicts a better prognosis than does location elsewhere,[135,136] but this location did not have independent prognostic influence in the one large multifactorial analysis.[98]

Histologic Parameters

Eskelinen et al. performed a retrospective clinicopathologic study of quantitative histologic parameters on 111 patients with a mean follow-up period of 6 years. Most of the patients did not have curative resections and the tissue studied consisted of needle biopsy and surgical biopsy specimens. A multifactor regression analysis of survival identified the volume-corrected mitotic index as the most important histologic prognosticator ($p = 0.009$), with other histologic factors having no independent prognostic value.[137] This parameter should be included in future studies of resected specimens to evaluate whether it remains an independent prognostic factor when compared with extrapancreatic spread, perineural invasion outside the pancreas, and lymph node metastasis. Percentage of Ki-67–positive cells by immunohistochemistry, another measure of mitotic activity, has been independently found to be the most important determinant of survival (long survival correlating with low positivity).[138] Overexpression of tissue plasminogen activator type 2 is associated with significantly longer survival than is negative or weak expression.[139]

DNA Ploidy and Proliferative Index

DNA diploidy and proliferative index are found to predict survival in some studies,[140] but not in others,[141,142] but the technical methodologies used to determine ploidy varied. Some authors contend that DNA diploid tumors represent a less aggressive subset of pancreatic carcinoma.[140,143,144] Allison and colleagues[140] found that cancer cell DNA content (measured by absorption cytometry on Feulgen-stained nuclei) correlated with survival. Their patients with diploid tumors had a median survival time of 25 months, compared with 10.5 months for those with aneuploid tumors. Tetraploid tumors also had a more favorable prognosis than did nontetraploid aneuploid tumors.[144] Hyoty et al. found, however, that neither aneuploidy nor synthesis phase fraction correlated significantly with size, stage, or differentiation and the survival (median, 9 months) of the patients with DNA-aneuploid tumors, when compared with survival of the patients with diploid tumors (median, 14 months). They concluded that DNA analysis by flow cytometry is not helpful in selecting patients with resectable pancreatic carcinoma who will benefit from resection.[136] These flow cytometry results are mutually incompatible and vividly demonstrate to nonexperts the problems encountered when treatment decisions are based on flow cytometric analysis of solid neoplasms. Weger et al. assessed pancreatic carcinomas and chronic pancreatitis cases by both flow cytometry and by image cytometry.[145] The patients with carcinomas whose cell nuclei showed a triploid DNA distribution survived a significantly shorter time than did those with tumor cell populations of nontriploid DNA distribution patterns.

Treatment-Related Factors

Treatment-related factors undoubtedly play a role in survival, and the extent and successfulness of resection are important variables. Resections in which surgical margins are free of disease (R0) give much better prognosis than do those with residual disease (R1 or R2).[113,135] Surgeon-related factors undoubtedly play an important role, too, and studies have shown that centers with higher surgical volumes of pancreatic resection had lower mortality rates and shorter mean lengths of stay associated with these procedures than did low-volume centers.[146–149]

Staging

There are two staging systems in use, the Union Internationale Contre le Cancer (UICC) or tumor-node-metastasis (TNM) system and the Japan Pancreas Society (JPS) system. The UICC (TNM) staging system (Table 7–5) is used widely in oncology practice throughout the West and is periodically modified to enhance its predictive capacity.[150] UICC staging is based on the proposition that the three factors of greatest import to prognosis are tumor size and extent, lymph node metastasis, and distant metastasis. UICC staging of pancreatic cancer assumes that lymph node metastasis is the most important prognostic factor. Thus, all tumors without lymph node metastasis are included in stages I and II, regardless of their size and whether they extend into peripancreatic tissue, the portal venous system, or adjacent organs. Unlike the Japanese system, the UICC system fails to take account of serosal, retroperitoneal, and venous invasion. T2 patients with extrapancreatic spread are still UICC stage I but are JPS

Table 7–5. TNM Staging of Pancreatic Carcinoma

Symbol	Description		
Primary tumor (T)			
pT1	Tumor limited to pancreas, ≤ 2 cm in greatest dimension		
pT2	Tumor limited to the pancreas, ≥ 2 cm in greatest dimension		
pT3	Tumor extends directly to any of the following: duodenum, bile duct, peripancreatic tissues (peripancreatic tissues include the surrounding retroperitoneal fat [retroperitoneal soft tissue or retroperitoneal space], including mesentery [mesenteric fat], mesocolon, greater and lesser omentum, and peritoneum; direct invasion to bile ducts and duodenum includes involvement of ampulla of Vater)		
pT3	Tumor extends directly into any of the following: stomach, spleen, colon, adjacent large vessels (adjacent large vessels are the portal vein, celiac artery, and superior mesenteric and common hepatic arteries and veins [not splenic vessels])		
Regional lymph nodes (N)			
NX	Regional lymph nodes cannot be assessed		
pN0	No regional lymph node metastases		
pN1	Regional lymph node metastases		
pN1a	Metastasis in a single regional lymph node		
pN1b	Metastasis in multiple regional lymph nodes		
Distant metastases (M)			
MX	Distant metastases cannot be assessed		
M0	No distant metastases		
M1	Distant metastases		
Stage Groupings			
Stage 0	Tis	N0	M0
Stage 1	T1	N0	M0
	T2	N0	M0
Stage II	T3	N0	M0
Stage III	T1	N1	M0
	T2	N1	M0
	T3	N1	M0
Stage IVA	T4	Any N	M0
Stage IVB	Any T	Any N	M1

stage III, and patients with venous involvement can be UICC stage II, whereas they are JPS stage IV. The TNM/pTNM-defined stage grouping is complemented by the R classification, which describes the presence or absence of residual tumor after treatment.[151]

The JPS staging system (Table 7–6) has better predictive capacity than UICC staging and relies on tumor size and local spread rather than on lymph node metastasis. The attributes assessed are tumor size, lymph node metastasis (N), serosal invasion (S), retroperitoneal invasion (Rp), and invasion of the portal venous system (V). Nagakawa et al. found that there was no significant survival difference between JPS stages I, II, and III but that there was a significant difference for stage IV in patients who underwent resection.[122] Zerbi et al. found no significant difference in survival between UICC stages in a multivariate analysis, but they did find a significant survival difference for JPS stage.[114] UICC staging was retrospectively compared with JPS staging by Tsunoda et al., using 229 consecutive patients.[124] They concluded that the UICC system understaged some tumors with a poor prognosis.

Table 7–7 shows the correlation of UICC and JPS stage classifications in patients who have undergone resection. By UICC staging, 7% of the patients were stage IV and 65% stage III, but by JPS, 39% of the patients belonged to stage IV and 42% to stage III. Thus, by UICC, patients were classified to a less advanced stage than by JPN. Curative resection rates in JPS stages II and III were significantly higher than those in UICC. For 60 patients who underwent surgical resection, postoperative cumulative survival (PCS) curves and rates by each staging criterion were calculated by the Kaplan–Meier method. The factors examined were tumor size,

Table 7–6. Japan Pancreas Society Staging

Stage I	T_1 (0–2 cm)	N_0	S_0	Rp_0	V_0
Stage II	T_2 (2.1–4.0 cm)	N_1	S_1	Rp_1	V_1
Stage III	T_3 (4.1–6.0 cm)	N_2	S_2	Rp_2	V_2
Stage IV*	T_4 (> 6.1 cm)	N_3	S_3	Rp_3	V_3

N_0: No lymph node involvement
N_1: Involvement of primary group of nodes situated close to the tumor
N_2: Involvement of secondary group of lymph nodes between N_1 and N_3
N_3: Involvement of tertiary group of lymph nodes regarded as juxtaregional lymph nodes

S = serosal invasion. RP = retroperitoneal invasion. V = invasion of the portal venous system

S_0	Rp_0	V_0	Absence of invasion
S_1	Rp_1	V_1	Suspected invasion
S_2	Rp_2	V_2	Definite invasion
S_3	Rp_3	V_3	Severe invasion

* Distant metastasis, including liver metastasis or peritoneal dissemination, is allocated to stage IV.

Adapted from: Tsunoda T, Ura K, Eto T, et al. UICC and Japanese stage classifications for carcinoma of the pancreas. Int J Pancreatol 8:205–214, 1991.

lymph node metastasis, distant metastasis, serosal invasion, retroperitoneal invasion, and invasion of the portal venous system. Among these prognostic factors, significant differences in the PCS curves were demonstrated between patients with two specific features—retroperitoneal involvement and portal venous invasion—and those with negative findings for those features. In UICC staging, these factors are not taken into account. This explains why cancers are assigned to a less advanced UICC stage than in JPS staging.

Zerbi et al. staged cancers in 74 Italian patients, who underwent resection, according to both UICC and JPS classifications.[114] Table 7–8 illustrates the superior predictive capacity of the JPS system. A radical resection was possible in 48 patients (65%); the survival was significantly worse in the nonradical resection group. The survival difference among UICC stages was not significant in a multivariate analysis, whereas among JPS stages a significant survival difference was found by both univariate and multivariate analysis. Tumor invasion of the retroperitoneal tissues and the presence of distant metastasis were indicators of a significantly worse prognosis. Lymph node involvement, tumor size, and serosal invasion had no significant effect on survival. Peritoneal cytology and liver biopsies did not provide further prognostic information.

Tannapfel et al. used the UICC staging only and found that in 81 patients tumor stage was the most important prognostic factor: In UICC stages I, II, and III, the median survival times were 13, 16, and 8 months, respectively.[112]

Table 7–7. Correlation of UICC and JPS Staging Classes

	JPS I	JPS II	JPS III	JPS IV	Total
UICC I	2	4	4	1	11
UICC II	0	0	3	3	6
UICC III	0	6	18	15	39
UICC IV	0	0	0	4	4
Total	2	10	25	23	60

Key: JPS, Japanese Pancreas Society; UICC, Union Internationale Contra le Cancer.
Adapted from Tsunoda T, Ura K, Eto T, et al.: UICC and Japanese stage classifications for carcinoma of the pancreas. Int J Pancreatol 8:205–214, 1991.

Table 7–8. Median Survival in Months According to UICC and JPS Stages

	Stage I	Stage II	Stage III	Stage IV
UICC/TNM	17	10	12	6
JPS		29	14	7

Key: JPS, Japanese Pancreas Society; TNM, tumor-node-metastasis; UICC, Union Internationale Contra le Cancer.

SPREAD AND METASTASIS

The duodenum and stomach are often directly invaded by carcinomas of the head of pancreas. The spleen, left adrenal, and left kidney can be involved by carcinomas of the tail. The transverse colon is mainly involved by cancers of the body of pancreas. Peritoneal metastases are commonly found at presentation in primary carcinomas of the body and tail but less often in tumors of the head of pancreas. These secondary tumors involve the intestines, stomach, gallbladder, pouch of Douglas, and diaphragm. Peritoneal metastases are present in about 50% of patients with pancreatic cancer at the time of death and are the second most common site of involvement, following the liver. The small size of peritoneal metastases precludes their identification by CT scan; they have to be identified by direct inspection, either at laparotomy or laparoscopy. Adding laparoscopy to the staging protocol permits preoperative identification of patients who will not benefit from surgery. Malignant cells are also found in peritoneal washings in 20% to 30% of patients who otherwise have no peritoneal or liver metastases and is an adverse prognostic indicator.[152,153] Laparoscopy can also detect liver metastases that are missed by CT, ultrasound, and angiography, thus avoiding unnecessary laparotomy.[154] In 13% of patients at autopsy, the amount of ascites was disproportionate to the severity of peritoneal dissemination, vessel invasion, or liver disease in chronic pancreatitis.[155]

Hematogenous metastasis to the liver was found in 31.3% of patients at laparotomy.[156] The incidence was 22.9% in patients with carcinoma of the head of pancreas and 47.3% in those with cancer of the pancreas body or tail. All patients with a tumor size of < 2 cm were free of liver metastasis, but 37.5% of those with tumors > 6 cm in diameter had liver metastasis. Of patients with no lymph node involvement, 6.3% had liver metastasis, but 50% of patients with distant lymph node metastasis had liver metastasis, too. The mean survival of patients with liver metastasis was 3.1 months, less than half that of patients free of liver metastasis.[156] Liver metastases can uncommonly form thin, flat lesions on the surface of the liver that are not amenable to diagnosis by imaging but can be found by laparoscopy. When a patient has no local recurrence and a solitary metastasis in the liver, surgical resection of the liver metastasis should be performed.[157] With longer patient survival, there may be an increasing rate of metastasis to various organs. One study found metastasis to the liver in 72.3%, to the lungs in 52.1%, to the adrenals in 24.5%, to the small intestine in 21.1%, to the kidneys in 9.6%, and to the abdominal wall in 3.2% of the patients.[158]

Para-aortic lymph node metastasis can be found even in small cancers, and these nodes should be dissected en bloc during radical resections of pancreatic cancer.[119] Tian et al. concluded that use of anticytokeratin monoclonal antibody to study lymph nodes for occult metastasis was not warranted as a routine measure, although it did increase the pickup rate for nodal metastasis.[159]

Cutaneous metastasis from pancreatic carcinoma is uncommon and presents as umbilical nodules of adenocarcinoma that may stain for CA 19-9.[22] Micrometastasis in bone marrow has been detected in cytologic bone marrow preparations using anticytokeratin antibodies.[153] Cells were detected in 25 (52%) of 48 patients. On follow-up examination, tumor relapse was found to be significantly associated with positive cells in the bone marrow.

AUTOPSY FINDINGS

Autopsies of patients who died of pancreatic cancer show intrapancreatic metastasis or multicentric cancers in 8%.[155] In 20% of patients, pancreatic cancer skips the primary lymph node filter to metastasize to the secondary chain of nodes. Pulmonary metastasis occurs without liver metastasis in 8% of patients. Carcinoma of the body and/or tail of the pancreas is more likely to evince transperitoneal as well as hematogenous dissemination than is carcinoma of the head of the pancreas. Small tumors (< 2 cm in diameter) may be associated with remote metastasis in up to 64% of patients. Chronic obstructive pancreatitis may complicate pancreatic carcinoma in up to 12% of patients, whereas, in 5% of patients, pancreatic carcinoma probably develops in preexisting chronic pancreatitis. In 13% of patients, the amount of ascites may be disproportionate to the severity of peritoneal dissemination, vessel invasion, or liver disease. Systemic complications that often contribute to death are thromboembolic disease, severe infection, stress ulcer, acute hemorrhagic erosive gastritis, and cachexia.[155] Thrombosis has long been recognized as a complication of pancreatic carcinoma, especially carcinoma of the body or tail of pancreas. In one autopsy series, the incidence of thrombosis was 24%.[17]

TREATMENT

The only chance of cure, and a faint one, is surgical excision by pancreatoduodenectomy. Extended clearance of lymph nodes and connective tissue and dissection of autonomic nerves around the celiac and superior mesenteric arteries has been used since the 1980s by Japanese surgeons and is now the standard of treatment in specialist centers in the West. The clearance should include even the para-aortic lymph nodes and the nodes around the superior mesenteric artery.[132] The very high morbidity rates of earlier years have been lowered by preserving the pylorus.[160] Modern surgical techniques, in the hands of specialists, have resulted in a steep decline in mortality from the procedure itself. Trede et al. reported 118 successive pancreatoduodenectomies (for a variety of indications) without a hospital death.[97] This contrasts with a 5% mortality among 201 patients who had cancer of the pancreas and underwent resection at Johns Hopkins Hospital between 1970 and 1994 but only 1 death in the most recently resected 149 patients.[99,161] Nagakawa et al. reported a 60-day mortality of 15% since 1973 for patients having extended pancreatic resection by their translateral retroperitoneal en bloc technique.[132] Patients with both negative margins and negative lymph nodes had a median survival of 32 months and a 5-year survival of 40%,[161] or 43%.[132] Fifty percent of patients have tumor extension to the margins of pancreatectomy specimens, and this justifies the trials of preoperative or intraoperative radiotherapy and postoperative chemoradiation that are in progress.[70]

Local failure after pancreatic resection is a significant problem that could be addressed by adjuvant radiotherapy and chemotherapy.[126] Seventy-three percent of recurrences after curative resection of pancreatic carcinoma had a component of local failure and 19% were local failures only. Forty-two percent of failures involved peritoneum and 62% involved liver metastases. Adjuvant postoperative radiation is an independent predictor of long survival.[126]

The frequency of retroperitoneal involvement and of spread to para-aortic lymph nodes suggests that extended retroperitoneal resection, including nerve plexi and para-aortic lymph nodes, should be included in curative resections for patients with stage I or II pancreatic cancer.[129,131]

A new cytidine analogue, gemcitabine, was recently shown to be superior to 5-fluorouracil (5-FU) and to slightly prolong survival.[162] It has been approved by the U.S. Food and Drug Administration for chemotherapy for pancreatic carcinoma. There are ongoing trials of the combination of gemcitabine and 5-FU and of various doses and methods of delivery of gemcitabine.[163]

MORPHOLOGIC VARIANTS OF DUCTAL ADENOCARCINOMA

Mucinous Noncystic (Colloid) Carcinoma

This tumor displays copious extracellular mucin, exceeding 50% of the tumor volume, similar to mucinous carcinomas of the stomach or colon, but does not have a cystic component. It may be combined with usual-type duct carcinoma. It should be distinguished from carcinoma arising in mucinous cystic tumors and papillary mucinous tumors. The average size of the tumor is 4.3 cm.[164] The cut surface is gelatinous but not cystic. Microscopically, the mucinous lakes are bordered by a layer of neoplastic epithelium, often well differentiated, and clumps of tumor cells float in the mucin (Fig. 7–10). There may be a minor component of signet ring cells. The stroma may be collagenous. This tumor constitutes 1% to 2% of pancreatic carcinomas. It can be diagnosed by FNAC.[165] The principal location for this tumor is the head of pancreas. The demographics are no different from those for usual ductal adeno-

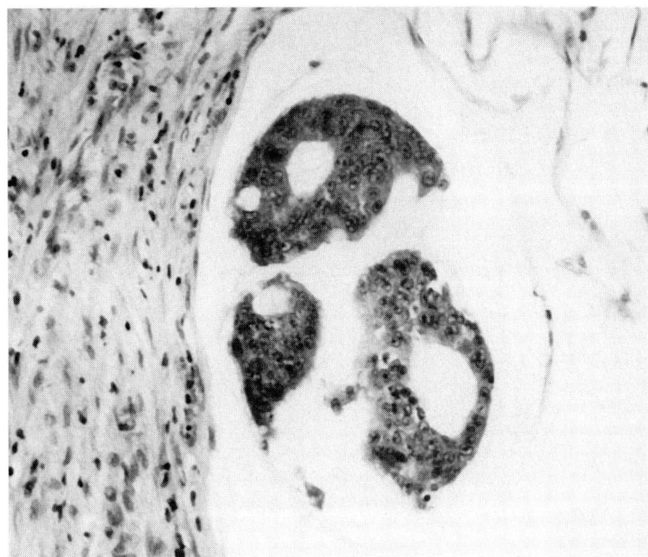

Figure 7–10. Colloid carcinoma of the pancreas with tumor cells "floating" in a pool of mucin.

carcinoma. Prognostic data from the Johns Hopkins Hospital showed a 14% 5-year survival in patients who underwent resection. The differential diagnosis is both papillary mucinous tumor and mucinous cystic neoplasm (see Chapter 8), which predominates in women and has an ovarian-like stroma.

Signet Ring Cell Carcinoma

Signet ring cell carcinoma is rare when rigorously defined as a tumor that is predominately composed of cells that each contain a discrete cytoplasmic mucinous vacuole. It has been referred to in major series[39,75] and textbooks[166] and in single-case reports[167] (Figs. 7–11 and 7–12). Signet ring cell carcinoma infiltrates the pancreas diffusely and may cause diffuse enlargement. One reported case involved strongly positive immunostaining for CEA and was associated with very high serum CEA levels.[167] This diagnosis should not be made unless the signet ring cell component exceeds 50% of the tumor area. The main differential diagnosis is metastatic gastric signet ring cell carcinoma.

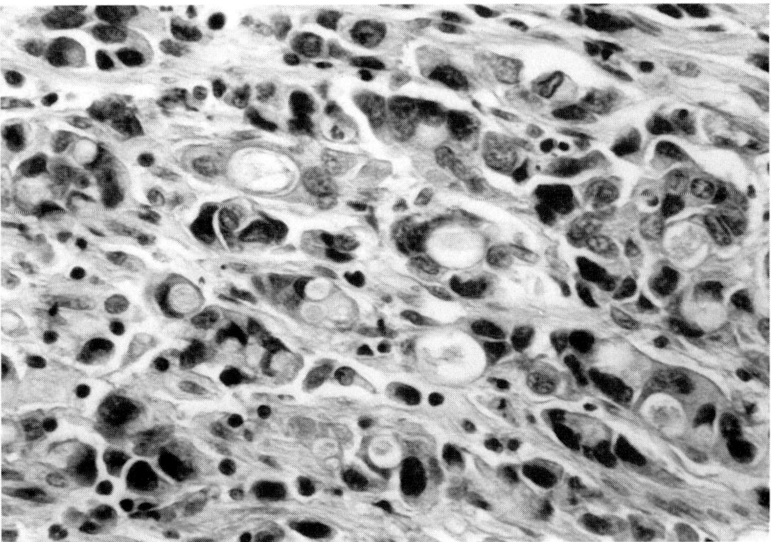

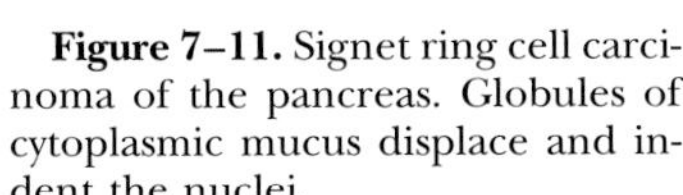

Figure 7–11. Signet ring cell carcinoma of the pancreas. Globules of cytoplasmic mucus displace and indent the nuclei.

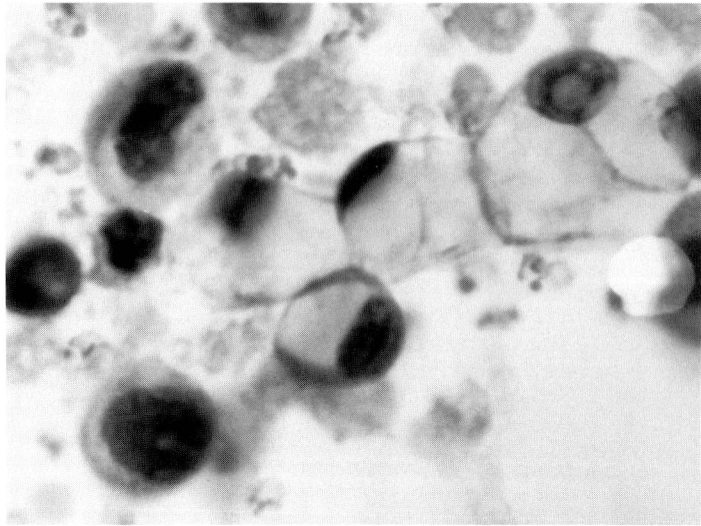

Figure 7–12. Fine-needle aspiration biopsy of a signet ring cell carcinoma. Care must be taken not to confuse this appearance with mucus vacuoles in goblet cells. Attention to nuclear size and details should prevent this mistake.

Adenosquamous Carcinoma

Adenosquamous carcinomas are tumors that contain unequivocally malignant glandular and squamous elements. The squamous component is diagnosed by finding keratinization and intercellular bridges (Fig. 7–13). The frequency of adenosquamous carcinomas is usually quoted at 3% to 4% of cases,[39,75,168,169] but a rate of 11% of cases was found in one series, after more extensive tumor sampling detected small squamous foci that might formerly have been overlooked.[170] If the designation of adenosquamous depends on the diligence with which a squamous component is searched for, it is not surprising that the incidence rises on review, but the World Health Organization (WHO) monograph sensibly recommends that the tumor be diagnosed only when the squamous component accounts for at least 30% of the tumor tissue.[37] In practice, this is not an easy quantitative assessment, because of variable differentiation.

The squamous cell component in adenosquamous carcinoma of the pancreas is generally considered as metaplasia of the preexisting adenocarcinoma, although rare collision tumors are encountered.[171] A case that arose in a mucinous cystadenoma has been reported.[172] In one series of eight patients, the mean age was 56 years, 9 years younger than the mean for other

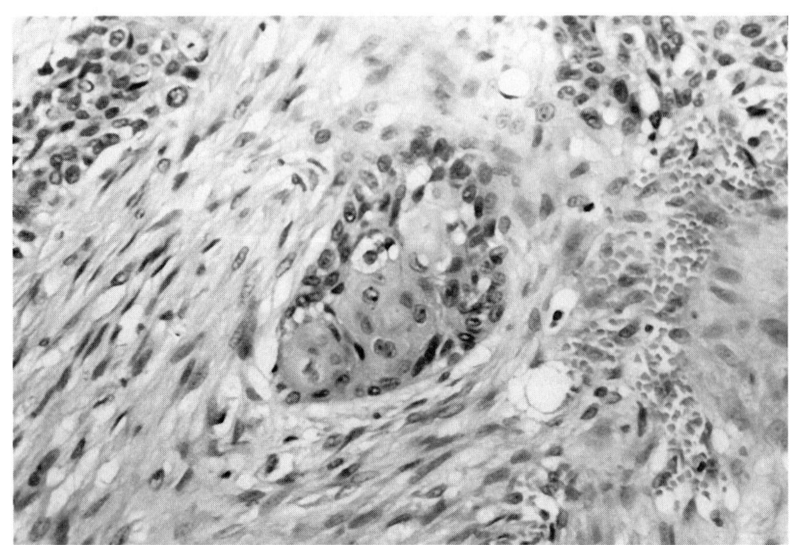

Figure 7–13. Adenosquamous carcinoma of the pancreas. This island of tumor cells shows squamoid differentiation without the presence of keratin.

pancreatic carcinomas.[173] Adenosquamous carcinomas constituted 9% of pancreatic cancers in that series. The site of origin and size of the tumors were similar to those of usual pancreatic carcinoma. Histologically, all eight tumors showed an abrupt transition between adenocarcinoma and squamous cell carcinoma. Squamous cell elements were located at the periphery of the tumors.

The prognosis of adenosquamous tumors is poor, and patients with them exhibit shorter survivals and higher frequency of liver metastases than do patients with adenocarcinoma.[171] The cumulative 1-year survival rate was 21.4%, compared with 42.1% of 72 with adenocarcinoma.[173] Metastasis can be predominantly glandular or squamous or can show a pleomorphic appearance.[169]

Squamous Cell Carcinoma

Pure squamous cell carcinoma of the pancreas is rare and accounts for < 0.5% of all pancreatic carcinomas. Any squamous cell carcinoma of the pancreas must be examined carefully and sampled thoroughly to exclude adenocarcinomatous elements.[169] Squamous cell carcinoma is usually a solid mass but can be cystic. The cyst formation in squamous carcinomas has been ascribed to hemorrhage or ischemia in the center of the tumor rather than to tumor arising in a preexisting pseudocyst.[174] Rarely, hypercalcemia complicates squamous carcinoma.[175] Prognostic data are not available, because of the rarity of pure squamous carcinoma.

Composite Ductal-Endocrine Cell Tumors, Acinar-Endocrine Cell Tumors, and Amphicrine Cell Tumors

Also called ductuloinsular tumors, mixed ductal-endocrine cell tumors are rare tumors in which neoplastic ducts and islet cells are intermingled in fairly even proportions.[176] The WHO monograph states that the endocrine cell component should comprise at least 30% of the tumor tissue.[37] The islet cell component may have an insular, trabecular, or ribbonlike arrangement and may appear to arise out of the ductal elements. The endocrine cells show characteristic dense core granules ultrastructurally. They may contain immunostainable hormones, such as glucagon, insulin,[177] or chromogranin A. Ductal differentiation can be confirmed by mucin staining or by immunostaining for CEA. In the cases reported by Reid et al.,[177] the ducts appeared to be normal morphologically, suggesting that they may be normal entrapped ducts that underwent proliferation and not dysplastic or carcinomatous ducts. The occurrence of these tumors is understandable by consideration of the embryonic pancreas and cases of chronic pancreatitis, where islet cells are seen to arise from terminal ducts. The distinction from a collision tumor is based on the demarcation of the two components in a collision tumor, compared with the intermingling of elements seen in a mixed tumor.

An amphicrine cell is one that contains two differentiating elements, such as mucin and endocrine granules, or exocrine granules and endocrine granules. Amphicrine cells may show bidirectional differentiation in single neoplastic cells. An amphicrine tumor, with features of both acinar and endocrine cell neoplasms, has been reported.[178] Ultrastructurally, both types of granules were identified within the same cell. The immunostains available at that time for endocrine differentiation were negative, but lipase test results were positive. The tumor arose in a 30-year-old woman and was 9.3 cm in diameter, replacing most of the pancreas. It grew as solid nests, ribbons, or acini and was composed of cells with abundant eosinophilic cytoplasm and basal nuclei. There is insufficient data to predict the behavior of these tumors, but any element of ductal carcinoma is likely to impart the usual dire prognosis.

Small Cell Undifferentiated Carcinoma

About 1% of primary carcinomas of the pancreas resemble small cell carcinoma of the lung, both morphologically and functionally.[1,41,179] They probably arise from endocrine cells present within the pancreatic ductal system rather than from the islet cells themselves. This tumor may produce corticotrophin,[179] neuron-specific enolase,[180] or hypercalcemia.[181] Grossly, the tumor is whitish-gray with areas of necrosis that are soft and creamy. Before making a diagnosis of a primary pancreatic tumor, it is mandatory to exclude metastasis from a small cell carcinoma of lung. Small cell carcinoma is usually seen in elderly men who have a history of cigarette smoking. It progresses rapidly and metastasizes widely, as does its pulmonary equivalent.[182] The tumor may, however, respond to chemotherapy regimens used for small cell carcinomas of the lung.[183]

Pleomorphic, Sarcomatoid, and Anaplastic Carcinoma

Pleomorphic, sarcomatoid, and anaplastic tumors have been reported as pleomorphic giant cell carcinomas, pleomorphic large cell carcinomas, sarcomatoid carcinomas, carcinosarcomas, and spindle cell carcinomas. Some of these pleomorphic tumors have both tumor giant cells and an osteoclastic reaction, so there is some overlap with osteoclastic giant cell tumors. A clear-cut distinction between these two types of pleomorphic neoplasm is not always possible.[184–186] Sarcomatoid carcinomas are virtually pure spindle cell neoplasms that express cytokeratins or epithelial membrane antigen, revealing their epithelial origin (Fig. 7–14). Anaplastic carcinomas are composed of dyscohesive tumor giant cells and often show a dense inflammatory infiltrate of neutrophils. Pleomorphic and anaplastic carcinomas have an age and sex distribution similar to that of usual pancreatic carcinomas and constitute about 2% of pancreatic cancers when the criteria for diagnosis are stringent, requiring most of the neoplasm to have sarcomatoid features.[187] The incidence figure might be three times this number if tumors having small areas with pleomorphic features were included.

Grossly, pleomorphic and anaplastic carcinomas tend to be large tumors with hemorrhage and necrosis. They may measure up to 15 cm in diameter. Microscopically, they are characterized by a loose sarcomatoid growth pattern of mononuclear and multinuclear tumor giant cells (Fig. 7–15). Tschang et al. considered the mononuclear tumor giant cell to be the most characteristic histologic feature of these tumors.[184] The cell in question

> [. . . is a large, ovoid or irregular cell, varying from 20 μm to 60 μm in diameter. The nucleus varies from round to angulated or irregular, is bizarre in shape, sometimes extremely large, forming a grotesque, multilobulated nuclear mass. Very often, the nuclei are pushed to the edge of the cells, resulting in bent, reniform, eccentric nuclei. The nuclear chromatin is coarse, hyperchromatic and condensed peripherally along the nuclear membrane. An intranuclear space is a prominent feature in many cells. Occasionally, eosinophilic intranuclear inclusion-like focus is seen. Nucleoli vary in number (none to more than one; usually one or two), prominence (from inconspicuous to large and prominent), and color (from eosinophilic to basophilic). Mitotic figures are numerous including many abnormal forms [Fig. 7–16]. The cytoplasm is usually abundant, eosinophilic and granular. Intracytoplasmic vacuoles, which sometimes stained positively with mucicarmine, may be seen. Phagocytosis of erythrocytes or leukocytes is not observed, but convincing "cannibalism" (one tumor cell being completely surrounded by another) is consistently present[184] (Fig. 7–17).

These authors also say of the giant cells:

> Multinucleate tumor giant cells were seen in every case of pleomorphic carcinoma in our series. The multinucleated tumor giant cells have all the features of the mononuclear tumor giant cells described

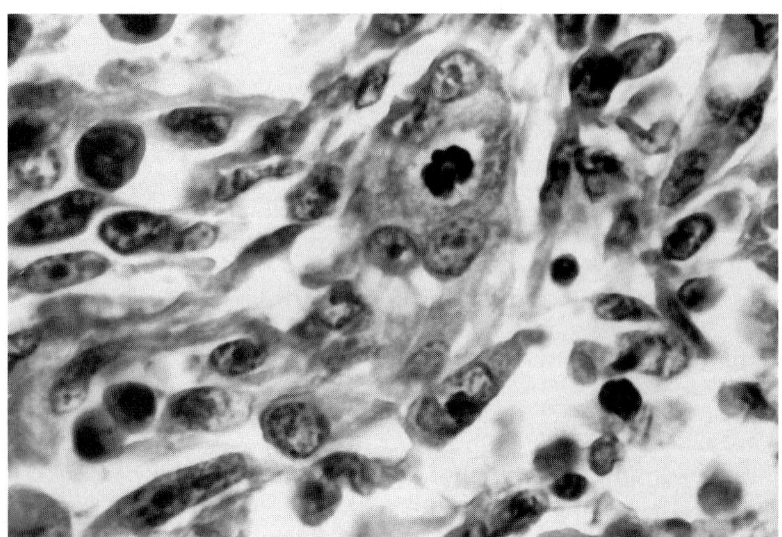

Figure 7–14. Sarcomatoid carcinoma (spindle cell carcinoma) of the pancreas.

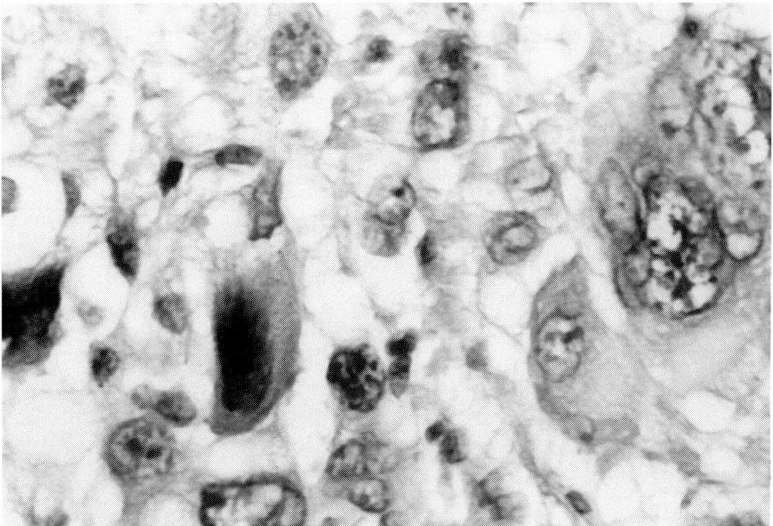

Figure 7–15. Pleomorphic carcinoma of the pancreas with a tumor giant cell.

above, except they are larger, about 40 μm to 140 μm in diameter. They contain multiple ragged, hyperchromatic nuclei, usually two to five in number. None of the multinucleated tumor giant cells had more than 10 nuclei, and none resembled the giant cells seen in giant cell tumor which have many (50 or more) centrally located, round to oval, benign appearing nuclei.[184]

Pleomorphic tumors commonly contain foci of adenocarcinoma, which stain positively for one or more keratin subtypes and, in most cases, for cytokeratins 7, 8, 18, and 19, like usual ductal adenocarcinomas. Likewise, more than half of these tumors show K-*ras* mutations at codon 12 typical of ductal adenocarcinomas.[188,189] These tumors are therefore believed to be of ductal origin but to have undergone what Sommers and Meissner benignly called "a late anaplastic flowering."[168] Loss of heterozygosity is not found for $p16^{INK4}$, *DPC4, APC,* or p53, suggesting that progression of this tumor may be different from that to usual adenocarcinoma.[189] The sarcomatoid areas are generally positive for vimentin and are variably cytokeratin positive. The pleomorphic giant cells also often show dual staining.[189] Pleomorphic carcinomas can arise in mucinous cystadenomas.[168,190,191] A case has also been reported as a malignant fibrous

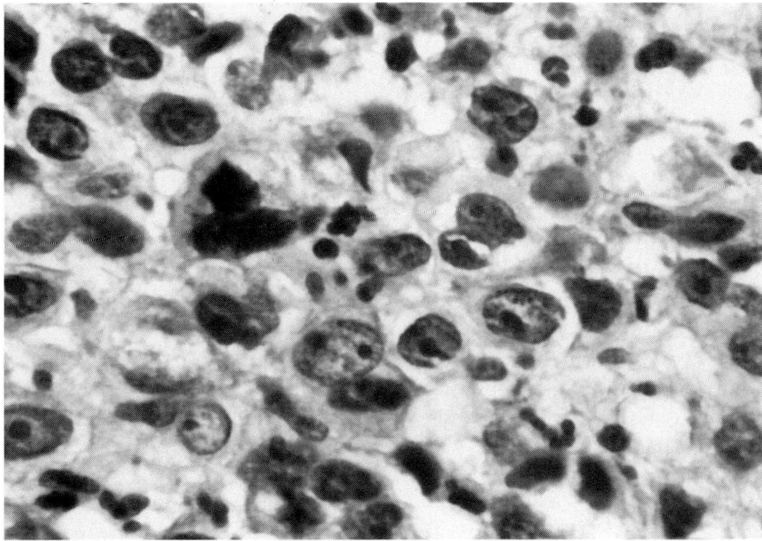

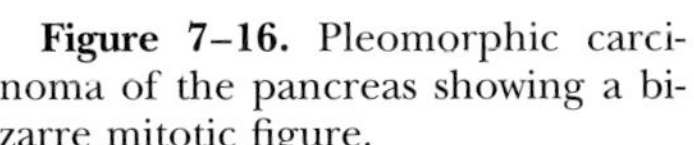

Figure 7–16. Pleomorphic carcinoma of the pancreas showing a bizarre mitotic figure.

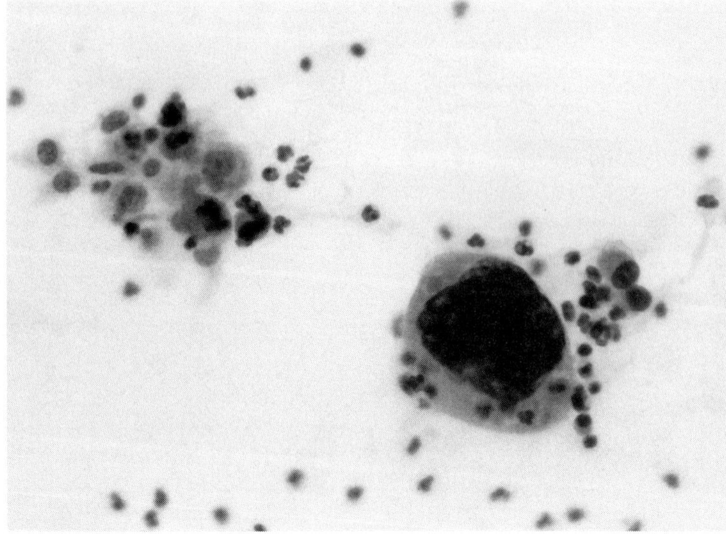

Figure 7–17. Fine-needle aspiraton biopsy of pancreatic pleomorphic carcinoma. Note the giant cell containing phagocytosed neutrophils.

histiocytoma, giant cell type, where there was no evidence of epithelial differentiation.[192] A pancreatic tumor displaying areas of both adenocarcinoma and leiomyosarcoma has been reported. The adenocarcinomatous areas localized to the tumor within the head of the pancreas, whereas the leiomyosarcomatous areas localized to regions of the tumor infiltrating the duodenal wall. Both the adenocarcinomatous and the leiomyosarcomatous areas showed evidence of monoclonality and clonal identity.[193]

Undifferentiated Carcinoma with Osteoclast-like Giant Cells

Rare undifferentiated carcinomas with osteoclast-like giant cells have been reported as pleomorphic, giant cell, or sarcomatoid carcinomas, as well as carcinomas that simulate giant cell tumor of bone.[184,187,194,195] Their distinctiveness suggests that they merit recognition as a separate class of tumor. They are undifferentiated carcinomas that show an osteoclastic giant cell reaction. They may also display metaplastic mesenchymal elements, such as osteoid, bone, or cartilage.[196] If thoroughly sampled, they may also contain foci of conventional adenocarcinoma. The giant cells have the immunophenotype of osteoclastic giant cells, whereas the carcinomatous areas, and often the spindle cells, are positive for cytokeratin. As in many pleomorphic carcinomas, the spindle cells may contain vimentin, in addition to epithelial markers. Even if the tumor spindle cell components are negative for epithelial markers by immunohistochemistry or electron microscopy, they are believed to be of epithelial origin. However, the location, the immunohistochemical confirmation of epithelial differentiation in most cases, and the presence of mutated K-*ras* in the mononuclear cells,[197,198] support an epithelial origin. In rare examples, a definite malignant component of the neoplasm is not identified; the question then arises as to whether a component of carcinoma has been overlooked, as the quantity of carcinoma can be trivial by contrast to the volume of giant cells.[199] It is contingent on the pathologist who encounters a giant cell tumor of the pancreas to search for carcinoma by blocking the entire tumor if necessary.

Grossly, osteoclast-like giant cell tumors range from 3.5 to 14 cm in greatest dimension, averaging 9 cm.[196] The cut surface is firm and grayish white in color, with extensive hemorrhage and prominent central necrosis.[184,186] These tumors have also been reported in the walls of pancreatic mucinous cystadenomas.[166,196,200]

Microscopically, osteoclast-like giant cell tumors display two components, which are intimately intermingled: nonneoplastic osteoclast-like giant cells are usually the more plentiful component; malignant elements are the second component and they include pleomorphic bizarre cells, carcinoma cells with a spindle-cell sarcomatoid appearance, and adenocarcinomatous elements exhibiting varying degrees of differentiation[201] (Fig. 7–18). Fine-needle aspira-

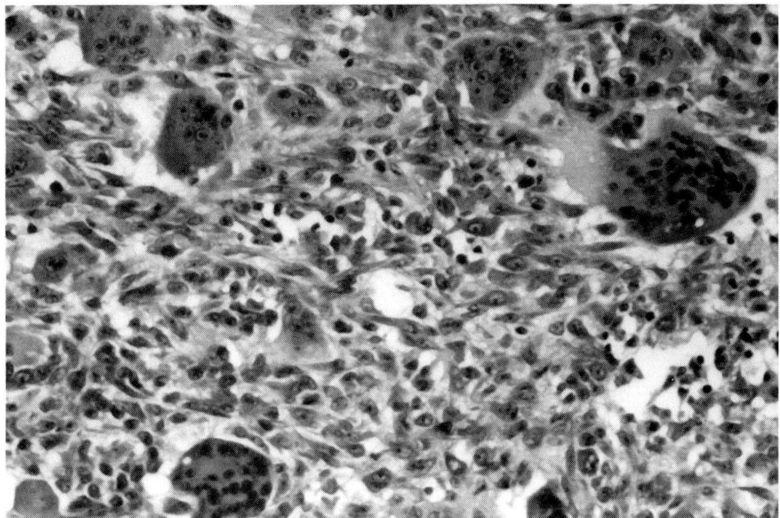

Figure 7–18. Undifferentiated carcinoma with osteoclast-like giant cells. Note the background spindle and inflammatory component.

tion of these tumors commonly permits an accurate diagnosis, with the identification of multinucleated tumor cells (Fig. 7–19). The osteoclast-like giant cells are frequently located around sites of necrosis, hemorrhage, and hemosiderin deposition.[187,201] Bone or osteoid is sometimes present.[187,194,196,202] The weight of evidence now points to the truly osteoclastic nature of the giant cells and it is assumed that they are recruited and stimulated to differentiate by secretory products of the primary tumor, such as osteocalcin. Individual osteoclastic giant cells have been microdissected and found to contain K-*ras* oncogene mutations, and this has been interpreted as being due to phagocytosis of tumor cells.[198]

Immunohistochemically, most sarcomatoid tumor cells and some anaplastic giant cells are positive for vimentin and cytokeratin; the mononuclear cells may also be positive for CD68, leukocyte common antigen (LCA), and α_1-antichymotrypsin. Both CEA and CA 19-9 may be detected in tumor cells that form ducts or glands but not in pleomorphic elements. In contrast, the osteoclast-like giant cells show strong immunoreactivity with vimentin, CD68,

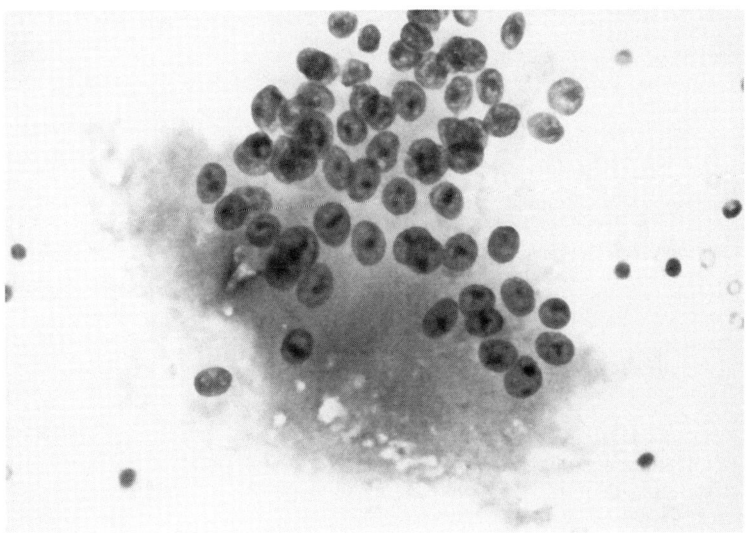

Figure 7–19. Undifferentiated carcinoma with osteoclast-like giant cells. Fine-needle aspiration biopsy shows the multiple nuclei that have spread over the slide as the smear was prepared.

and LCA but no reaction with any epithelial markers. Other positive markers in the giant cells include CD4, CD13, CD45, and CD71. The mononuclear cells show similar staining. Thus, the osteoclast-like giant cells are of histiocyte-macrophage lineage and probably induced by paraneoplastic cytokine or chemokine production.[195]

The largest review of osteoclast-like giant cell tumors reported to date describes 20 cases involving 12 women and 8 men.[203] The average age of the patients was 59.5 years. A smaller series confirmed the female preponderance and showed an average age of 67 years.[196] Most tumors are located in the head or body of the pancreas, with only 10% occurring in the tail. The mean reported survival time is 12 months, with some patients surviving up to 15 years after diagnosis. These results suggest a marginally better prognosis than for conventional duct car-

Table 7–9. Checklist for Pathology Reports on Resected Pancreatic Carcinomas

- Gross description
  - How the specimen was received
  - How the specimen was identified
  - Part(s) of stomach, duodenum, pancreas, and bile ducts included and dimensions
  - Tumor description
    - Site
    - Proximity to nearest margin
    - Gross morphology
    - Dimensions
  - Status of stomach, bowel, ampulla, and common bile duct
  - Lymph nodes identified
  - Tissue submitted for special investigation
- Diagnostic information
  - Site of tumor
  - Histologic type
    - Adenocarcinoma not otherwise specified
    - Mucinous carcinoma (> 50%)
    - Mucinous cystic tumor
    - Adenosquamous carcinoma
    - Pleomorphic carcinoma
    - Small cell undifferentiated carcinoma
    - Solid and cystic carcinoma
    - Acinar cell carcinoma
    - Pancreatoblastoma
    - Small cell carcinoma
  - Histological grade
  - TNM status
    - T1: Tumor limited to pancreas
      - T1a: Tumor ≤ 2 cm in greatest dimension
      - T1b: Tumor > 2 cm in greatest dimension
    - T2: Tumor extends directly to any of the following: duodenum, bile duct, peripancreatic tissues
    - T3: Tumor extends directly to any of the following: stomach, spleen, colon, adjacent large vessels
    - Regional lymph node metastases—N1
  - Perineural infiltration.
  - Presence of omental or mesenteric deposits
  - Other sites biopsied for metastatic disease
  - Adequacy of local excision—peripancreatic margins
  - Other significant disease
- Optional features
  - Stage
  - Results of ancillary investigations
  - Specific lymph nodes
  - Lymph vessel infiltration
  - Venous infiltration
  - Inflammatory infiltrate
  - In situ carcinoma/papillomatosis/ductal dysplasia
  - Other pathology (pancreatitis, gallstones, etc.)

cinoma but a decidedly better prognosis than for pleomorphic or anaplastic carcinoma without osteoclastic giant cells.[203]

Microadenocarcinoma

Microadenocarcinoma was described by Cubilla and Fitzgerald in 1975 as a variant that exhibited nests of small to intermediate-size cells without intervening stroma, generally with small glandular lumina within the solid nests.[39] It was found to have a very poor prognosis. However, doubting its distinctiveness, Lonardo et al. revisited the topic in 1996 and employed immunocytochemistry for acinar, endocrine, and ductal differentiation to further classify the tumors.[204] They identified two morphologic patterns: microglandular and solid-cribriform. The microglandular tumors were not distinguishable from typical ductal adenocarcinomas, either morphologically or by immunocytochemistry. However, the solid-cribriform tumors proved to be heterogeneous: Three of their six cases were acinar cell carcinomas, one an endocrine cell carcinoma, one a mixed ductal-endocrine carcinoma, and one a ductal adenocarcinoma. Therefore, microadenocarcinoma is best regarded as a tumor pattern that is associated with an aggressive clinical course rather than a distinct entity.

Clear Cell Carcinoma

Primary clear cell carcinoma of the pancreas is a rare tumor that resembles renal cell carcinoma.[205,206] One reported case was associated with a small intraductal papillary component, indicating local origin in the pancreas. It also had the common K-*ras* point mutation at codon 12 that is seen in pancreatic carcinomas.[205] The growth pattern of clear cell tumor is predominantly solid, with a few scattered tubular structures. Immunocytochemically, the tumor expresses cytokeratins but not vimentin or neuroendocrine markers. Luttges et al.[205] concluded that only three cases of acceptable clear cell carcinoma have been described in pancreas. The differential diagnostic considerations are all rare: metastatic renal cell carcinoma, a tumor that often contains vimentin as well as cytokeratin; clear cell endocrine tumor,[207] which may be immunopositive for chromogranin and/or synaptophysin; solid serous cystadenoma,[208] which lacks CEA; sugar tumor, which displays a sinusoidal network of vessels and HMB45 positivity.[209] Solid-cystic-papillary tumor has characteristic morphology and may be positive for neuron-specific enolase, α_1-antitrypsin, and vimentin. It may occasionally be confused with a clear cell carcinoma.

REPORTING PANCREATIC CARCINOMA

Table 7–9 is a checklist of features that may be incorporated into a surgical pathology report of a resected pancreatic carcinoma. It also lists features that may be required for further disease management.

REFERENCES

1. Morohoshi T, Held G, Klöppel G: Exocrine pancreatic tumours and their histological classification. A study based on 167 autopsy and 97 surgical cases. Histopathology 645–661, 1983.
2. National Cancer Institute of Canada: Canadian Cancer Statistics 1996.
3. Parkin DM, Pisani P, Ferlay J: Global cancer statistics. CA Cancer J Clin 49:33–64, 1999.
4. Parkin DM, Muir C, Whelan SL, et al.: Cancer incidence in five continents. IARC Scientific Publications No.120. IARC Sci Publ 1–1033, 1992.
5. Yamamoto M, Ohashi O, Saitoh Y: Japan Pancreatic Cancer Registry: Current status. Pancreas 16:238–242, 1998.
6. Davis DL, Hoel D, Fox J, Lopez A: International trends in cancer mortality in France, West Germany, Italy, Japan, England and Wales, and the USA. Lancet ii:905–906, 1990.
7. Fontham ETH, Correa P: Epidemiology of pancreatic cancer. Surg Clin North Am 69:551–567, 1989.
8. MacMahon B, Yen S, Trichopoulos D, et al.: Coffee and cancer of the pancreas. N Engl J Med 304:630–633, 1981.
9. Niederhuber JE, Brennan MF, Menck HR: The National Cancer Data Base report on pancreatic cancer. Cancer 76:1671–1677, 1995.
10. Kato I, Tajima K, Kuroishi T, et al.: Latitude and pancreatic cancer. Jpn J Clin Oncol 15:403–413, 1985.
11. Wynder EL: An epidemiological evaluation of the causes of cancer of the pancreas. Cancer Res 35:2228–2233, 1975.
12. Morgan RGH, Wormsley KG: Progress report. Cancer of the pancreas. Gut 18:580–592, 1977.
13. Mills PK, Beeson WL, Abbey DE, et al.: Dietary habits and past medical history as related to past fatal pancreas cancer risk among Adventists. Cancer 61:2578–2585, 1988.
14. Levin DL, Connelly RR, Devesa SS: Demographic characteristics of cancer of the pancreas: Mortality, incidence and survival. Cancer 47:1456–1468, 1981.
15. MacMahon B: Risk factors for cancer of the pancreas. Cancer 50:2676–2680, 1982.

16. Greenberg RE, Bank S, Stark B: Adenocarcinoma of the pancreas producing pancreatitis and pancreatic abscess. Pancreas 5:108–113, 1990.
17. Lafler CJ, Hinerman DL: A morphologic study of pancreatic carcinoma with reference to multiple thrombi. Cancer 14:944–952, 1961.
18. Min KW, Gyorkey F, Sato C: Mucin-producing adenocarcinomas and nonbacterial thrombotic endocarditis: Pathogenic role of tumor mucin. Cancer 45:2374–2382, 1980.
19. Ishikawa O, Ohhigashi H, Wada A, et al.: Morphological characteristics of pancreatic carcinoma with diabetes mellitus. Cancer 64:1107–1112, 1989.
20. Diasio RB, Eanes RZ, Chen ML, et al.: Adenocarcinoma of the pancreas associated with hypoglycemia: Case report and review of the literature. Cancer 43:2457–2464, 1979.
21. Monno AR, Nagata A, Bittner CA, et al.: Exocrine pancreatic carcinoma with humoral hypercalcemia. Am J Gastroenterol 79:128–132, 1984.
22. Taniguchi S, Hisa T, Hamada T: Cutaneous metastases of pancreatic carcinoma with unusual clinical features. J Am Acad Dermatol 31:877–880, 1994.
23. Gudjonsson B: Cancer of the pancreas. 50 years of surgery. Cancer 60:2284–2303, 1987.
24. Gloor B, Todd KE, Reber HA: Diagnostic workup of patients with suspected pancreatic carcinoma: The University of California–Los Angeles approach. Cancer 79:1780–1786, 1997.
25. Aoki K, Okada S, Moriyama N, et al.: Accuracy of computed tomography in determining pancreatic cancer tumor size. Jap J Clin Oncol 24:85–87, 1994.
26. Vahldiek G, Roemel T, Klapdor R: MR-cholangiopancreatography (MRCP) and MR-angiography: Morphologic changes with magnetic resonance imaging. Anticancer Res 19:2451–2458, 1999.
27. Johnson PT, Outwater EK: Pancreatic carcinoma versus chronic pancreatitis: Dynamic MR imaging. Radiology 212:213–218, 1999.
28. Kaneko T, Nakao A, Harada A, et al.: Intraportal endovascular ultrasonography in pancreatic cancer—a new technique for the diagnosis of portal vein invasion: A preliminary report. Surgery 115:438–444, 1994.
29. Snady H, Bruckner H, Siegel J, et al.: Endoscopic ultrasonographic criteria of vascular invasion by potentially resectable pancreatic tumors. Gastrointest Endoscopy 40:326–333, 1994.
30. Keogan MT, Tyler D, Clark L, et al.: Diagnosis of pancreatic cancer: Role of FDGPET. Am J Roentgenol 171:1565–1570, 1998.
31. Kiriyama S, Hayakawa T, Kondo T, et al.: Usefulness of a new tumor marker, Span-1, for the diagnosis of pancreatic cancer. Cancer 65:1557–1561, 1990.
32. Zhou W, Sokoll LJ, Bruzek DJ, et al.: Identifying markers for pancreatic cancer by gene expression analysis. Cancer Epidemiol Biomarkers Prev 7:109–112, 1998.
33. Mulcahy HE, Lyautey J, Lederrey C, et al.: A prospective study of K-*ras* mutations in the plasma of pancreatic cancer patients. Clin Cancer Res 4:271–275, 1998.
34. Furukawa T, Chiba R, Kobari M, et al.: Varying grades of epithelial atypia in the pancreatic ducts of humans. Classification based on morphometry and multivariate analysis and correlated with positive reactions of carcinoembryonic antigen. Arch Pathol Lab Med 118:227–234, 1994.
35. Brat DJ, Lillemoe KD, Yeo CJ, et al.: Progression of pancreatic intraductal adenocarcinoma of the pancreas. Am J Surg Pathol 22:163–169, 1998.
36. Apple SK, Hecht JR, Lewin DN, et al.: Immuno-histochemical evaluation of K-*ras*, p53, and HER-2/*neu* expression in hyperplastic, dysplastic, and carcinomatous lesions of the pancreas: Evidence for multistep carcinogenesis. Hum Pathol 30:123–129, 1999.
37. Klöppel G, Solcia E, Longnecker DS, et al., eds.: Histologic typing of tumours of the exocrine pancreas. 2nd ed. (World Health Organization). New York: Springer-Verlag, 1996.
38. Klöppel G, Bommer G, Ruckert K, et al.: Intraductal proliferation in the pancreas and its relationship to human and experimental carcinogenesis. Virchows Arch Pathol Anat 387:221–233, 1980.
39. Cubilla AL, Fitzgerald PJ: Morphological patterns of primary non-endocrine human pancreatic carcinoma. Cancer Res 35:2234–2248, 1975.
40. Cubilla AL, Fitzgerald PJ: Morphological lesions associated with human primary invasive nonendocrine pancreas cancer. Cancer Res 36:2690–2698, 1976.
41. Chen J, Baithun SI: Morphological study of 391 cases of exocrine pancreatic tumours with special reference to the classification of exocrine pancreatic carcinoma. J Pathol 146:17–29, 1985.
42. Obara T, Saitoh Y, Maguchi H, et al.: Multicentric development of pancreatic intraductal carcinoma through atypical papillary hyperplasia. Hum Pathol 23:82–85, 1992.
43. Moskaluk CA, Hruban RH, Kern SE: *p16* and dK-*ras* gene mutations in the intraductal precursors of human pancreatic carcinoma. Cancer Res 57:2140–2143, 1997.
44. Tada M, Ohashi M, Shiratori Y, et al.: Analysis of K-*ras* gene mutation in hyperplastic duct cells of the pancreas without pancreas disease. Gastroenterology 110:227–231, 1996.
45. Yanagisawa A, Ohtake K, Ohashi K, et al.: Frequent c-Ki-*ras* oncogene activation in mucous cell hyperplasias of pancreas suffering from chronic inflammation. Cancer Res 53:953–956, 1993.
46. Z'graggen K, Rivera JA, Compton CC, et al.: Prevalence of activating K-*ras* mutations in the evolutionary stages of neoplasia in intraductal papillary mucinous tumors of the pancreas. Ann Surg 226:491–500, 1997.
47. Rivera JA, Rall CJ, Graeme-Cook F, et al.: Analysis of K-*ras* mutations in chronic pancreatitis with ductal hyperplasia Surgery 121:42–49, 1997.
48. Schutte M, Hruban RH, Geradts J, et al.: Abrogation of the *RB/p16* tumor-suppressive pathway in virtually all pancreatic carcinomas. Cancer Res 57:3126–3130, 1997.
49. Boschman CR, Stryker S, Reddy JK, et al.: Expression of p53 protein in precursor lesions and adenocarcinoma of the human pancreas. Am J Pathol 145:1291–1295, 1994.
50. DiGiuseppe JA, Yeo CJ, Hruban RH: Review article. Molecular biology and the diagnosis and treatment of adenocarcinoma of the pancreas. Adv Anat Pathol 3:139–155, 1996.
51. Hameed M, Marrero AM, Conlon KC, et al.: Expression of p53 nucleophosphoprotein in in situ pancreatic ductal adenocarcinoma: An immunohistochemical analysis of 100 cases (abstract). Lab Invest 70:132, 1994.
52. Kozuka S, Sassa R, Taki T, et al.: Relation of pancreatic duct hyperplasia to carcinoma. Cancer 43:1418–1428, 1979.
53. Tillou A, Schwartz MR, Jordan PH Jr: Percutaneous needle biopsy of the pancreas: When should it be performed? World J Surg 20:283–287, 1996.

54. Moussa AR: Invited commentary. World J Surg 20:287, 1996.
55. Tao LC, Ho CS, McLoughlin MJ, et al.: Percutaneous fine needle aspiration biopsy of the pancreas. Cytodiagnosis of pancreatic carcinoma. Acta Cytol 22:215–220, 1978.
56. Hancke S, Holm HH, Koch F: Ultrasonically guided puncture of solid pancreatic mass lesions. Ultrasound Med Biol 10:613–615, 1984.
57. Kocjan G, Rode J, Lees WR: Percutaneous fine needle aspiration cytology of the pancreas: Advantages and pitfalls. J Clin Pathol 42:341–347, 1989.
58. Mitchell ML, Bittner CA, Wills JS, et al.: Fine needle aspiration cytology of the pancreas. A retrospective study of 73 cases. Acta Cytol 32:447–451, 1988.
59. Soudah B, Fritsch RS, Wittekind C, et al.: Value of the cytologic analysis of fine needle aspiration biopsy specimens in the diagnosis of pancreatic carcinomas. Acta Cytol 33:875–880, 1989.
60. Johnson DE, Pendurthi TK, Balshem AM, et al.: Implications of fine-needle aspiration in patients with resectable pancreatic cancer. Am Surg 63:675–679, 1997.
61. Gupta RK: Value of image guided fine-needle aspiration cytology in the diagnosis of pancreatic malignancies. Diagn Cytopathol 13:120–123, 1995.
62. Saez A, Catala I, Brossa R, et al.: Intraoperative fine needle aspiration cytology of pancreatic lesions. A study of 90 cases. Acta Cytol 39:485–488, 1995.
63. Earnhardt RC, McQuone SJ, Minasi JS, et al.: Intraoperative fine needle aspiration of pancreatic and extrahepatic biliary masses. Surg Gynecol Obstet 177:147–152, 1993.
64. Fritscher-Ravens A, Schirrow L, Atay Z, et al.: Endoscopically controlled fine needle aspiration cytology—indications and results in recent diagnosis. Z Gastroenterol 37:343–351, 1999.
65. Fornari F, Buscarini L: Ultrasonically-guided fine-needle biopsy of gastrointestinal organs: Indications, results and complications. Dig Dis Sci 10:121–133, 1992.
66. Weiss SM, Skibber JM, Mohiuddin M, et al.: Rapid intraabdominal spread of pancreatic cancer. Arch Surg 120:415–416, 1985.
67. Pinto MM, Emanuel JR, Chaturvedi V, et al.: Ki-*ras* mutations and the carcinoembryonic antigen level in fine needle aspirates of the pancreas. Acta Cytol 41:427–434, 1997.
68. Iwao T, Hanada K, Tsuchida A, et al.: The establishment of a preoperative diagnosis of pancreatic carcinoma using cell specimens from pancreatic duct brushing with special attention to p53 mutations. Cancer 82:1487–1494, 1998.
69. Warshaw AL: Implications of peritoneal cytology for staging of early pancreatic cancer. Am J Surg 161:26–30, 1991.
70. Willett CG, Rattner DW, Fernandez-del Castillo C: Implications of peritoneal cytology for pancreatic management. Arch Surg 133:361–365, 1998.
71. Martin JK Jr, Goellner JR: Abdominal fluid cytology in patients with malignant lesions. Mayo Clin Proc 61:467–471, 1986.
72. Balen FG, Little A, Smith AC, et al.: Biopsy of inoperable pancreatic tumors does not adversely influence patient survival time. Radiology 193:753–755, 1994.
73. Lee Y-T N: Tissue diagnosis for carcinoma of the pancreas and periampullary structures. Cancer 49:1035–1039, 1982.
74. Böttger TC, Junginger T: Treatment of tumors of the pancreatic head with suspected but unproved malignancy: Is a nihilistic approach justified? World J Surg 23:158–163, 1999.
75. Cubilla AL, Fitzgerald PJ: Pancreas cancer. 1. Duct adenocarcinoma. A clinical-pathological study of 380 patients. Pathol Annu 13:241–289, 1978.
76. Cubilla AL, Fitzgerald PJ: Pancreas cancer—duct cell adenocarcinoma: Survival in relation to site, size, stage and type of therapy. J Surg Oncol 10:465–482, 1978.
77. Kloppel G, Maillet B: Histologic typing of pancreatic and periampullary carcinoma. Eur J Surg Oncol 17:139–152, 1991.
78. Goggins M, Offerhaus GJ, Hilgers W, et al.: Pancreatic adenocarcinoma with DNA replication errors (RER+) are associated with wild-type K-*ras* and characteristic histopathology. Poor differentiation, a syncytial growth pattern, and pushing borders suggest RER+. Am J Pathol 152:1501–1507, 1998.
79. Al-Nafussi A, O'Donnell M: Poorly differentiated adenocarcinoma with extensive rhabdoid differentiation: Clinicopathological features of two cases arising in the gastrointestinal tract. Pathol Int 49:160–163, 1999.
80. Takasaki H, Uchida E, Tempero MA, et al.: Correlative study on expression of CA 19-9 and DU-PAN-2 in tumor tissue and serum of pancreatic cancer patients. Cancer Res 48:1435–1438, 1988.
81. Moll R, Robine S, Dudouet B, et al.: Villin: A cytoskeletal protein and a differentiation marker expressed in some human adenocarcinomas. Virchows Arch B 54:155–169, 1987.
82. Schüssler MH, Skoudy A, Ramaekers F, et al.: Intermediate filaments as differentiation markers of normal pancreas and pancreas cancer. Am J Pathol 140:559–568, 1992.
83. Osborn M, vanLessen G, Weber K, et al.: Differential diagnosis of gastrointestinal carcinomas by using monoclonal antibodies specific for individual keratin polypeptides. Lab Invest 55:497–504, 1986.
84. Iwase K, Kato K, Nagasaka A, et al.: Immunohistochemical study of neuron-specific enolase and Ca19-9 in pancreatic disorders. The value of neuron-specific enolase as a marker for islet cell and nerve tissue. Gastroenterology 91:576–580, 1986.
85. Eusebi V, Capella C, Bondi A: Endocrine-paracrine cells in pancreatic exocrine carcinomas. Histopathology 5:599–613, 1981.
86. Pour PM, Permert J, Mogaki M, et al.: Endocrine aspects of exocrine cancer of the pancreas. Their patterns and suggested biologic significance. Am J Clin Pathol 100:223–230, 1993.
87. Tot T: Adenocarcinomas metastatic to the liver: The value of cytokeratins 20 and 7 in the search for unknown primary tumors. Cancer 85:171–177, 1999.
88. Guarda L: Gastrointestinal tract, pancreas, and liver. *In* Silva EG, Kramer BB: Intraoperative Pathologic Diagnosis: Frozen Section and Other Techniques. Baltimore: Williams & Wilkins, 1987, pp 145–165.
89. Hyland C, Kheir SM, Kashlan MB: Frozen section diagnosis of pancreatic carcinoma. A prospective study of 64 biopsies. Am J Surg Pathol 5:179–191, 1981.
90. Loquvam GS, Russell WO: Accessory pancreatic ducts of the major duodenal papilla. Normal structures to be differentiated from cancer. Am J Clin Pathol 20:305–313, 1950.
91. Costa J: Epithelial inclusions in pancreatic nerves. Am J Clin Pathol 67:306–307, 1976.

92. Bartow SA, Mukai K, Rosai J: Pseudoneoplastic proliferation of endocrine cells in pancreatic fibrosis. Cancer 47:2627–2633, 1981.
93. Hedberg M, Borgstrom A, Genell S, et al.: Survival following pancreatic carcinoma: A follow-up study of all cases recorded in Malmö, Sweden, 1977–1991. Br J Surg 85:1641–1644, 1998.
94. Conlon KC, Klimstra DS, Brennan MF: Long-term survival after curative resection for pancreatic ductal adenocarcinoma. Ann Surg 223:273–279, 1996.
95. Bramhall SR, Allum WH, Jones AG, et al.: Treatment and survival in 13,560 patients with pancreatic cancer, and incidence of the disease, in the West Midlands: An epidemiological study. Br J Surg 82:111–115, 1995.
96. Fabre JM, Houry S, Manderscheid JC, et al.: Surgery for left-sided pancreatic cancer. Br J Surg 83:1065–1070, 1996.
97. Trede M, Schwall G, Saeger HD: Survival after pancreatoduodenectomy: 118 consecutive resective resections without an operative mortality. Ann Surg 211:447–458, 1990.
98. Geer RJ, Brennan MF: Prognostic indicators for survival after resection of pancreatic adenocarcinoma. Am J Surg 165:68–73, 1993.
99. Cameron JL, Crist DW, Sitzmann JV, et al.: Factors influencing survival after pancreatoduodenectomy for pancreatic cancer. Am J Surg 161:120–124, 1991.
100. Pedrazzoli S, DiCarlo V, Dionigi R, et al.: Standard versus extended lymphadenectomy associated with pancreatoduodenectomy in the surgical treatment of adenocarcinoma of the head of the pancreas: A multicenter, prospective, randomized study. Lymphadenectomy study group. Ann Surg 228:508–517, 1998.
101. Huguier M, Baumel H, Manderscheid JC, et al.: Surgical palliation for unresected cancer of the exocrine pancreas. Eur J Surg Oncol 19:342–347, 1993.
102. Bakkevold KE, Kambestad B: Staging of carcinoma of the pancreas and ampulla of Vater. Tumor (T), lymph node (N), and distant metastasis (M) as prognostic factors. Int J Pancreatol 17:249–259, 1995.
103. Yamaguchi K, Enjoji M, Tsuneyoshi M: Pancreatoduodenal carcinoma: A clinico-pathologic study of 304 patients and immunohistochemical observation for CEA and CA19-9. J Surg Oncol 47:148–154, 1991.
104. Yamaguchi K, Nishihara K, Tsuneyoshi M: Non-icteric pancreas head carcinoma fares worse than icteric pancreas head carcinoma. J Surg Oncol 49:253–258, 1992.
105. Thompson LDR, Becker RC, Przygodzki RM, et al.: Mucinous cystic neoplasm (mucinous cystadenocarcinoma of low-grade malignant potential) of the pancreas. A clinico-pathological study of 130 cases. Am J Surg Pathol 23:1–16, 1999.
106. Connolly MM, Dawson PJ, Michelassi F, et al.: Survival in 1001 patients with carcinoma of the pancreas. Ann Surg 206:366–373, 1987.
107. Rickaert F, Cremer M, Deviere J, et al.: Intraductal mucin-hypersecreting neoplasms of the pancreas. A clinicopathologic study of eight patients. Gastroenterology 101:512–519, 1991.
108. Brower ST, Newman RM, Pertsemlidis D, et al.: Histopathological determinants of survival in resected cases of pancreas cancer. HPB Surgery 7:1–14, 1993.
109. Sperti C, Bonadimani B, Pasquali C, et al.: Ductal adenocarcinoma of the pancreas: Clinicopathologic features and survival. Tumori 79:325–330, 1993.
110. Mannell A, Weiland LH, van Heerden JA, et al.: Factors influencing survival after resection for ductal adenocarcinoma of the pancreas. Ann Surg 203:403–407, 1986.
111. Boettger TC, Maschek H, Lobo M, et al.: Prognostic value of immunohistochemical expression of beta-1 integrin in pancreatic carcinoma. Oncology 56:308–313, 1999.
112. Tannapfel A, Wittekind C, Hunefeld G: Ductal adenocarcinoma of the pancreas. Histopathological features and prognosis. Int J Pancreatol 12:145–152, 1992.
113. Yamamoto M, Saitoh Y, Hermanek P: Exocrine pancreatic carcinoma. *In* Hermanek P, Godspodarowicz MK, Henson DE, Hutter RVP, Sobin JH (eds): Prognostic Factors in Cancer. New York: Springer, 1995, pp 105–117.
114. Zerbi A, Balzano G, Bottura R, et al.: Reliability of pancreatic cancer staging classifications. Int J Pancreatol 15:13–18, 1994.
115. Nix GA, Dubbelman C, Wilson JH, et al.: Prognostic implications of tumor diameter in carcinoma of the head of the pancreas. Cancer 67:529–535, 1991.
116. Baumel H, Huguier M, Manderscheid JC, et al.: Results of resection for cancer of the exocrine pancreas: A study from the French Association of Surgery. Br J Surg 81:102–107, 1994.
117. Fortner JG, Klimstra DS, Senia RT, et al.: Tumor size is the primary prognosticator for pancreatic cancer after regional pancreatectomy. Ann Surg 223:147–153, 1996.
118. Manabe T, Miyashita T, Ohshio G, et al.: Small carcinoma of the pancreas: Clinical and pathologic evaluation of 17 patients. Cancer 62:135–141, 1988.
119. Ohta T, Nagakawa T, Ueno K, et al.: The mode of lymphatic and local spread of pancreatic carcinomas less than 4.0 cm in size. Int Surg 78:208–212, 1993.
120. Takao S, Shinchi H, Sha K, et al.: Clinical and biological features of T1 ductal adenocarcinoma of the pancreas. Hepatogastroenterol 46:498–503, 1999.
121. Sellner F, Machacek E: The importance of tumour volume in the prognosis of radically treated periampullary carcinomas. Eur J Surg 159:95–100, 1993.
122. Nagakawa T, Nagamori M, Futakami F, et al.: Results of extensive surgery for pancreatic carcinoma. Cancer 77:640–645, 1996.
123. Nagakawa T, Mori K, Nakano T, et al.: Perineural invasion of carcinoma of the pancreas and biliary tract. Br J Surg 80:619–621, 1993.
124. Tsunoda T, Ura K, Eto T, et al.: UICC and Japanese stage classifications for carcinoma of the pancreas. Int J Pancreatol 8:205–214, 1991.
125. Willett CG, Lewandrowski K, Warshaw AL, et al.: Resection margins in carcinoma of the head of the pancreas. Implications for radiation therapy. Ann Surg 217:144–148, 1993.
126. Griffin JF, Smalley SR, Jewell W, et al.: Patterns of failure after curative resection of pancreatic carcinoma. Cancer 66:56–61, 1990.
127. Takahashi T, Ishikura H, Kato H, et al.: Intra-pancreatic, extra-tumoral perineural invasion (nex). An indicator for the presence of retroperitoneal neural plexus invasion by pancreas carcinoma. Acta Pathol Jpn 42:99–103, 1992.
128. Bockman DE, Buchler M, Beger HG: Interaction of pancreatic ductal carcinoma with nerves leads to nerve damage. Gastroenterology 107:219–230, 1994.
129. Kayahara M, Nagakawa T, Ohta T, et al.: Analysis of paraaortic lymph node involvement in pancreatic carcinoma: A significant indication for surgery. Cancer 85:583–590, 1999.

130. Fuhrman GM, Leach SD, Staley CA, et al.: Rationale for en bloc vein resection in the treatment of pancreatic adenocarcinoma adherent to the superior mesenteric-portal vein confluence. Ann Surg 223:154–162, 1996.
131. Nagakawa T, Kayahara M, Ueno K, et al.: A clinicopathologic study on neural invasion in cancer of the pancreatic head. Cancer 69:930–935, 1992.
132. Nagakawa T, Kobayashi H, Ueno K, et al.: Clinical study of lymphatic flow to the paraaortic lymph nodes in carcinoma of the head of the pancreas. Cancer 73:1155–1162, 1994.
133. Nagakawa T, Konishi I, Ueno K, et al.: A clinical study on lymphatic flow in carcinoma of the pancreatic head area—peripancreatic regional lymph node grouping. Hepatogastroenterol 40:457–462, 1993.
134. Nagakawa T, Kobayashi H, Ueno K, et al.: The pattern of lymph node involvement in carcinoma of the head of the pancreas. A histologic study of the surgical findings in patients undergoing extensive nodal dissections. Int J Pancreatol 13:15–22, 1993.
135. Gall FP, Kessler H, Hermanek P: Surgical treatment of ductal pancreatic carcinoma. Eur J Surg Oncol 17:173–181, 1991.
136. Hyoty M, Visakorpi T, Kallioniemi OP, et al.: Prognostic value of analysis of DNA in pancreatic adenocarcinoma by flow cytometry. Eur J Surg 157:595–600, 1991.
137. Eskelinen M, Lipponen P, Marin S, et al.: Prognostic factors in human pancreatic cancer, with special reference to quantitative histology. Scand J Gastroenterol 26:483–490, 1991.
138. Ferrara C, Tessari G, Poletti A, et al.: Ki-67 and *c-jun* expression in pancreatic cancer: A prognostic marker? Oncol Rep 6:1117–1122, 1999.
139. Takeuchi Y, Nakao A, Harada A, et al.: Expression of plasminogen activators and their inhibitors in human pancreatic carcinoma: Immuno-histochemical study. Am J Gastroenterol 88:1928–1933, 1993.
140. Allison DC, Bose KK, Hruban RH, et al.: Pancreatic cancer cell DNA content correlates with long-term survival after pancreatoduodenectomy. Ann Surg 214:648–656, 1991.
141. Park CS, Wiebke EA, Sidner RA, et al.: The role of flow cytometric DNA analysis in determining prognosis of resectable ductal adenocarcinoma of the pancreas. Ann Surg 62:609–615, 1996.
142. Herrera MF, van Heerden JA, Katzman JA, et al.: Evaluation of DNA nuclear pattern as a prognostic determinant in resected pancreatic ductal adenocarcinoma. Ann Surg 215:120–124, 1992.
143. Linder S, Falkmer U, Hagmar T, et al.: Prognostic significance of DNA ploidy in pancreatic carcinoma. Pancreas 9:764–772, 1994.
144. Eskelinen M, Lipponen P, Marin S, et al.: DNA ploidy, S-phase fraction, and G2 fraction as prognostic determinants in human pancreatic cancer. Scand J Gastroenterol 27:39–43, 1992.
145. Weger AR, Lindholm JL: Discrimination of pancreatic adenocarcinomas from chronic pancreatitis by morphometric analysis. Pathol Res Pract 188:44–48, 1992.
146. Glasgow RE, Mulvihill SJ: Hospital volume influences outcome in patients undergoing pancreatic resection for cancer. West J Med 165:294–300, 1996.
147. Lieberman MD, Kilburn H, Lindsey M, et al.: Relation of perioperative deaths to hospital volume among patients undergoing pancreatic resection for malignancy. Ann Surg 222:638–645, 1995.
148. Gordon TA, Burleyson GP, Tielsch JM, et al.: The effects of regionalisation on cost and outcome for one general high-risk surgical procedure. Ann Surg 221:43–49, 1995.
149. Simunovic M, To T, Theriault M, et al.: Relation between hospital surgical volume and outcome for pancreatic resection for neoplasm in a publicly funded health care system. Can Med Assoc J 160:643–648, 1999.
150. Sobin LH, Wittekind CH, eds.: TNM Classification of Malignant Tumours. 5th ed. New York: John Wiley & Sons, 1997.
151. Hermanek P: Staging of exocrine pancreatic carcinoma. Eur J Surg Oncol 17:167–172, 1991.
152. del Castillo CF, Warshaw L: Peritoneal metastases in pancreatic carcinoma. Hepatogastroenterol 40:430–432, 1993.
153. Thorban S, Roder JD, Siewert JR: Detection of micrometastasis in bone marrow of pancreatic cancer patients. Ann Oncol 10(suppl 4):111–113, 1999.
154. Nishizaki T, Matsumata T, Adachi E, et al.: Laparoscopy preferable to imaging procedures in detecting metastases of a pancreas carcinoma to the liver. Report of two cases. Surg Endosc 8:1340–1342, 1994.
155. Mao C, Domenico DR, Kim K, et al.: Observations on the developmental patterns and the consequences of pancreatic exocrine adenocarcinoma. Findings of 154 autopsies. Arch Surg 130:125–134, 1995.
156. Matsuno S, Kato S, Kobari M, et al.: Clinicopathological study on hematogenous metastasis of pancreatic cancer. Jpn J Surg 16:406–411, 1986.
157. Takamori H, Hiraoka T, Kanemitsu K, et al.: Treatment strategies for hepatic metastases from pancreatic cancer in patients previously treated with radical resection combined with intraoperative radiation therapy. HPB Surgery 8:107–110, 1994.
158. Kishi K, Hirota T, Nakamura K, et al.: Carcinoma of the pancreas: A review of 94 autopsy cases. Jpn J Clin Oncol 10:273–279, 1980.
159. Tian F, Myles JL, Appert HE, et al.: Detection of occult metastases in pancreatic adenocarcinoma with anticytokeratin antibody. Pancreas 7:159–164, 1992.
160. Nimura Y: Pancreatic surgery: Cutting-edge developments and technology. Pancreas 16:227–232, 1998.
161. Yeo CJ, Cameron JL, Lillemoe KD et al.: Pancreatoduodenectomy for cancer of the head of the pancreas. Ann Surg 221:721–733, 1995.
162. Burris HA III, Moore MJ, Andersen J, et al.: Improvements in survival and clinical benefit with gemcitabine as first-line therapy for patients with advanced pancreas cancer: A randomized trial. J Clin Oncol 15:2403–2413, 1997.
163. Berlin J: Gemcitabine. Clin Perspect Gastroenterol 106–111, 1999.
164. Talamini MA, Pitt HA, Hruban RH, et al.: Spectrum of cystic tumors of the pancreas. Am J Surg 163:117–123, 1992.
165. Gupta RK, alAnsari AG: Needle aspiration cytology in the diagnosis of mucinous cystadenocarcinoma of pancreas. A study of five cases with an emphasis on utility and differential diagnosis. Int J Pancreatol 15:149–153, 1994.
166. Solcia E, Capella, Klöppel G: Tumors of the pancreas. Atlas of tumor pathology, Third Series Fascicle 20. Washington, DC: Armed Forces Institute of Pathology, 1997.
167. Tracey KJ, O'Brien J, Williams LF, et al.: Signet ring carcinoma of the pancreas, a rare variant with very

high CEA values. Immunohistologic comparison with adenocarcinoma. Dig Dis Sci 29:573–576, 1984.
168. Sommers SC, Meissner WA: Unusual carcinomas of the pancreas. Arch Pathol 58:101–111, 1954.
169. Cihak RW, Kawashima T, Steer A: Adenoacanthoma (adenosquamous carcinoma) of the pancreas. Cancer 29:1133–1140, 1972.
170. Ishikawa O, Matsui Y, Aoki I, et al.: Adenosquamous carcinoma of the pancreas: A clinicopathologic study of three cases. Cancer 46:1192–1196, 1980.
171. Motojima K, Tomioka T, Kohara N, et al.: Immunohistochemical characteristics of adenosquamous carcinoma of the pancreas. J Surg Oncol 49:58–62, 1992.
172. Campman SC, Fajardo MA, Rippon MB, et al.: Adenosquamous carcinoma arising in a mucinous cystadenoma of the pancreas. J Surg Oncol 64:159–162, 1997.
173. Yamaguchi K, Enjoji M: Adenosquamous carcinoma of the pancreas: A clinicopathologic study. J Surg Oncol 47:109–116, 1991.
174. Serafini F, Rosemurgy AS, Carey L: Squamous cell carcinoma of the pancreas. Am J Gastroenterol 91:2621–2622, 1996.
175. Brayko CM, Doll DC: Squamous cell carcinoma of the pancreas associated with hypercalcemia. Gastroenterology 83:1297–1299, 1982.
176. Lewin K: Carcinoid tumors and the mixed (composite) glandular-endocrine cell carcinomas. Am J Surg Pathol 11(suppl):71–86, 1987.
177. Reid JD, Yuh S-L, Petrelli M, et al.: Ductuloinsular tumors of the pancreas. A light electron microscopic and immunohistochemical study. Cancer 49:908–915, 1982.
178. Ulich T, Cheng L, Lewin KJ: Acinar-endocrine cell tumor of the pancreas. Report of a pancreatic tumor containing both zymogen and neuroendocrine granules. Cancer 50:2099–2105, 1982.
179. Corrin B, Gilby ED, Jones NF, et al.: Oat cell carcinoma of the pancreas with ectopic ACTH secretion. Cancer 31:1523–1527, 1973.
180. O'Connor TP, Wade TP, Sunwoo YC, et al.: Small cell undifferentiated carcinoma of the pancreas. Cancer 70:1514–1519, 1992.
181. Hobbs RD, Stewart AF, Ravin ND, et al.: Hypercalcemia in small cell carcinoma of the pancreas. Cancer 53:1552–1554, 1984.
182. Chetty R, Clark SP, Pitson GA: Primary small cell carcinoma of the pancreas. Pathology 25:240–242, 1993.
183. Wahid NA, Neugut AI, Hibshoosh H, et al.: Response of small cell carcinoma of pancreas to a small cell lung cancer regimen. A case report. Cancer Invest 14:335–339, 1996.
184. Tschang T-P, Garza-Garza R, Kissane JM: Pleomorphic carcinoma of the pancreas. Cancer 39:2114–2126, 1977.
185. Watanabe M, Miura H, Inoue H, et al.: Mixed osteoclastic/pleomorphic-type giant cell tumor of the pancreas with ductal adenocarcinoma: Histochemical and immuno-histochemical study with review of the literature. Pancreas 15:201–208, 1997.
186. Deckard-Janatpour K, Kraegel S, Teplitz R, et al.: Tumors of the pancreas with osteoclast-like and pleomorphic giant cells: An immunohistochemical and ploidy study. Arch Pathol Lab Med 122:266–272, 1998.
187. Alguacil-Garcia A, Weiland LH: The histologic spectrum, prognosis, and histogenesis of the sarcomatoid carcinoma of the pancreas. Cancer 39:1181–1189, 1977.
188. Hoorens A, Prenzel K, Lemoine NR, et al.: Undifferentiated carcinoma of the pancreas: Analysis of intermediate filament profile and Ki-*ras* mutations provides evidence of a ductal origin. J Pathol 185:53–60, 1998.
189. Imai Y, Morishita S, Ikeda Y, et al.: Immunohistochemical and molecular analysis of giant cell carcinoma of the pancreas: A report of three cases. Pancreas 18:308–315, 1999.
190. Marinko A, Nogueira R, Schmitt F, et al.: Pancreatic mucinous cystadenocarcinoma with a mural nodule of anaplastic carcinoma. Histopathology 26:284–287, 1995.
191. Lane RB Jr, Sangueza OP: Anaplastic carcinoma occurring in association with mucinous cystic neoplasm of the pancreas. Arch Pathol Lab Med 121:533–535, 1997.
192. Suster S, Phillips M, Robinson MJ: Malignant fibrous histiocytoma (giant cell type) of the pancreas. A distinctive variant of osteoclast-type giant cell tumor of the pancreas. Cancer 64:2303–2308, 1989.
193. Millis JM, Chang B, Zinner MJ, et al.: Malignant mixed tumor (carcinosarcoma) of the pancreas: A case report supporting organ-induced differentiation of malignancy. Surgery 115:132–137, 1994.
194. Rosai J: Carcinoma of pancreas simulating giant cell tumor of bone. Electron-microscopic evidence of its acinar cell origin. Cancer 22:333–344, 1968.
195. Goldberg RD, Michelassi F, Montag AG: Osteoclast-like giant cell tumor of the pancreas: Immunophenotypic similarity to giant cell tumor of bone. Hum Pathol 22:618–622, 1991.
196. Molberg KH, Heffess C, Delgado R, et al.: Undifferentiated carcinoma with osteoclast-like giant cells of the pancreas and periampullary region. Cancer 82:1279–1287, 1998.
197. Gocke CD, Dabbs DJ, Benko FA, et al.: K-*ras* oncogene mutations suggest a common histogenetic origin for pleomorphic giant cell tumor of the pancreas, osteoclastoma of the pancreas, and pancreatic duct adenocarcinoma. Hum Pathol 28:80–83, 1997.
198. Westra WH, Sturm P, Drillenburg P, et al.: K-*ras* oncogene mutations in osteoclast-like giant cell tumors of the pancreas and liver. Clinical evidence to support origin from the duct epithelium. Am J Surg Pathol 22:1247–1254, 1998.
199. Martin A, Texier P, Bahnini JM, et al.: An unusual epithelial pleomorphic giant cell tumour of the pancreas with osteoclast-type cells. J Clin Pathol 47:372–374, 1994.
200. Mentes A, Yuce G: Osteoclast-type giant cell tumor of the pancreas associated with mucinous cystadenoma. Eur J Surg Oncol 9:84–86, 1993.
201. Nojima T, Nakamura F, Ishikura M, et al.: Pleomorphic carcinoma of the pancreas with osteoclast-like giant cells. Int J Pancreatol 14:275–281, 1993.
202. Newbould MJ, Benbow EW, Sene A, et al.: Adenocarcinoma of the pancreas with osteoclast-like giant cells: A case report with immunocytochemistry. Pancreas 7:611–615, 1992.
203. Dworak O, Wittekind C, Koerfgen HP, et al.: Osteoclastic giant cell tumor of the pancreas. An immunohistological study and review of the literature. Pathol Res Pract 189:228–234, 1993.
204. Lonardo F, Cubilla AL, Klimstra DS: Microadenocarcinoma of the pancreas—morphological pattern or pathological entity? A reevaluation of the original series. Am J Surg Pathol 20:1385–1393, 1996.

205. Luttges J, Vogel I, Menke M, et al.: Clear cell carcinoma of the pancreas: An adenocarcinoma with ductal phenotype. Histopathology 32:444–448, 1998.
206. Kanai N, Nagari S, Tanaka T: Clear cell carcinoma of the pancreas. Acta Pathol Jpn 37:1521–1526, 1987.
207. Guarda LA, Silva EG, Ordonez NG, et al.: Clear cell islet cell tumor. Am J Clin Pathol 79:512–517, 1983.
208. Perez-Ordonez B, Naseem A, Lieberman PH, et al.: Solid serous adenoma of the pancreas. The solid variant of serous cystadenoma? Am J Surg Pathol 20:1401–1405, 1996.
209. Zamboni G, Pea M, Martignoni G, et al.: Clear cell "sugar" tumor of the pancreas. A novel member of the family of lesions characterized by the presence of perivascular epithelioid cells. Am J Surg Pathol 20:722–730, 1996.

Chapter

8

OTHER NONENDOCRINE TUMORS

A classification of neoplasms of the pancreas is given in Table 8–1. This excludes islet cell tumors, which are dealt with in Chapter 9, and ductal adenocarcinomas, which are discussed in Chapter 7.

MICROCYSTIC ADENOMA

Microcystic adenoma has also been called serous cystadenoma and glycogen-rich cystadenoma. The first synonym is appropriate, as the tumor contains a watery fluid. However, it shares no histologic features with serous cystadenoma of the ovary and does not show serous acinar differentiation. This can be a cause of confusion. The second synonym is also appropriate. Most such tumors do have glycogen-rich cells, although these can be sparse and poorly granulated. *Microcystic adenoma* is the most commonly used name and is appropriate to describe the vast majority of neoplasms. However, there are macrocystic and even solid variants described. There are also rare malignant examples.

Microcystic adenomas account for between 1% and 2% of exocrine pancreatic neoplasms and about 25% of cystic neoplasms. The average age at diagnosis is 65 years (range, 34 to 91 years),[1] with most of these tumors occurring in women. In some series, the female predominance is marked (70%),[1,2] but in others it is only slight.[3] Smaller tumors may be discovered incidentally on routine physical examination or ultrasound investigation. These account for about one third of cases. Patients with the larger neoplasms generally present with vague upper abdominal pain or discomfort, as adjacent organs are compressed. Symptoms may also include nausea, vomiting, and weight loss, although obstructive jaundice is rare. Occasionally, the tumors are multiple,[3–5] and there is a weak association with von Hippel–Lindau syndrome.[6–8] In patients with von Hippel–Lindau syndrome, the mean age at presentation is lower than in sporadic disease. The tumors also tend to be oligocystic.

Associated clinical findings include gallstones, diabetes, and extrapancreatic neoplasms.[9,10] It is probable that these are coincidental and may actually be the reason the microcystic adenoma was first discovered. Plain x-rays of the abdomen may show flecks of calcification within the tumor and computed tomography (CT) scan demonstrates a well-circumscribed multilocular cyst, with a characteristic central stellate scar.[11]

Microcystic adenomas may be found anywhere within the pancreas, although they are most common within the body and tail. The average diameter is between 7 and 10 cm, with a range of 1 to 25 cm. Externally, they are well circumscribed, have a bosselated appearance, and may be covered by a thin capsule. The cut surface shows multiple small cysts, separated by thin, fibrous septa, and resembles a sponge (Fig. 8–1). The cysts vary in size: Some are microscopic; others are as large as 2 cm in diameter. They have a smooth lining and contain clear fluid. Hemorrhage may be present, although necrotic foci are unusual. In the center of the tumor, there may be a stellate scar with

Table 8–1. Neoplasms of the Pancreas

Epithelial Tumors
Microcystic adenoma (serous cystadenoma)
Oligocystic variant
Solid variant
Serous cystadenocarcinoma
Mucinous cystic neoplasm
Benign
Borderline
Malignant
Papillary mucinous tumor
Benign
Borderline
Malignant
Solid-cystic-papillary tumor (solid-pseudopapillary tumor)
Solid, infiltrating variant
Malignant variant
Acinar cell carcinoma
Mixed acinar-endocrine tumor
Pancreatoblastoma
Connective Tissue Tumors
Benign tumors
Fibrous histiocytoma
Schwannoma
Lipoma
Granular cell tumor
Vascular tumors
Hemangioma
Hemangioendothelioma
Lymphangioma
Sarcomas
Malignant fibrous histiocytoma
Malignant nerve sheath tumor
Leiomyosarcoma
Liposarcoma
Rhabdomyosarcoma
Primitive neuroectodermal tumor
Desmoplastic small round cell tumor
Solitary fibrous tumor
Lymphomas
Primary non-Hodgkin's lymphoma
Secondary lymphomas
Hodgkin's disease
Plasmacytoma
Non-Hodgkin's lymphoma
Miscellaneous Tumors
Teratoma
Sugar tumor
Tumorlike Masses
Hamartoma
Inflammatory pseudotumor

radiating fibrous bands.[1,2,6,12] In larger tumors (> 5 cm diameter), the fibrous tissue may contain flecks or denser deposits of calcified material.

Microscopic appearances are uniform throughout the tumor (Fig. 8–2). The cysts are lined by a single layer of flattened or cuboidal cells that may be invaginated to form tiny papillae, with no central fibrous core. Within the cyst, a small quantity of lightly eosinophilic material may be present. The cells have central rounded nuclei, with inconspicuous nucleoli and cytoplasm that varies from clear to lightly eosinophilic (Fig. 8–3A). Pleomorphic nuclei are not usually encountered and there is no mitotic activity. Periodic acid–Schiff (PAS) stains with and without prior diastase digestion demonstrate that the clear cytoplasm is due to the presence of glycogen (Fig. 8–3B). The stroma is hyalinized and contains a delicate capillary network. Hemosiderin-laden macrophages, cholesterol clefts, and dystrophic calcification may be encountered in those patients in whom there has been previous hemorrhage.[2]

Fine-needle aspiration (FNA) can be useful in preoperative diagnosis and serves to distinguish microcystic adenomas from carcinomas and mucinous cystic tumors.[13–15] Aspiration samples tend to be hypocellular with scattered clumps and strips of uniform polygonal or cuboidal cells (Fig. 8–4). These have a clear nonmucinous cytoplasm and regular oval nuclei, with an even distribution of chromatin. The smear background is also nonmucinous.

Immunohistochemistry shows positive staining with epithelial membrane antigen (EMA) and cytokeratins 7, 8, 18, and 19.[1,2] Fifty percent of tumors also stain positively for neuron-specific enolase (NSE). Negative results are obtained with immunostains for carcinoembryonic antigen (CEA), p53, chromogranin, and pancreatic hormones and enzymes.[2] Fifteen percent of tumors stain positively for CA19-9. K-*ras* oncogene mutations have not been detected.[16] Mucin stains for epithelial acid mucin, using alcian blue at pH 2.5 and 1.0, are negative, although traces of neutral mucin may be demonstrated by PAS staining after diastase digestion and by mucicarmine staining.[17] Ultrastructural examination reveals a thin basement membrane. On the luminal surface of the cysts, the cells have small blunted microvilli with no microfilaments. The cytoplasm contains glycogen granules and occasional fat droplets but with few mitochondria and only short profiles of endoplasmic reticulum.[2]

The clinical behavior of microcystic adenomas is that of benign slow-growing expansile masses. They have an excellent prognosis and require treatment only if they become bulky and cause symptoms. There are rare reports of a malignant variant, termed serous cystadenocarcinoma.[4,18–22] These have metastasized to the wall of the stomach, to the liver, and to regional

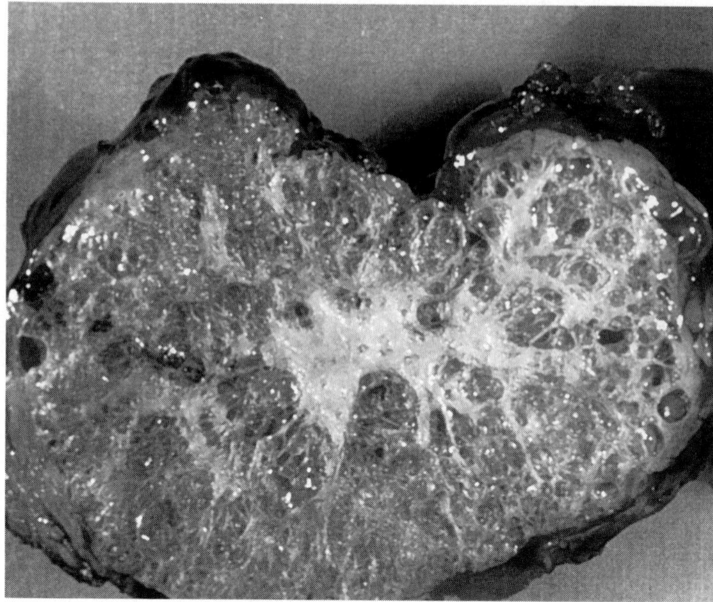

Figure 8–1. Gross appearances of a microcystic adenoma. The tumor is well demarcated with a central scar and numerous microcysts.

nodes.[20,21] Because of the small number of cases reported, it is difficult to draw general conclusions. However, malignant serous tumors tend to occur at an older age, tend to be symptomatic, and tend to be larger in size when compared with a typical microcystic adenoma. Metastases have been encountered in the liver and lymph nodes. Invasion of peripancreatic fat and perineural invasion are also recorded. In these reports, the pancreatic tumor demonstrated focal mild cytologic atypia with some nuclear enlargement and hyperchromatism but was otherwise identical to nonmetastasizing tumors. In neither of the reported cases did the patients have von Hippel–Lindau syndrome or a primary renal tumor. In one reported case,[18] the patient died of surgical complications during tumor removal. In a second case, the patient is alive and well 5 years after removal of the primary tumor and liver metastases.[19] A cystadenoma has been described[22] in which part of the tumor had the usual bland cytologic appearance and part had mild nuclear atypia. The atypical foci showed a tendency to form papil-

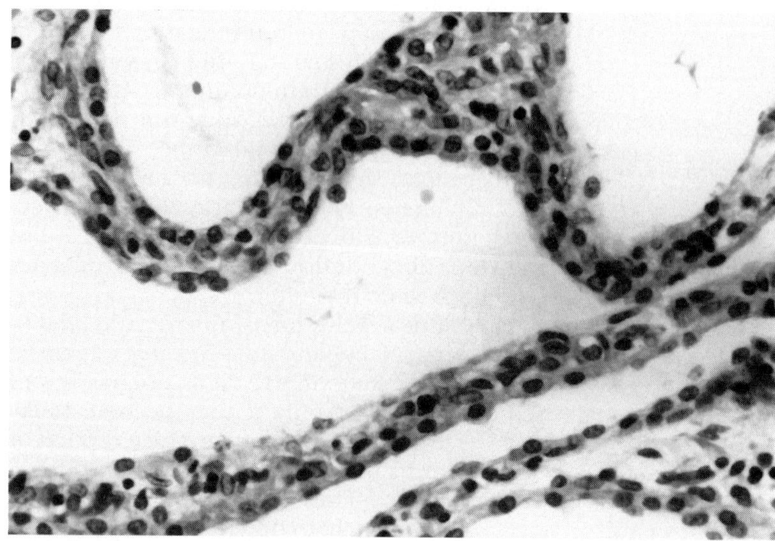

Figure 8–2. Microcystic adenoma with a uniform honeycomb appearance.

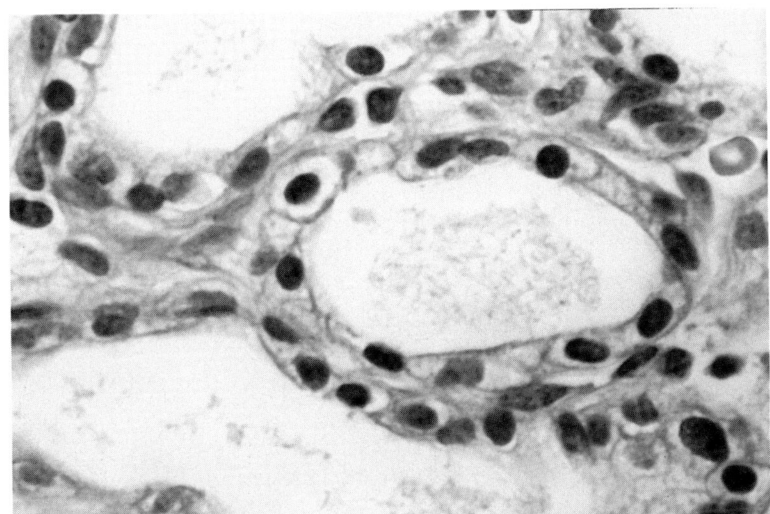

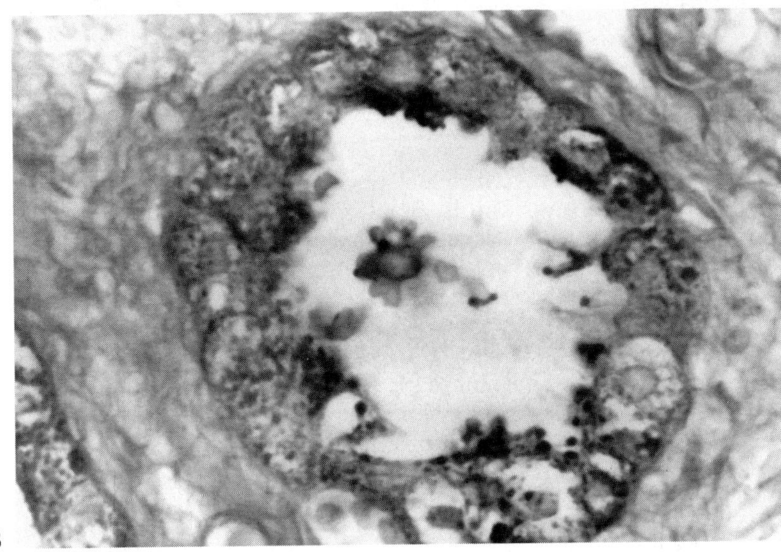

Figure 8–3. *A,* The cells lining the microcysts are flattened and have inconspicuous cytoplasm with central rounded nuclei. *B,* Cytoplasmic granularity is demonstrated. (PAS.)

lary structures with a central fibrovascular core. The cytoplasm was nonmucinous and glycogen poor. Focal vascular and perivascular invasion was identified. Although metastases were not observed, this neoplasm was appropriately labeled serous cystadenoma with focal malignant changes. It is reasonable to accept that rare examples of nonmucinous microcystic tumors may metastasize locally but are still very low grade and do not appear to kill the patient.

Three histologic variants of microcystic adenoma have been described. The first of these is one that contains myoepithelial cells.[23] On light microscopic examination, the myoepithelial cells appear as spindle cells "hugging" the lining cuboidal cells. The biologic significance of this finding is not clear. Typical microcystic adenomas show ultrastructural evidence of a centroacinar derivation with no myoepithelial layer.[6,16] The second variant is one in which macrocysts are present.[12,24] In two of the nine adult cases described, the cysts were unilocular. In the other cases, several cysts were present, ranging in size from 1.5 to 8.0 cm (so-called oligocystic variant). Isolated cases have been described in children.[25–27] Two of these pediatric cases occurred in infants with cytomegalovirus infection. The significance of this finding is unclear. Oligocystic adenomas lack the characteristic central scar of the multicystic adenomas and are also much less well circumscribed grossly, with no distinct capsule.[12] The lining of the cysts is otherwise typical of microcystic adenoma, with a tendency for more flattened

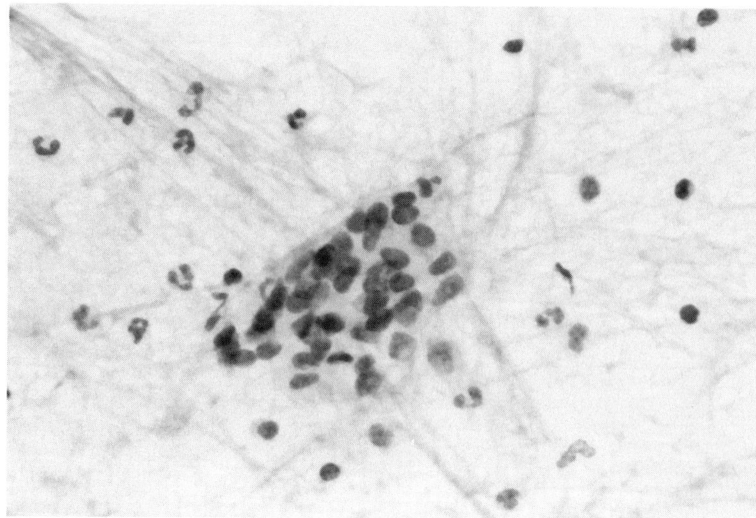

Figure 8–4. Aspiration cytology showing a hypocellular sample with a cluster of uniform polygonal cells.

cells to be present at the expense of cuboidal cells. The third variant has been termed a solid serous adenoma.[28] This consists of nests, sheets, and trabeculae of glycogen-rich clear cells, separated by thick fibrous bands. Small glandular spaces may be seen, but cysts are absent. Foci of solid growth pattern may be occasionally encountered in otherwise typical microcystic tumors.

Rare examples of a combination of microcystic adenoma with other pancreatic tumors, particularly malignancies, have been described.[29,30] These associations may be fortuitous. Multifocal microcystic adenomas are rarely described[3–5] and include examples in which only two tumors are present[5] and examples in which there are large numbers of tumors, ranging in size from 2 to 4 cm in diameter.[3] In most cases, multifocal tumors are histologically unremarkable, although one example had cytologic atypia and perineural invasion.[4]

Factors influencing the occurrence of microcystic adenomas are unknown. However, there has been a study of this tumor examining cases occurring sporadically[10] and another study of cases occurring in conjunction with von Hippel–Lindau syndrome.[2] Loss of heterozygosity at the von Hippel–Lindau gene locus on chromosome 3p25 was detected in 7 of 10 sporadically occurring tumors and a somatic mutation of exon 2 was documented in an additional sporadic case.[31] Both von Hippel–Lindau tumors showed loss of heterozygosity (LOH) with at least one of the microsatellite markers tested. Currently, it is thought that in von Hippel–Lindau syndrome there is a germline mutation of one allele with an acquired deletion of the other wild-type allele.[32] In sporadic microcystic adenoma, it is postulated that acquired alterations to the von Hippel–Lindau gene play a role in tumorigenesis.[31]

The differential diagnosis of microcystic adenomas is limited. It is important to exclude mucinous tumors, which, although histologically benign, have significant malignant potential. A mucin stain (usually PAS with diastase) will be helpful here. Another possible source of diagnostic confusion is acinar cell cystadenocarcinoma.[33] Grossly, this neoplasm closely mimics the honeycomb appearance of microcystic adenoma, but microscopically, the cystic spaces are seen to be lined by tall columnar cells, in which fine PAS-/diastase-positive granules are easily recognized in the apical cytoplasm. The granules of a microcystic adenoma are PAS positive but PAS/diastase negative.

MUCINOUS CYSTIC NEOPLASM

The 1996 World Health Organization (WHO) classification of pancreatic tumors has subdivided mucinous cystic tumors according to histologic appearance as cystadenoma, borderline tumor, or cystadenocarcinoma, with or without invasion.[34] However, this subdivision may not be advisable, or even possible, in all cases, as mucinous cystic neoplasms may show a spectrum of histologic grades and appearances within the same tumor. This may lead to the misclassification of small unrepresentative biopsy specimens, with serious clinical consequences.[35] Resected neoplasms should be thoroughly sampled to ensure that small foci of invasive malignancy are not missed. No rules based on scientific evidence exist to mandate exactly how many sections should be taken, but it is recommended that reliance be placed on naked-eye appearances, with sampling of any unusually firm, nodular, or papillary areas. As a minimum, one section per 1 cm of tumor diameter should be obtained. Ideally, all mucinous cystic neoplasms should be excised surgically to remove foci of carcinoma and permit histologic evaluation.

Mucinous cystic neoplasms account for about 30% of all cystic pancreatic neoplasms and about 7% of all pancreatic cysts. However, they are relatively rare and account for only 2% of all pancreatic neoplasms. They occur predominately in adult women.[35] In two recent large series, comprising 136 cases and 56 cases, respectively, no examples were encountered in men.[36,37] The average age of patients is 44.6 years, with a range of 20 to 95 years.[36] However, if cases are subdivided according to histologic appearances, the mean age of patients with adenomas is 48; with borderline tumors, 40; with noninvasive carcinoma, 50; and with invasive carcinoma, 55.8 years.[37] This age differential raises the possibility of an adenoma–carcinoma sequence. Men with this tumor tend to be older than women who have it (mean age for men, 64 years). Histologically, benign tumors are twice as common as malignant ones (adenoma, 39%; borderline, 21%; carcinoma, 39%).[37] Almost all tumors (93% to 95%) involve the tail of the pancreas, although the larger ones can affect the body and head also.[36–39]

The major clinical symptom is pain and discomfort, usually located in the epigastric region or left upper quadrant. Pain is experienced by 62% to 72% of individuals.[36,37] Patients describe a dull aching or a sharp stabbing or cramping pain that occasionally radiates through to the back. This may be continuous or intermittent. Weight loss is noted in between 7% and 10% of patients. In 5% to 34% of patients, a palpable upper abdominal mass is detected.[36,37] Smaller tumors are discovered incidentally by ultrasonography or CT examination, which reveals a circumscribed hypoechoic or low-density mass, in which separate locules may be recognized.[40] Spiral CT is the examination of choice for correct preoperative determination of tumor type.

On gross examination, mucinous tumors are irregular in shape with a smooth, glistening capsule covered by prominent vessels. The larger neoplasms are frequently adherent to adjacent organs.[41] Sectioning reveals a fibrous capsule of varying thickness, which may contain flecks of calcification. Viscous mucus exudes from the center of the tumor, which may be uni- or multilocular (Fig. 8–5). Occasionally, the mucus may be turbid or hemorrhagic. Generally, the lining of the locules is smooth, although in the more proliferative tumors, papillary excrescences may be seen on the cyst wall lining. The cysts only rarely communicate with the lumen of the pancreatic duct.[42] The average size is between 7 and 10 cm, although sometimes they are considerably larger (≤ 30 cm). As a general rule, the larger neoplasms are more likely to be malignant,[37] although in an individual case, size is

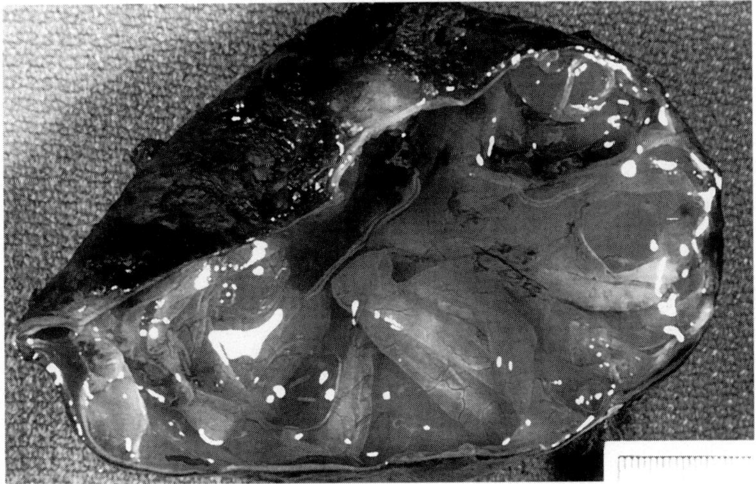

Figure 8–5. Cut surface of mucinous cystic tumor. The locules exude mucus and have thin walls with no solid areas or papillary excrescences (cystadenoma).

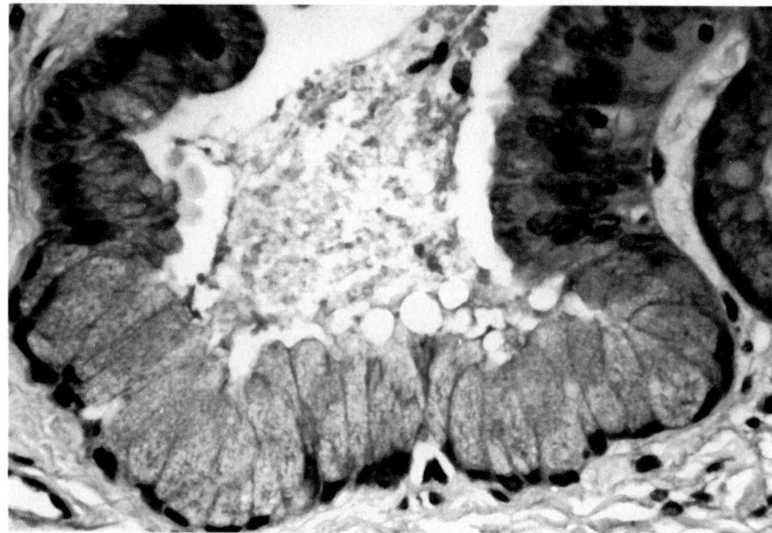

Figure 8–6. Lining of cystadenoma. Some cells resemble gastric foveolar epithelium. Others are non–mucus secreting.

not a useful predictor of malignancy. Frankly malignant tumors may show obvious invasion of the surrounding structures.

Histologically, the cysts are lined by mucus-secreting epithelium, which in benign tumors may resemble that of gastric foveolar epithelium (Fig. 8–6). In some areas, nonmucinous epithelium may be present, along with mucin-secreting columnar cells and goblet cells (Fig. 8–7). Because of nuclear atypia and crowding, the cyst lining may resemble a large bowel adenoma. Occasional endocrine cells and Paneth's cells are common (Fig. 8–8). In large locules, the epithelium may become flattened or even partly denuded. The degree of differentiation of the lining epithelium may vary from locule to locule. Some locules tend to be lined by an extremely well differentiated epithelium with small, regular, basally located nuclei and abundant cytoplasmic mucin (Fig. 8–8). Other locules or parts of locules may be denuded of epithelium. If the tumor consists entirely of this bland epithelium, then it may reasonably be labeled as a mucinous cystadenoma. Locules

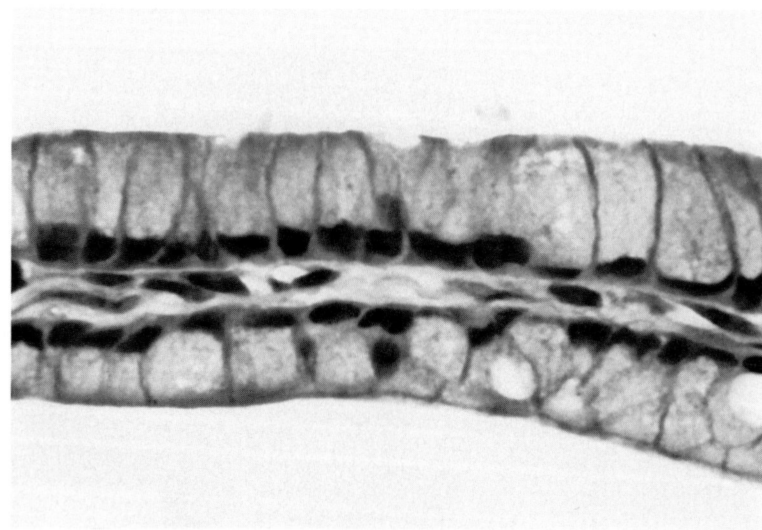

Figure 8–7. Simple mucus-secreting epithelium lining a mucinous cystadenoma.

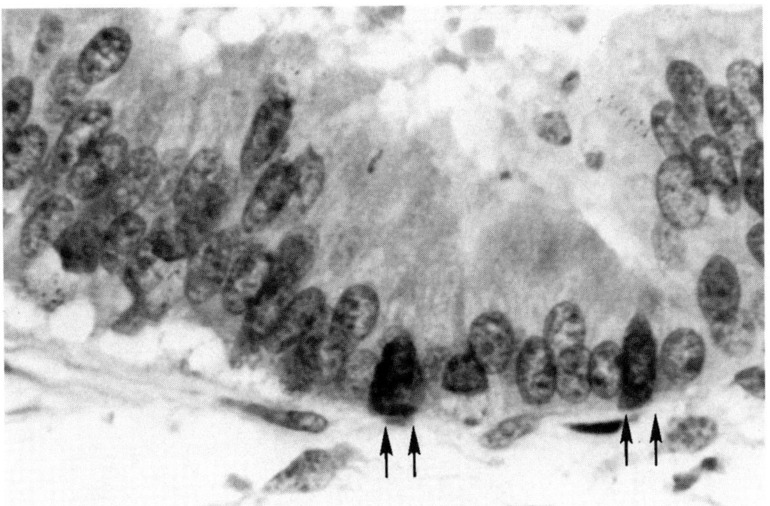

Figure 8–8. Endocrine cells in a mucinous cystadenoma. (Immunostain for synaptophysin.)

with papillary excrescences tend to have more poorly differentiated cells, with larger irregular nuclei showing loss of polarity and increased mitotic activity. A papillary or cribriform arrangement may be present (Fig. 8–9). The epithelium may be multilayered; such moderately differentiated neoplasms have been called borderline mucinous tumors. Areas with very poorly differentiated epithelium resembling colonic adenocarcinoma may be called mucinous cystadenocarcinoma (Fig. 8–10). Where stromal infarction has occurred, this may be appreciated grossly by the finding of solid necrotic areas in the stroma between locules. Occasionally, the invasive component of the tumor may be adenosquamous in type[43] or may contain osteoclast giant cells and choriocarcinomatous differentiation.[44] It is characteristic for benign-appearing epithelium to be present immediately adjacent to noninvasive carcinoma, with no gradation of atypia.[36] Rupture of locules with extravasation of mucus into the stroma may occur. Free-floating cells may be benign, borderline, or malignant.

Although not prominent in every case, it is quite common for mucinous cystic tumors to have a stroma composed of plump spindle cells that have a close resemblance to ovarian

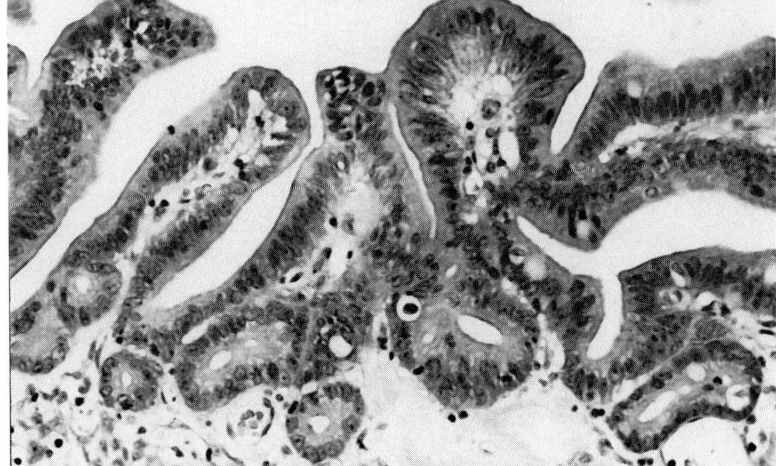

Figure 8–9. Borderline mucinous tumor with papillary areas.

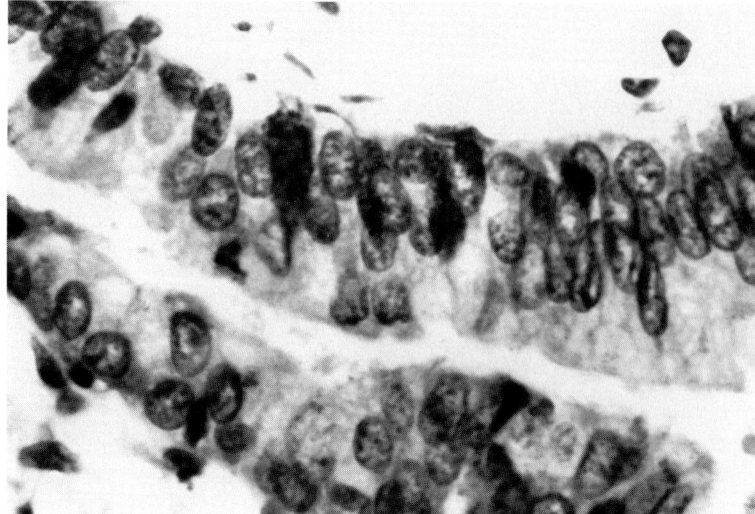

Figure 8–10. High-grade mucinous cystic neoplasm (cystadenocarcinoma).

stroma[35–39] (Fig. 8–11). This specialized stroma consists of two layers: a subepithelial zone of mesenchyme that is moderately to densely cellular and an outer zone that is less cellular and more fibrous. This outer layer may contain scattered, normal-appearing ducts with lymphoid tissue and large vessels. Interestingly, this phenomenon occurs predominately in women with cystic mucinous tumors. Only rare tumors with "ovarian stroma" have been described in men.[45] Within this stroma, structures resembling a corpus albicans may be encountered.[36,46] Stromal luteinization occurs in up to 28% of cases.[36] It is interesting to note that mucinous cystadenomas arising from the bile duct and occurring in the retroperitoneum may also display this ovarian-type stroma.[47]

In common with ovarian mucinous tumors, mucinous pancreatic neoplasms may develop spindle cell nodules or masses in the wall of the cysts.[48–53] Both cystadenomas and cystadenocarcinomas may develop this complication. These nodules are of three types: reactive fibrous nodules (pseudosarcoma),[48] spindle cell carcinoma[49–51] or true sarcoma resembling leiomyosarcoma, or malignant fibrous histiocytoma.[52,53] Distinguishing these types of nodule is not always easy but relies on both traditional light microscopy and immunohistochemistry. Pseudosarcomatous nodules lack cellular pleomor-

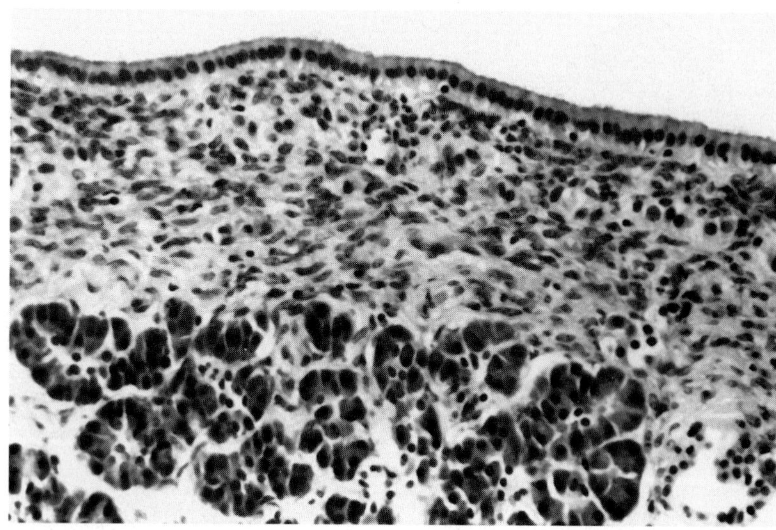

Figure 8–11. Specialized "ovarian" stroma in the wall of a mucinous cystic tumor.

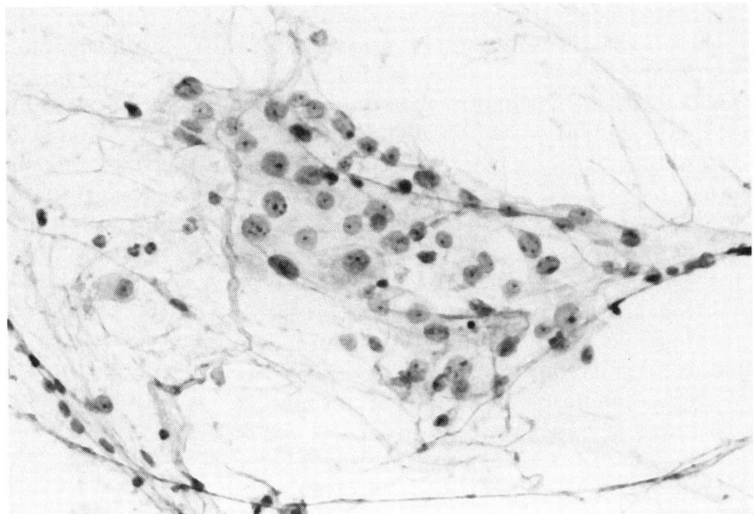

Figure 8–12. Fine-needle aspiration biopsy of mucinous cystic neoplasm. Note the regular cells in a mucinous background.

phism and abundant mitotic activity. They may be derived from myofibroblasts.[48] Carcinomatous nodules may be cytokeratin, epithelial membrane antigen, and vimentin positive but are negative for actin and desmin.[49] In contrast, the sarcomatous nodules are keratin negative but are positive with vimentin and actin (muscle-specific and smooth muscle types).[53] This distinction between pseudosarcoma and true spindle cell neoplasia is crucial, as the presence of poorly differentiated carcinoma or sarcoma is associated with a poor prognosis.

On fine-needle aspiration biopsy (FNAB), the key to the diagnosis of mucinous cystic tumors is the recognition of large quantities of mucus, both within the cell cytoplasm and in the smear background.[14,54] (Fig. 8–12). Nuclear pleomorphism is variable (Fig. 8–13), depending on the area sampled, but it should be reemphasized that the finding of benign cytology does not necessarily imply that this is representative of the neoplasm as a whole and that the tumor's clinical behavior will be benign. Large sheets, clumps, or even papillary configurations of cells are found sometimes with a honeycomb appearance. In malignant tumors, necrotic debris may be identified.[53]

With the use of immunohistochemical stains, endocrine cells are seen in up to 65% of mucinous cystic neoplasms[39] (see Fig. 8–8). Serotonin-

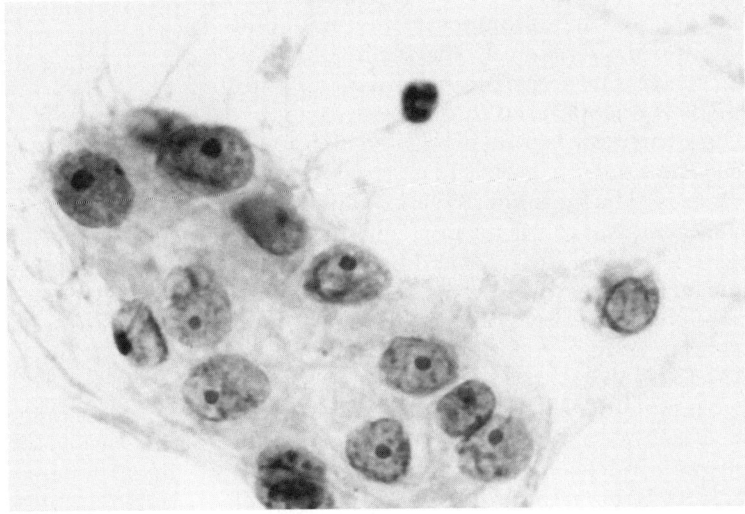

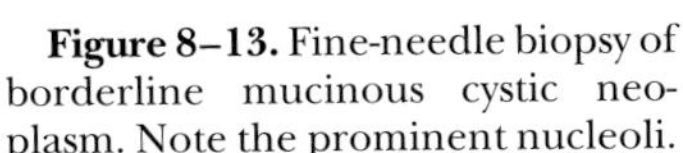

Figure 8–13. Fine-needle biopsy of borderline mucinous cystic neoplasm. Note the prominent nucleoli.

positive cells tend to be concentrated in the more poorly differentiated components of the neoplasm and have focal strong positivity. Weak positivity for somatostatin, pancreatic polypeptide, and gastrin is also seen and there are no differences between benign and malignant tumors. As with adenocarcinomas of the large bowel, the presence of small numbers of scattered endocrine cells should not lead to a diagnosis of mixed carcinoid/carcinoma. Immunostaining for CEA shows negative results in histologically benign areas of the tumor but positive results in borderline areas and in areas of frank mucinous cystadenocarcinoma.[55] Cytokeratins 7, 8, 18, and 19 and EMA are also positive[56,57] and there is focal positivity for p53 and c-*erb*B-2.[57] More than 10% of nuclei positive for p53 is highly suggestive of malignancy. Heterogeneous staining is also observed with CA 19-9, DUPAN-2, and B72.3.[36,37] Stromal cells are uniformly positive with vimentin, smooth muscle actin, and muscle-specific actin. Approximately 25% of both benign and malignant tumors have estrogen receptors.[36] Eighty-three percent of benign tumors and 63% of malignant tumors have progesterone receptors.[36] The positive cells are luteinized epithelioid stromal cells.[37] Positivity is also observed with TE-101 (tyrosine hydroxylase, calretinin, and α-inhibitin).[37] Interestingly, a case of mucinous cystic tumor has been described in a man in which the "ovarian stroma" was positive for both estrogen and progesterone receptors.[37]

Histochemical evaluation of the intracytoplasmic mucin reveals that it consists of neutral mucin, sialomucin, and sulfomucin. It stains positively with PAS/diastase and alcian blue at pH 1.0 and 2.5.[17] Normal pancreatic ducts are rich in sulfomucin, but this highly acidic mucin is relatively sparse in mucinous cystic neoplasms. Considerable variation in mucin type is encountered in different tumors.[58]

Ultrastructural examination[39] reveals appearances very similar to gastric foveolar and mucus neck cells. The columnar cells contain mucin vacuoles in the apical portion and have long and short microvilli on the luminal border. Some of the microvilli show actin filaments, which extend to the apical cytoplasm as long anchoring rootlets.

Mucinous cystic tumors are all negative for K-*ras* mutations. Flow cytometry reveals that 90% of tumors are diploid, including some with high-grade nuclear abnormalities. These have a uniformly good prognosis. Ten percent of tumors are aneuploid and these carry a general unfavorable prognosis.[36]

It should be emphasized that thorough histologic sampling of these tumors is extremely important because small foci of invasive carcinoma may coexist with large areas of histologically benign tumor. Making a diagnosis of mucinous cystadenoma on the basis of biopsy findings or even incomplete resection is ill advised; for this reason, the term *mucinous cystic neoplasm* may be preferred.[24,36] Serious undertreatment may occur if a unilocular tumor is misdiagnosed clinically as a pseudocyst[59] and marsupialized to the bowel. The surgeon may be reluctant to proceed to appropriate radical excision if the pathologist has rendered a diagnosis of cystadenoma on a small biopsy. Furthermore, it has been suggested, but not confirmed, that even tumors with histologically benign appearing epithelium may have metastatic potential. Occasional cases have been encountered in which the lymph node metastases have appeared histologically bland.[60] The recommended treatment for this tumor is complete surgical excision if technically feasible. Even if frank invasive carcinoma is present, complete surgical excision may be curative, especially if only superficial stromal invasion is encountered. If the whole tumor has been excised and has been thoroughly analyzed histologically, it seems reasonable to break down the diagnosis of mucinous cystic tumor into more specific subgroups as outlined in the WHO classification.[34] This is justified, as it relates to prognosis.[37,38] All patients with adenomas, borderline tumors, and noninvasive carcinomas are cured by cystectomy. Fifty percent of patients with invasive tumors die of their disease, with a median survival of 11 months.[37] Factors associated with a poor prognosis are age $>$ 50 years, invasive tumor in the outer wall of the cyst (relative risk, 9.7; confidence interval, 1.8 to 52.3), and nuclear positivity for p53.[37]

The differential diagnosis of mucinous cystic tumor includes pseudocyst, papillary mucinous tumors, and colloid carcinoma. Papillary mucinous tumor has many histologic similarities but differs in that it is predominately a tumor that affects men and generally occurs in the head of the pancreas, where, unlike mucinous cystic tumor, it expands and fills major ducts. It, too, may show benign, borderline, and malignant cytologic features. Mucinous cystic tumor only rarely communicates with the pancreatic ductal system. As the name suggests, papillary mucinous tumor has papillary growth as a major feature, whereas occasional examples of mucinous cystic tumors typically have only a minor papillary component. Colloid carcinoma of the pancreas resembles mucinous carcinomas that may occur elsewhere in the colon and stomach. It is regarded as a variant of ductal carcinoma. Colloid carcinoma is characterized by large quantities of extravasated mucin, in which tumor cells may be floating. Poorly differentiated colloid carcinomas may have signet ring cells present. Usually, thorough sampling of a colloid carcinoma will reveal areas typical of pancreatic ductal carcinoma and will not demonstrate foci of cystadenocarcinoma. Distinguishing mucinous cystic tumors from pseudocysts can be a major problem on frozen section. The difficulty is magnified if only a small crushed fragment of tissue is submitted by the surgeon from a unilocular mucinous tumor. Not all pseudocysts are preceded by a clear-cut history of chronic pancreatitis. Caution is advised, as it is seldom possible to make a definitive diagnosis of pseudocyst under these circumstances.

INTRADUCTAL PAPILLARY-MUCINOUS TUMOR

Intraductal papillary-mucinous tumor has only recently been defined and separated from mucinous cystic tumor. In the literature, it is referred to by a wide variety of names, which include papillary hyperplasia,[61] intraductal papillary neoplasm,[62] villous adenoma,[63–65] mucinous ductal ectasia,[66] intraductal carcinoma,[67–69] and papillary mucin-producing (or mucinous) tumor.[70–74] The designation as intraductal papillary-mucinous tumor is now the most widely accepted.[34,75] It has many histologic similarities to mucinous cystic tumor but arises within and expands the major duct system rather than forming cysts. It also may be subclassified into benign, borderline, and malignant variants,[34] but otherwise it is rather homogeneous with regard to incidence, clinical findings, and morphologic appearance. The incidence of papillary mucinous tumor is not accurately known, but it seems to be about half as common as mucinous cystic tumors.

Papillary mucinous tumor predominately affects men (59% to 60% in large series,[74,76,77]) with a mean age of 65 years (range, 41 to 87 years). There is no age differential for benign and malignant tumors. Rare examples have been recorded in children.[78] Seventy percent to 86% of tumors involve the head of the pancreas and a further 25% to 14% involve the head plus body, or the body alone.[77] Clinically,[70,72,77,79] patients present with epigastric discomfort and pain (50%), jaundice (23%), weight loss (23%), steatorrhea (18%), nausea and vomiting (18%), diarrhea (14%), and fever (14%). Many tumors are, however, discovered incidentally during CT or ultrasound examination of the upper abdomen performed for unrelated causes. Pain can be chronic or episodic and may well be the result of transient episodes of localized acute pancreatitis, following obstruction of major ducts. Elevated amylase levels may be found in some individuals. CEA and CA 19-9 levels are usually normal but can be moderately elevated in a minority of patients. Large elevations suggest a malignant papillary mucinous tumor.[76] Individuals with long-standing disease may ultimately develop diabetes mellitus or steatorrhea, secondary to chronic pancreatitis. By CT scan and ultrasound examination, dilation of ducts in the head of the pancreas may be demonstrated and intraductal polypoid lesions may be seen.[74,80] At endoscopy, the ampulla of Vater typically has a wide-open orifice and exudes mucus into the duodenum.[62,72,81] Polypoid filling defects may be identified by pancreatography.[77,82]

The histogenesis of papillary mucinous tumor is interesting and highly controversial. It has been suggested that a hyperplasia–adenoma–carcinoma sequence exists.[74,83–88] There is considerable histologic evidence to support this concept, in that in some patients, obviously neoplastic lesions are surrounded by dilated ducts containing hyperplasic lesions. The hyperplasia may appear atypical but may also be quite regular and histologically benign. This observation by itself does not, however, exclude the possibility that the hyperplasia is reactive in nature and secondary to the adjacent neoplastic growth. Significantly, K-*ras* oncogene mutations have been demonstrated in cells covering the entire morphologic spectrum of neoplasia and hyperplasia, suggesting that regular hyperplasia may be the earliest lesion of the neoplastic sequence.[87,89] Microsatellite analysis to detect LOH reveals widespread allelic losses, with evidence of clonal progression.[88] The significance of these findings may be considerable. It is a common observation that benign-appearing ductal epithelial hyperplasia, without evidence of neoplasia, may accompany chronic pancreatitis. The hyperplasia may be papillary or nonpapillary in type and may demonstrate goblet cell and gastric pyloric metaplasia. It is also accompanied by K-*ras* mutations.[90,91] At present, therefore, the whole relationship between chronic pancreatitis, ductal hyperplasia, and neoplasia remains in question, not only in papillary mucinous tumors but also in the usual type of pancreatic ductal carcinomas.

As might be anticipated, the gross size and appearance of papillary mucinous tumor varies, depending on the histologic differentiation, with carcinomas being larger than adenomas and borderline tumors. The average size of hyperplasias is 2.0 cm, of adenomas is 3.0 cm, and of carcinomas is 4.8 cm.[74] On gross inspection, the pancreas is hard and nodular with a thickened capsule. The cut surface reveals multilocular (80%), or unilocular (20%) cysts, which discharge thick mucus. Occasional examples of this tumor are not grossly cystic.[77] Not uncommonly, the whole proximal duct system is dilated, even measuring up to 8.0 cm in diameter. Malignant tumors contain soft, friable tissue within the cyst and the wall. Benign tumors typically have cysts lined by overtly papillary material, with the wall being densely fibrotic. Distal dilation of the pancreatic ducts is particularly common, and these may be filled with mucin. The ductectatic variant of the tumor contains only multiple extremely dilated ducts, with no definite tumor visible on gross inspection. On rare occasions, the tumor may form fistulas into the duodenum[71,92] or grow in a diffuse fashion.[93]

Histologically, the tumors are characterized by dilation of the main pancreatic duct and its major tributaries. The lining epithelium shows a variety of appearances, ranging from frank invasive carcinoma through highly atypical but noninvasive tumor (borderline) (Fig. 8–14) to low-grade adenomatous epithelium (Fig. 8–15). It is characteristic to find a variety of types of epithelium within the same tumor, with a gradual gradation of appearances. In adenomatous lesions, the ducts show papillary proliferation to varying degrees, but a cribriform and glandular architecture may be present in up to 24% of tumors. The individual cells are crowded with nuclear hyperchromasia and loss of polarity. Cytoplasmic mucin production is abundant. In most areas of the tumor, this is noted within columnar cells; however, goblet cells may be present to a minor degree in up to 67% of tumors. Cytoplasmic mucin is most abundant in low-grade adenomatous epithelium, where the nuclei occupy less than half the cell volume. In high-grade adenomas with larger nuclei, there are smaller quantities of apical mucus present. In borderline and frankly invasive tumors, there are progressive degrees of nuclear abnormality with piling up of cells to produce a multilayered appearance. In these areas, relatively sparse mucin production is encountered. In invasive carcinomatous areas, nuclear polarity is lost and the nuclei contain prominent nucleoli. Papillary mucinous tumors have a fibrous stroma. "Ovarian" type stroma is not described. Some grossly identifiable "tumors" have been designated as examples of hyperplasia, rather than neoplasia, because of the absence of epithelial atypia[74] (Fig. 8–16).

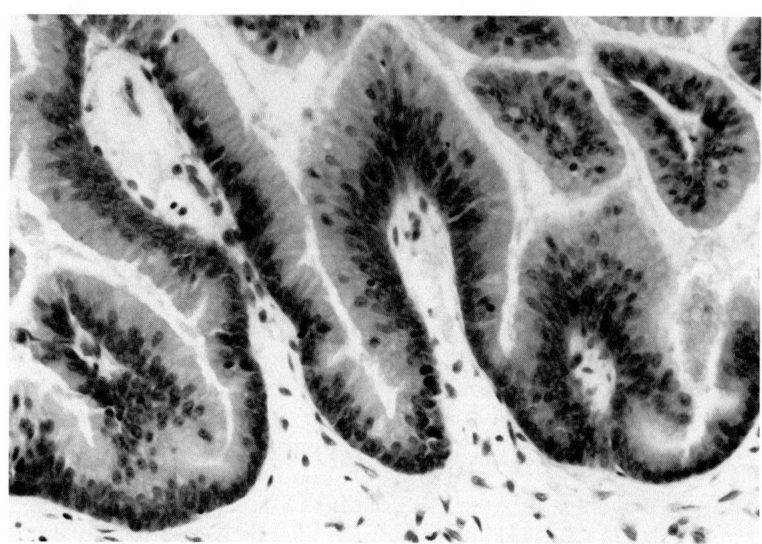

Figure 8–14. Borderline papillary mucinous tumor.

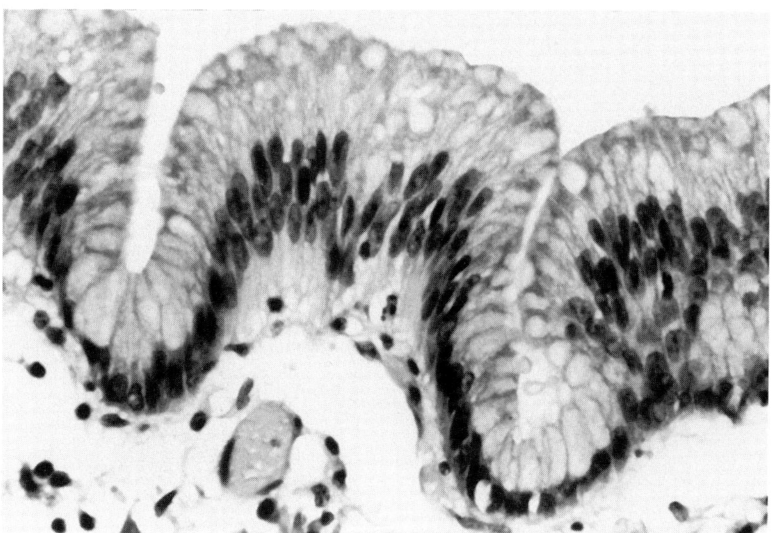

Figure 8–15. Low-grade papillary mucinous tumor (adenoma).

However, it remains to be seen whether these lesions are truly nonneoplastic. Similar benign-appearing epithelium may be found alongside obviously neoplastic epithelium in other tumors.

Papillary mucin-secreting tumors show progressively less mucin content with increasing loss of differentiation. In adenomatous areas, the columnar cells contain predominantly neutral mucin, with smaller amounts of sialomucin and virtually no sulfomucin (Fig. 8–17). In contrast, carcinomas are rich in sulfomucin, with only small amounts of neutral mucin. When goblet cells are present, these contain sialomucin.[76]

Few studies of the cytologic appearances of this neoplasm have been made.[94] Endoscopic brush biopsies, made via the ampulla of Vater, demonstrate cohesive sheets of cells, with evenly spaced nuclei in an orderly distribution, with little overlap. The nuclei are enlarged, with a prominent nuclear membrane, coarse and uneven chromatin distribution, and distinct nucleoli. Variation in nuclear abnormalities is present, probably reflecting differences in differentiation within the same tumor.

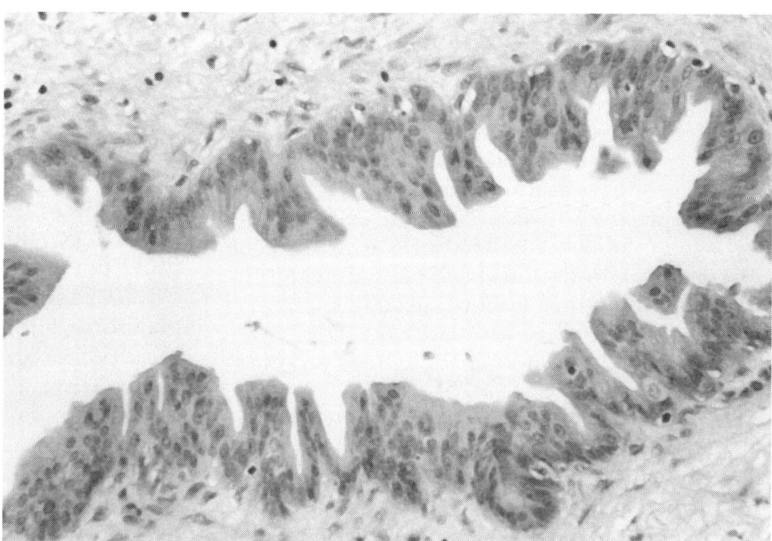

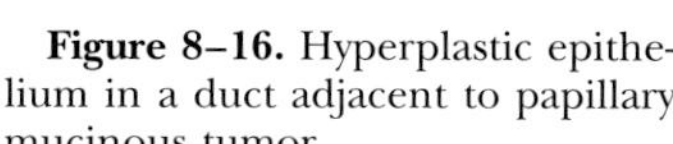

Figure 8–16. Hyperplastic epithelium in a duct adjacent to papillary mucinous tumor.

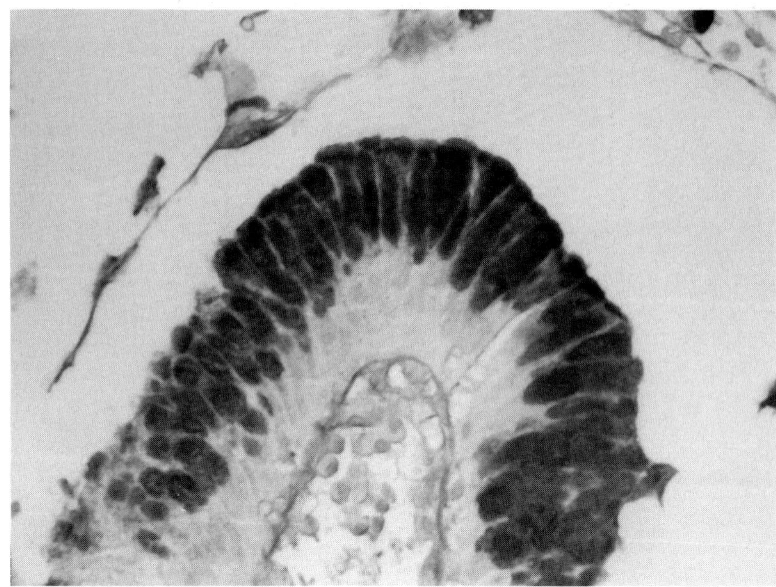

Figure 8–17. Sialomucin production in a mucinous cystic neoplasm. (Alcian blue at pH 2.5.)

By immunohistochemical staining, scattered small numbers of endocrine cells may be present. Predominately, these contain serotonin, with smaller numbers of somatostatin-, insulin-, and PP-secreting cells.[95] Immunostaining for CAM 5.2 is present in all tumors. Positivity for cytokeratins 7 and 20 is present in 80% of tumors, with no obvious preferential distribution between columnar cell and goblet cell areas.[77] Staining for DUPAN-2 (8% of cases), CA 19-9 (65% of cases) and CEA (100% of cases) is heterogeneous but has a general tendency for negative or weakly positive results in very well differentiated tumors, with strongly positive results in carcinomas.[62,72,74,77] Proliferating cell nuclear antigen positivity is present in all tumors and is considered useless in tumor discrimination.[77] Ki-67 (MIB-1) and p53 show variable results from tumor to tumor and even considerable variability within individual tumors.[74,76,87] There is a tendency for p53 to show greater positivity in the more poorly differentiated neoplasms.[77] In some series, c-*erb*-B-2 staining is completely negative, but it is positive in others.[87] K-*ras* mutations have been detected in papillary mucinous tumors, usually in malignant examples.[77,87] At the present time, however, it is not clear whether these have prognostic implications.

Ultrastructural examination adds little to the diagnosis of papillary mucinous tumors. Well-developed microvilli are present on the luminal cell surface and the cytoplasm contains mucin vacuoles measuring up to 300 nm in diameter.[62]

The prognosis of papillary mucinous tumors is rather similar to mucinous cystic tumor. Only 10% to 20% are invasive at the time of surgical excision. They are relatively indolent and can remain as intraductal growth with a favorable prognosis for long periods.[96,97] Nevertheless, when invasive carcinoma does develop, survival is only in the range of 6 to 63 months.[68,73,81,98] Histologically benign tumors should be removed by proximal pancreaticoduodenectomy, if this is technically feasible.[99] The risk of recurrence appears to be related to the depth of invasion at the time of diagnosis. Preoperative assessment is rather poor at predicting which tumors contain areas of invasion.[98] Attention should be paid to the resection margins to ensure that these are free of tumor extending microscopically along minimally dilated ducts. A negative surgical margin does not, however, guarantee cure, as the neoplasm can be multifocal. Malignant tumors may also benefit from radical treatment, because their prognosis appears to be substantially better than that of the usual ductal adenocarcinoma.[74]

Rare examples of papillary-mucinous tumors may show oncocytic differentiation.[100,101] These tumors tend to be large and more obviously cystic. When compared with the usual type of papillary-mucinous tumor, the oncocytic variant has a more complex branching pattern and may have mucin-filled intracytoplasmic lumina. As might be anticipated, ultrastructural examination reveals large numbers of mitochondria.

The differential diagnosis of papillary-mucinous tumors includes mucinous cystic neoplasm, ductal adenocarcinoma, and intraductal papillary hyperplasia.[73] Usually, there is little trouble in excluding mucinous cystic tumors, which occur most commonly in women and are located in the tail of the pancreas. Mucinous cystic tumors are usually multicystic and do not communicate with the main pancreatic duct. Unlike papillary-mucinous tumors, the lining of the cysts is not extensively papillary. No doubt, in the past, many papillary-mucinous tumors were misdiagnosed as adenocarcinoma. However, the usual ductal adenocarcinoma is not cystic. If it does produce excessive quantities of mucus (colloid carcinoma), this occurs as pools within the stroma. Colloid carcinoma is characterized by the presence of "free floating" tumor cells, frequently signet ring in type, but not by cystlike spaces lined by tumor cells. Ductal hyperplasia can be extremely difficult to distinguish microscopically from low-grade papillary-mucinous tumor but generally does not present as a tumorlike mass. It may be discovered incidentally in portions of pancreas resected for chronic pancreatitis. In problem cases, reliance has to be placed on the greater nuclear atypia present in neoplastic intraductal proliferations, although there is no doubt that overlap exists. Some authors[74] believe that hyperplasia forms the earliest component of a hyperplasia–adenoma–carcinoma sequence.

SOLID-CYSTIC-PAPILLARY TUMOR

Solid-cystic-papillary tumor is also known by a variety of other names, including *papillary-cystic tumor,*[102–107] *solid and cystic tumor,*[108] *solid and papillary tumor,*[109] and, more recently, *solid-pseudopapillary tumor.*[34,75] The designation *solid-cystic-papillary tumor*[110,111] is preferred because this most completely describes the tumor's morphologic appearances. Nevertheless, it should be recognized that the basic original architecture of this tumor is a solid growth pattern, with the cystic and papillary areas representing an artifact of degeneration.

This tumor appears to be rare. In one series,[108] there were only 10 cases among 1,459 surgical pancreatic resections (0.7%). Many cases have been reported from Japan, where a slightly higher incidence (2.7%) has been recorded.[109,111] This tumor has a strong female preponderance, ranging in different series from 80%[107] to 100%.[109,112] Nevertheless, cases occurring in men are well recognized.[113] Many patients are young and in the pediatric age group, with the four largest series[105–108] recording an average patient age of 27 years and a range of 12 to 67 years. No significant differences in age exist between men and women with this tumor. The manner of patient presentation is variable, but most individuals complain of an abdominal mass with or without associated epigastric pain.[107] Jaundice or hormonal disturbances are not a feature. A sizeable percentage of patients (in the range of 20% to 25%) are asymptomatic and the tumor is discovered incidental to physical or radiologic examination.

Overall, solid-cystic-papillary tumors have a tendency to involve either the body or the tail of the pancreas, although in about 30% of instances, the tumor involves the head, either in isolation or in continuity with other parts of the pancreas. Occasional examples of multifocal tumors have been described.[114,115] In most cases, the tumors are well circumscribed and have a peripheral pseudocapsule. The average size is 9 cm in diameter, with a range of 3 to 18 cm.[75] Unencapsulated neoplasms that show extrapancreatic spread and attachment to adjacent organs have been referred to as the solid infiltrating variety of solid-cystic-papillary tumor.[116] Malignant variants exist and may demonstrate metastases to local lymph nodes, liver, or peritoneum. There is no difference in size between tumors that are benign and those that are malignant.[107] On the cut surface of the tumor, it is common to find cystic spaces containing thin mucoid material, necrotic foci, hemorrhage, and calcification (Fig. 8–18). In the solid areas, this tumor has a soft grayish brown to yellowish appearance. Extensive degeneration may produce tumors that are almost completely cystic.

Preoperative radiologic examination of these tumors reveals well-circumscribed nodular lesions containing multiple cysts and solid areas. Larger neoplasms located in the head of the pancreas may cause displacement of the duodenum. Calcification may be detected in 30% of cases and, with magnetic resonance imaging, fluid-debris levels may be found within cysts.[116]

On histologic examination, the tumor cells are remarkably uniform from area to area. They are cuboidal or polygonal in shape and contain ovoid nuclei that can be indented or grooved (Fig. 8–19). The nuclear chromatin is widely dispersed with only inconspicuous nucleoli. The cytoplasm is moderately abundant and can vary in color from lightly eosinophilic to clear. Rare tumors may have an oncocytic cyto-

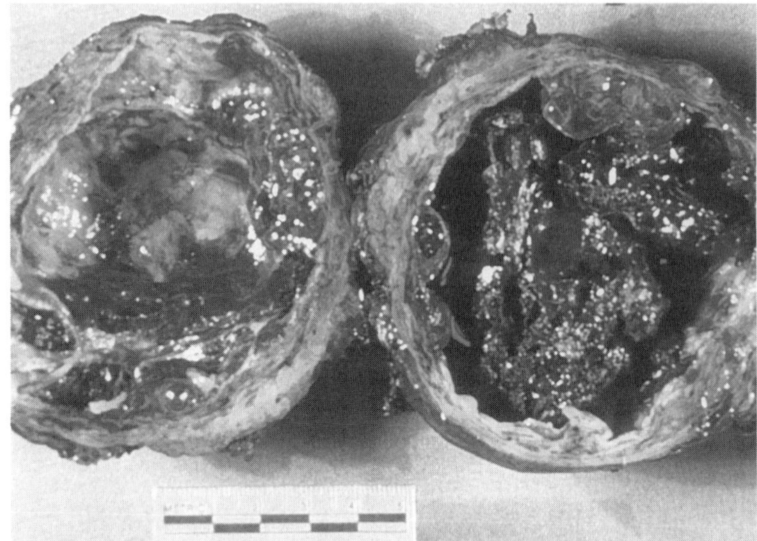

Figure 8–18. Solid-cystic-papillary tumor of the pancreas.

plasm.[117] Focal areas of mild nuclear pleomorphism are common and up to five mitoses per high-power field may be present, even in nonmetastasizing tumors.[107] In the solid areas of tumor (Fig. 8–20), the cells grow in featureless sheets with intervening delicate fibrovascular septa. Cysts and papillae (Fig. 8–21) form by degeneration as cells become discohesive, a change that is most marked in areas distant from the fibrous septa. In addition, myxoid degeneration may occur around the vessels. Epithelial mucus is not present, but the cytoplasm may contain dense PAS-/diastase-positive hyaline granules of varying diameter (Fig. 8–22). In the areas of degeneration, debris and foamy macrophages may be identified. Occasional tumors also show hemorrhage and cholesterol granulomas and foamy macrophages.[106] At the periphery of almost every tumor, there are entrapped normal ducts and acini. Capsular infiltration by small tongues of tumor cells may be identified in up to 60% of cases.[106]

The FNA cytopathologic appearances of this tumor are characteristic.[106,118–121] The cells are bland appearing and monotonous (Fig. 8–23), but the aspirate also contains numerous thin-walled capillaries, which may be straight or branching. Sleeves of cells may surround the

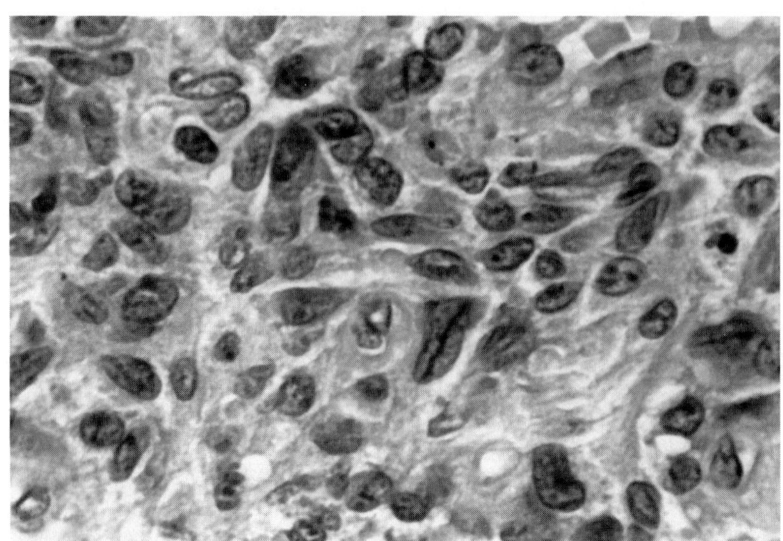

Figure 8–19. Solid-cystic-papillary tumor consisting of ovoid nuclei, which are indented and grooved.

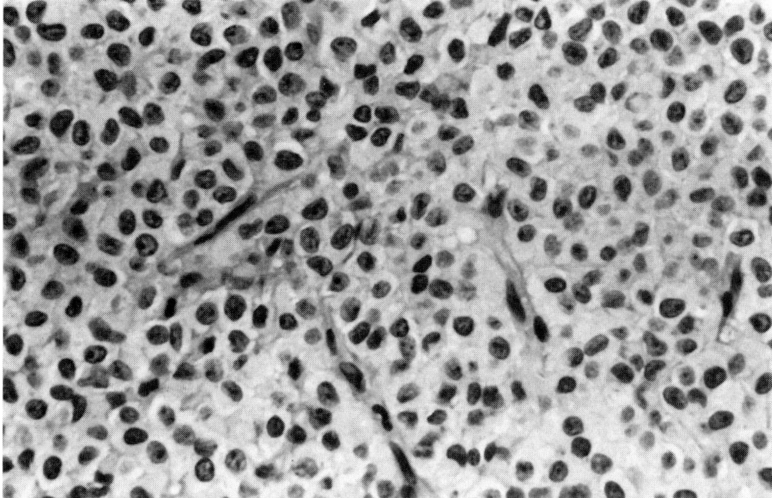

Figure 8–20. Solid architecture in a solid-cystic-papillary tumor.

capillaries forming a rosettelike pattern or they may occur as naked vessels (Fig. 8–24).

Ultrastructural examination of solid-cystic-papillary tumors[104,106,108,109,122] has produced differing results. All authors found rough endoplasmic reticulum, mitochondria, and intermediate filaments. Some authors found zymogen-type granules measuring 500 to 3,000 nm,[108,109,122] whereas others did not.[104,106] Degenerate granules, in the form of vesicles and lipid droplets, may be encountered, however. Neurosecretory granules may also be found,[122] as well as annulate lamellae.[106,108]

There are a number of immunohistochemical studies of this neoplasm,[104,106,108,112] most of which are in agreement that the majority of examples are positive for vimentin, α_1-antitrypsin and NSE. The eosinophilic globules seen on routine hematoxylin and easin sections represent the cytoplasmic accumulation of α_1-antitrypsin. In some studies, most tumors are also positive for α_1-antichymotrypsin.[107] In one study, 50% of tumors were positive for S100,[107] but in another, all tumors were negative.[104] Occasional tumors are positive with cytokeratins AE1/AE3 and CAM.[107] Specific endocrine markers, such as synaptophysin and chromogranin, are usually, but not invariably, negative, as are markers for pancreatic hormones, such as insulin, glucagon, gastrin, PP, bombesin, adrenocortico-

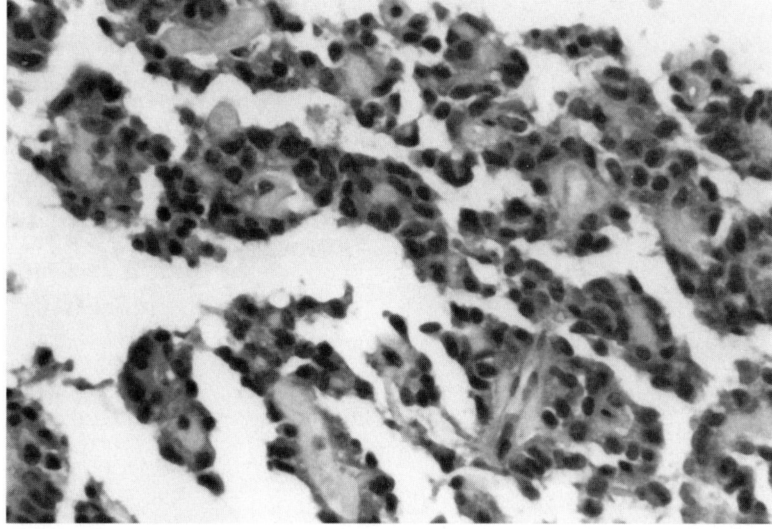

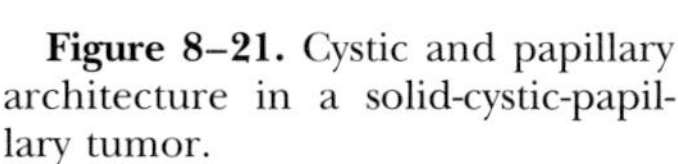

Figure 8–21. Cystic and papillary architecture in a solid-cystic-papillary tumor.

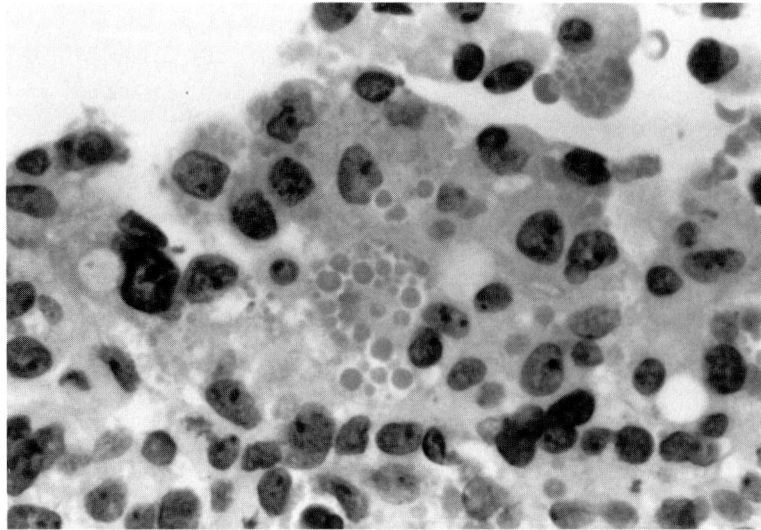

Figure 8–22. Hyaline granules in a solid-cystic-papillary tumor.

tropic hormone, and calcitonin.[107,108] Antigens, such as EMA, CEA, alphafetoprotein (AFP), and CA 19-9, are invariably negative.[104,106,113] One study has shown positivity for trypsin and chymotrypsin.[106] Estrogen and progesterone receptors have been demonstrated by biochemical methods,[123,124] but only progesterone receptors have been demonstrated immunohistochemically.[125] These findings support the concept of a ductuloacinar derivation of the tumor,[110] with some neoplasms demonstrating evidence of both acinar and islet cell differentiation.

The clinical behavior of solid-cystic-papillary tumors has been the subject of considerable discussion. In the 1996 WHO classification, the neoplasm is assigned to a category of uncertain malignant potential.[34] Some quite large series record no cases with metastasis or postoperative recurrence.[106] In other series,[107] 14% of such tumors were considered malignant. A comprehensive review of the literature determined a figure of 16% malignancy,[126] when malignancy is defined as having either histologic blood vessel invasion or gross tumor extension to adjacent organs. However, only 7% of tumors in this review series had liver metastases. These figures probably overestimate the true numbers of malignant tumors because of an understand-

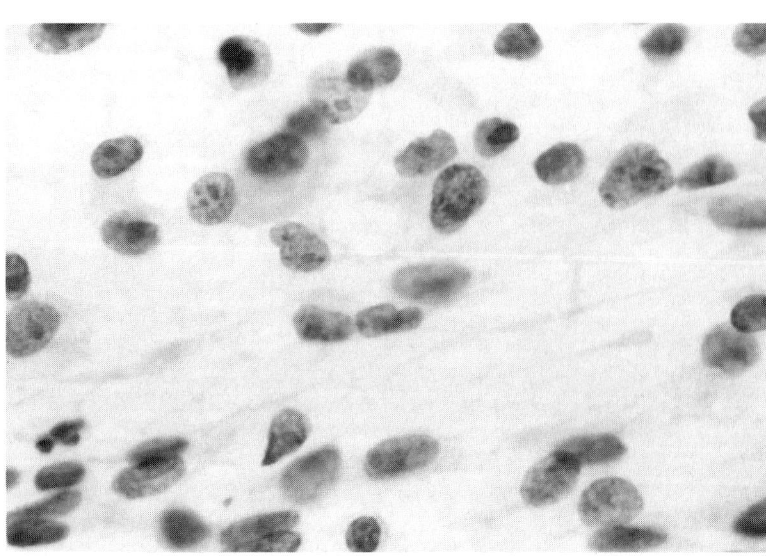

Figure 8–23. Solid-cystic-papillary tumor with bland monotonous cytologic appearance.

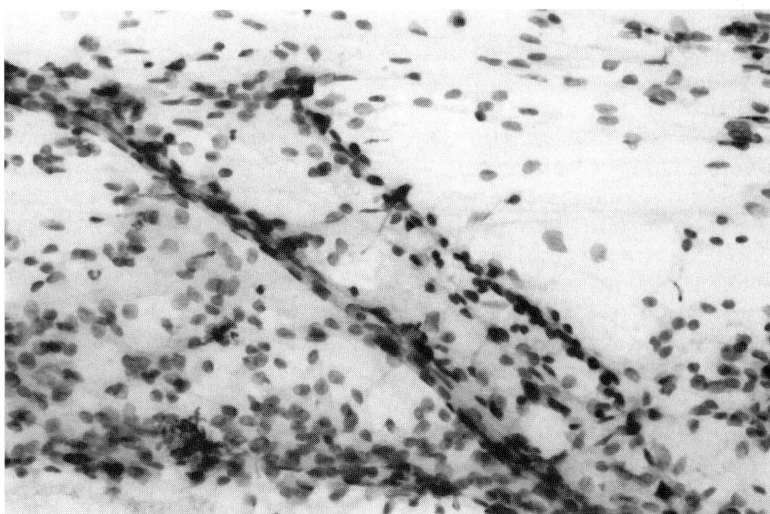

Figure 8–24. Distinctive vascular pattern encountered in fine-needle aspiration biopsy of solid-cystic-papillary tumor.

able tendency among authors to publish reports of unusual cases. Furthermore, many of the patients who did develop metastases are alive and well up to 14 years after surgery,[107] although some fatalities are recorded.[127] There is an intermediate category of solid-cystic-papillary tumor characterized by local spread outside of the pancreas to involve adjacent organs, such as duodenum and celiac axis. However, this locally aggressive behavior does not necessarily imply metastatic potential, nor does it mean that death will invariably occur because of local tumor growth. These locally spreading tumors have been labeled as the infiltrating variant of solid-cystic-papillary neoplasm,[115] but histologically they appear identical to the usual encapsulated neoplasms. There are also no histologic features that serve to identify with certainty malignant from benign or locally infiltrating tumors, although, as might be anticipated, malignant neoplasms tend to be more pleomorphic and mitotically active with a higher nuclear grade.[108] Venous invasion has been suggested as a valuable diagnostic feature of malignant solid-cystic-papillary tumors[75] but may be demonstrated in neoplasms that have not metastasized and that are cured by total local excision. Presumably, these benign behaving angioinvasive tumors are so slow growing that surgical excision proves curative before metastases occur. Retrospective studies measuring nuclear DNA content[128] and measuring nuclear morphology[129] show that metastasizing solid-cystic-papillary tumors are likely to have a higher proliferation index, DNA index, nuclear diameter, and nuclear volume than do nonmetastasizing tumors, but it is not clear if these parameters carry prognostic significance in an individual case. Flow cytometry studies demonstrate that most tumors are diploid[104,106] but that 1 in 10 is aneuploid. Aneuploid tumors do not appear different on light microscopy and aneuploidy does not appear to predict an unfavorable prognosis. Karyotypic analysis of one pleomorphic tumor showed an unbalanced translocation.[130] Another tumor showed a double loss of X chromosomes and trisomy 3.[131] It is not clear whether these observations have any general practical value. Care should be taken not to confuse oncocytic change in solid-cystic-papillary neoplasm[117] with acinar cell carcinoma, as the cytoplasmic granules may have a superficial similarity.[132]

The major differential diagnoses of solid-cystic-papillary neoplasm include acinar cell carcinoma, islet cell tumor, and pancreatoblastoma. Acinar cell carcinomas are most common in middle-aged to elderly men but can also occur in younger individuals. Their cytologic appearances may be relatively monotonous and they may occasionally lack abundant mitotic activity, thus mimicking solid-cystic-papillary neoplasms. If immunostains for trypsin or lipase are not available, their characteristic fine cytoplasmic acinar granules may be adequately identified using simply a PAS/diastase stain. These differ from the coarse α_1-antitrypsin granules of solid-cystic-papillary tumor, which are also PAS/diastase positive. Both solid-cystic-papillary tumors and islet cell tumors may be

NSE positive, but solid-cystic-papillary tumors do not display widespread positivity for chromogranin or synaptophysin. Islet cell tumors are not usually strongly positive for α_1-antitrypsin, which is common in solid-cystic-papillary neoplasms. Pancreatoblastoma is common in children and teenagers and therefore overlaps, to a certain extent, the age group of solid-cystic-papillary neoplasm. However, pancreatoblastoma almost invariably shows some acinar differentiation and lacks the delicate fibrovascular stroma characteristic of solid-cystic-papillary neoplasms. Thorough sampling of a pancreatoblastoma will reveal squamoid corpuscles, a finding never encountered in solid-cystic-papillary tumors.

ACINAR CELL CARCINOMA

Acinar (also called acinic) cell carcinomas account for about 1% to 5% of all malignant neoplasms in the pancreas.[112,133–135] The mean age at presentation is 62 years, with a range from childhood to old age.[135] Eighty-six percent occur in men, with the majority in whites. The usual presenting symptoms are weight loss, abdominal pain, nausea, and vomiting. These appear to be related to local expansion or regional metastatic spread. Jaundice is uncommon (12% of patients), even when the tumor was located in the head of the pancreas.[135] Small numbers of patients have diarrhea, anorexia, fever, anemia, and constipation. About 15% of patients may develop symptoms referable to excess lipase production by the tumor and an increased serum lipase.[135–137] These consist of subcutaneous fat necrosis and panniculitis, together with polyarthralgia/polyarthritis. This group of systemic complications may occur in patients with and without disseminated disease. Occasionally, patients with acinar cell carcinoma may have an asymptomatic elevation of pancreatic enzymes. Peripheral blood eosinophilia may also occur.

More than 50% of acinar cell carcinomas occur in the head of the pancreas. The remainder are found in the tail (36%) and body (8%). Occasional multifocal tumors are encountered. Tumors tend to be large at presentation, averaging 10 cm in diameter.[112,135] They may be well circumscribed, or even encapsulated, although some tumors have an irregular edge and invade adjacent organs. On the cut surface, acinar cell carcinomas are pink to tan colored and fleshy with division into lobules by fine fibrous strands. Minor cystic changes and foci of necrosis are commonly seen but are generally not extensive.[135] Calcification is usually not present.

Microscopically, acinar carcinomas are markedly cellular with only a scanty stroma containing thin-walled vessels. The two major histologic patterns are acinar (Fig. 8–25) and solid (Fig. 8–26), with many neoplasms containing a mixture of both.[134,135] Minor histologic patterns that can be encountered include glandular (Fig. 8–27) and trabecular areas (Fig. 8–28). The acinar pattern resembles the normal pancreatic structure, with well-formed, tightly packed acini containing centrally located lumina and basally oriented nuclei. The solid pattern demon-

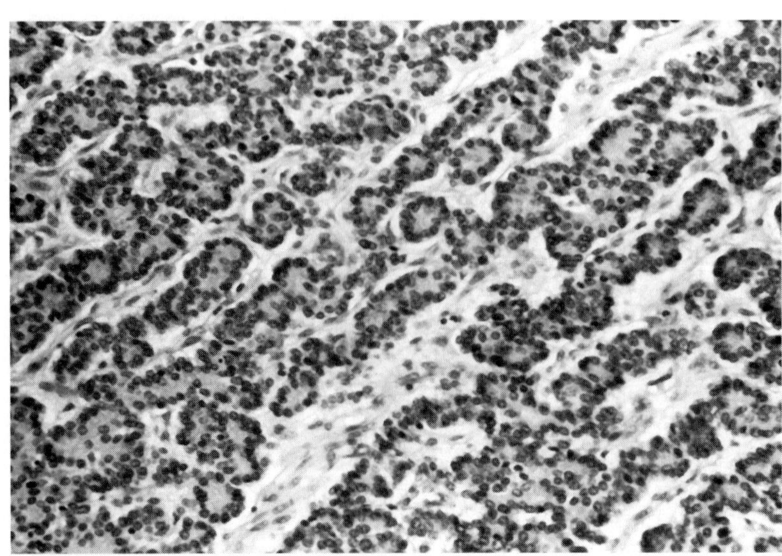

Figure 8–25. Acinar cell carcinoma of the pancreas—acinar growth pattern.

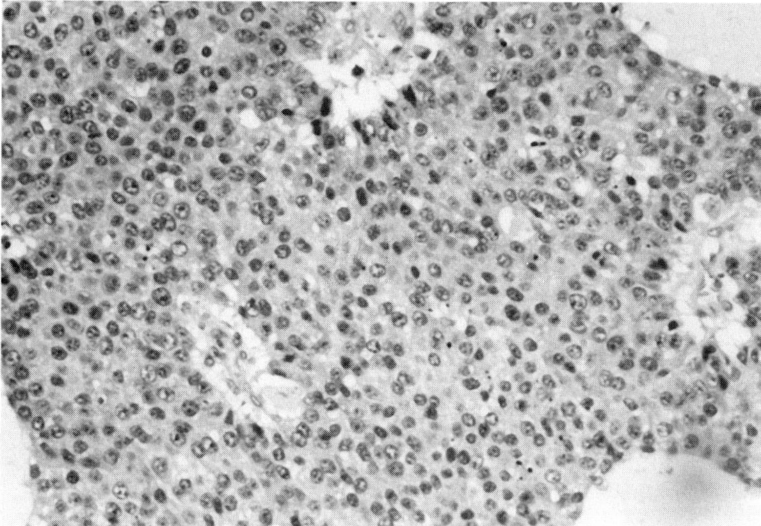

Figure 8–26. Acinar cell carcinoma of the pancreas—solid growth pattern.

strates sheets of rounded or boxlike cells with a centrally placed nucleus. Where fibrous septa are present, the nucleus may be located close to the cell border in contact with the septum. The rare glandular pattern of tumor growth is probably a variant of acinar differentiation, in which the acinar lumen becomes dilated and irregular. Eosinophilic secretion may be present within the lumen. The trabecular pattern resembles an islet cell tumor, with ribbons of cells often occurring in two layers with the nuclei oriented toward the outer margin of the ribbon (see Fig. 8–28). In all of these gross growth patterns, the cytoplasm is granular. Granules located close to the nuclei are basophilic (ribosomes), whereas apical granules are eosinophilic (zymogen granules). This distribution is most obvious in areas of the tumor with an acinar pattern. In other patterns, distinction between the two types of granule is lost and all may appear purplish (amphophilic). Zymogen granules are usually positive with PAS stain after diastase digestion, and this finding is an important diagnostic feature because the granules are present to a greater or lesser extent in up to 96% of acinar cell carcinomas.

In spite of the apparent gross encapsulation of some neoplasms, microscopic examination generally reveals focal capsular invasion. Vascular invasion may be identified in 60% of tumors,

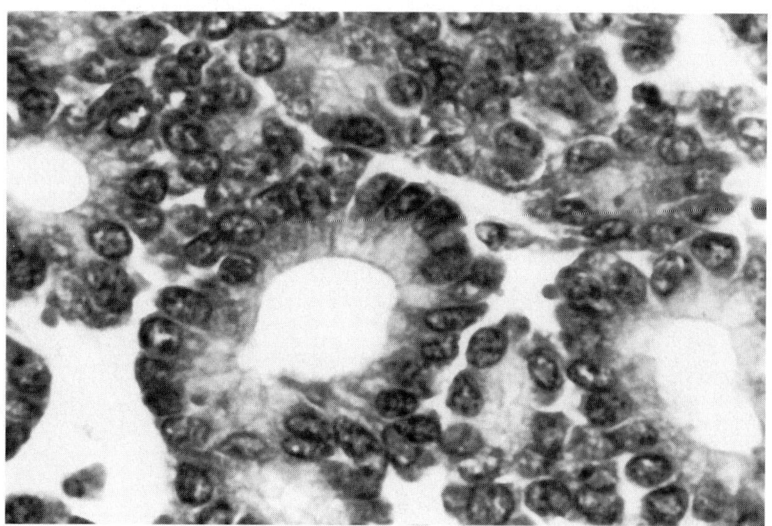

Figure 8–27. Glandular growth pattern of acinar carcinoma, showing centrally located lumina and basally oriented regular-appearing nuclei.

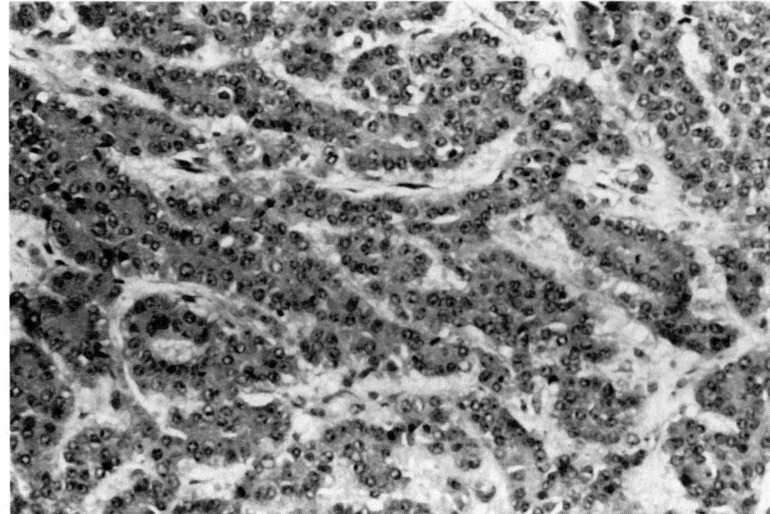

Figure 8–28. Trabecular growth pattern of acinar carcinoma, showing regular boxlike cells with a centrally located nucleus.

and perineural infiltration in 32% of tumors.[135] Acinar cell carcinomas generally do not have pleomorphic nuclei and mitotic activity is quite variable (0 to 50 mitoses per 10 high-power fields, with a mean of 14).[135] There is no correlation between mitotic activity and histologic subtype.

FNAC of these tumors characteristically reveals a cellular aspirate, with cohesive or discohesive groups of cells having a uniform appearance. There is little pleomorphism. The cytoplasm is abundant and contains numerous fine granules, which are PAS positive after diastase digestion[138] (Fig. 8–29). The nuclei may be central or eccentrically located and are hyperchromatic, with prominent nucleoli.[139] The appearances closely mimic those of an islet cell tumor, apart from the characteristic PAS-/diastase-positive cytoplasmic granules.

Ultrastructural examination[135,140] demonstrates the presence of zymogen granules. These are round, measure 200 to 700 nm in diameter, and show apical polarity. In some neoplasms, a more pleomorphic population of granules is encountered, some of which measure up to 3,500 nm in diameter. In addition, the cells show well-developed rough endoplasmic reticulum and microvilli on the cell surface. Endocrine granules are not usually seen, even in small numbers. It is difficult to reconcile the

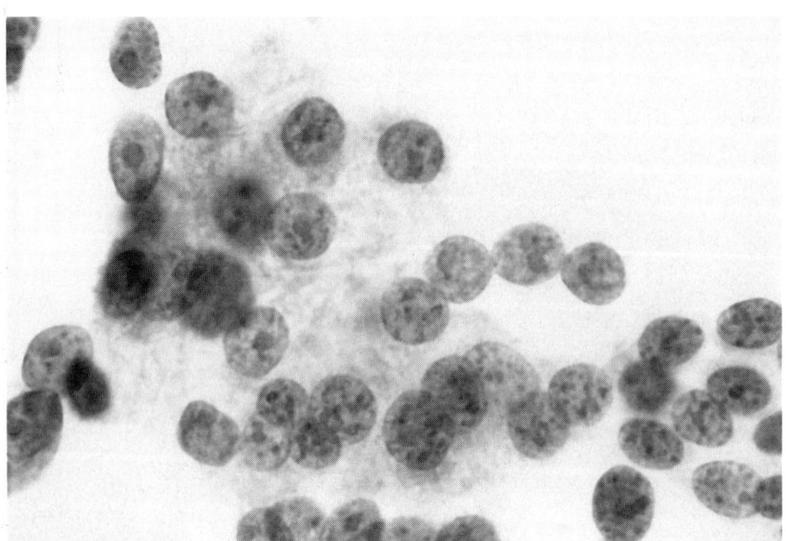

Figure 8–29. Fine-needle aspiration biopsy of acinar carcinoma. Note the granular cytoplasm.

absence of endocrine granules with the immunohistochemical findings, but this may be a sampling problem, with only very small numbers of cells containing granules.[140] Some tumors also contain pleomorphic membrane-bound granules that contain filaments.[141] These filaments may become an important diagnostic feature in some acinar cell carcinomas, where the zymogen granules cannot be distinguished morphologically from endocrine granules.

As would be expected, acinar tumors may contain a wide variety of enzymes and other proteins that are normally produced in the pancreatic acini.[135,139,142] With the use of immunohistochemical techniques, almost all tumors are positive for trypsin. About three quarters of the tumors are diffusely or focally positive for lipase and about half are diffusely or focally positive for chymotrypsin, phospholipase A2, and amylase. Positivity tends to be localized to the apical region of the cells, where enzyme granules are normally located. One third of tumors are positive for synaptophysin, α_1-antitrypsin, CA 19-9 and B72.3.[134,135,140] Neuroendocrine markers, such as chromogranin, are positive in widely scattered cells in only about 50% of cases.[135,140] Interestingly, three of three tumors that were tested for the presence of prostate-specific antigen were found to be positive.[134] Mucin stains may reveal that the luminal membrane is positive, but the cytoplasm is generally negative. Cytokeratin CAM 5.2 is positive in virtually all tumors.[134] Histochemical staining for butyrate esterase is positive in 73% of cases.[134] Surprisingly, this enzyme activity may be retained after prolonged storage of tissue in a paraffin block. Unlike the usual pancreatic ductal carcinomas, acinar cell carcinomas show mutations in K-*ras* and p53 tumor suppressor genes in < 5% of cases.[140,143,144] These results suggest that although acinar cell carcinoma differentiates predominately along acinar lines, it also retains the potential for islet cell and ductular differentiation.[135]

The prognosis for patients with acinar cell carcinoma is uniformly poor and 50% of patients have metastases at presentation. However, the prognosis is marginally better than that of the usual ductal pancreatic carcinoma. The mean survival for all adult patients is 18 months, the 3-year survival is 25%, and the 5-year survival is 6%.[133] Particularly adverse prognostic factors are age at presentation of > 60 years, tumor size > 10 cm, and the presence of an elevated serum lipase. Histologic factors, such as mitotic activity, atypical mitoses, and growth pattern, do not seem relevant.

The differential diagnosis of acinar cell carcinoma includes ductal adenocarcinoma, islet cell tumor, solid-cystic-papillary epithelial neoplasm, and pancreatoblastoma. Ductal carcinoma is typically characterized by a prominent glandular growth pattern, the presence of at least moderate pleomorphism, and the absence of fine cytoplasmic granules that are PAS/diastase positive. However, oncocytic variants of ductal carcinoma can have a granular cytoplasm that superficially resembles exocrine differentiation, although oncocytic tumors are not PAS/diastase positive.[145,146] Islet cell tumors can be difficult to distinguish from acinar cell carcinoma, especially those which have a trabecular or glandular pattern. An islet cell tumor is favored in a patient younger than 50 years of age, in which the tumor has no PAS-/diastase-positive granules and in which immunohistochemistry does not reveal the presence of digestive enzymes. The presence of scanty immunopositivity for pancreatic hormones is, however, compatible with the usual type of acinar cell carcinoma. There are a small number of tumors in which both the acinar and endocrine differentiation may be encountered. Where these components each exceed 25% of the neoplasm, a mixed tumor should be diagnosed.[147–149] These rare neoplasms occur in elderly adults with an approximately equal sex incidence. They have no clinical evidence of hormone or enzyme production, although immunohistochemically, two separate cell populations may be identified. Some cells may be amphicrene in type (endocrine and exocrine granules within the same cell). Although acinar–endocrine combinations are interesting, it is not clear whether the mixed tumor behaves any differently from the usual type of acinar cell carcinoma. Rare examples of oncocytic acinar cell carcinoma have been described. These can be extremely difficult to distinguish from oncocytic islet cell tumors,[150] with reliance having to be placed on immunohistochemical markers.

Solid-cystic-papillary epithelial neoplasm and pancreatoblastoma are mainly tumors of adolescence and childhood, so confusion with acinar cell carcinoma is less likely. Acinar carcinomas may, however, rarely occur in this age group.[132] Histologically, they are similar to adult acinar carcinomas, although clinically they have a considerably better prognosis and they closely resemble pancreatoblastoma in their clinical features. The only sure histologic way to distinguish juvenile acinar cell carcinoma from pancreatoblastoma is the presence of "squamoid corpuscles" in pancreatoblastoma. Clinically, this may be an artificial distinction, however, because both tumors in children have a similar prognosis. Authorities have suggested that they may even be the same tumor.[151] Case reports have described a cystic variant of acinar cell carcinoma, termed *acinar cell cystadenocarcinoma*.[152,153] This may grossly resemble—and has microscopic similarity to—solid-cystic-papillary tumor but is cytologically more atypical with prominent mitotic activity. The growth pattern is usually cystic in type, although there may be some solid areas. This tumor also has the usual abundant fine PAS-/diastase positive cytoplasmic granules, so diagnostic confusion is unlikely.

PANCREATOBLASTOMA

As might be anticipated, pancreatoblastomas are predominately tumors of children, although a small number do occur in adults.[151,154–156] They are rare neoplasms, even in children's hospitals,[110,157–160] and must be distinguished from other childhood pancreatic neoplasms, such as ductal adenocarcinoma, acinar carcinoma, and solid-cystic-papillary epithelial neoplasm.[158] Pancreatoblastomas are so rare that most reports are of single cases. The largest series is from Klimstra et al.,[158] who collected data on 14 cases of their own and comprehensively reviewed the literature. In their series, they found 9 cases in infants and children, with the remainder occurring in adults, one of whom was 56 years old. In the pediatric group, most tumors are found in the first decade of life, with an average age of 4 years. The male to female ratio is 1.3:1.

The majority of patients present with incidental abdominal masses, although some children experience weight loss, abdominal pain, diarrhea, vomiting, and jaundice. No instance of excess production of either exocrine enzymes or hormones has been recorded, although in about 30% of cases, the AFP levels are raised in serum.[161,162] Rare cases have occurred in association with Beckwith–Weidemann syndrome (omphalocele, macroglossia, visceromegaly, Leydig cell hyperplasia, and enlarged kidneys with perilobar nephrogenic rests).[158,163,164]

Pancreatoblastomas are found equally in the head and body/tail of the pancreas. They range in size from 1.5 to 20 cm, with a mean of 10.6 cm.[157] Grossly, they are poorly circumscribed solid masses that may extend into adjacent soft tissues. The cut surface is generally tan to yellowish in color, soft, and fleshy, with occasional focal areas of necrosis and cyst formation. Fibrous septa may be present and there may be foci of calcification.

Histologically, pancreatoblastomas are predominately epithelial neoplasms. Stromal elements are present but in most instances are clearly reactive rather than neoplastic. The epithelial component is usually highly cellular and separated into lobules by thin fibrous septa. The pattern may be as solid sheets of cells, variably differentiated acinar structures, as well differentiated ducts, or as squamoid corpuscles. These architectural patterns generally merge imperceptibly. Acinar areas are frequently located at the edge of solid areas at the epithelial–stromal interface. Secretion is usually absent from the acinar lumina. The cells in the solid and acinar areas are regular, with little pleomorphism (Fig. 8–30). They have a high nuclear–cytoplasmic ratio, with rounded or ovoid nuclei and prominent nucleoli. The cytoplasm is amphophilic and finely granular. Mitoses can be quite variable in extent but average 10 per high-power field.[158] Ductular structures are uncommon. They consist of regular columnar cells, often containing mucin in the apical cytoplasm. Squamoid corpuscles are usually abundant and are present in every case, where they form an important differential diagnostic feature. Their appearance is somewhat variable: In some cases, they are very sharply defined (Fig. 8-31), but in others they merge gradually with the solid and acinar areas (Fig. 8–32). They vary in size from 10 to 15 cells and in diameter up to 1.0 mm. The squamoid cells have more abundant and lightly eosinophilic cytoplasm and have larger and more vesicular nuclei than do the background cells. They show a swirling growth pattern, typical of squamous epithelium, although central keratinization is quite uncommon. The stromal component of pancreatoblastoma generally consists of hypercellular areas containing bands of bland spindle cells that are orientated parallel to the long axis of the band. Pleomorphism and mitotic activity is usually not seen and there is a clear demarcation between epithelial and stromal areas. In occasional cases, the stroma can be more atypical and disorganized, with heterologous bone and cartilage present.

FNAC yields a highly cellular aspirate, consisting of oval to cuboidal cells with a moderate

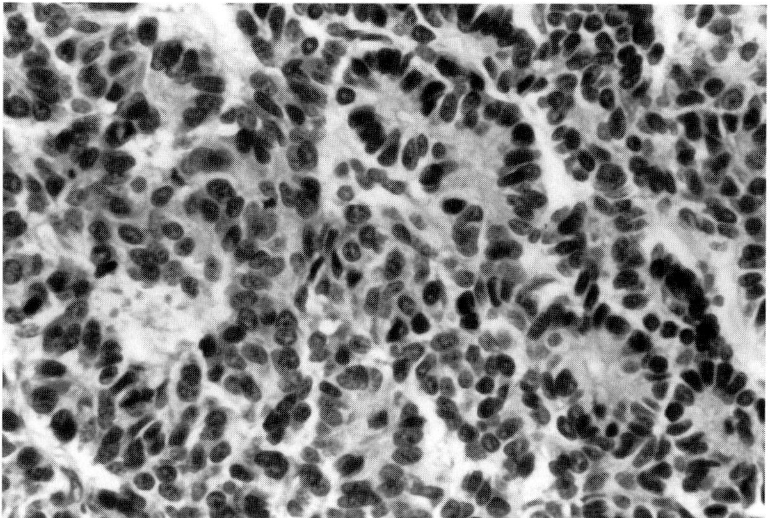

Figure 8–30. Solid and acinar areas of a pancreatoblastoma with regular cells displaying little pleomorphism.

amount of cytoplasm. Occasional spindle-shaped and triangular cells are also noted. Portions of stroma may also be found within the aspirated material.[165]

Electron microscopic examination of pancreatoblastomas confirms the presence of features expected in an epithelial malignancy. Abundant desmosomes are present and on the acinar luminal surface there are blunt microvilli with tight junctions between adjacent cells. All cases show extensive cytoplasmic zymogen-like electron dense granules with some tumors also containing mucin granules and neurosecretory granules.[158,166,167]

Immunohistochemical staining reveals that in the solid and acinar areas, all tumors are positive for trypsin and a majority of tumors are positive for chymotrypsin, NSE, and CEA. About half the tumors are positive for lipase, chromogranin, and CA19.9. Rare tumors are positive for synaptophysin and AFP[158] or for NSE and for various pancreatic polypeptide

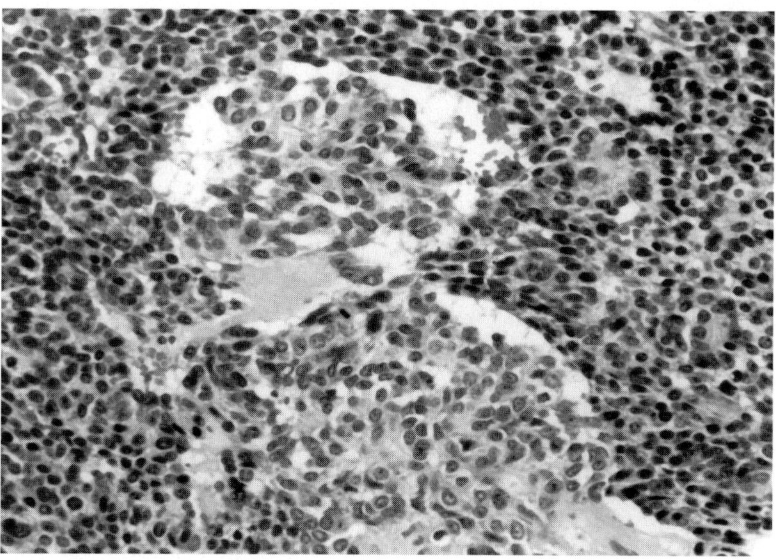

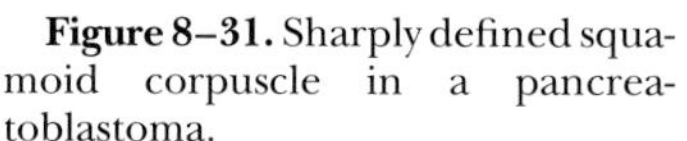

Figure 8–31. Sharply defined squamoid corpuscle in a pancreatoblastoma.

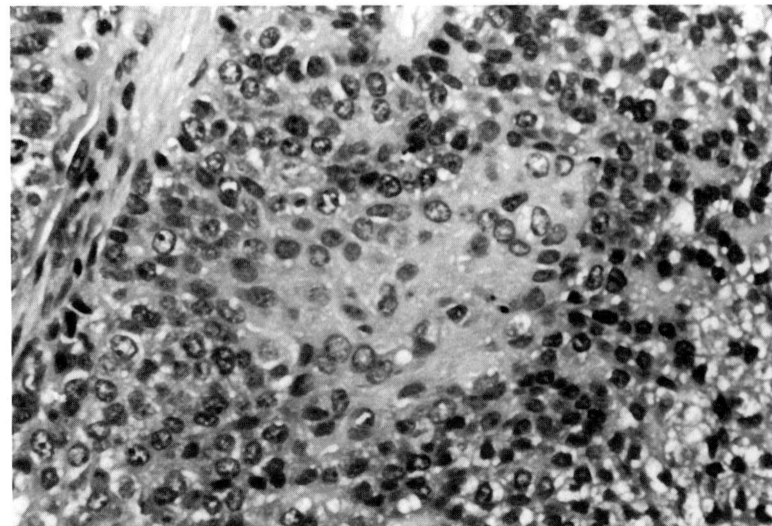

Figure 8–32. Ill-defined squamoid corpuscle in a pancreatoblastoma.

hormones.[168] All tumors are also positive with PAS after diastase digestion, reflecting the presence of zymogen granules. The squamoid areas are generally immunohistochemically nonreactive.

The prognosis of this tumor differs substantially in adults versus children. In the series of Klimstra et al.,[158] 60% of adults (three of five) died after a mean survival of 17 months. In children, the mortality was only 17% (one of six) and three individuals were alive and well 5 years after the initial diagnosis. Tumors in the head of the pancreas were more likely to be fatal than were tumors occurring elsewhere, but there was no obvious correlation between survival and histologic features.

Pancreatoblastoma is a distinctive neoplasm and should not cause confusion with other pancreatic tumors if the diagnostic criteria are applied fully. Acinar carcinoma is the closest mimic, but this tumor does not have squamoid corpuscles. Ductal carcinomas may also occur in childhood but are quite similar to ductal carcinomas in adults: They do not have the acinar pattern and fine PAS with diastase cytoplasmic granularity. A word of caution is in order here, however. The designation pancreatoblastoma was not used until the mid-1980s; prior to that time, pancreatic neoplasms of whatever histology in children tended to be lumped together as "infantile or childhood pancreatic carcinoma."[166] Many cases so described are in fact pancreatoblastomas, but some are not. Currently, for prognostic reasons, it is recommended that a sharp distinction be made between the different types of pancreatic neoplasms occurring in childhood.

CONNECTIVE-TISSUE TUMORS

Connective-tissue tumors are all rare neoplasms and most reports are of single cases. As a general rule, the clinical features of these neoplasms closely mimic those of similar tumors arising within the retroperitoneum.

Benign soft-tissue tumors include schwannoma,[169,170] granular cell tumor,[171,172] fibrous histiocytoma,[60] and lipoma.[173] Schwannoma is by far the most common of these, with 20 cases reported in the 20-year period between 1975 and 1995.[169] Schwannomas < 5.0 cm in diameter tend to be solid, but larger ones may be cystic. This may cause confusion at ultrasound or CT examination with cystic epithelial neoplasms. FNAC may suggest the diagnosis, but surgical excision is generally required for confirmation.

A variety of primary malignant soft-tissue neoplasms have been described within the pancreas. These includes malignant fibrous histiocytoma,[174–178] malignant nerve sheath tumors,[179,180] leiomyosarcoma,[181–184] undifferentiated sarcoma,[185] liposarcoma,[186] rhabdomyosarcoma,[187] primitive neuroectodermal tumor,[188] intra-abdominal desmoplastic small round cell tumor,[189] and solitary fibrous tumor.[190] One malignant fibrous histiocytoma occurred in association with a mucinous cystadenoma.[178] Poorly differentiated sarcomas may be difficult to distinguish from spindle cell carcinomas and reliance may have to be placed on a battery of immunostains. As a general rule, carcinomas will be cytokeratin positive and sarcomas will be cytokeratin negative. There are, however, exceptions to this rule.

Vascular tumors are also rare in the pancreas. Most examples are lymphangiomas, but occasional cases of hemangioma,[191] hemangiopericytoma,[192] and juvenile hemangio-endothelioma[193,194] have been recorded. Lymphangiomas in the region of the pancreas are usually regarded as developmental abnormalities rather than true neoplasms.[195–198] However, in the majority of cases, they present in adults [average age, 29 years; 80% in women] and may be difficult to distinguish from true cystic neoplasms by radiologic or ultrasound examination. The majority occur in the tail of the pancreas. Lymphangiomas are multilocular, with cavities measuring 0.7 to 20 cm in diameter (average, 12.7 cm), separated by thin, curvilinear septa. They are sonolucent and contain serous fluid (lymph) or altered blood. Histologically, they have thin, fibrous walls, lined by flattened endothelium. The endothelial lining cells are immunoreactive for factor VIII antigen and CD31.[198] A distinction has been made between cystic and cavernous lymphangiomas.[195] Lymphangiomas arise as a result of abnormal development of fetal lymphatic sacs during the second to third month of intrauterine life. Cystic lymphangiomas are considered to arise from primary buddings of the lymphatic sacs, which become separated and lose their connection to the sac. This occurs at the same time as the development of the dorsal mesoduodenum, which later gives rise to the visceral peritoneum covering the pancreas, as well as the retroperitoneal fascia of Treitz and Toldt. The cystic lymphangiomas therefore arise from the extralobular connective tissue of the pancreas and can, at least in theory, be completely excised by a surgical procedure that spares the pancreatic substance. In contrast, cavernous lymphangiomas are considered to arise secondary to sequestration into the pancreatic substance of lymphatics more peripheral than the buddings of the primary lymphatic sacs. This implies that some form of pancreatectomy is required for curative excision.

LYMPHOMA

Primary lymphoma of the pancreas is a rare disease. The presenting signs and symptoms are generally nonspecific and consist of abdominal pain, weight loss, and a palpable mass.[199] Jaundice may also be present.[200] Most patients are adults (average age, 68 years), with a reported male-to-female ratio of 2:5.[200] The mean size of the mass at presentation is 8.1 cm and most individuals are assumed, at least initially, to have inoperable carcinoma. FNAB may not reveal the correct diagnosis, so an open biopsy may be required.[200] This is potentially highly significant, because of a favorable response to chemotherapy or radiotherapy. Individuals who do not receive this treatment survive only an average of 5 months.[200]

A variety of lymphoma subtypes has been described, mostly non-Hodgkin's lymphoma of B-cell lineage. Occasional T-cell lymphomas[201] and anaplastic Ki-1 lymphomas are recorded.[202] Interestingly, primary pancreatic lymphoma has also been described during immunosuppression, both acquired immunodeficiency syndrome[203] and post-transplantation related,[204] as well as a complication of chronic malabsorption and short bowel syndrome.[205] Familial pancreatic lymphoma is also recorded.[206]

MISCELLANEOUS TUMORS

Miscellaneous tumors include those of germ-cell origin, both mature teratoma[207–209] and choriocarcinoma,[210] as well as hamartoma.[211] Mature teratomas resemble ovarian dermoid cysts and consist predominately of cystic structures, lined by mature stratified squamous epithelium or ciliated columnar epithelium. Sebaceous glands may be present and solid areas can contain bone, cartilage, and glia. Immature teratomas, embryonal carcinomas, and yolk-sac tumors have not been recorded in the pancreas. The one recorded instance of hamartoma occurred in a 20-month-old child and consisted of a 9-cm-diameter mass, comprising well-formed pancreatic acini, dilated ductlike structures, fibrous tissue, and fat.[211]

A single instance of the extremely rare "sugar tumor" has been described in the pancreas.[212] These neoplasms, which have an unknown histogenesis, have a clear cytoplasm and may microscopically mimic a clear cell carcinoma. However, they are negative with immunohistochemical stains for epithelial markers, although they are typically HMB45 positive.

REFERENCES

1. Shorten SD, Hart WR, Petras RE: Microcystic adenomas (serous cystadenomas) of pancreas: A clinicopathologic investigation of eight cases with immunohistochemical and ultrastructural studies. Am J Surg Pathol 10:365–372, 1986.
2. Alpert LC, Truong LD, Bossart MI, et al.: Microcystic adenoma (serous cystadenoma) of the pancreas. A study of 14 cases with immunohistochemical and electron microscopic correlation. Am J Surg Pathol 12:251–263, 1988.
3. Kim YI, Seo JW, Suh JS, et al.: Microcystic adenomas of the pancreas. Report of three cases with two of multicentric origin. Am J Clin Pathol 94:150–156, 1990.
4. Kamei K, Funabiki T, Ochiai M, et al.: Multifocal pancreatic serous cystadenoma with atypical cells and focal perineural invasion. Int J Pancreatol 10:161–162, 1991.
5. Tanno S, Obara T, Sohma M, et al.: Multifocal serous cystadenoma of the pancreas. A case report and review of the literature. Int J Pancreatol 24:129–132, 1998.
6. Compagno J, Oertel JE: Microcystic adenomas of the pancreas (glycogen-rich cystadenomas). A clinicopathologic study of 34 cases. Am J Clin Pathol 69:289–298, 1978.
7. Beerman MH, Fromkes JJ, Carey LC, et al.: Pancreatic cystadenoma in von Hippel–Lindau disease: An unusual cause of pancreatic and common bile duct obstruction. J Clin Gastroenterol 4:537–540, 1982.
8. Horton WR, Wong V, Eldridge R: von Hippel–Lindau disease. Clinical and pathological manifestations in nine families with 50 affected members. Arch Intern Med 136:769–777, 1976.
9. Hodgkinson DJ, ReMine WH, Weiland LH: Pancreatic cystadenoma. A clinicopathologic study of 45 cases. Arch Surg 113:512–519, 1978.
10. Pyke CM, van Heerden JA, Colby TV, et al.: The spectrum of serous cystadenoma of the pancreas. Clinical, pathological and surgical aspects. Ann Surg 215:132–139, 1992.
11. Mathieu D, Guigui B, Valette PJ, et al.: Pancreatic cystic neoplasms. Radiol Clin North Am 27:163–176, 1989.
12. Egawa N, Maillet B, Schroeder S, et al.: Serous oligocystic and ill-demarcated adenoma of the pancreas: A variant of serous cystic adenoma. Virchows Archiv 424:13–17, 1994.
13. Jones EC, Suen KC, Grant DR, et al.: Fine-needle aspiration cytology of neoplastic cysts of the pancreas. Diagn Cytopathol 3:238–243, 1987.
14. Laucirica R, Schwartz MR, Ramzy I: Fine needle aspiration of pancreatic cystic epithelial lesions. Acta Cytologica 36:881–886, 1992.
15. Nguyen G-K, Vogelsang PJ: Microcystic adenoma of the pancreas. A report of two cases with fine needle aspiration cytology and differential diagnosis. Acta Cytologica 37:908–910, 1993.
16. Ishikawa T, Nakao A, Nomoto S, et al.: Immunohistochemical and molecular biological studies of serous cystadenoma of the pancreas. Pancreas 16:40–44, 1998.
17. Bogomoletz WV, Adnet JJ, Widgren S, et al.: Cystadenoma of the pancreas: A histological, histochemical and ultrastructural study of seven cases. Histopathology 4:309–320, 1980.
18. George DH, Murphy F, Michalski R, et al.: Serous cystadenocarcinoma of the pancreas: A new entity? Am J Surg Pathol 13:61–66, 1989.
19. Yoshimi N, Sugie S, Tanaka T, et al.: A rare case of serous cystadenocarcinoma of the pancreas. Cancer 69:2449–2453, 1992.
20. Widmaier U, Mattfeldt T, Siech M, et al.: Serous cystadenocarcinoma of the pancreas. Internat J Pancreatol 20:135–139, 1996.
21. Abe H, Kubota K, Mori M, et al.: Serous cystadenoma of the pancreas with invasive growth: Benign or malignant? Am J Gastroenterol 93:1963–1966, 1998.
22. Ohta T, Nagakawa T, Itoh H, et al.: A case of serous cystadenoma of the pancreas with focal malignant changes. Int J Pancreatol 14:283–289, 1993.
23. Nyongo A, Huntrakoon M: Microcystic adenoma of the pancreas with myoepithelial cells. Am J Clin Pathol 84:114–120, 1985.
24. Lewandrowski K, Warshaw A, Compton C: Macrocystic serous cystadenoma of the pancreas. A morphologic variant differing from microcystic adenoma. Hum Pathol 23:871–875, 1992.
25. Chang CH, Perrin EV, Hertzler J, et al.: Cystadenoma of the pancreas with cytomegalovirus infection in a female infant. Arch Pathol Lab Med 104:7–8, 1980.
26. Amir G, Hurvitz H, Neeman Z, et al.: Neonatal cytomegalovirus infection with pancreatic cystadenoma and the nephrotic syndrome. Pediatr Pathol 6:393–401, 1986.
27. Warfel KA, Faught PR, Hull MT: Pancreatic cystadenoma in an infant: Ultrastructural study. Pediatr Pathol 8:559–565, 1988.
28. Perez-Ordonez B, Naseem A, Lieberman PH, et al.: Solid serous adenoma of the pancreas. The solid variant of serous cystadenoma? Am J Surg Pathol 20:1401–1405, 1996.
29. Montag AG, Fossati N, Michelassi F: Pancreatic microcystic adenoma coexistent with pancreatic ductal carcinoma. A report of two cases. Am J Surg Pathol 14:352–355, 1990.
30. Keel SB, Zukerberg L, Graeme-Cook F, et al.: Pancreatic endocrine tumor arising within a serous cystadenoma of the pancreas. Am J Surg Pathol 20:471–475, 1996.
31. Vortmeyer AO, Lubensky IA, Fogt F, et al.: Allelic deletion and mutation of the von Hippel–Lindau (VHL) tumor suppressor gene in pancreatic microcystic adenomas. Am J Pathol 151:951–956, 1997.
32. Knudson AG: Genetics of human cancer. Annu Rev Genet 20:231–251, 1986.
33. Stamm B, Burger H, Hollinger A: Acinar cell cystadenocarcinoma of the pancreas. Cancer 60:2542–2547, 1987.
34. Kloppel G, Solcia E, Longnecker DS, et al.: Histological typing of tumors of the exocrine pancreas. 2nd Ed. World Health Organization, International Histological Classification of Tumors. Berlin: Springer, 1996.
35. Compagno J, Oertel JE: Mucinous cystic neoplasms of the pancreas with overt and latent malignancy (cys-

tadenocarcinoma and cystadenoma). A clinicopathologic study of 41 cases. Am J Clin Pathol 69:573–580, 1978.
36. Thompson LDR, Becker RC, Przygodzki RM, et al.: Mucinous cystic neoplasm (mucinous cystadenocarcinoma of low malignant potential) of the pancreas. Am J Surg Pathol 23:1–16, 1999.
37. Zamboni G, Scarpa A, Bogina G, et al.: Mucinous cystic tumors of the pancreas. Clinicopathologic features, prognosis and relationship to other mucinous cystic tumors. Am J Surg Pathol 23:410–422, 1999.
38. Wilentz RE, Albores-Saavedra J, ZAhurak M, et al.: Pathologic examination accurately predicts prognosis in mucinous cystic neoplasia of the pancreas. Am J Surg Pathol 23:1320–1327, 1999.
39. Albores-Saavedra J, Angeles-Angeles A, Nadji M, et al.: Mucinous cystadenocarcinoma of the pancreas. Am J Surg Pathol 11:11–20, 1987.
40. Buelow PC, Rao P, Thompson LD: From the archives of the AFIP. Mucinous cystic neoplasms of the pancreas: Radiologic-pathologic correlation. Radiographics 18:433–449, 1998.
41. LeBorgne J, de Calan L, Partensky C: Cystadenomas and cystadenocarcinomas of the pancreas: A multi institutional retrospective study of 398 cases. French Surgical Association. Ann Surg 230:152–161, 1999.
42. Herrera L, Glassman CI, Komins JI: Mucinous cystic neoplasm of the pancreas demonstrated by ultrasound and endoscopic retrograde pancreatography. Am J Gastroenterol 73:512–515, 1980.
43. Campman SC, Fajardo MA, Rippon MB, et al.: Adenosquamous carcinoma arising in a mucinous cystadenoma of the pancreas. J Surg Oncol 64:159–162, 1997.
44. Zamboni G, Bonetti F, Gastelli P, et al.: Mucinous cystic tumor of the pancreas recurring after 11 years as cystadenocarcinoma with foci of dioriocarcinoma and osteoclast-like giant cell tumor. Surg Pathol 5:253–256, 1994.
45. Wouters K, Ectors N, Van Steenbergen W, et al.: A pancreatic mucinous cystadenoma in a man with mesenchymal stroma expressing oestrogen and progestogen receptors. Virchows Archiv 432:187–189, 1998.
46. Mozan AA: Cystadenoma of the pancreas. Am J Surg 81:204–214, 1951.
47. Weihing RR, Shintaku IP, Geller SA, et al.: Hepatobiliary and pancreatic mucinous cystadenomas with mesenchymal stroma: Analysis of estrogen receptors/progestogen receptors and expression of tumor associated antigens. Mod Pathol 10:372–379, 1997.
48. Garcia Rego JA, Valbuena Ruvira L, Alvarez Garcia A, et al.: Pancreatic mucinous cystadenocarcinoma with pseudosarcomatous mural nodules. Cancer 67:494–498, 1991.
49. Marinho A, Nogueira R, Schmitt F, et al.: Pancreatic mucinous cystadenocarcinoma with a mural nodule of anaplastic carcinoma. Histopathology 26:284–287, 1995.
50. Lane RB Jr, Sangueza OP: Anaplastic carcinoma occurring in association with mucinous cystic neoplasm of the pancreas. Arch Pathol Lab Med 121:533–535, 1997.
51. Nishihara K, Katsumoto F, Kurokawa Y, et al.: Anaplastic carcinoma showing rhabdoid features combined with mucinous cystadenocarcinoma of the pancreas. Arch Pathol Lab Med 121:1104–1107, 1997.
52. Bergman S, Medeiros LJ, Radr T, et al.: Giant cell tumor of the pancreas arising in ovarian-like stroma of a mucinous cystadenocarcinoma. Int J Pancreatol 18:71–75, 1995.
53. Wenig BM, Albores-Saavedra J, Buetlow PC: Pancreatic mucinous cystic neoplasm with sarcomatous stroma. Am J Surg Pathol 21:70–80, 1997.
54. Dodd LG, Farrell TA, Layfield LJ: Mucinous cystic tumor of the pancreas: An analysis of FNA characteristics with an emphasis on the spectrum of malignancy associated features. Diagn Cytopathol 12:113–119, 1995.
55. Ohta T, Nagakawa T, Fukushima W, et al.: Immunohistochemical study of carcinoembryonic antigen in mucinous cystic neoplasm of the pancreas. Eur Surg Res 24:37–44, 1992.
56. Yamaguchi K, Enjoji M: Cystic neoplasms of the pancreas. Gastroenterology 92:1934–1943, 1987.
57. Helpap B, Vogel J: Immunohistochemical studies on cystic pancreatic neoplasms. Pathol Res Pract 184:39–45, 1989.
58. Wouters K, Ectors N, Van Steenbergen W, et al.: A pancreatic mucinous cystadenoma in a man with mesenchymal stroma, expressing oestrogen and progesterone receptors. Virchows Arch 432:187–189, 1998.
59. Sachs JR, Deren JJ, Sohn M, et al.: Mucinous cystadenoma. Pitfalls of differential diagnosis. Am J Gastroenterol 84:811–816, 1989.
60. Cubilla AL, Fitzgerald PJ: Tumors of the exocrine pancreas. *In* Atlas of Tumor Pathology, second series, fascicle 19. Washington, DC: Armed Forces Institute of Pathology, 1984, p 287.
61. Shimizu M, Itoh H, Okumura S, et al.: Papillary hyperplasia of the pancreas. Hum Pathol 20:806–807, 1989.
62. Morohoshi T, Kanda M, Asanuma K, et al.: Intraductal papillary neoplasm of the pancreas. A clinicopathologic study of six patients. Cancer 64:1329–1335, 1989.
63. Rogers PN, Seywright MM, Murray WR: Diffuse villous adenoma of the pancreatic duct. Pancreas 2:727–730, 1989.
64. Warshaw AL, Berry J, Garg DL: Villous adenoma of the duct of Wirsung. Dig Dis Sci 32:1311–1313, 1987.
65. Payan M-J, Xerri L, Moncada K, et al.: Villous adenoma of the main pancreatic duct: A potentially malignant tumor. Am J Gastroenterol 85:459–463, 1990.
66. Bastid C, Bernard JP, Sarles H, et al.: Mucinous ductal ectasia of the pancreas: A premalignant disease and cause of obstructive pancreatitis. Pancreas 6:15–22, 1991.
67. Conley CR, Scheithauer B, Weiland LH, et al.: Diffuse intraductal papillary adenocarcinoma of the pancreas. Am J Gastroenterol Surg 205:246–249, 1987.
68. Milchgrub S, Campuzano M, Casillas J, et al.: Intraductal carcinoma of the pancreas. Cancer 69:651–656, 1992.
69. Tian FZ, Myler J, Howard JM: Mucinous pancreatic duct ectasia of latent malignancy: An emerging clinicopathologic entity. Surgery 111:109–113, 1992.
70. Obara T, Maguchi H, Saitoh Y, et al.: Mucin-producing tumor of the pancreas: A unique clinical entity. Am J Gastroenterol 86:1619–1625, 1991.
71. Yamada M, Kozuka S, Yamao K, et al.: Mucin-producing tumor of the pancreas. Cancer 68:159–168, 1991.
72. Rickaert F, Cremer M, Deviere J, et al.: Intraductal mucin-hypersecreting neoplasms of the pancreas. Gastroenterology 101:512–519, 1991.
73. Loftus EV, Olivares-Pazkad BA, Batts KP, et al.: Intraductal papillary-mucinous tumors of the pancreas:

Clinicopathologic features, outcome and nomenclature. Gastroenterology 110:1909–1918, 1996.

74. Nagai E, Ueki T, Chijiiwa K, et al.: Intraductal papillary mucinous neoplasms of the pancreas associated with so called "mucinous ductal ectasia." A histochemical and immunohistochemical analysis of 29 cases. Am J Surg Pathol 19:576–589, 1995.
75. Solcia E, Capella C, Kloppel G: Tumors of the pancreas. *In* Rosai J (Ed): Atlas of Tumor Pathology, third series, fascicle 19. Washington, DC: Armed Forces Institute of Pathology, 1997, pp 53–64.
76. Fukushima N, Mukai K, Kanai Y, et al.: Intraductal papillary tumors and mucinous cystic tumors of the pancreas: Clinicopathologic study of 38 cases. Hum Pathol 28:1010–1017, 1997.
77. Paal E, Thompson LDR, Przygodzki RM, et al.: A clinicopathologic and immunohistochemical study of 22 intraductal papillary mucinous neoplasms of the pancreas, with a review of the literature. Am J Surg Pathol 12:518–528, 1999.
78. Koyanagi S, Miyahara T, Migita Y, et al.: Case report: Mucin-producing cystic neoplasm of the pancreas in a child. J Gastroenterol Hepatol 11:768–770, 1996.
79. Azar C, Van de Stadt J, Rickaert F, et al.: Intraductal papillary mucinous tumours of the pancreas. Clinical and therapeutic issues in 32 patients. Gut 39:457–464, 1996.
80. Cellier C, Cuillerier E, Palazzo L, et al.: Intraductal papillary and mucinous tumors of the pancreas: Accuracy of pre-operative computed tomography, endoscopic retrograde pancreatography and endoscopic ultrasound, and long-term outcome in a large surgical series. Gastrointest Endosc 47:42–49, 1998.
81. Pavone E, Mehta SN, Hilzenrat N, et al.: Role of ERCP in the diagnosis of intraductal papillary mucinous neoplasms. Am J Gastroenterol 92:887–890, 1997.
82. Itai Y, Ohhashi K, Nagai H, et al.: "Ductectatic" mucinous cystadenoma and cystadenocarcinoma of the pancreas. Radiology 161:697–700, 1986.
83. Nickl NJ, Lawson JM, Cotton PB: Mucinous pancreatic tumors: ERCP findings. Gastrointest Endosc 37:133–138, 1991.
84. Santani D, Campione O, Salerno A, et al.: Intraductal papillary mucinous neoplasm of the pancreas: A clinicopathologic entity. Arch Pathol Lab Med 119:209–212, 1995.
85. Obara T, Saitoh Y, Maguchi H, et al.: Multicentric development of a pancreatic intraductal carcinoma through atypical papillary hyperplasia. Hum Pathol 28:82–85, 1992.
86. Kozuka S, Sassa R, Taki T, et al.: Relation of pancreatic duct hyperplasia to carcinoma. Cancer 43:1418–1428, 1979.
87. Sessa F, Solcia E, Capella C, et al.: Intraductal papillary mucinous tumors represent a distinct group of pancreatic neoplasms: An investigation of tumor cell differentiation and k-*ras*, p53 and c-*erb*B-2 abnormalities in 26 patients. Virchows Archiv 427:357–367, 1994.
88. Fujii H, Inagaki M, Kasai S, et al.: Genetic progression and heterogeneity in intraductal papillary-mucinous tumors of the pancreas. Am J Pathol 151:1447–1454, 1997.
89. Z'graggen K, Rivera JA, Compton CC, et al.: Prevalence of activating K-*ras* mutations in the evolutionary stages of neoplasia in intraductal papillary tumors of the pancreas. Ann Surg 226:491–500, 1997.
90. Yanagisawa A, Ohtake K, Ohashi K, et al.: Frequent K-*ras* oncogene activation in mucinous cell hyperplasias of pancreas suffering from chronic inflammation. Cancer Res 53:953–956, 1993.
91. Rivera JA, Rall CJ, Graeme-Cook F, et al.: Analysis of K-*ras* oncogene mutations in chronic pancreatitis with ductal hyperplasia. Surgery 121:42–49, 1997.
92. Furuta K, Watanabe H, Ikeda S: Differences between solid and duct-ectatic types of pancreatic ductal carcinoma. Cancer 69:1327–1333, 1992.
93. Conley CR, Scheithauer BW, van Heerden JA, et al.: Diffuse intraductal papillary adenocarcinoma of the pancreas. Ann Surg 205:246–249, 1987.
94. Stewart CJ, Carter R, Imrie CW, et al.: Brush cytology of papillary mucinous neoplasm of the pancreas. Cytopathology 431:31–36, 1997.
95. Terada T, Ohta T, Kitamura Y, et al.: Endocrine cells in intraductal papillary-mucinous neoplasms of the pancreas. A histochemical and immunohistochemical study. Virchows Archiv 431:31–36, 1997.
96. Rivera JA, Fernández-del Castillio C, Pins M, et al.: Pancreatic mucinous ductal ectasia and intraductal papillary neoplasms. A single malignant clinical entity. Ann Surg 225:637–646, 1997.
97. Karawada Y, Yano T, Yamamoto T, et al.: Intraductal mucin-producing tumors of the pancreas. Cancer 69:651–656, 1992.
98. Stommer P, Gebhardt C, Schultheiss KH: Adenocarcinoma of the pancreas with a predominant intraductal component: A special variety of ductal adenocarcinoma. Pancreas 5:114–118, 1990.
99. Longnecker DS: Intraductal papillary mucinous tumors of the pancreas. Arch Pathol Lab Med 119:197–198, 1995.
100. Adsay NV, Adair CF, Heffess CS, et al.: Intraductal oncocytic papillary neoplasms of the pancreas. Am J Surg Pathol 20:980–994, 1996.
101. Jyotheeswaran S, Zotalis G, Penmetsa P, et al.: A newly recognised entity: Intraductal "oncocytic" papillary neoplasm of the pancreas. Am J Gastroenterol 93:2539–2543, 1998.
102. Boor PJ, Swanson MR: Papillary-cystic neoplasm of the pancreas. Am J Surg Pathol 3:69–75, 1979.
103. Learmonth GM, Price SK, Visser AE, et al.: Papillary and cystic neoplasm of the pancreas—an acinar cell tumor? Histopathology 9:63–79, 1985.
104. Miettinen M, Partanen S, Fraki O, et al.: Papillary cystic tumor of the pancreas. An analysis of cellular differentiation by electron microscopy and immunohistochemistry. Am J Surg Pathol 11:855–865, 1987.
105. Yamaguchi K, Hirakata R, Kitamura K: Papillary cystic neoplasm of the pancreas: Radiological pathological characteristics in 11 cases. Br J Surg 77:1000–1003, 1990.
106. Pettinato G, Manivel JC, Ravetto C, et al.: Papillary cystic tumor of the pancreas. A clinicopathologic study of 20 cases with cytologic, ultrastructural and flow cytometric observation, and a review of the literature. Am J Clin Pathol 98:478–488, 1992.
107. Nishihara K, Nagoshi M, Tsuneyoshi M, et al.: Papillary cystic tumors of the pancreas. Assessment of their malignant potential: Cancer 71:82–92, 1993.
108. Stommer P, Kraus J, Stolte M, et al.: Solid and cystic pancreatic tumors. Clinical, histochemical and electron microscopic features in ten cases. Cancer 67:1635–1641, 1991.
109. Lieber MR, Lack EE, Roberts JR, et al.: Solid and papillary epithelial neoplasm of the pancreas. An ultrastructural and immunocytochemical study of six cases. Am J Surg Pathol 11:85–93, 1987.

110. Kissane JM: Pancreatoblastoma and solid and cystic papillary tumor. Two tumors related to pancreatic ontogeny. Semin Diagn Pathol 11:152–164, 1994.
111. Merkle EM, Weber CH, Siech M, et al.: Papillary cystic and solid tumor of the pancreas. Z Gastroenterol 34:743–746, 1996.
112. Morohoshi T, Held G, Kloppel G: Exocrine pancreatic tumors and their histological classification: A study based on 167 autopsy and 97 surgical cases. Histopathology 7:645–661, 1983.
113. Kloppel G, Maurer R, Hofmann E, et al.: Solid-cystic (papillary-cystic) tumors within and outside the pancreas in men: Report of two patients. Virchows Archiv A 418:179–183, 1991.
114. Orlando CA, Bowman RL, Loose JH: Multicentric papillary-cystic neoplasm of the pancreas. Arch Pathol Lab Med 115:958–960, 1991.
115. Matsunou H, Konishi F, Yamamichi N, et al.: Solid infiltrating variety of papillary cystic neoplasm of the pancreas. Cancer 65:2747–2757, 1990.
116. Kobayashi T, Kimura T, Takabayashi N, et al.: Two synchronous solid and cystic tumors of the pancreas. J Gastroenterol 33:439–442, 1998.
117. Goldstein J, Benharroch D, Sion-Vardy N, et al.: Solid cystic and papillary tumor of the pancreas with oncocytic differentiation. J Surg Oncol 56:63–67, 1994.
118. Katz LB, Ehya H: Aspiration cytology of papillary cystic neoplasm of the pancreas. Am J Clin Pathol 94:328–333, 1990.
119. Naresh KN, Borges AM, Chinoy RF, et al.: Solid and papillary epithelial neoplasm of the pancreas. Diagnosis by fine needle aspiration cytology in four cases. Acta Cytol 39:489–493, 1995.
120. Remadi S, MacGee W, Doussis-Anagnostopoulou I, et al.: Papillary-cystic tumor of the pancreas. Diagn Cytopathol 15:398–402, 1996.
121. Kashima K, Hayashida Y, Yokoyama S, et al.: Cytologic features of solid and cystic tumors of the pancreas. Acta Cytol 41:443–449, 1997.
122. Jorgensen LJ, Hansen AB, Burcharth F, et al.: Solid and papillary neoplasm of the pancreas. Ultrastruct Pathol 16:659–666, 1992.
123. Ladanyi M, Mulay S, Arsenau J, et al.: Estrogen and progesterone receptor determination in the papillary cystic neoplasms of the pancreas. With immunohistochemical and ultrastructural observations. Cancer 60:1604–1611, 1987.
124. Wrba F, Chott A, Ludvik B, et al.: Solid and cystic tumor of the pancreas. A hormonal dependent neoplasm. Histopathology 12:338–340, 1988.
125. Zamboni G, Bonetti F, Scarpa A, et al.: Expression of progesterone receptor in solid cystic tumor of the pancreas: A clinicopathological, immunohistochemical and ultrastructural study of 10 cases. Virchows Arch [A] 423:425–431, 1993.
126. Sclafani LM, Reuter VE, Coit DG, et al.: The malignant nature of papillary and cystic neoplasm of the pancreas. Cancer 68:153–158, 1991.
127. Shimizu M, Matsumoto T, Hirokawa M, et al.: Solid-pseudopapillary carcinoma of the pancreas. Pathol Int 49:231–234, 1999.
128. Kamei K, Funabiki T, Ochiai M, et al.: Three cases of solid and cystic tumor of the pancreas. Analysis comparing the histopathological findings and DNA histograms. Int J Pancreatol 10:269–278, 1991.
129. Nishihara K, Tsuneyoshi M: Papillary cystic tumors of the pancreas: An analysis by nuclear morphometry. Virchows Archiv [A] 422:211–217, 1993.
130. Grant LD, Lauwers GY, Meloni AM, et al.: Unbalanced chromosomal translocation, der(17)t(13,17)(q14;p11) in a solid and cystic papillary epithelial neoplasm of the pancreas. Am J Surg Pathol 20:339–345, 1996.
131. Matsubara K, Nigami H, Harigaya H, et al.: Chromosome abnormality in solid and cystic tumor of the pancreas. Am J Gastroenterol 92:1219–1221, 1997.
132. Lee W-Y, Tzeng C-C, Jin Y-T, et al.: Papillary cystic tumor of the pancreas: A case indistinguishable from oncocytic carcinoma. Pancreas 8:127–132, 1993.
133. Chen J, Baithun SI: Morphological study of 391 cases of exocrine pancreatic tumors with special reference to the classification of exocrine pancreatic carcinoma. J Pathol 146:17–29, 1985.
134. Kuopio T, Ekfors TO, Nikkanen V, et al.: Acinar cell carcinoma of the pancreas. APMIS 103:69–78, 1995.
135. Klimstra DS, Heffess CS, Oertel JE, et al.: Acinar cell carcinoma of the pancreas. A clinicopathologic study of 28 cases. Am J Surg Pathol 16:815–837, 1992.
136. Burns WA, Matthews MJ, Hamosh M, et al.: Lipase-secreting acinar cell carcinoma of the pancreas with polyarthropathy. Cancer 33:1002–1009, 1974.
137. Van Klaveren RJ, de Mulder PH, Boerbooms AM, et al.: Pancreatic carcinoma with polyarthritis, fat necrosis and high serum lipid and trypsin activity. Gut 31:953–955, 1990.
138. Villanueva RR, Nguyen-Ho P, Nguyen G-K: Needle aspiration cytology of acinar-cell carcinoma of the pancreas. Report of a case with diagnostic pitfalls and unusual ultrastructural findings. Diagn Cytopathol 10:362–364, 1994.
139. Samuel LH, Frierson HF: Fine needle aspiration cytology of acinar cell carcinoma of the pancreas: Report of two cases. Acta Cytologica 40:585–591, 1996.
140. Hoorens A, Lemoine NR, McLennan et al.: Pancreatic acinar cell carcinoma. An analysis of cell lineage markers, p53 expression and Ki-*ras* mutation. Am J Pathol 143:685–698, 1993.
141. Tucker JA, Shelburne JD, Benning TL, et al.: Filamentous inclusions in acinar cell carcinoma of the pancreas. Ultrastruct Pathol 18:279–286, 1994.
142. Morohoshi T, Kanda M, Horie A, et al.: Immunocytochemical markers of uncommon pancreatic tumors: Acinar cell carcinoma, pancreatoblastoma and solid-cystic (papillary-cystic) tumor. Cancer 59:739–747, 1987.
143. Pellegata NS, Sessa F, Renault B, et al.: K-*ras* and p53 gene mutations in pancreatic cancer. Ductal and nonductal tumors progress through different genetic lesions. Cancer Res 54:1556–1560, 1994.
144. Terhune PG, Heffess CS, Longnecker DS: Only wild-type c-ki-*ras* codons 12, 13 and 61 in human pancreatic acinar cell carcinomas. Mol Carcinog 10:110–114, 1994.
145. Huntrakoon M: Oncocytic carcinoma of the pancreas. Cancer 51:332–336, 1983.
146. Nozawa Y, Abe M, Sakuma H, et al.: A case of pancreatic oncocytic tumor. Acta Pathol Jpn 40:367–370, 1990.
147. Ulich T, Cheng L, Lewin KJ: Acinar-endocrine cell tumor of the pancreas. Cancer 50:2099–2105, 1982.
148. Klimstra DS, Rosai J, Heffess CS: Mixed acinar-endocrine carcinomas of the pancreas. Am J Surg Pathol 18:765–778, 1994.
149. Hassan MO, Gogate PA: Malignant mixed exocrine-endocrine tumor of the pancreas with unusual intracy-

toplasmic inclusions. Ultrastruct Pathol 17:483–493, 1993.
150. Gotchall J, Traweek ST, Stenzel P: Benign oncocytic endocrine tumor of the pancreas in a patient with polyarteritis nodosa. Hum Pathol 18:967–969, 1987.
151. Hoorens A, Gebhard F, Fraft K, et al.: Pancreatoblastoma in an adult: its separation from acinar cell carcinoma. Virchows Arch [A] 424:485–490, 1994.
152. Cantrell BB, Cubilla AL, Erlandson RA, et al.: Acinar cell cystadenocarcinoma of the human pancreas. Cancer 47:410–416, 1981.
153. Stamm B, Burger H, Hollinger A: Acinar cell cystadenocarcinoma of the pancreas. Cancer 60:2542–2547, 1987.
154. Palosaari D, Clayton F, Seaman J: Pancreatoblastoma in an adult. Arch Pathol Lab Med 110:650–652, 1986.
155. Dunn JL, Longnecker DS: Pancreatoblastoma in an older adult. Arch Pathol Lab Med 119:547–551, 1995.
156. Levey JM, Banner BF: Adult pancreatoblastoma: A case report and review of the literature. Am J Gastroenterol 91:1841–1844, 1996.
157. Kissane JM: Tumors of the exocrine pancreas in childhood. Cancer Treat Res 8:99–129, 1982.
158. Klimstra DS, Wenig BM, Adair CF, et al.: Pancreatoblastoma: A clinicopathologic study and review of the literature. Am J Surg Pathol 19:1371–1389, 1995.
159. Chun Y, Kim W, Park K, et al.: Pancreatoblastoma. J Pediatr Surg 32:1612–1615, 1997.
160. Willnow U, Willberg B, Schwamborn D, et al.: Pancreatoblastoma in children. Eur J Pediatr Surg 6:369–372, 1996.
161. Iseki M, Suzuki T, Koizumi Y, et al.: Alpha-fetoprotein producing pancreatoblastoma: A case report. Cancer 57:1833–1835, 1986.
162. Morohoshi T, Sagawa F, Mitsuya T: Pancreatoblastoma with marked elevation of serum alpha-fetoprotein. An autopsy case report with immunocytochemical study. Virchows Archiv [A] 416:265–270, 1990.
163. Drut R, Jones MC: Congenital pancreatoblastoma in the Beckwith–Wiedemann syndrome: An emerging association. Pediatr Pathol 8:331–337, 1988.
164. Koh TH, Cooper JE, Newman CL, et al.: Pancreatoblastoma in a neonate with Wiedemann–Beckwith syndrome. Eur J Pediatr 145:435–438, 1986.
165. Silverman JF, Holbrook CT, Pories WJ, et al.: Fine needle aspiration cytology of pancreatoblastoma with immunocytochemical and ultrastructural studies. Acta Cytol 34:632–640, 1990.
166. Lack EE, Cassady JR, Levey R, et al.: Tumors of the exocrine pancreas in children and adolescents. A clinical and pathologic study of eight cases. Am J Surg Pathol 7:319–327, 1983.
167. Horie A, Morohoshi T, Kloppel G: Ultrastructural comparison of pancreatoblastoma, solid cystic tumor and acinar cell carcinoma. J Clin Electron Microscopy 20:353–362, 1987.
168. Hua C, Shu XK, Lei C: Pancreatoblastoma, a histochemical and immunohistochemical analysis. J Clin Pathol 49:952–954, 1996.
169. Brown SJ, Owen DA, O'Connell JX, et al.: Schwannoma of the pancreas. Report of two cases and a review of the literature. Mod Pathol 11:1178–1182, 1998.
170. Feldman L, Philpotts LE, Reinhold C, et al.: Pancreatic schwannoma: Report of two cases and a review of the literature. Pancreas 15:99–105, 1997.
171. Seidler A, Burstein S, Orweiga W, et al.: Granular cell tumor of the pancreas. J Clin Gastroenterol 8:207–209, 1986.
172. Sekas G, Talamo TS, Julian TB: Obstruction of the pancreatic duct by a granular cell tumor. Dig Dis Sci 33:1334–1337, 1988.
173. Merli M, Fossati GS, Alessiani M, et al.: A rare case of pancreatic lipoma. Hepatogastroenterology 43:734–736, 1996.
174. Pascal RR, Sullivan L, Hauser L, et al.: Primary malignant fibrous histiocytoma of the pancreas. Hum Pathol 20:1215–1217, 1989.
175. Allen KB, Skandalakis LJ, Brown BC, et al.: Malignant fibrous histiocytoma of the pancreas. Am Surg 56:364–368, 1990.
176. Haba R, Kobayashi S, Hirakawa E, et al.: Malignant fibrous histiocytoma of the pancreas. Pathol Int 46:515–519, 1996.
177. Bastien D, Ramaswamy A, Barth PJ: Malignant fibrous histiocytoma of the pancreas: A case report with genetic analysis. Cancer 85:2352–2358, 1999.
178. Tsujimura T, Kawano K, Taniguchi M, et al.: Malignant fibrous histiocytoma co-existent with mucinous cystadenoma of the pancreas. Cancer 70:2792–2796, 1992.
179. Moller-Pederson VM, Hedes A, Graem N: A solitary malignant schwannoma mimicking a pancreatic pseudocyst. Acta Chir Scand 148:697–698, 1982.
180. Eggermont A, Vuzenski V, Huisman M, et al.: Solitary malignant schwannoma of the pancreas: Report of a case. J Surg Oncol 36:21–25, 1987.
181. Ishikawa O, Matsui Y, Aoki Y, et al.: Leiomyosarcoma of the pancreas. Report of a case and review of the literature. Am J Surg Pathol 5:597–602, 1981.
182. DeAlva E, Torramadé J, Vazquez JJ: Leiomyosarcoma of the pancreas. Virchows Archiv [A] 422:419–422, 1993.
183. Sato T, Asanuma Y, Nanjo H, et al.: A resected case of giant leiomyosarcoma of the pancreas. J Gastroenterol 29:223–227, 1994.
184. Aranha GV, Simples PE, Veselik K: Leiomyosarcoma of the pancreas. Int J Pancreatol 17:95–97, 1995.
185. Neibling HA: Primary sarcoma of the pancreas. Am Surg 34:690–693, 1968.
186. Elliott TE, Albertazzi VJ, Danto LA: Pancreatic liposarcoma: A case report and a review of retroperitoneal liposarcomas. Cancer 45:1720–1723, 1980.
187. Grosfeld JL, Clatworthy HW Jr, Hamoudi AB: Pancreatic malignancy in children. Arch Surg 101:370–375, 1970.
188. Danner DB, Hruban RH, Pitt HA, et al.: Primitive neuroectodermal tumor arising in the pancreas. Mod Pathol 7:200–204, 1994.
189. Gerald WL, Miller HK, Battifora H, et al.: Intra-abdominal desmoplastic small round-cell tumor. Report of 19 cases of a distinctive type of high-grade polyphenotypic malignancy affecting young individuals. Am J Surg Pathol 15:499–513, 1991.
190. Luttges J, Mentzel, T, Hubner G, et al.: Solitary fibrous tumor of the pancreas: A new member of the small group of mesenchymal pancreatic tumors. Virchows Arch 435:37–42, 1999.
191. Kobayashi H, Itoh T, Murata R, et al.: Pancreatic cavernous hemangioma: CT, MRI, US and angiography characteristics. Gastrointest Radiol 16:307–310, 1991.
192. Bardaxogon E, Manganas D, Landen S, et al.: Hemangiopericytoma of the pancreas: Report of a case and review of the literature. Hepatogastroenterology 42:172–174, 1995.
193. Tunell WP: Hemangioendothelioma of the pancreas obstructing the common bile duct and duodenum. J Pediatr Surg 11:827–830, 1976.

194. Horie H, Iwasaki I, Iida H, et al.: Benign hemangioendothelioma of the pancreas with obstructive jaundice. Acta Pathol Jpn 35:975–979, 1985.
195. Khandelwal M, Lichtenstein GR, Morris JB, et al.: Abdominal lymphangioma masquerading as a pancreatic cystic neoplasm. J Clin Gastroenterol 20:142–144, 1995.
196. Daltrey IR, Johnson CD: Cystic lymphangioma of the pancreas. Postgrad Med J 72:564–566, 1996.
197. Abe H, Kubota K, Noie T, et al.: Cystic lymphangioma of the pancreas: A case report with special reference to embryological development. Am J Gastroenterol 92:1566–1567, 1997.
198. Paal E, Thompson LD, Heffess CS: A clinicopathologic and immunohistochemical study of ten pancreatic lymphangiomas and a review of the literature. Cancer 82:2150–2158, 1998.
199. Behrns KE, Sarr MG, Strickler JG: Pancreatic lymphoma. Is it a surgical disease? Pancreas 9:662–667, 1994.
200. Tuchek JM, De Jong SA, Pickelman J: Diagnosis, surgical intervention and prognosis of primary pancreatic lymphoma. Am Surg 59:513–518, 1993.
201. Satake K, Arimoto Y, Fujimoto Y, et al.: Malignant T cell lymphoma of the pancreas. Pancreas 6:120–124, 1991.
202. Maruyama H, Nakatsuji N, Sugihara S, et al.: Anaplastic Ki-1-positive large cell lymphoma: A case report and review of the literature. Jpn J Clin Oncol 27:51–57, 1997.
203. Jones WF, Sheikh MY, McClave SA: AIDS-related non-Hodgkin's lymphoma of the pancreas. Am J Gastroenterol 92:335–338, 1997.
204. Cario E, Runzi M, Metz K, et al.: Diagnostic dilemma in pancreatic lymphoma. Case report and review. Int J Pancreatol 22:67–71, 1997.
205. Keung YK, Cobos E, Trowers E: Primary pancreatic lymphoma associated with the short bowel syndrome: Review of carcinogenesis of gastrointestinal malignancies. Leuk Lymph 26:405–408, 1997.
206. James JA, Milligan DW, Morgan GJ, et al.: Familial pancreatic lymphoma. J Clin Pathol 51:80–82, 1998.
207. Iacono C, Zamboni G, DiMarcello R, et al.: Dermoid cyst of the head of pancreas area. Int J Pancreatol 14:269–273, 1993.
208. Mester M, Trajber H, Compton CC, et al.: Cystic teratomas of the pancreas. Arch Surg 125:1215–1218, 1990.
209. Fernandez-Cebrian JM, Carda P, Morales V, et al.: Dermoid cyst of the pancreas: A rare cystic neoplasm. Hepatogastroenterology 45:1874–1876, 1998.
210. Childs CC, Korsten MA, Choi HS: Pancreatic choriocarcinoma presenting as inflammatory pseudocyst. Gastroenterology 89:426–431, 1985.
211. Flaherty MJ, Benjamin DR: Multicystic pancreatic hamartoma: A distinctive lesion with immunohistochemical and ultrastructural study. Hum Pathol 23:1309–1312, 1992.
212. Zamboni G, Pea M, Martignoni G, et al.: Clear cell "sugar" tumor of the pancreas. A novel member of the family of lesions characterized by the presence of perivascular epithelioid cells. Am J Surg Pathol 20:722–730, 1996.

Chapter

9

PANCREATIC ENDOCRINE TUMORS AND TUMORLIKE LESIONS

Clinically significant islet cell (endocrine) tumors of the pancreas are rare. The prevalence is estimated at approximately 1 per 100,000[1]; however, small clinically insignificant tumors are detected in between 1.5% and 10% of unselected autopsy cases, depending on how thoroughly the pancreas is examined.[2,3] Clinically significant endocrine tumors represent between 1% and 6% of all pancreatic neoplasms included in surgical series.[4] Endocrine tumors may be functional or nonfunctional. A designation as ''functional'' implies that the tumor gives rise to a clinical syndrome, secondary to specific hormone overproduction. Immunohistochemical or biochemical demonstration of hormonal activity within cells does not, in this context, imply that a tumor is functional. Nonfunctional tumors are most frequently encountered by chance at autopsy or may be discovered at upper abdominal radiographic or sonographic examination performed for investigation of a mass lesion, pain, or discomfort.

The majority (> 90%) of all islet cell tumors occur in individuals older than 30 years of age, with the mean age at occurrence being 58 years.[5] They are extremely rare in infants and small children. No major sex difference has been observed and no geographic differences in prevalence have been recorded.

No significant etiologic agents are identified for islet cell tumors, other than the multiple endocrine neoplasia syndrome type I (MEN I). This syndrome is considered to be the result of a mutation of a gene located on the long arm of chromosome 11 at locus 11q13[6] (see discussion under Multiple Endocrine Neoplasia Syndrome Type I). There is some evidence that sporadic insulinoma may be more common in persons with diabetes than it is in the general population; however, it is still exceptionally rare in both groups. Occasionally, individuals with the von Hippel–Lindau syndrome may have islet tumors.[7]

Some controversy exists about the histogenesis of endocrine tumors. Two major possibilities need to be considered: Either the tumors are derived directly from islet cells or they originate from pleuripotential terminal ductular (intra-acinar) stem cells. Evidence favors the second theory. Terminal ductular origin is suggested by the rare finding of mixed endocrine-acinar neoplasms and the more common occurrence of scattered endocrine cells throughout what is otherwise a typical ductal adenocarcinoma. The ductal origin theory is also supported by studies of pancreatic embryology, which reveal that islet cells, intra-acinar terminal duct cells, and acinar cells are all derived from primitive peripheral ducts.[8] Nesidioblastosis, not uncommonly, occurs at the edge of insulinomas in the surrounding nonneoplastic pancreas. This is characterized by the presence of (1) hypertrophic B cells within otherwise normal-appearing islets, (2) small scattered endocrine cell clusters, and (3) ductulo–islet cell complexes. The presence of nesidioblastosis raises the possibility that insulinomas are derived from ductulo-islet nesidioblastic foci but obviously does not exclude the alternative possibility that nesidioblastosis is a reactive—not preneoplastic—change occurring secondary to tumor formation. Evidence of an origin from preexistent islets is scanty. In animal models, it has been observed that tumors induced in transgenic mice may, during the course of growth, switch from production of one hormone to multihormone expression. However, such transformation of intraductal cells is not observed.[9]

Outside of the MEN I syndrome, islet cell tumors are generally solitary, although this varies to some extent, depending on the type of hormonal activity. For example, only 10% of insulinomas are multiple, whereas multiplicity is a common finding with gastrinomas. Where multiple tumors are encountered, it may occasionally be found that different tumors produce a different set of hormones.

A classification of islet cell tumors based on major hormonal activity is given in Table 9–1. The relative frequency of these neoplasms varies somewhat in different published series. Specialized endocrinology centers record a majority of functional neoplasms, 85% of which are insulinomas. Series from surgical centers record more nonfunctional tumors. Clearly, the detection of functionality varies, depending on how extensively the patient is examined. On gross inspection of a tumor and simple microscopic appearances, it is mostly impossible to determine which hormone, if any, is being produced. Certain histologic characteristics are more common in some tumors than in others, but this is not absolute and cannot be relied on. Identification of a tumor as one of islet cell origin is not always straightforward, and for this reason, immunohistochemical staining is highly desirable to obtain the correct diagnosis. Of great clinical importance is the ability to determine which islet cell tumors are benign and which are malignant. Unfortunately, this, too, can be extremely difficult from routine histologic appearances. Information assisting in this important distinction can, however, be obtained by identifying the hormone being produced, further emphasizing the utility of immunostaining.

Table 9–1. Classification of Pancreatic Islet Cell Tumors

Insulinoma
PP-oma (neoplasm secreting pancreatic polypeptide)
VIP-oma (neoplasm secreting vasoactive intestinal polypeptide)
Glucagonoma
Gastrinoma
Somatostatinoma
Carcinoid tumor (enterochromaffin)
Tumors producing growth hormone
Adrenocorticotropic hormone– and parathormone-secreting tumors
Small cell carcinoma
Nonfunctioning tumors

GROSS FEATURES (GENERAL)

Islet cell tumors occur throughout the pancreas, with approximately equal frequency. However, different subtypes may occur more frequently in some areas than in others. For example, gastrinomas tend to occur in the head of the pancreas, whereas insulinomas are more frequent in the pancreatic body and tail. At gross inspection, islet cells tumors are firmer in consistency than the surrounding pancreatic parenchyma, with a homogeneous consistency lacking the fine lobular structure of normal pancreas (Fig. 9–1). They generally have a well-demarcated border and have a grayish, pinkish, or white color, in contrast to the normal pancreas, which is light tan. Necrosis and hemorrhage should raise a suspicion of malignancy, as should foci with a softer texture and a more yellowish or cream-colored appearance. Cystic degeneration may occur in both benign and malignant islet cell tumors, as well as in certain low-grade ductally derived tumors, such as solid-cystic-papillary epithelial neoplasms. This is therefore not a critical gross diagnostic feature. The overall size of an islet cell tumor may vary considerably: Insulinomas are generally small and glucagonomas are often large. Some clinically significant tumors—for example, gastrinomas—may be < 0.5 cm in diameter, so that careful palpation and visual inspection is necessary to detect them in resection specimens.

MICROSCOPIC FEATURES (GENERAL)

As a general rule, islet cell tumors are composed of monomorphic, medium-size cells. They are usually round or polygonal and only rarely spindle shaped. The nuclei are round or oval, with small distinct nucleoli, but otherwise the chromatin distribution is even (Fig. 9–2). Bizarre nuclei, or multinucleated cells, are uncommon. The cytoplasm is moderately plentiful and is typically lightly granular or eosinophilic.

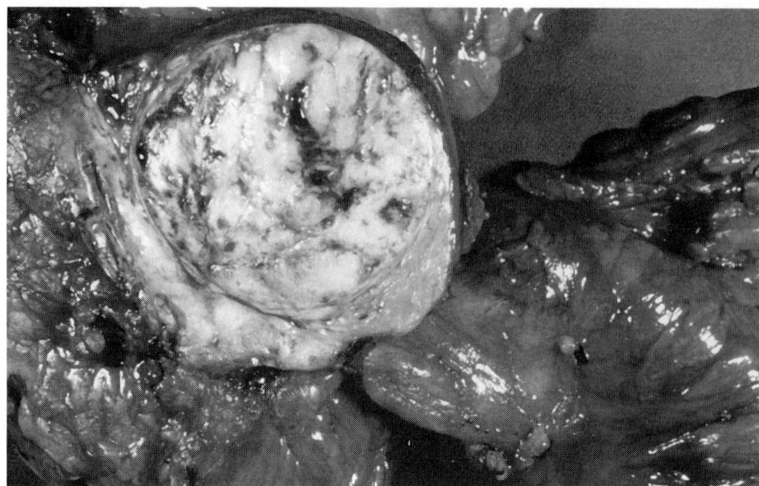

Figure 9–1. Gross appearance of a typical islet cell tumor. Note the homogeneous appearance and demarkation from the surrounding pancreatic parenchyma.

Occasionally, the cytoplasm is basophilic or clear (Fig. 9–3), and rarely, an oncocytic appearance is observed. Three basic architectural patterns are found: solid (Fig. 9–4), trabecular (or gyriform) (Fig. 9–5), and glandular (tubular) (Fig. 9–6). Variants of these patterns may demonstrate vascular pseudorosettes, or acini (lobules). Mixtures of patterns are not uncommonly encountered within the same tumor. As a general rule, a trabecular pattern is associated with a benign prognosis, whereas malignant tumors tend to have a solid or glandular pattern. However, this association is weak and cannot be relied on in individual cases.

General immunohistochemical markers that may be used to establish whether a pancreatic tumor is of islet cell origin include chromogranin,[10] synaptophysin,[11] and neuron-specific enolase (NSE).[10,12] Staining results will of course vary, depending on the method and duration of fixation employed; however, all well-differentiated tumors should be diffusely NSE positive. If this marker is negative, the diagnosis of islet cell tumor is suspect. The converse is not, however, true, because not all NSE-positive neoplasms are islet cell tumors. Chromogranin positivity varies and may be focal or diffuse. It works best for cells secreting glucagon and most poorly in insulinomas and somatostatinomas.[10] Negative results for chromogranin may be obtained with pure insulinomas. This surprising finding is related to the fact that although some

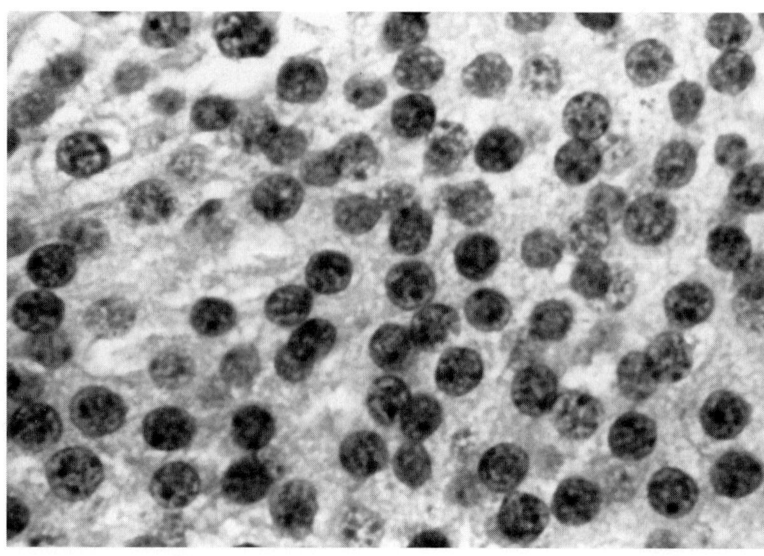

Figure 9–2. Typical appearance of a well-differentiated islet cell tumor with regular nuclei containing evenly dispersed chromatin. The cytoplasm is inconspicuous.

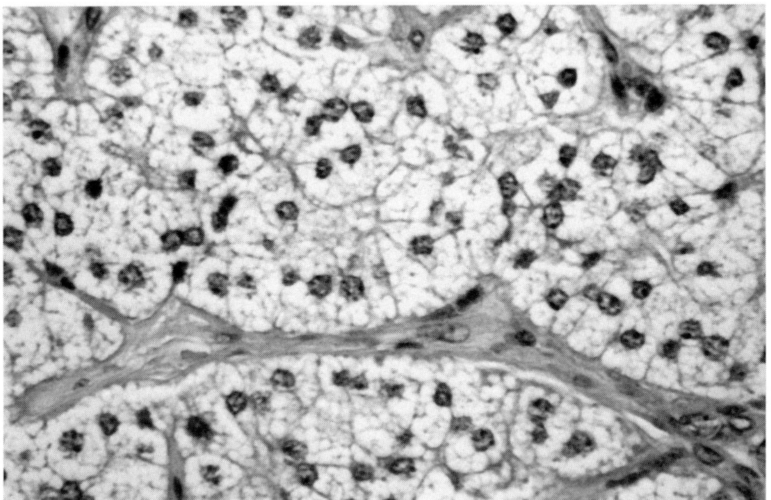

Figure 9–3. Clear cell change in an islet cell tumor. Lipid is present within the cytoplasm.

endocrine tumors may avidly secrete hormone, many do not store enough cytoplasmic granules to retain positive staining. Overall, approximately 70% of islet cell tumors are positive for chromogranin.[10] Low-grade islet cell tumors are all positive for synaptophysin. These markers are not, however, specific for islet cell tumors; isolated cells, positive for chromogranin and synaptophysin, may be encountered in other histologically low-grade neoplasms, especially solid-cystic-papillary tumors and acinar cell carcinomas. NSE stains may be diffusely positive in solid-cystic-papillary tumors[13] (see Distinguishing Benign from Malignant Islet Cell Tumors, below). For these reasons, it is recommended that in difficult cases, tumor tissue be examined ultrastructurally. Silver stains (such as Grimelius) for the diagnosis of islet cell tumors are now outmoded and of historical interest only.

ULTRASTRUCTURAL FINDINGS

All islet cell tumors contain dense core granules. The morphologic features of the granules vary, depending on the hormone secreted, and, especially in well-differentiated neoplasms, they

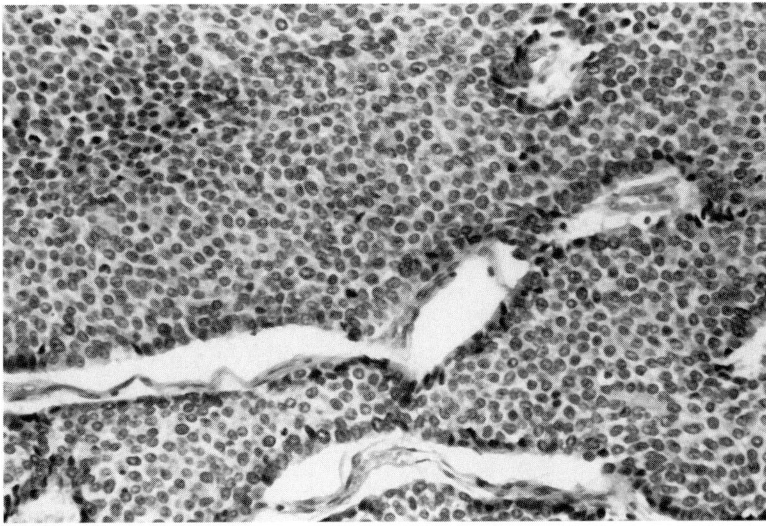

Figure 9–4. Solid pattern of islet cell tumor.

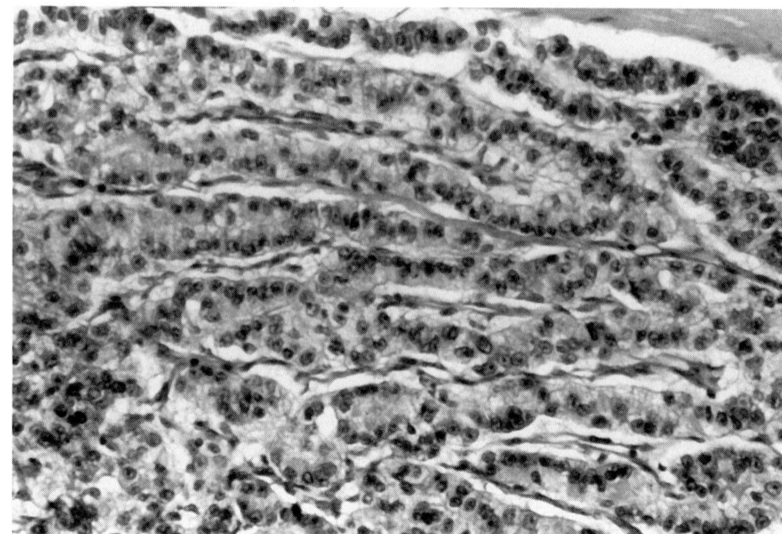

Figure 9–5. Trabecular pattern of islet cell tumor.

tend to resemble normal nonneoplastic granules[14,15] (see Chapter 1). B-cell granules (containing insulin) are typically crystalline and pleomorphic in appearance. They are surrounded by a clear halo and have a distinct limiting membrane. Their size is generally not > 300 nm. In addition, insulinomas may contain sparsely granulated cells and cells with unusual-appearing granules. These atypical granules are smaller in size than typical B granules, with rounded dark or light cores and a less conspicuous halo, or even an absent halo. Occasionally, atypical granules have an inconspicuous or absent core. On the basis of the type of granules present, four categories of insulinoma may be recognized[14,15]: type 1, containing typical B-cell granules only; type 2, containing typical and atypical granules; type 3, with atypical granules only; and type 4 tumors, which are virtually agranular. Tumors of types 1 and 2 are strongly immunopositive for insulin and have a trabecular histiologic pattern. They usually respond well to treatment. In contrast, tumors of types 3 and 4 show sparse immunopositivity for insulin and have a solid growth pattern histologically. By chemical analysis, type 3 and

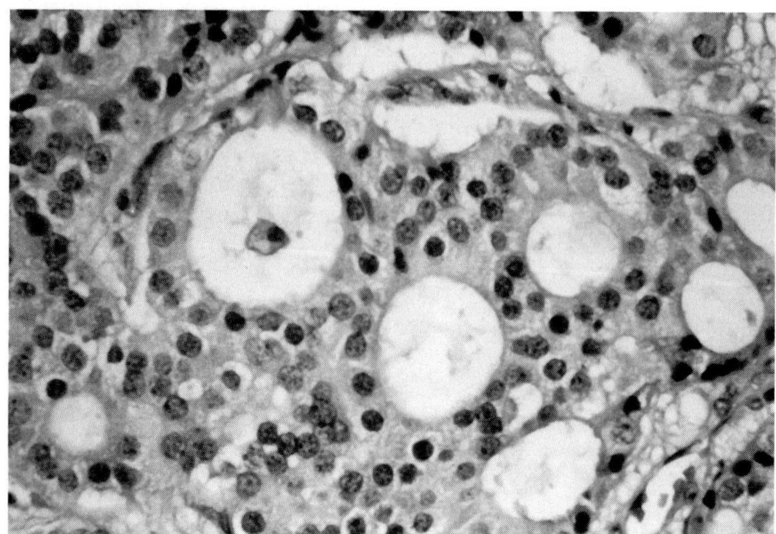

Figure 9–6. Glandular pattern of islet cell tumor.

4 tumors contain more proinsulin than they do insulin. They respond poorly to standard drug therapy.

Ultrastructural analysis of glucagonomas reveals that a variety of granules are present.[16,17] Typical A-cell granules are 180 to 300 nm in diameter and have an inner dark-staining core, separated from the membrane by a lighter grayish mantle. Atypical granules include two types of small granule, one measuring 130 to 250 nm, with a uniform core of various densities, and a second type of medium size (150 to 260 nm), resembling fetal A cells. These have a low-density core with a higher-density mantle. Most glucagonomas contain predominantly atypical granules.

Gastrinomas contain granules that have nonspecific ultrastructural features.[18] These are small and rounded, measuring 170 to 190 nm in diameter with a variable density. Some have a dark core with a clear halo and some have a dark core with no halo.

VIP-omas, or tumors that secrete vasoactive intestinal polypeptide, are usually sparsely granulated, but the cells have a well developed Golgi complex and rough endoplasmic reticulum.[19] Endocrine granules present are varied. The typical VIP-producing granule is 120 to 160 nm in size, with a moderately dense core and a thin clear halo. PP-cell (pancreatic polypeptide–secreting) granules are also commonly encountered in VIP-omas. These are slightly larger (140 to 190 nm) and may be round, ovoid, or comma shaped.[20] Morphologically, these resemble the granules located normally in F-type PP cells derived from PP-rich islets of the posterior pancreatic head.[20] PP-omas also have cells in which the endoplasmic reticulum becomes dilated and filled with secretory material. Elongated electron-dense bodies may be present, which are immunopositive for α_1-antitrypsin.[19]

Ultrastructural examination of somatostatinomas reveals a dual population of cells. The most common are typical D cells, in which the granules are approximately 300 nm in diameter (range, 250 to 450 nm), with granular electron-dense cores and no surrounding halo.[21] A smaller population of cells is also present, in which the granules are smaller (150 to 300 nm), with dense cores and a thin halo. Some of the discrepancy in granule morphology may be explained on the basis of granule immaturity, but some may reflect the elaboration of different hormones, such as PP and calcitonin.[22]

Rare examples of enterochromaffin cell (EC) tumors are encountered within the pancreas. These produce a variety of hormones, including serotonin, substance P, prostaglandins, and kallikreins, any of which may give rise to a clinical carcinoid syndrome. Ultrastructurally, the EC granules are irregularly shaped with a dense core and a thin peripheral halo. Depending on the degree of differentiation of the tumor, more or less granules are present within the cytoplasm.

CYTOLOGIC FINDINGS

Fine-needle aspiration biopsy (FNAB) of pancreatic tumors can be a useful method of securing a tissue diagnosis of a mass in the pancreas. Aspirations may be performed percutaneously or intraoperatively. The method does, however, carry the theoretical possibility of tumor implantation along the needle track.

Aspirates from islet cell tumors are usually highly cellular and have a monomorphic appearance.[23–27] Generally, the cells are dispersed singly, but clumps may be present in which it is possible to identify a trabecular or acinar arrangement. The individual cells are small to medium in size, with regular rounded or oval nuclei. The chromatin is evenly dispersed, although small nucleoli may be encountered. The cytoplasm is abundant but is generally pale staining (Fig. 9–7). A fine granularity may be noted. Occasional larger cells may be encountered, with a more irregular coarse chromatin distribution in eccentric nuclei.[27] Immunohistochemical staining may be useful in confirming the endocrine nature of the tumor.[27] However, care has to be taken to avoid nonspecific false positive staining. It is also important to remember that NSE stains may also be positive in solid-cystic-papillary neoplasms. Chromogranin or synaptophysin positivity is more specific for endocrine differentiation, but scattered positivity is also encountered in acinar cell carcinomas and solid-cystic-papillary neoplasms. Occasional examples of islet cells tumors with oncocytic differentiation have been described.[28] Cytologic preparations from these neoplasms have demonstrated cells with abundant eosinophilic cytoplasm, so that a differential diagnosis of hepatocellular carcinoma has to be considered.

It is generally agreed that it is rarely possible to distinguish benign from malignant islet cell tumors purely on cytologic grounds. Cytologic features that raise a suspicion of malignancy include the presence of mitotic figures, nuclear

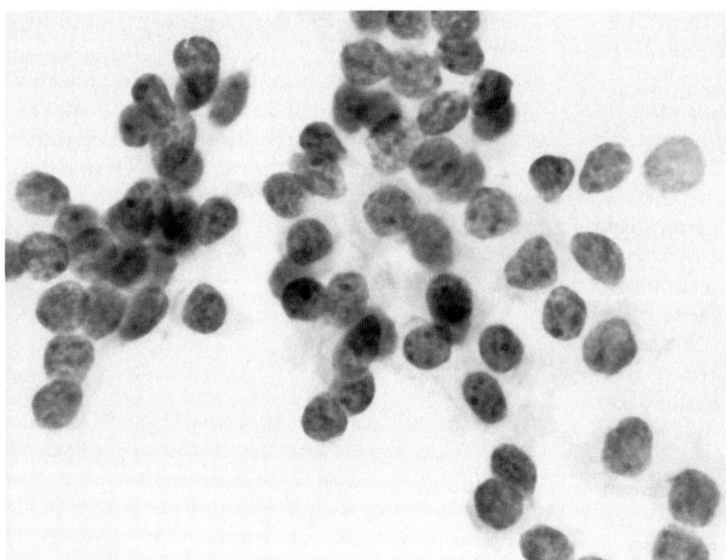

Figure 9–7. Cytologic appearances of an islet cell tumor. The cells are mainly dispersed, although small clumps may be present.

pleomorphism, macronucleoli, and tumor necrosis.[29]

The differential diagnosis of pancreatic endocrine tumors includes well-differentiated adenocarcinoma, acinar cell carcinoma, solid-cystic-papillary epithelial neoplasms, and reactive islet cell hyperplasia. A summary of the important distinguishing features is given in Table 9–2. Reactive and hyperplastic islets may occur in areas of chronic pancreatitis and at the edge of neoplasms of all kinds. Cytologically, these closely resemble well-differentiated islet cell tumors but may be distinguished by the finding of an aspirate of low cellularity containing small clusters of islet cells mixed with acinar cells and ductal cells.[30] Low-grade ductal and acinar carcinomas usually produce imprints with clearly defined cell clusters having irregular contours. The cells are typically slightly more pleomorphic than islet cell tumors and have more prominent nucleoli. Ductal carcinoma cells may contain mucus vacuoles; acinar carcinoma cells may have a prominent granular cytoplasm with the granules demonstrating

Table 9–2. Cytologic Features Distinguishing Islet Cell Tumors from Other Low-Grade Pancreatic Neoplasms

	Islet Cell Tumors	Acinar Carcinoma	Ductal Carcinoma	Solid-Cystic Papillary Tumor
Cellularity of aspirate	Highly cellular; dispersed individual cells; occasional clumps	Defined irregular clusters; uniform appearance	Defined irregular clusters; glands may be present	Uniform cells; pseudopapillae
Chromatin pattern	Evenly dispersed; small nucleoli	Prominent nucleoli	Prominent nucleoli	Dispersed small nucleoli
Cytoplasm	Pale staining; finely granular; PAS/D negative	Prominent granularity; PAS/D positive	Variable; mucin may be present	Pale staining; nongranular
Neuron-specific enolase	Always positive	Scattered positive cells		Mostly positive
Synaptophysin	Nearly always positive	Positive in 30% of cases	Very rarely positive in scattered cells	Commonly scattered positivity
Vessels	Not present	Not present	Not present	Fine capillaries in the cores of papillae

Key: PAS, periodic acid–Schiff.

periodic acid–Schiff/diastase positivity. The key to the recognition of solid-cystic-papillary neoplasms is the finding of delicate straight or branching capillary-size vessels in the cores of papillary-like structures.[31]

DISTINGUISHING BENIGN FROM MALIGNANT ISLET CELL TUMORS

In many cases, it is impossible to determine with certainty whether an islet cell tumor is going to behave in a benign or malignant fashion. For this reason, some neoplasms are best assigned to a borderline category. A number of factors need to be considered in this evaluation: these include clinical features, hormone production, gross size, and histology (Table 9–3). However, it must be recognized that the criteria quoted here are derived from collected data specific to tumors at the time of diagnosis and surgical excision. These may not be applicable to tumors diagnosed and left in place. Thus, for example, certain tumors < 2.0 cm in diameter have a favorable prognosis if excised and are considered to be benign. However, this does not exclude the possibility that they have a capacity for metastasis if allowed to remain in place to grow larger.

Malignancy in islet cell tumors may be diagnosed unequivocally only when, at the time of surgery, a tumor is metastatic to liver or regional lymph nodes, when there is infiltration of adjacent organs, or when vascular invasion is subsequently demonstrated histologically. In diagnosing vascular invasion, great caution must be exercised to avoid overinterpreting retraction artefact. Ideally, the presence of an endothelial lining should be confirmed by demonstrating immunopositivity for factor VIII or CD31. The tumor embolus must either be attached to the vessel wall or seen to be infiltrating through it[32] (Fig. 9–8). Irregular fragments of tumor lying within a vascular space without attachment may have been implanted at the time of surgical pathology dissection and might not represent true invasion.

Functional activity of a tumor, if it is known, is a useful guide to subsequent clinical behavior. Ninety percent to 95% of insulinomas are benign at the time of diagnosis.[33] In contrast, 55% of VIP-omas,[34] 80% of glucagonomas,[35] 64% to 80% of gastrinomas,[36,37] and 75% of somatostatinomas[38] are malignant. As insulinomas comprise a majority of all islet cell tumors, it may be seen immediately that when considered as a group, most islet cell tumors behave in a benign fashion.

In common with many other slow-growing neoplasms, gross size at initial diagnosis of islet cell tumors is an important determinant of metastatic potential.[39–42] Neoplasms < 2.0 cm in diameter are usually benign, tumors > 6.0 cm in diameter are almost invariably malignant, and tumors between 3.0 and 6.0 cm in diameter are commonly malignant. Tumors measuring 2.0 to 3.0 cm in diameter fall into a borderline category. It must be emphasized, however, that there are a small number of exceptions to the above statements and that gross size alone cannot be used as an absolute criterion to determine malignancy.[5,42]

Tumor necrosis is not present in benign or borderline tumors. If it is found, it is usually in larger tumors and is a confirmation of probable malignant behavior (Fig. 9–9). However, necrosis is absent in 94% of malignant tumors, so that this negative finding is of little prognostic significance.[42]

Table 9–3. Characteristics of Benign and Malignant Islet Cell Tumors

	Benign	Borderline	Malignant
Hormonal activity	Most insulinomas		Most glucagonomas, VIP-omas, and somatostatinomas
Gross size	< 2.0 cm	2.0–3.0 cm	> 3.0 cm
Tumor necrosis	Never present	Never present	Rare
Mitotic activity (per 10 high-power fields)	Always < 2	Always < 2	60% > 2
Microscopic architecture	Variable	Variable	Variable
Vascular invasion	Absent	Usually absent	May be present
Nuclear anaplasia	Absent	Rare	Rare
AgNOR cells[44]	Few (2.5) but large		Many (5.0) but small
Ki-67[32]	0%–2% of cells labeling		1%–10% of cells labeling

Key: AgNOR, silver-stained nucleolar organizer region; VIP-oma, vasoactive intestinal polypeptide–secreting tumor.

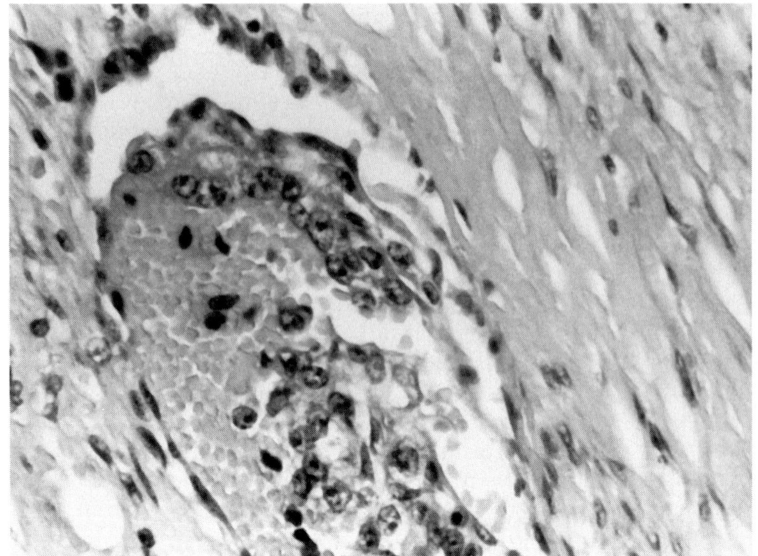

Figure 9–8. Tumor embolus in a vein adjacent to a malignant islet cell tumor.

Mitotic activity may also be useful in confirming that an islet cell tumor is malignant. Eighty percent of tumors with a mitotic count of 2 or more per 10 high-power fields will behave in a malignant fashion.[32,42] A mitotic count of 0 or 1 per 10 high-power fields cannot, however, be relied on to predict a benign behavior. All benign and borderline tumors fall into this group, but so do 42% of malignant neoplasms.[32]

Histologic architectural features (solid, trabecular, or glandular) cannot be used to predict subsequent clinical behavior.[42] The vast majority of islet cell tumors, even malignant ones, are well differentiated; however, there is a small subset of tumors that display a high grade of cellular anaplasia, necrosis, and high mitotic activity (Fig. 9–10). These neoplasms, which may easily be recognized as being poorly differentiated, are malignant. It is important to appreciate, however, that in common with endocrine tumors occurring at other locations, nuclear pleomorphism is, by itself, an unreliable criterion of malignant potential.[42]

Much attention has been paid recently to the possibility of further refining islet cell tumor prognosis by the use of modern markers. Sug-

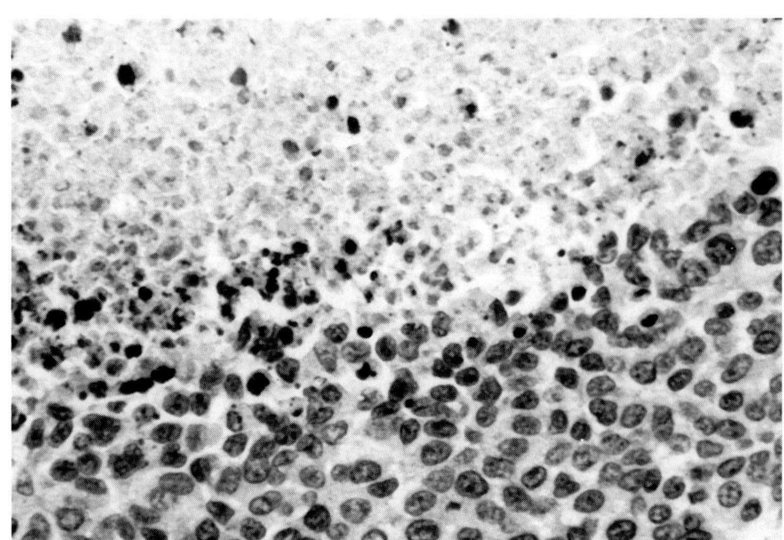

Figure 9–9. Tumor necrosis in a malignant islet cell tumor.

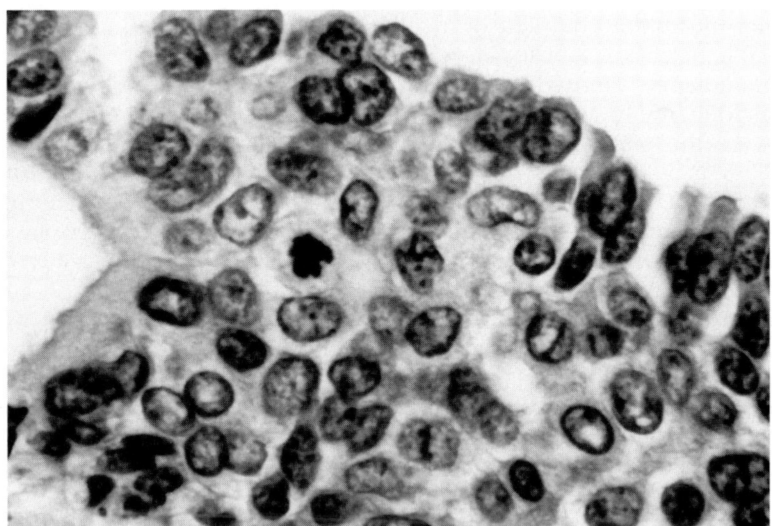

Figure 9–10. Pleomorphism in a high-grade islet cell carcinoma.

gested techniques include morphometry;[41] flow cytometry;[43] proliferation index, as measured by silver-stained nucleolar organizer region (AgNOR)–rich cells;[44] or Ki-67,[32] Ha-*ras* oncogene overexpression,[45] and presence of human chorionic gonadotropin (HCG)–secreting cells.[46] It is probably fair to conclude that, at the present time, use of these markers has proved disappointing.

Alanen et al.[43] tested 17 islet cell tumors by flow cytometry. Eight were aneuploid, 2 multiploid, and 7 diploid. In particular, seven of eight insulinomas had an abnormal DNA content. At follow-up examination, it was found that 3 patients had developed metastases; 2 of these tumors were multiploid and 1 was diploid. It appears, therefore, that the finding of aneuploidy or diploid status is not particularly useful prognostically.[47,48]

AgNORs in malignant islet cell tumors are small but multiple, whereas in benign tumors, they are few and large.[44] Ninety-six percent of malignant tumors had more than six AgNORs per cell in > 5% of cells, giving this test a high positive predictive value. In contrast, a low AgNOR score had a poor predictive value for benign behavior. It is not clear, however, whether the AgNOR score has a prognostic significance independent of more traditional criteria for tumor assessment. Similar comments apply to the Ki-67 proliferative index and proliferating cell nuclear antigen (PCNA), which have also shown a statistical correlation with tumor prognosis.[32,49] Ki-67 seems to be the best discriminator, with 0% to 2% of cells labeling in benign tumors and 1% to 10% of cells labeling in malignant tumors.[32] The comparable figures for PCNA are 0% to 8.5% labeling for benign tumors and 1% to 10% for malignant tumors.[49]

Immunohistochemical detection of α-HCG may be positive in both benign and malignant islet cells tumors; however, there are differences. Early reports of positivity in 59% of malignant tumors versus 1.2% positivity in benign tumors[46] have not been confirmed. More recent results suggest positivity in 66% of malignant tumors and in 18% of benign tumors.[44] This discrepancy may be explained by technical differences. The current general consensus appears to be that α-HCG detection is not useful in practice.[50]

On the basis of the above criteria, it is possible to subdivide islet cell tumors into adenomas, borderline tumors, low-grade carcinomas, and high-grade carcinomas (see Table 9–3). Adenomas are, therefore, tumors < 2 cm in diameter, with fewer than 2 mitoses per 10 high-power fields and a low proliferative index (< 2% of cells labeling with Ki-67). Within this group, it is possible to subclassify adenomas into those > 0.5 cm (macroadenomas) and those < 0.5 cm (microadenomas) in diameter. Macroadenomas may be functioning or nonfunctioning. The majority produce insulin. In examples where other hormones are being produced, benign behavior is less certain, so it is better not to refer to these as macroadenomas but instead place them into the borderline category. Macroadenomas are commonly encapsulated. The capsule may be complete or incomplete. Capsular penetration is not considered evidence of malignancy. Microadenomas may be discovered incidentally in autopsy specimens, particularly when the pancreas is examined meticulously. They may also occur in the MEN I syndrome, where they may be present in conjunction with larger neoplasms. Microadenomas are well demarcated, often with a thin, fibrous capsule, and are homogenous morphologically. Immunohistochemically, they frequently produce PP or glucagon. They must be distinguished from giant or so-called dysplastic islets, which are nonhomogeneous and contain a variety of different hormone-secreting cells.

Borderline islet cell tumors are an ill-defined group. The category may be used for neoplasms 2 to 3 cm in diameter, with three or fewer mitoses per 10 high-power fields and an increased proliferative index. These tumors are commonly cellular, with a high nuclear-to-cytoplasmic ratio, nuclear pleomorphism, and prominent nucleoli, but lack additional features that would definitely categorize them as malignant. Bland-appearing functional tumors, other than insulinoma, should be placed in this category.

Low-grade carcinomas are > 3.0 cm in diameter, with an average size of 6.0 cm. Histologically, they tend to grow in sheets, rather than narrow trabeculae. The mitotic rate may be quite variable but is often higher than three per 10 high-power fields. These tumors, too, are cellular and have a high nuclear-to-cytoplasmic ratio, pleomorphism, and prominent nucleoli. Proliferative markers show higher levels of cell labeling. Low-grade carcinomas not uncommonly show peripancreatic extension, and a careful histologic evaluation of the capsular region may demonstrate blood vessel invasion. Some larger insulinomas may fall into this category, as may tumors > 2.0 cm in diameter with other hormonal activity (especially glucagonomas, VIP-omas, and gastrinomas).

High-grade endocrine carcinomas are quite uncommon. They are characterized by poor demarcation and areas of necrosis. Histologically, they are highly mitotic (usually more than 10 mitoses per high-power field), with a high proliferative index (usually exceeding 10% of cells). The growth pattern is usually as diffuse sheets with no trabecular pattern. These carcinomas include large cell (atypical carcinoid) or small cell types.

Functional Islet Cell Tumors

By convention, tumors producing a clinical syndrome due to excess hormone secretion are referred to as insulinomas, glucagonomas, somatostatinomas, and so forth (Table 9–4). Each type of neoplasm generally has fairly distinct clinical and pathologic features, varying with the hormone being produced. Tumors in which hormone production may be demonstrated immunohistochemically, or by bioassay, but where there is no associated clinical syndrome are by convention named according to the cell of origin—B-cell tumors (or insulin cell tumors), D-cell tumors (somatostatin cell tumors), and so on.

Table 9–4. Major Clinical and Morphologic Features of Functional Islet Cell Tumors*

	Insulinoma	Glucagonoma	Gastrinoma	VIP-oma	Somatostatinoma
Age (y)	Mainly 30–60	40–70	Mainly 30–50	Average, 50	30–84
Sex ratio	Slight female predominance	Slight female predominance	Slight male predominance	Slight female predominance	Slight female predominance
Major symptom	Hypoglycemia	Skin rash	Zollinger–Ellison syndrome	Watery diarrhea	Diabetes
Size	95% < 2 cm	Wide range; average, 7.5 cm	Usually > 2 cm	1.5–2.0 cm	3.5–11 cm
Multiplicity	Rare	Approximately 10%	≤ 50%	Usually solitary	Usually solitary
Histology	Mainly trabecular	Variable	Usually trabecular	Variable	Variable
Malignancy	5%–10%	50%–80%	68%%–84%	55%–65%	75%
Frequency	80%–85%	3%–8%	4%–10%	4%	1%

* Refers to non–multiple endocrine neoplasia type I tumors.
Key: VIP-oma, vasoactive intestinal polypeptide–secreting tumor.

Insulinoma

Overproduction of insulin results in a clinical syndrome characterized by weakness, dizziness, headache, and dysarthria. Not uncommonly, patients have bizarre personality changes, anxiety attacks, or focal paralysis and may first present to a psychiatric clinic. In severe examples, there may be coma, convulsions, and even death. Symptoms disappear with prompt administration of glucose.[51] Investigation reveals profound hypoglycemia (< 40 mg/dL) with hyperinsulinemia (> 6 μU/mL) and hyperproinsulinemia.[15,52] There is no relationship between the size of the tumor and the severity of clinical symptoms, although most symptomatic tumors weigh more than 2 g.

Insulinomas are by far the most common type of islet cell neoplasm.[42,33,53] Estimates of its frequency range from 46% to 84% of all islet tumors. Patients of all ages may be affected, although insulinoma is most frequent between ages 30 and 60 years. Rare examples occurring in children and infants have been described.[54–56] Women are affected slightly more commonly than are men.[33]

Insulinomas may involve any area of the pancreas but are more common in the body and tail simply because a larger percentage of islets are present at these locations. One percent occur at extrapancreatic sites, including the duodenum, stomach, small bowel, lung, and cervix.[42] Most insulinomas are solitary. Multiple tumors are, however, characteristic of MEN I syndrome. Insulinomas tend to be small benign tumors, with 50% measuring < 1.5 cm in diameter and 85% to 90% measuring < 2.5 cm in diameter. On gross inspection, they are well demarcated, often with an incomplete thin, fibrous capsule. They range in color from gray-white through pinkish tan to red. Generally, the consistency is soft. Occasional cystic insulinomas have been described.[57] Enucleation is the preferred surgical treatment, but distal pancreatectomy may be performed if the neoplasm is located in the tail.[52]

Histologic examination of insulinomas reveals that most tumors have a trabecular arrangement (Fig. 9–11). However, a mixed architectural pattern is not uncommon, and many tumors show solid or glandular areas. Most insulinomas have uniform nuclei, with a fine chromatin pattern and only small nucleoli. Occasional larger irregular nuclei may be encountered, but these do not indicate a poor prognosis. The general rules for determining malignant potential of islet cell tumors should be followed for insulinomas, recognizing that 90% to 95% are benign. One histologic feature observed more commonly in insulinomas than in other islet cell tumors is the presence of amyloid. This is located within the fibrous stroma and displays the characteristic apple-green birefringence when viewed under polarized light (Fig. 9–12). By biochemical analysis, this insulinoma amyloid polypeptide is 40% homologous to calcitonin-gene related polypeptide.[42]

Immunohistochemical study of insulinomas reveals that when they are compared to normal

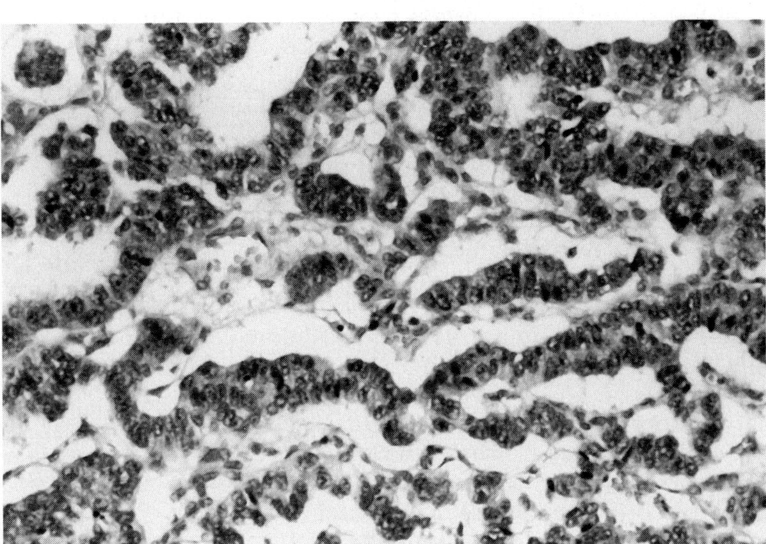

Figure 9–11. Trabecular histologic pattern of a typical insulinoma.

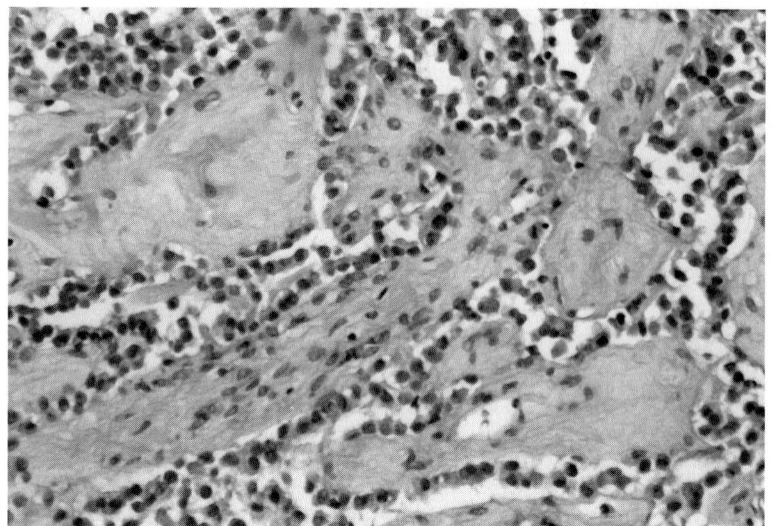

Figure 9–12. Insulinoma with a densely hyalinized stroma containing amyloid.

islets, there are reduced amounts of insulin but increased levels of proinsulin.[15] This is reflected, ultrastructurally, by the presence of atypical B-cell granules, some of which may have deficient dense cores. This suggests that the tumors have a defective insulin storage capability. In most insulinomas, insulin and proinsulin are distributed in an abnormal pattern within B cells.[58] The pattern in normal B cells is diffuse cytoplasmic staining. In many insulinomas, however, insulin staining is abnormally distributed throughout the cell, with intense perinuclear positivity. This finding suggests abnormal prohormone processing.[58] By specific immunostaining, about 50% of insulinomas may be demonstrated as multihormonal. Hormones found may include glucagon, somatostatin, PP, gastrin, adrenocorticotropic hormone (ACTH), and calcitonin.[59]

Ultrastructurally, four categories of insulinoma are recognized: type 1, with normal B-cell granules; type 2, with a mixture of normal granules and atypical granules; type 3, containing only atypical granules; and type 4, agranular neoplasms.[14,15] As a rule, the fewer typical granules present, the less intense the staining for insulin.

Study of the nontumorous pancreas alongside insulinomas reveals changes that may be regarded as an adaptive response to the presence of prolonged hyperinsulinemia.[60] These consist of a decrease in insulin-reactive areas and a corresponding expansion of the glucagon and somatostatin areas. Ultrastructural examination confirms the depression of B-cell granulation, which increases with the duration of hypoglycemia. Nesidioblastosis may also be found on light microscopy.

Glucagonoma

Overproduction of glucagon may result in a variety of clinical findings, not all of which are present in every patient with a glucagonoma (Table 9–5). These consist of skin rashes, stomatitis, glossitis, vaginitis, weight loss, mental depression, and deep vein thrombosis.[17,61–63] The skin rash is highly characteristic and has been described as necrolytic migratory erythema. It is symmetric, first appearing on the buttocks, groin, perineum, thighs, and distal extremities. It may be migratory, with healing at the initial sites of involvement. In the early stages, there are macules and small papules, which are light brown in color and resemble

Table 9–5. Clinical Manifestations of the Glucagonoma Syndrome

Necrolytic migratory erythema
Stomatitis/glossitis/vaginitis
Thromboembolic disease
Diarrhea
Weight loss
Abdominal pain
Diabetes/glucose intolerance
Psychiatric disturbance
Anemia
Hypocholesterolemia/hypoaminoacidemia

eczema. Later, there is intraepidermal bulla formation, which progresses to crusting and healing with hyperpigmentation. The lesional cycle is 7 to 10 days. Other epidermal manifestations include alopecia, cheilitis glandularis, and ungual dystrophy. Experienced dermatologists are aware of these highly specific skin manifestations and may be the first to suspect an underlying pancreatic neoplasm. Venous thrombosis occurs in 30% of patients and may be fatal.

Laboratory testing will reveal hyperglycemia and a normochromic normocytic anemia. Plasma glucagon levels are elevated. Hypoaminoacidemia occurs and is thought to result from increased hepatic gluconeogenesis and ureogenesis.[42] This latter finding may be responsible for the skin rash. In spite of having elevated blood sugar levels, patients with glucagonomas do not develop diabetic ketoacidosis.

Glucagonomas account for between 3% and 8% of functional islet cell tumors.[64] The average age at presentation is 55 years (range, 40 to 70 years) and tumors are marginally more common in women (55% of cases).[42] Rarely (13%), they occur as part of the MEN I syndrome, but they are mostly sporadic.[64,65]

Characteristically, glucagonomas are located in the body and tail of the pancreas (72%). The remainder occur in the pancreatic head, except for rare examples at extrapancreatic sites, including the duodenum[66] and lung.[67] Most (88%) are solitary lesions, with an average diameter of 7.6 cm. However, 29% measure ≤ 2.0 cm in diameter.[64] Fifty percent to 80% of tumors are malignant, with direct extrapancreatic extension or metastases to the liver or regional nodes present in up to 70% at the time of diagnosis.

At gross inspection, most glucagonomas are soft, fleshy tumors of a creamy-tan color. Foci of necrosis may be present, but cyst formation is distinctly uncommon.[68] At routine microscopy, it is impossible to positively identify a glucagonoma, and the usual islet cell pattern of trabecular, glandular, and solid growth patterns are encountered. The individual cells are polyhedral and regular in appearance. Amyloid deposition is unusual. Immunohistochemical findings are variable, depending on the degree of granulation and the differentiation of the granules. Again, defective granule storage in tumors may account for this finding. In addition to positivity for glucagon and proglucagon, it may be possible to demonstrate the presence of glicentin and glucagon-like peptides (GLPs) 1 and 2.[17,69] Proglucagon is a large molecule, consisting of glycentin, GLP1 and GLP2. Glucagon is a component of glicentin. It appears that GLP2 is the most reliable immunomarker for glucagonoma, with positivity located mainly in the portion of the cell adjacent to capillary blood vessels.[35] Occasional tumors have been reported where glucagon is cosecreted with VIP.[70]

Examination of nonneoplastic pancreas alongside a glucagonoma may reveal complete loss of A cells with a concomitant reduction in immunoreactive B cells.[71] PP- and somatostatin-secreting cells are increased in number. These changes are accompanied by nesidioblastosis. The loss of B-cell activity is explained by accelerated insulin secretion with loss of immunoreactive granules.

Gastrinoma

Pancreatic gastrinomas give rise to Zollinger–Ellison syndrome[72–75] and are the most common, but not the only, cause of the syndrome. The excess gastrin produced directly stimulates parietal cells present in the body of the stomach to produce large quantities of hydrochloric acid. The hyperacidity causes peptic ulceration. Peptic ulcers may occur not only in the first part of the duodenum and prepyloric region but also in the second part of the duodenum or even more distally, in the small bowel. The ulcers are not uncommonly multiple and are larger than the usual type of peptic ulcer. They have a high incidence of complications, including perforation and hemorrhage. In addition, the excess unneutralized acid entering the small bowel may cause a profound diarrhea, with resulting hypokalemia.[76] The mechanism of diarrhea production is unclear. Possibilities include a simple increased osmotic (electrolyte) load, irritation of jejunal mucosa, and inactivation of pancreatic enzymes. Within the stomach, the gastric body mucosa becomes hyperplastic and may develop giant folds.[77]

Patients with Zollinger–Ellison syndrome usually have unstimulated acid secretory rates greater than 15 mEq/h. In many cases, the rate exceeds 150 mEq/h. However, in about 10% of cases, the amount of acid produced falls into the normal range or into the range encountered in patients with the usual type of peptic ulcer. Many patients have clear-cut hypergastrinemia. The level of serum gastrin in normal individuals is in the range of 50 to 60 pg/mL, with an upper range of normal at 150 pg/mL.

Individuals with gastrinoma and Zollinger–Ellison syndrome have values often as high as 1,000 pg/mL. Unfortunately, however, approximately half of all patients with a gastrinoma have serum gastrin levels that are elevated but not at a sufficient level to be diagnostic.[74] For these patients, a secretin provocation test is indicated, and 95% of individuals with a gastrinoma will have a serum gastrin in excess of 200 pg/mL.[80] The magnitude of gastrin elevation may be a good indication of the biologic behavior of the tumor, with the higher levels being associated with malignant behavior. It is important to remember that elevated serum levels of gastrin are not confined to individuals with a gastrinoma and may be encountered, for example, in patients with pernicious anemia and achlorhydria, where they are secondary to longstanding achlorhydria. For this reason, therefore, the diagnosis of gastrinoma is not based solely on serum gastrin measurements.

Gastrinomas occur with a frequency similar to that of glucagonomas: between 0.5 and 1.5 cases/100,000 persons.[78,79] They are most common between the ages of 30 and 50 years but have been recorded in individuals as young as 7 and as old as 92 years.[81] There is a slight male predominance. Approximately 55% of gastrinomas occur in the pancreas, with a further 10% located within the duodenum. In many instances, localizing the tumor may be difficult, even using advanced techniques such as computed tomography scans, ultrasonography, and magnetic resonance imaging. At explorative surgery, 35% to 45% of tumors prove undetectable, although selective arteriography may reduce this number.[82] The basic problem is that the tumors are small, generally < 1.5 cm in diameter and, in many instances, only 1 to 2 mm in size. Reports of "primary" lymph node gastrinomas are thought to represent metastases from small undetectable primaries. Another possibility to be considered in instances where there is a lymph node metastasis of a gastrinoma but where no obvious primary can be found is the possibility that the primary was excised previously. Before the advent of powerful acid-inhibitory drugs, the standard treatment for peptic ulcer was distal gastrectomy to include a cuff of proximal duodenum. In instances where the surgical specimen was not examined thoroughly, a small tumor in the excised duodenal cuff could easily have been missed. When they can be located, 90% of gastrinomas are found within an area referred to as the gastrinoma triangle.[83] This may be defined anatomically. The apex is the junction of the neck and body of the pancreas and its base is a line joining the junction of the cystic and common bile ducts superiorly to the junction of the second and third portions of the duodenum inferiorly. Although gastrin is not normally secreted by the pancreatic islets, prograstrin is.[84]

Approximately 75% to 80% of gastrinomas occur sporadically. The remainder are found as part of the MEN I syndrome or Wermer's syndrome.[85–97] In comparing the two groups, it may be stated that the MEN I–associated neoplasms tend to be small, multiple, and extrapancreatic. Patients with MEN I have a better survival than do those with sporadic gastrinomas.

Gastrinomas located with the pancreas are generally functional. Grossly, they are well circumscribed but unencapsulated. They may have a variable texture, depending on the amount of fibrous tissue present. Sporadic tumors in individuals who do not have MEN I syndrome are generally > 2.0 cm in diameter. Gastrinomas arising within the duodenum are nonfunctional in 40% of patients and are functional, but only to a minor degree, in a further 20% of patients. Functional tumors (40%) generally occur at an earlier age than do nonfunctioning ones and are more likely to be malignant. Grossly, they resemble pancreatic gastrinomas but are smaller (generally ≤ 1.0 cm in diameter). Locations of gastrinomas outside of the pancreas and duodenum include gallbladder and biliary tree (including an intrahepatic location), distal stomach, jejunum, kidney, and ovary.[42]

The microscopic findings in pancreatic and extrapancreatic gastrinomas have some differences. Pancreatic tumors are generally trabecular in appearance with a minor component of solid growth. Acinar or glandular growth is not a feature. The individual cells are bland with an evenly distributed nuclear chromatin and moderate amounts of pale eosinophilic cytoplasm. Pleomorphism is generally absent and mitoses are sparse. Malignant potential is therefore hard to predict, except in those uncommon examples where blood vessel or lymphatic permeation may be demonstrated. A proportion of these tumors, which are obviously gastrin secreting because they are occurring in patients with Zollinger–Ellison syndrome, may be immunohistochemically negative for gastrin. This may be explained by their elaboration of variants of gastrin that are biologically active but immunohistochemically negative to the standard antigastrin. In highly specialized laboratories, antibodies directed against different components of the gastrin molecule may be used to stain these tumors (*C*-terminus gastrin-17, non–*C*-terminus gastrin-17, *N*-terminus gastrin-34, etc.). It is also possible to detect gastrin m-RNA, by in situ hybridization.[42] Pancreatic gastrinomas may also produce small quantities of PP, insulin, somatostatin, and glucagon.[5,18,59] Rarely, these tumors may contain calcitonin,[89] ACTH,[18] and growth hormone–releasing factor.[90] Because of abnormal synthesis and hormone storage, not all cells within the tumor have positive immunostaining.

In contrast to pancreatic gastrinomas, gastrin-secreting tumors, arising within the duodenum, are more likely to have a prominent glandular or pseudorosette pattern. Broad trabeculae may be seen, but the thin trabeculae of pancreatic tumors are not a feature. The tumors are located within the submucosa and appear as sessile nodules. MEN I–associated tumors are smaller and have a greater tendency for multiplicity than do non–MEN I tumors. By immunohistochemistry, somatostatin-secreting cells are found to be present and intimately mixed with gastrin-secreting cells. There may be occasional insulin-, serotonin-, and cholecystokinin-secreting cells also present.[88]

Approximately 50% of patients with gastrinoma will die of metastatic disease if the neoplasm is not surgically resected. Malignancy rates are higher for pancreatic gastrinomas than for gastrinomas arising within the duodenum (68% to 84% versus 25% to 57%).[42,83] A major part of this difference is in the rate and pattern of metastasis. Gastrinomas at both sites are equally likely to spread to lymph nodes, but duodenal tumors have a much lower rate (3%) of hepatic metastases than do pancreatic neoplasms (30%).[18,83,88,91–93] Because gastrinomas are slow growing, metastatic spread to lymph nodes has little influence on survival, provided that both primary tumor and nodal metastases are surgically excised. In a long-term follow-up study of 185 patients with Zollinger–Ellison syndrome, there were 30 deaths related to gastrinoma.[93] Patients with solitary gastrinoma had a 20-year survival of 68%, whereas those with MEN I had a close to 100% survival. Patients with liver metastases at the time of diagnosis had a 10-year survival of only 30%, whereas for those without liver metastases, the 15-year survival was 83%. However, when patients with metastases to the liver at the time of diagnosis were excluded from consideration, the survival of patients with MEN I and those without it was similar.

In the nontumorous pancreas, adjacent to a gastrinoma, there may be chronic pancreatitis and nesidioblastosis.[18] Islet cell hyperplasia is not a recognized cause of Zollinger–Ellison syndrome, and tumors apparently showing this abnormality have now been reinterpreted as examples of microadenomas.[18,89]

Gastrinoma is not the only cause of gastric acid hypersecretion and Zollinger–Ellison syndrome, although it does account for the majority of cases. Other rare causes include systemic mastocytosis,[94] non–gastrin-secreting pancreatic islet cell tumors,[95] gastrin cell hyperplasia in the gastric antrum,[96] and massive resection of the small bowel.[97] Acid hypersecretion is present in up to one third of individuals with systemic mastocytosis. The levels are not usually as great as those seen in a gastrinoma but may nevertheless result in Zollinger–Ellison syndrome. The mechanism of action is probably direct stimulation of parietal cells by histamine liberated from tumor mast cells. Occasional pancreatic[95] and duodenal[98] tumors have caused Zollinger–Ellison syndrome but have not been demonstrated to secrete gastrin. The nature of the secretagogue is not known but is thought to be a low-molecular-weight peptide that is destroyed by trypsin. Antral gastrin (G) cell hyperplasia may produce serum gastrin levels that are usually less than 1,000 pg/mL. The cause has not been identified but may be a loss of G-cell regulation by intragastric pH. Nontumorous Zollinger–Ellison syndrome may be distinguished from gastrinoma syndrome by its lack of elevated gastrin production after secretin stimulation. The cause of hypergastrinemia occurring after small bowel resection remains obscure. It is most likely due to the loss of an intestinal hormone or substance that is normally inhibitory to gastrin release from the antral G cells. This hypergastrinemia is transitory, presumably the result of adaption by the remaining small bowel.

Two types of gastric lesion may be encountered in Zollinger–Ellison syndrome. The first of these is a hyperplasia of parietal cells, located within the fundic (corpus) mucosa. Grossly, the fundic mucosal folds are thickened and thrown into a cerebriform pattern. Microscopically, the mucosal thickness is expanded 1.5 to 2.0 times normal. The glands contain hypertrophic and hyperplastic parietal cells that crowd out chief cells and mucus neck cells. These changes are considered to arise simply as a direct result of the trophic action of excess gastrin. The second gastric lesion encountered is the presence of endocrine cell hyperplasia and carcinoid tumors. In this condition, the antral G cells are normal, but hyperplasia and neoplasia involves the enterochromaffin-like (ECL) cells of the fundic mucosa. The trigger for ECL cell growth is not, however, simply the presence of hypergastrinemia, as the proliferation is present only in examples of Zollinger–Ellison syndrome occurring as part of the MEN I syndrome. Sporadic pancreatic gastrinomas do not result in ECL neoplasia. Gastric carcinoid tumors, arising in this situation, are similar morphologically to those present in long-standing pernicious anemia but are more commonly larger and have a greater metastatic potential.

Somatostatinoma

Somatostatinomas are rare neoplasms. A majority (75% to 76%) occur in the pancreas, with the most of the remaining tumors being located in the periampullary region of the duodenum. Small numbers may be found in the jejunum or cystic duct.

Clinically, somatostatinomas are characterized by the finding of diabetes mellitus, gallbladder disease, weight loss, diarrhea, steatorrhea, and hypochlorhydria.[22] These findings may be explained by known physiologic actions of the hormone, which include the inhibition of release of various other gastrointestinal hormones and the inhibition of absorption of amino acids, sugars, and calcium. Somatostatin may have either an inhibitory or stimulatory effect on intestinal and biliary tract smooth muscle.

Diabetes mellitus is present in > 50% of patients with somatostatinomas. Only a mild elevation of blood glucose is seen, and this generally responds to oral hypoglycemic agents. Ketoacidosis is unusual.[99] Diabetes likely occurs secondarily to inhibition of insulin release and many cases have depressed serum concentrations of both insulin and glucagon.

Abnormalities of smooth muscle function may result in gallbladder disease, caused by delayed emptying, which leads to bile stasis with the formation of biliary sludge and ultimately gallstones. This is thought to occur because increased somatostatin levels result in inhibition of smooth muscle contraction. Diarrhea and steatorrhea are common in patients with a pancreatic somatostatinoma. The usual explanation for these findings is the ability of excess somatostatin to inhibit pancreatic enzyme and bicarbonate secretion, leading to an interference with digestive function. Impaired gallbladder emptying doubtless also has implications for lipid digestion and absorption.

Hypochlorhydria is present in > 70% of patients with a pancreatic somatostatinoma.[100] Both basal and stimulated gastric acid secretion are impaired.[99] This action of somatostatin is thought to be related to its ability to suppress release of gastrin.

Laboratory findings in the somatostatinoma syndrome include elevated serum levels of somatostatin-like immunoreactive material (SLI). This finding is present in 94% of advanced somatostatinomas, many of which have metastases at the time of diagnosis.[38] The prevalence of elevated SLI levels in small tumors has not been established, so that in some cases SLI may not be elevated to diagnostic levels. At the present time, therefore, the preoperative diagnosis of somatostatinoma depends heavily on clinical acumen and searching for a pancreatic mass in patients with mild diabetes, gallbladder disease, and unexplained diarrhea. Chemical analysis of tumors has demonstrated that in 70% of cases, SLI is present in the usual tetradecapeptide form, whereas in the remaining neoplasms, it is present in a high-molecular-weight form. Somatostatinoma is not the only cause of elevated SLI levels. This finding has also been recorded in patients with medullary thyroid carcinoma, small cell carcinoma, pheochromocytoma, and extra-adrenal paraganglioma.

Somatostatinomas account for < 1% of all functional pancreatic endocrine neoplasms. They occur in adults between the ages of 30 and 84 years, with an average age of 54 years.[38] There is a slight female preponderance.[21] Simultaneous somatostatinomas of the pancreas and duodenum have been described,[100] but this neoplasm only rarely occurs in MEN I syndrome.[99] Isolated cases of pancreatic somatostatinoma have been associated with von Hippel–Lindau disease,[101] the carcinoid syndrome,[102] and hypercalcemia.[103]

Most (56%) pancreatic somatostatinomas are located within the head of the pancreas, with the majority of the remainder (30%) present in the tail. At the time of diagnosis, they are large, ranging in size from 3.5 to 11 cm in diameter, with an average size of 6.7 cm.[38] Grossly, the tumors tend to be circumscribed but not encapsulated and are soft in consistency.[42] Histologically, they are difficult to distinguish from other islet cell tumors and may have a solid, trabecular, or acinar arrangement. In distinguishing benign from malignant tumors, the usual rules have to be applied. However, overall, approximately 75% will behave in a malignant fashion, with either local invasion or metastatic spread to liver and lymph nodes.[21,38] In some individuals, distant metastases to various sites have been described.[104] Somatostatinomas are usually readily identified by immunohistochemical staining, where the majority of cells are positive. In addition, there may be minor populations of calcitonin, ACTH, and gastrin-secreting cells.[22]

Pancreatic somatostatinomas must be distinguished from similar tumors occurring within the duodenum. In the majority of cases, however, this distinction is obvious, because of the different anatomic location. Duodenal somatostatinomas are somewhat more common than pancreatic tumors but are much less likely (only 25% of cases) to express the characteristic symptoms of diabetes mellitus, gallbladder disease, diarrhea, and weight loss. On specific investigation, patients with these tumors are also much less likely to have steatorrhea and hypochlorhydria.[99,105] They characteristically present with only local symptoms, usually vague upper abdominal discomfort.[105] There is, however, a relatively strong association with von Recklinghausen's neurofibromatosis.[106,107] Typically, duodenal somatostatinomas arise at or close to the ampulla of Vater. They measure 1 to 4 cm in diameter and often deeply invade the duodenal wall. About 50% are metastatic at the time of diagnosis, but they tend to have a better prognosis than that of pancreatic tumors, because they do not develop symptoms related to somatostatin overproduction.

Histologically, duodenal somatostatinomas tend to have a rather characteristic appearance.[107] The dominant pattern is glandular, with a minor solid or trabecular component. Many of the glands contain eosinophilic secretion. Scattered throughout the tumor but particularly within the gland lumina are psammoma bodies (Fig. 9–13). These have the typical lamellated appearance. Unlike many other tumors associated with the presence of psammoma bodies, duodenal somatostatinomas do not have papillary epithelial formations.

VIP-oma

Pancreatic islet cell tumors secreting the hormone VIP give rise to a clinical syndrome characterized by watery diarrhea, hypochlorhydria, and hypokalemia. The terms *Verner–Morrison syndrome,*[108] *pancreatic cholera,*[109] and *WDHA* (watery diarrhea with hypokalemia and achlorhydria)[110] have also been used to describe the clinical effects of excess VIP secretion.

VIP-omas are tumors of adults, except for very rare tumors occurring in children.[111] The average age at the time of diagnosis is 50 years,[112–114] with a slight female preponderance. Diarrhea, dehydration, and hypokalemia are

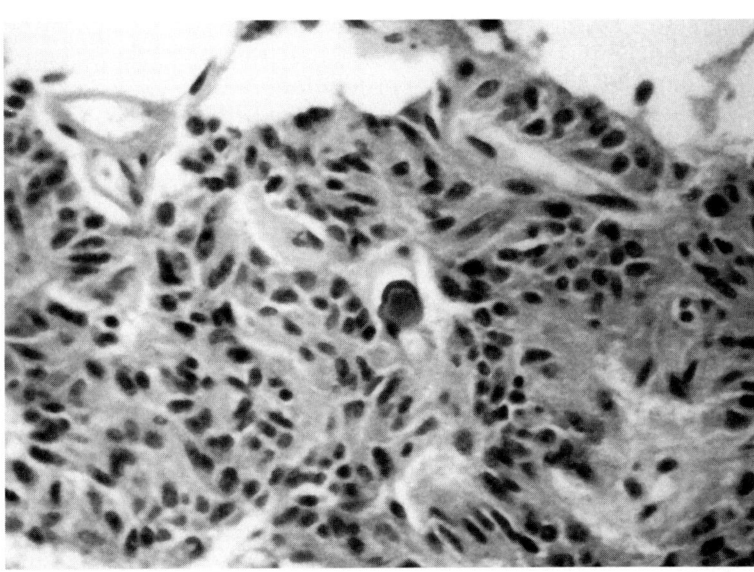

Figure 9–13. Duodenal somatostatinoma with psammoma bodies.

present in all cases. Initially, the diarrhea may be episodic, but later in the course of the disease it becomes continuous and is present every day.[108–110] The volume of diarrhea is large. In all cases, it exceeds 1 L/24 h, and in many cases, it is > 3 L/d. As a rule of thumb, it has been suggested that where the volume of diarrhea is < 700 mL/24 h, the diagnosis of VIP-oma is effectively excluded.[115] The diarrhea has been described as grossly resembling weak tea, and it persists during periods of fasting.[109,115] Not surprisingly, weight loss is also characteristic of the VIP-oma syndrome and is generally within the range of 7 to 27 kg.[112] Inconsistent findings include cramping abdominal pain and cutaneous flushing, usually involving the head and trunk areas.[116] Steatorrhea is not a feature.

Investigations usually reveal severe hypokalemia, with serum levels < 2.5 mmol/L in 93% of patients.[112] Hypercalcemia may be found in up to 8% of patients but is generally mild, with serum levels not exceeding 3 mmol/L. Hyperglycemia may be present but is also mild. Occasional patients develop tetany attributable to hypomagnesemia.[116] Differentiation of a VIP-oma from other causes of watery diarrhea depends on the measurement of plasma VIP levels. Absolute values cannot be quoted, as this is a highly specialized investigation with different laboratories having different reference ranges. In general, however, it may be stated that in cases of VIP-oma, the plasma VIP is usually between 6 and 12 times the upper limit of normal and that all VIP-omas produce plasma levels at least 1.3 to 3.0 times normal.

In adults, most (80% to 90%) VIP-producing neoplasms are derived from the pancreas.[19,112] Occasional VIP-omas are found at other sites, including the jejunum, retroperitoneum, and mediastinum.[117] Nongut tumors producing VIP-oma syndrome include pheochromocytomas,[19,117] ganglioneuromas, and ganglioneuroblastomas.[118] VIP-omas occurring at any location are rare, and in the pancreas, they constitute only 8% of all endocrine neoplasms.[42] They are commonly solitary, with only rare examples described in MEN 1 syndrome.[59,118] Tumors are most likely to be present in the tail of the pancreas (50%), with smaller numbers found in the head (20%), the body (20%), and the body and tail combined (10%).[19,108,118] The average size at diagnosis is 4.5 cm in diameter, with a range of between 1.5 and 20 cm. VIP-omas are typically well circumscribed but have no characteristic gross features to distinguish them from islet cell tumors with other hormonal activity.

Microscopically, VIP-omas are typical islet cell tumors, with a variable growth pattern that may be solid, trabecular, or tubuloacinar. Cystlike degenerative spaces containing pale eosinophilic material may be seen within the solid areas. VIP-oma cells are regular and polygonal in shape. They have light eosinophilic cytoplasm, which may contain fine granules. The nuclei are mildly hyperchromatic and display a mild degree of pleomorphism. In about 15% of cases, there is abundant mitotic activity and occasional atypical mitoses may be noted. Rare examples of massive tumor amyloid deposition have been described.[119]

Immunohistochemical findings have been extensively studied.[18,117] VIP-positive cells are found in 87% of clinical VIP-omas, but the number of cells that stain is small. This sparse granularity indicates defective storage and rapid release of the hormone into the circulation shortly after synthesis. Other hormones that may be encountered include the VIP precursor PHM (peptide, histidine, and carboxyl terminal methionine), present in 57% of cases; PP, present in 53% of cases; α–human chorionic gonadotrophin, present in 48% of cases; and growth hormone–releasing hormone (GRH) present in 50% of cases. Other hormones that are less commonly detected include neurotensin, insulin, somatostatin, glucagon, and metencephalin. The generic endocrine cell markers NSE, synaptophysin, and chromogranin are found in 95%, 93%, and 61% of cases, respectively. Approximately one third of cases are positive for α_1-antitrypsin. Immunohistochemical staining for VIP does not provide an absolute criterion for the diagnosis of VIP-oma, however, as small numbers of VIP-positive cells may also be detected within duct-derived mucinous adenocarcinomas[120] and even within amphicrine neoplasms.[121]

Ultrastructural studies have confirmed that VIP-omas are sparsely granulated but have well developed Golgi bodies and rough endoplasmic reticulum.[19] Typical granules measure 120 to 160 nm in size, with a moderately dense core and a thin, clear halo. Other granules have features of PP production (F type) and may be round, ovoid, or comma shaped and measure 140 to 190 nm.[20] In a few tumors, elongated electron dense bodies resembling endosomal tubulovesicles may be encountered.[19]

It is now established that excessive VIP secretion is the major chemical mediator of the VIP syndrome. Receptors for VIP are present on intestinal epithelial cells and activate adenylate cyclase and cyclic adenosine monophosphate activity, leading to increased electrolyte and fluid secretion. The precursor hormone PHM is also secreted by VIP-omas, and this, too, can induce intestinal chloride secretion. Hypokalemia in VIP-oma syndrome develops as a consequence of two physiologic mechanisms. The most important is fecal loss of potassium,[116] but there is also renal potassium loss through renin release and secondary hyperaldosteronism.[116] Hypercalcemia probably originates from VIP activity, stimulating the action of osteoblasts.[116] Hyperglycemia has been attributed to the gluconeogenic activity of VIP on the liver.[116] VIP is known to directly affect vessels and cause cutaneous flushing. Patients will, with time, become refractory to this action, which is postulated to be the reason that it is not encountered in every case.[116]

More than 50% of VIP-omas are obviously malignant at the time of diagnosis.[42] After follow-up examination, this increases to 67%.[19] Liver is the most common (86%) location for metastases, followed by regional lymph nodes (31%). Factors determining malignant behavior in tumors that have not metastasized at the time of diagnosis are similar to other hormonally active islet cell tumors and are listed in Table 9–3.

Extrapancreatic VIP-secreting neoplasms fall into two major groups: neurogenic tumors and epithelial tumors. The neurogenic tumors are mainly ganglioneuromas or ganglioneuroblastomas,[117,122,123] but may also include some pheochromocytomas.[124] They occur predominately in children, with the earliest recorded example diagnosed at 2 weeks of age.[123] Two thirds of tumors are located within the abdomen, whereas most of the remainder involve the mediastinum. About 40% of VIP-producing neurogenic tumors are malignant. Up to 25% of all ganglioneuromas/ganglioneuroblastomas are associated with VIP production and may give rise to watery diarrhea (Fig. 9–14). VIP production occurs predominately in the neuronal cells but is also found, to a lesser extent, in nonneuronal cells. In addition to VIP, this tumor group of neurogenic tumors may also elaborate PHM, neuropeptide Y, methionine-encephalin, somatostatin, substance P, corticotropin-releasing hormone and tyrosine-hydroxylase.[125] A rare example of VIP overproduction was recognized in a case of ganglioneuromatosis affecting the entire colon and rectum.[126]

Epithelial tumors are also occasionally associated with VIP production and watery diarrhea. These neoplasms may be primary in the small bowel,[19,127] lung,[128] large bowel,[129] esophagus,[130] kidney,[131] and liver.[132,133] Presumably, they are derived from either gastrointestinal endocrine cells or ectopic paraganglia.

Rare examples of watery diarrhea syndrome, occurring as a result of pancreatic islet cell hyperplasia, have been described. Instances apparently secondary to excess VIP[134] and PP production[135] have been recorded. Others[42] have challenged the possibility of VIP secretion by pancreatic hyperplasia, pointing out that the

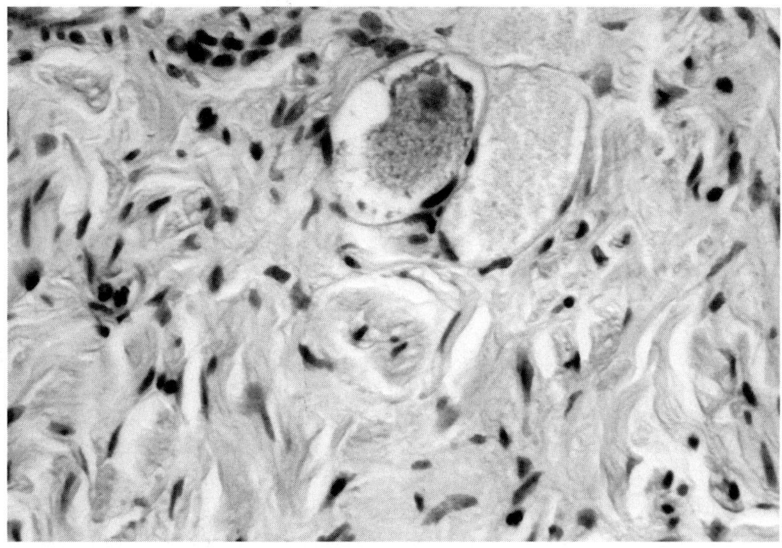

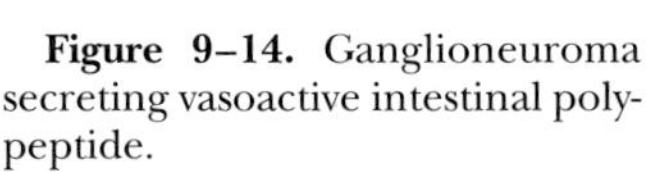

Figure 9–14. Ganglioneuroma secreting vasoactive intestinal polypeptide.

normal pancreas does not contain VIP-producing cells.

GRH-omas

Pancreatic tumors secreting growth hormone releasing factor (or hormone) (GRH-omas) are rare. They tend to occur in younger patients than do other islet cell tumors, with an average age of 38 years and a range of 15 to 63 years.[136] Seventy-eight percent occur in women.[136] Symptomatology has been divided into three major categories: acromegaly, local mass effect of the neoplasm, and systemic effects due to the corelease of other hormones.[136,137] When acromegaly occurs, it appears entirely similar to acromegaly arising secondary to a pituitary neoplasm.[138] It is characterized by enlargement of the hands and feet, coarse facial features, macroglossia, headache, peripheral nerve entrapment, and thickening and furrowing of the skin due to hypertrophy of the skin and subcutaneous tissues. Other hormones that may be produced by GRH-omas include gastrin, ACTH, and insulin. Any of these may be produced in sufficient quantities to be symptomatic. The diagnosis of GRH-oma is usually suspected on clinical grounds, particularly if the patient is known to have MEN I[139] syndrome. The diagnosis may be confirmed by demonstrating increased plasma growth hormone and GRH levels.

GRH-omas are very rare and responsible for only 1.7% of cases of acromegaly.[139] Only 30% of GRH-omas arise in the pancreas. The remainder arise either in the lung (53%), the small bowel (10%), or miscellaneous sites.[136] Most pancreatic tumors occur in the tail, but in up to 30% of cases, they are multiple and associated with MEN I syndrome.[140] Approximately 40% of GRH-omas occur in individuals with gastrinomas and 40% occur in individuals with Cushing's syndrome. The average size of the tumors is 6 cm in diameter, with a size range of 1.0 to 25 cm. Metastases, mainly present within the liver, are present at diagnosis in 30% of patients.

Histologically, GRH-omas are different from the usual islet cell tumor. A variety of appearances have been described.[136,140] Some tumors may have a whorl-like arrangement of oval or crescentic cells, resembling a meningotheliomatous meningioma,[140] a trabecular arrangement of tall columnar cells,[140] cell nests with a "Zellballen" pattern,[140] or areas more typical of islet cell neoplasms.[136] As a rule, the individual cells are small to medium in size, with a cytoplasm that usually contains fine, lightly eosinophilic granules. Ultrastructural examination reveals rounded granules 100 to 250 nm in diameter.[140,141] Immunohistochemical studies demonstrate GRH in up to 80% of patients.[136] Caution must be exercised, however, in interpreting this finding. GRH may also be demonstrated in up to 25% of pancreatic and up to 11% of gastrointestinal endocrine tumors, which are not associated with acromegaly.[142]

ACTH-omas

Pancreatic islet cell neoplasms are responsible for approximately 10% of cases involving ectopic Cushing's syndrome. They may be found as isolated neoplasms[143,144] or may be associated with gastrinoma as part of MEN I syndrome.[145] In patients with sporadic Zollinger–Ellison syndrome, Cushing's syndrome may be identified in 5%.[145] In patients with Zollinger–Ellison syndrome and MEN I, Cushing's syndrome may be present in 19%. Symptomatically, the sporadic gastrinomas are associated with the most severe Cushing's syndrome.[145] It has been suggested that all patients with either MEN I or Zollinger–Ellison syndrome should be screened for abnormal ACTH production.[145] ACTH-secreting tumors (ACTH-omas) may also produce melanocyte-stimulating hormone and opioid peptides, such as proopiomelanocortin.[146]

ACTH-omas can occur at a variety of ages; the average patient's age is 40 years (range, 16 to 61 years). In one series, there was a strong female preponderance.[143] Cushing's syndrome presents in the usual way, with weight gain, diabetes mellitus, acne, and a dorsal fat pad. About half the individuals also have cutaneous hyperpigmentation. Plasma corticosteroids are elevated and there may be an absence of the usual diurnal variation. ACTH serum levels are not suppressed by dexamethasone.[143]

Grossly, ACTH-omas present as firm gray to white nodular masses measuring 2 to 12 cm in diameter and may be found at any location within the pancreas. At the time of diagnosis, 88% have metastasized to the liver or local lymph nodes. There may also be more distant metastases to such sites as kidneys, thyroid, peritoneum, and bones.[143] Local spread may occur, with involvement of adjacent organs. The prognosis is worse if the patient also has Zollinger–

Ellison syndrome.[143,145] In patients with these tumors, only 40% survive 2 years.

Routine histologic sections demonstrate a growth pattern consisting predominantly of broad trabeculae, with intervening fibrous stroma. Some tumors may be poorly differentiated, with a pattern of growth consisting of narrow cords, with some spindle cells present. In most tumors, the cells are of three types. The predominant pattern is of small to medium-size cells with a finely granular amphophilic cytoplasm. The second pattern consists of larger cells with a granular eosinophilic cytoplasm. Occasional tumors may have many cells with a clear cytoplasm.[143]

In addition to recognizable islet cell tumors, significant ACTH production has also been reported in examples of pancreatoblastoma,[147] pancreatic small cell carcinoma,[148] and pancreatic exocrine carcinoma.[149]

Islet Cell Tumors with Hypercalcemia

Islet cell tumors with hypercalcemia are excessively rare. One review[150] identified reports of 19 cases published over 25 years. In a minority of cases, excess parathyroid hormone (PTH) is produced, but it is more usual that the tumors exert their biochemical effects via parathyroid hormone–related protein (PTHrP).[151–153] Occasional PTHrP-producing neoplasms occur as part of MEN I syndrome, although they are usually sporadic. Tumors producing PTHrP may also secrete somatostatin and VIP.

Islet cell tumors causing hypercalcemia may occur at any age and may affect children. A review of the recent literature[150] reveals that patients have an average age of 44.2 years at tumor diagnosis, with a range of 8 to 77 years. The sex ratio is approximately equal. The clinical presentation may be nonspecific and investigations primarily reveal a mass in the pancreas, with biochemical evidence of hypercalcemia discovered incidentally. In some instances, hypercalcemia may become manifest only several years after initial tumor diagnosis. Less commonly, the presenting symptoms may include some that are referable to hypercalcemia: anorexia, vomiting, muscular aches, twitching, and mental confusion.[150]

Gross pathologic findings are of a pancreatic mass averaging 10.0 cm in diameter. Seventy-five percent of tumors either are located in the pancreatic tail or involve both body and tail. Several accounts mention that the tumors are highly vascular and that this may give rise to problems in surgical removal. Histologic examination[154,155] reveals a typical endocrine neoplasm, growing either with thin cords of cells separated by fibrous stroma[154] or in a solid pattern without gland formation.[155] The individual cells may be irregular, with polymorphic hyperchromatic nuclei.[155] Electron microscopic examination reveals regular rounded secretory granules 120 to 180 nm in diameter, with fairly dense cores and a thin, clear halo.[156]

At the time of diagnosis, 85% of parathormone and PTHrP- secreting islet cell tumors have hepatic metastases.[150] Nevertheless, the tumors are relatively slowly progressive, so the 5-year survival is approximately 65%.[150]

In addition to neoplasms with islet cell differentiation, exocrine and ductal carcinomas of the pancreas may also rarely cause hypercalcemia, in the absence of bony metastases.[154,157,158] In at least one of the these cases, PTHrP immunoreactivity can be demonstrated.[154]

Neurotensinoma

Neurotensin is a 13–amino acid peptide that appears to have a role as a neurotransmitter and possibly as a hormone. Its biologic effects include inducing tachycardia, hypotension, cyanosis, intestinal motility, and intestinal electrolyte secretion. Although neurotensin production has been demonstrated within islet cell tumors,[99,159,160] it is not clear whether a distinct clinical syndrome of neurotensin overproduction exists.[5,160,161]

Many neurotensin-producing tumors also elaborate other hormones, including VIP,[160] gastrin,[159,161] and glucagon.[162] Routine light microscopic and ultrastructural examination of neurotensin-producing tumors does not reveal specific or distinctive features.[162]

Carcinoid Tumors

The term *carcinoid tumor* is used here in the classical sense, to indicate a neoplasm that is differentiated to enterochromaffin cells and is potentially capable of giving rise to the carcinoid syndrome (diarrhea, cutaneous flushing, hypotension, and bronchospasm).

These neoplasms are exceedingly rare as primary pancreatic tumors.[42] They mainly secrete serotonin but may also produce kallikreins, substance P, and prostaglandins. The diagnosis may be suspected clinically by a finding of raised levels of 5-hydroxyindole acetic acid in the urine.[163] Carcinoid tumors may be well differentiated (typical carcinoids) or poorly differentiated (atypical carcinoids, intermediate variant of small cell carcinoma). Typical carcinoids have a growth pattern that may be solid, trabecular, or glandular or a mixture of these types (Fig. 9–15). The cells are regular and polygonal in shape. The nuclei are vesicular and contain small nucleoli.[164] Fine cytoplasmic granularity may be present. A fibrous stroma is commonly seen. Ultrastructural examination demonstrates abundant EC granules, typically irregularly shaped with a thin halo. The atypical carcinoids tend to have a solid growth pattern, with areas of necrosis, nuclear irregularity and mitotic activity. Necrosis may or may not be present but is frequently a prominent feature. Atypical carcinoids often produce and secrete only scanty amounts of serotonin.

The behavior of these neoplasms is poor.[163–165] Overall, 88% have metastasized at the time of diagnosis and there is a high incidence of clinical carcinoid syndrome. Many neoplasms are unresectable.[163] The prognosis is better for typical carcinoids, where only 50% are metastatic at the time of diagnosis.[4]

Nonfunctioning Tumors and PP-omas

In the context of pancreatic islet cell tumors, the designation of nonfunctioning refers to the absence of any recognizable clinical syndrome. Tumors that have immunohistochemical evidence of hormone function or even of elevated serum hormone levels but no clinical evidence of increased hormonal activity are also included in this category. As well as PP-omas, many tumors containing principally A cells or D cells are also clinically nonfunctioning.[42] The percentage of nonfunctioning, clinically significant tumors in reported series of islet cell neoplasms has varied from 15% to 41%.[166,167] Doubtless, these differences reflect patient referral patterns at different institutions as well as differences in the intensity of disease investigation. At present, the average of quoted figures is 30% to 35% of all islet cell tumors, which rises to 65% if only patients with an islet cell tumor presenting as an expanding pancreatic mass are considered.[42]

It is possible to further subdivide nonfunctioning tumors into those that are symptomatic and those that are discovered incidentally, or at autopsy. If the pancreas is sampled microscopically by two or three random sections in unselected autopsies on elderly patients, tumors measuring 1.0 cm in diameter and smaller may be detected in 1.6% of cases. When the whole organ is examined microscopically, tumors are found in 10% of cases.[2]

Clinically significant nonfunctioning tumors occur in adults between the ages of 20 and 74 years, with an average age of 51 years.[99] Both sexes are equally affected. Thirty-six percent of patients present with upper abdominal pain and 28% with jaundice. In 16%, the tumors are discovered incidentally at surgery.[167] The major

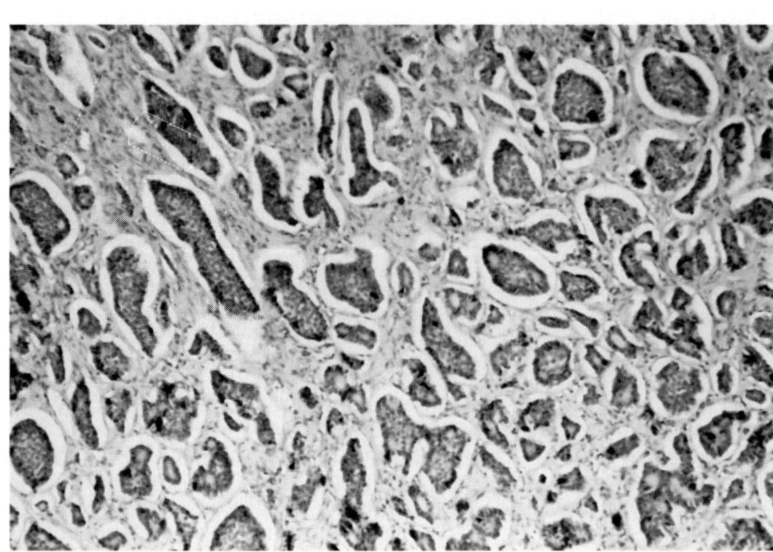

Figure 9–15. Solid nesting pattern of a pancreatic carcinoid tumor.

clinical challenge in such individuals is to determine whether their tumors are of islet cell origin or are ductal adenocarcinomas. Measurement of plasma levels of PP is of some help in this regard, as ductal adenocarcinomas do not secrete PP. However, high values of PP may also be found in a variety of functional islet cell tumors. High plasma PP levels are also present in patients with extrapancreatic carcinoid tumors, some older individuals, patients who have undergone a recent bowel resection, patients with alcoholism, patients with pancreatitis, and those with diabetes mellitus.[168–170]

Clinically significant nonfunctioning tumors are generally solitary and measure > 5.0 cm in diameter in 72% of cases.[171] If the patient has MEN I syndrome, multiple nonfunctioning tumors may be present, although they are usually accompanied by some functioning neoplasms.[172] Most tumors (74%) are located in the head of the pancreas. At the time of diagnosis, most nonfunctioning tumors are malignant, with the rate varying from 64% to 92%, depending on the series studied.[99,167,171,173]

There are no differences in histologic appearance between functional and nonfunctional islet cell tumors. PP-secreting tumors characteristically have a trabecular arrangement, often in a gyriform pattern. Ultrastructurally, a variety of granules may be detected. By immunohistochemistry, PP is detected in 35% of cases, glucagon in 30%, serotonin in 20%, calcitonin in 20%, somatostatin in 15%, neurotensin in 8%, and insulin in 2%. Gastrin and VIP production have not been detected.[174]

Criteria for predicting malignancy are outlined in Table 9–3. Tumors < 3.0 cm in diameter, with abundantly granulated cells, have a favorable prognosis. Larger tumors and those that are poorly granulated are all potentially malignant. When clinical and pathologic findings are comparable, the prognosis of nonfunctional tumors does not differ significantly from functional neoplasms.[175] However, as nonfunctioning tumors tend to be larger at the time of presentation, they have an overall worse prognosis. The 5-year survival rate for nonfunctioning tumors is 55%.[176]

Multiple Endocrine Neoplasia Syndrome Type I (Wermer's Syndrome)

Patients with MEN I typically develop hyperparathyroidism, pancreatic islet cell tumors, and pituitary lesions (Table 9–6). Parathyroid lesions are present in 88% to 97% of cases and usually consist of adenomas but rarely can be manifest as multiglandular hyperplasia. Pituitary lesions are present in 21% to 65% of cases and commonly present as adenomas, although hyperplasia is also described. Pituitary adenomas may be functional or nonfunctional, but most commonly are nonfunctional and present with local symptoms, such as headache or visual field defects. Functional tumors may be prolactin secreting (15% to 46%), growth hormone secreting (6% to 20%), or ACTH secreting (approximately 16%). Rarer manifestations of MEN I include adrenal cortical tumors (usually nonfunctional adenomas; 27% to 36% of cases), small intestinal and bronchial carcinoid tumors, schwannomas, lipomas, cutaneous leiomyomas, inclusion cysts, thymomas, and thyroid adenomas.

The cause of MEN I has now been traced to a defect on the long arm of chromosome 11 at the 11q13 locus, which is closely linked to the skeletal muscle glycogen phosphorylase locus.[177,178] It appears that a carcinogenic effect is exerted only when the inherited (or acquired) mutation on chromosome 11 is unmasked by a somatic deletion or mutation on the other normal chromosome, thereby removing the suppressor effect of the normal gene and leading to unrestricted proliferation. In most instances, the syndrome is inherited, but it may also occur after a new mutation.

Table 9–6. Clinical Manifestations of Multiple Endocrine Neoplasia Syndrome Type I

- Common
  - Parathyroid adenoma
  - Pituitary adenoma
    - Prolactin secreting
    - Growth hormone secreting
    - Adrenocorticotropic hormone–secreting
  - Pancreatic and duodenal gastrinoma
  - Zollinger–Ellison syndrome (gastric parietal cell hyperplasia)
- Rare
  - Pancreatic insulinoma, glucagonoma, vasoactive intestinal polypeptide–oma, growth hormone–releasing hormone–oma
  - Nonfunctional pancreatic tumor
  - Adrenal cortical adenoma (nonfunctional)
  - Thyroid follicular adenoma
  - Gastric enterochromaffin-like tumor
  - Multiglandular parathyroid hyperplasia
  - Small intestinal and bronchial carcinoids
  - Cutaneous leiomyomas, lipomas, and schwannomas
  - Thymomas

The frequency of MEN I syndrome in the general population is unknown, but features suggestive of the syndrome were noted in 2.5 per 1,000 unselected autopsies.[179] Pancreatic lesions are the second most common manifestation after hyperparathyroidism and are present in 80% of patients. Gastrinomas are the most common (54%) functional tumor identified: Insulinomas occur in 21%, glucagonomas in 3%, and VIP-omas in 1%.[180] Nonfunctional tumors are thought to be extremely common, but many are small (< 1.0 cm), benign, and not routinely searched for clinically, unless they are symptomatic. These small neoplasms may be detected in 100% of autopsied patients with MEN I.[181] The prevalence of MEN I among patients with a gastrinoma is approximately 20%.

As a general rule, patients who have MEN I with a functional tumor present at an earlier age than do patients with a similar tumor but without MEN I.[183] Also, as a general rule, patients with functional tumors and MEN I tend to have a better prognosis than do those with similar tumors occurring outside MEN I, although not all series have confirmed this finding. As a finding of multiple pancreatic tumors is usual in patients with MEN I, these individuals require closer clinical follow-up monitoring than do patients with sporadic pancreatic tumors. The diagnosis of MEN I in a patient may also have implications for other family members. Histologic examination of a single pancreatic tumor cannot predict whether it is occurring as part of MEN I.

Small Cell Carcinomas

Small cell carcinomas are now considered to represent poorly differentiated endocrine carcinomas. Morphologically and behaviorally, they are similar to small cell carcinomas of the lung. Numerically, they account for approximately 1% of all pancreatic malignancies and approximately 2% of all pancreatic endocrine neoplasms.[4,184] Typically, small cell carcinomas of the pancreas arise in elderly men, but they can occur between the ages of 40 and 75 years.[184,185] They are more common in cigarette smokers.[186] Patients generally present with advanced symptoms of malignancy, including weight loss, abdominal pain, and jaundice. Occasional tumors have been described that were functional, producing ACTH[148] and hypercalcemia.[187] In addition, some tumors may produce the carcinoid syndrome, but serotonin production has usually been confined to tumors that are somewhat better differentiated and described as atypical carcinoids.[188]

Small cell carcinomas of the pancreas are soft, bulky neoplasms, with areas of necrosis and hemorrhage. They are gray-white in color. The majority are located in the head and extend locally, to involve adjacent organs. Microscopically, they consist of the typical small to medium-size cells, with scanty cytoplasm and round to oval nuclei, with inconspicuous cytoplasm. Generally, the cells grow in a sheetlike arrangement, although there may be some areas with a ribbonlike or glandular pattern (Fig. 9–16). Mitoses are abundant. Ultrastructural examination reveals a granular cytoplasm, containing free ribosomes, intermediate filaments, and membrane-bound granules 100 to 200 nm in diameter.[189] Immunohistochemical examination may reveal positivity for NSE and synaptophysin. Intense staining for p53 is characteristic.

Small cell carcinoma usually presents at a stage when metastases are already present. If it is untreated, survival is only 1 to 2 months. However, chemotherapy may result in temporary remission, with prolongation of life. The best treatment results are obtained with the atypical carcinoid variant.[189]

TUMORLIKE LESIONS

Tumorlike lesions of pancreatic islets include hyperplasia, dysplasia, and nesidioblastosis. Hyperplasia has been further subdivided into nodular and diffuse variants. A complete discussion of these conditions is hampered by a lack of generally agreed definitions and by a paucity of carefully controlled clinicopathologic studies. In many publications, the terms are loosely applied or have been used differently by various authors.[42] The situation is further complicated by a wide variation in normal islet morphology and by differences that exist in islet size and number between children and adults.

Hyperplasia

On the basis of the work of Jaffe et al.[190] and Rahier et al.,[191] the 1995 Armed Forces Institute of Pathology fascicle on tumors of the pancreas has suggested criteria for the diagnosis of diffuse islet cell hyperplasia.[42] In adults, islets comprise 1% to 2% of the total pancreatic volume. In children, they comprise 10%.[191] Diffuse hy-

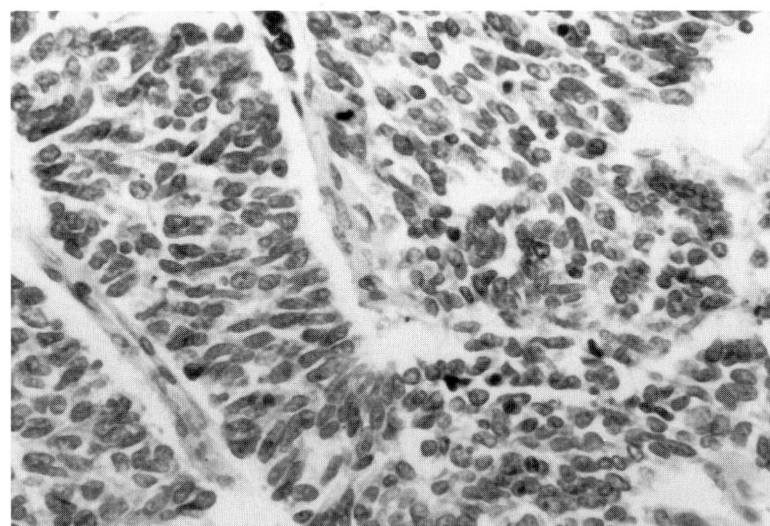

Figure 9–16. Small cell carcinoma of the pancreas.

perplasia in adults may be defined as the presence of individual compact (dorsal) islets measuring > 250 μm in diameter (normal, up to 225 μm). Diffuse hyperplasia of the compact islets in children is defined as being present when > 15% of islets measure > 200 μm in diameter.[190] As the authors of the fascicle point out, these definitions do not apply when chronic pancreatitis with exocrine atrophy and islet crowding is present. An additional major problem with these definitions is that they assume that islets contain a homogeneous cell population. Clearly, however, they do not and it is possible, for example, that clinically significant hyperinsulinemia and B-cell hyperplasia will not be detected microscopically unless measurements of individual cell types are performed. Such measurements are naturally time consuming and require that individual laboratories establish their own normal ranges. As a general guideline, within the adult compact islets, B cells comprise 60% to 70%; A cells, 15% to 20%; and D cells, < 10% of the total population.[192] The diffuse (ventral) islets, which are located in the posterior part of the head of the pancreas, comprise approximately 10% of the total islet volume. They frequently reach 450 to 500 nm in diameter, so care must be taken not to confuse them with hyperplastic dorsal islets. Within the adult diffuse islets PP-secreting cells comprise 70%; B cells, 20%; A cells, 5%; and D cells, 5%.[193,194]

Studies of proliferation rates of islet cells in non–tumor-related hyperinsulinemia have shown no increase over normal.[195] This suggests that although B cells are present in increased numbers and are oversecreting, they do not have increased proliferative activity characteristic of hyperplastic epithelium at other locations within the gastrointestinal tract.

The true incidence of diffuse islet cell hyperplasia is unknown, although it has been reported in a wide variety of clinical situations, as well as in asymptomatic individuals. In many of these examples, diffuse hyperplasia is accompanied by nesidioblastosis and it is unclear whether diffuse hyperplasia ever occurs as an isolated lesion.

In persistent hyperinsulinemic hypoglycemia of infancy (PHHI), some patients have insulin secreting neoplasms, some patients have focal (adenomatous) hyperplasia, and some patients have diffuse hyperplasia accompanied by nesidioblastosis[196–202] (see Chapter 3). However, careful measurements have demonstrated that in the infants with diffuse hyperplasia/nesidioblastosis, the extent of B-cell hyperplasia is no different from that encountered in control pancreata.[196] In children with clinical evidence of PHHI and no obvious neoplasm, the most important distinction to make is between pancreata with diffuse hyperplasia and those with focal hyperplasia. In clinical practice, this can be accomplished quite successfully using a combination of preoperative pancreatic venous catheterization with plasma insulin measurements and intraoperative frozen sections.[202] The treatment for focal hyperplasia is a localized resection; for diffuse abnormality, it is a near total pancreatectomy. The clinical outcome for infants with focal disease is much more favorable than for those with diffuse disease.[202] Focal hyperplasia is not detectable grossly and this distinguishes it from an adenoma. Microscopically, it shows one or more nodules measuring 2.5 to 7.5 mm in diameter, consisting of aggregated islets, separated by thin cords of acinar cells. These nodules tend to be located in the center of a pancreatic lobule.[202]

Other conditions in which islets containing diffusely hyperplastic islet cells are encountered include α_1-antitrypsin deficiency,[203] tyrosinemia,[204] erythroblastosis fetalis,[205] leprechaunism,[206] Beckwith–Wiedemann syndrome,[207] and Zollinger–Ellison syndrome.[208] In Zollinger–Ellison syndrome, it appears that A- and B-cell hyperplasia occurs secondary to hypergastrinemia.[208] Non–B cell diffuse hyperplasia has been described in chronic diarrhea, due to both excess VIP secretion[209] and excess PP secretion.[210,211]

Nesidioblastosis

As mentioned previously, many authors use the term *nesidioblastosis* interchangeably with *diffuse hyperplasia*. In the majority of instances, both lesions occur together. Traditionally, the term has been used to describe a more complex abnormality than a simple increase in islet size (hyperplasia). Grossly, no abnormality is recognized. Microscopically, as well as an increase in islet size, there is variability in islet size, scattered individual or small clusters of endocrine cells, and prominent ductulo-insular complexes.[42] The term *ductulo-insular complex* refers to the finding of islet cells budding off from a terminal ductule (Fig. 9–17).

Nesidioblastosis is the characteristic lesion encountered in infants with PHHI when there is no focal lesion or adenoma.[195–202] Nesidioblastosis is also encountered in adults with insular hyperfunction and hypoglycemia.[212–214]

Authoritative publications[195,202] have suggested that the term *nesidioblastosis* is obsolete and should be replaced by *diffuse hyperplasia*. This is entirely reasonable, as there is no evidence that it forms a separate clinical entity.

Dysplasia

Pancreatic islet dysplasia (also called nesidiodysplasia) has been defined as a lesion resembling nesidioblastosis, but with (1) a microarchitecture dissimilar to that of normal islets, usually with a ribbonlike appearance; (2) loss of the normal topographic and quantitative relationships among the four major islet cell subtypes; and (3) nuclear enlargement and atypia.[42] As defined, dysplasia is a common finding in the pancreata of individuals with MEN I.[215,216] However, similar changes have also been described in the pancreata of infants with PHHI.[217,218] This suggests that nesidiodysplasia is not a separate entity from diffuse hyperplasia. Indeed, cytologic atypia is a relatively common finding in diffuse hyperplasia. Many cells have nucleomegaly, with a diameter of up to 19

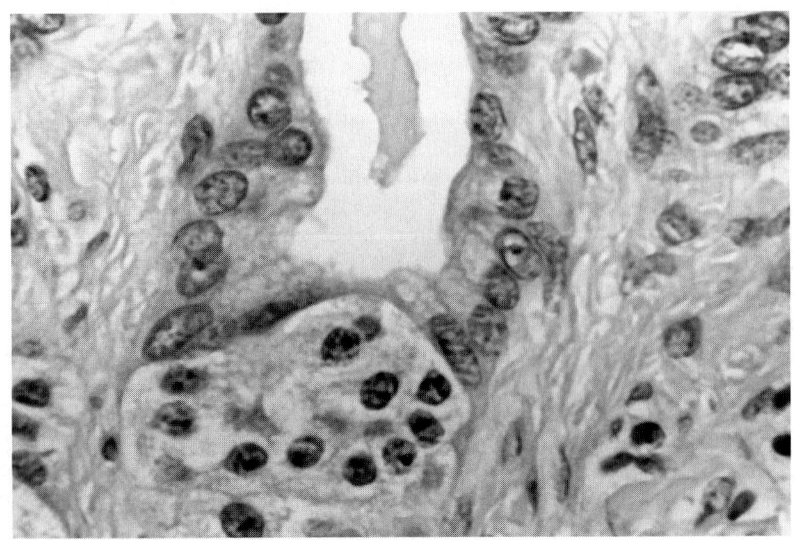

Figure 9–17. Ductulo-insular complex in diffuse endocrine cell hyperplasia.

nm.[202] The significance of islet cell dysplasia is as yet undetermined. In particular, there is no evidence that is a marker for the later development of islet cell neoplasia.

REFERENCES

1. Schein PS, De Lellis RA, Kahn CR, et al.: Islet cell tumors: Current concepts and management. Ann Intern Med 79:239–257, 1973.
2. Grimelius L, Hultquist G, Shenquist B: Cytological differentiation of asymptomatic pancreatic islet cell tumors in autopsy material. Virchows Arch [A] Pathol Anat Histol 365:278–288, 1975.
3. Kimura K, Kuroda A, Morioka Y: Clinical pathology of endocrine tumors of the pancreas. Dig Dis Sci 36:933–942, 1991.
4. Solcia E, Sessa F, Rindi G, et al.: Pancreatic endocrine tumors: General concepts; nonfunctioning tumors and tumors with uncommon function. *In* Dayal Y (ed): Endocrine Pathology of the Gut and Pancreas. Boca Raton, FL: CRC Press, pp 105–132, 1991.
5. Heitz PU, Kasper M, Polak JM, et al.: Pancreatic endocrine tumors. Hum Pathol 13:263–267, 1982.
6. Larsson C, Skogseid B, Oberg K, et al.: Multiple endocrine neoplasia maps to chromosome 11 and is lost in insulinoma. Nature 332:85–87, 1988.
7. Mount SL, Weaver DL, Taatjes DJ: Von Hippel–Lindau disease presenting as pancreatic neuroendocrine tumor. Virchows Arch 426:523–528, 1995.
8. Liu HM, Potter EL: Development of the human pancreas. Arch Pathol 74:439–452, 1962.
9. Madsen OD, Larsson LI, Rehfeld JF, et al.: Cloned cell lines from a transplantable islet cell tumor are heterogeneous and express cholecystokinin in addition to islet hormones. J Cell Biol 103:2025–2034, 1986.
10. Lloyd RV, Mervak T, Schmidt K, et al.: Immunohistochemical detection of chromogranin and neuron specific enolase in pancreatic endocrine neoplasms. Am J Surg Pathol 8:607–614, 1984.
11. Gould VE, Wiedenmann B, Lee I, et al.: Synaptophysin expression in neuroendocrine neoplasms as determined by immunocytochemistry. Am J Pathol 126:243–257, 1987.
12. Klöppel G, Girard J, Polak JM, et al.: Alpha human chorionic gonadotrophin and neuron-specific enolase as markers for malignancy and neuroendocrine nature of pancreatic endocrine tumors. Cancer Detect Prev 6:161–166, 1983.
13. Stommer P, Krans J, Stolte M, et al.: Solid and cystic pancreatic tumors. Clinical, histochemical and electron microscopic features in ten cases. Cancer 67:1635–1641, 1991.
14. Berger M, Bordi C, Cupper HY, et al.: Functional and morphologic characteristics of human insulinomas. Diabetes 32:921–931, 1983.
15. Creutzfeldt W, Arnold R, Creutzfeldt C, et al.: Biochemical and morphological investigations of 30 human insulinomas. Correlation between the tumor content of insulin and proinsulin-like components and the histological and ultrastructural appearance. Diabetologia 9:217–231, 1973.
16. Bordi C, Ravazzola M, Baetens D, et al.: A study of glucagonomas by light and electron microscopy and immunofluorescence. Diabetes 28:925–936, 1979.
17. Polak JM, Bloom SR: Glucagon-producing tumors and the glucagonoma syndrome. *In* Dayal Y (ed): Endocrine pathology of the gut and pancreas. Boca Raton, FL: CRC Press, pp 227–240, 1991.
18. Creutzfeldt W, Arnold R, Creutzfeldt C, et al.: Pathomorphologic, biochemical and diagnostic aspects of gastrinomas (Zollinger–Ellison syndrome). Hum Pathol 6:47–76, 1975.
19. Capella C, Polak JM, Buffa R, et al.: Morphologic patterns and diagnostic criteria of VIP-producing endocrine tumors. A histologic, histochemical, ultrastructural and biochemical study of 32 cases. Cancer 52:1860–1874, 1983.
20. Fiocca R, Sessa F, Tenti P, et al.: Pancreatic polypeptide (PP) cells in the PP-rich lobe of the human pancreas are identified ultrastructurally and immunocytochemically as F-cells. Histochemistry 77:511–523, 1983.
21. Dayal Y, Ganda OP: Somatostatin producing tumors. *In* Dayal Y (ed): Endocrine Pathology of the Gut and Pancreas. Boca Raton, FL: CRC Press pp 241–277, 1991.
22. Krejis GJ, Orci L, Conlon JM, et al.: Somatostatinoma syndrome. Biochemical, morphologic and clinical features. N Engl J Med 301:285–292, 1979.
23. Sneige N, Ordonez NG, Veanahukalathil S, et al.: Fine needle aspiration cytology in pancreatic endocrine tumors. Diagn Cytol 3:35–40, 1987.
24. Bell DA: Cytologic features of islet cell tumors. Acta Cytol 31:485–492, 1987.
25. Shaw JA, Vance RP, Geisinger KR, et al.: Islet cell neoplasms. A fine-needle aspiration cytology study with immunocytochemical correlations. Am J Clin Pathol 94:142–149, 1990.
26. Al-Kaisi W, Weaver MG, Abdul-Karim FW, et al.: Fine-needle aspiration cytology of neuroendocrine tumors of the pancreas. A cytologic, immunocytochemical and electron microscopic study. Acta Cytol 36:655–660, 1992.
27. Collins BT, Cramer HM: Fine-needle aspiration cytology of islet cell tumors. Diagn Cytopathol 15:37–45, 1996.
28. Pacchioni D, Papotti M, Macri L, et al.: Pancreatic oncocytic endocrine tumors. Cytologic features of two cases. Acta Cytol 40:742–746, 1996.
29. Hsiu JG, D'Amato NA, Sperling MH, et al.: Malignant islet cell tumor of the pancreas diagnosed by fine-needle aspiration biopsy. A case report. Acta Cytol 29:576–579, 1985.
30. Nguyen GK, Rayani NA: Hyperplastic and neoplastic endocrine cells of the pancreas in aspiration biopsy. Diagn Cytopathol 2:204–211, 1986.
31. Remadi S, MacGee W, Doussis-Anagnostopoulou I, et al.: Solid and papillary neoplasm of the pancreas. Diagn Cytopathol 15:398–402, 1996.
32. La Rosa, Sessa F, Capella C, et al.: Prognostic criteria in non-functioning pancreatic endocrine tumors. Virchows Arch 429:323–333, 1996.
33. Stefanini P, Carboni M, Patrassi N, et al.: Beta-islet cell tumors of the pancreas: Results of a study on 1,067 cases. Surgery 75:597–609, 1974.
34. Morrison AB: Islet cell tumors and the diarrheogenic syndrome. *In* Fitzgerald PJ, Morrison AB (eds): The Pancreas. Baltimore: Williams & Wilkins, 1978, pp 185–207.

35. Ruttman E, Klöppel G, Klehn M, et al.: Pancreatic glucagonoma with and without the syndrome. Immunocytochemical study of 5 tumor cases and review of the literature. Virchows Arch [Anat Pathol] 388:51–67, 1980.
36. Ellison EH, Wilson SD: The Zollinger–Ellison syndrome updated. Surg Clin North Am 47:1115–1124, 1967.
37. Stabile BE, Morrow DJ, Passaro E Jr: The gastrinoma triangle: Operative implications. Am J Surg 147:25–31, 1984.
38. Konomi K, Chijiiwa K, Katsuta T, et al.: Pancreatic somatostatinoma. Biochemical, morphologic and clinical features. J Surg Oncol 43:259–265, 1990.
39. Broder LE, Carter SK: Pancreatic islet cell carcinoma. I. Clinical features of 52 patients. Ann Intern Med 79:101–107, 1973.
40. Cubilla AL, Hajdu SI: Islet cell carcinoma of the pancreas. Arch Pathol 99:204–207, 1975.
41. Kenny BD, Sloan JM, Hamilton PW, et al.: The role of morphometry in predicting prognosis in pancreatic islet cell tumors. Cancer 64:460–465, 1989.
42. Solcia E, Capella C, Klöppel G: Tumors of the pancreas. *In* Atlas of Tumor Pathology, fascicle 20, third series. Washington, DC: Armed Forces Institute of Pathology, 1995, pp 145–209.
43. Alanen KA, Joensun H, Klemi PJ, et al.: DNAploidy in pancreatic neuroendocrine tumors. Am J Clin Pathol 93:784–788, 1990.
44. Rüschoff J, Willemer S, Brunzel M, et al.: Nucleolar organizer regions and glycoprotein-hormone alpha chain reaction as markers of malignancy in endocrine tumors of the pancreas. Histopathology 22:51–57, 1993.
45. Höfler H, Ruhri C, Putz B, et al.: Oncogene expression in endocrine pancreatic tumors. Virchows Arch B Cell Pathol Inc Mol Pathol 55:355–361, 1988.
46. Heitz PU, Kasper M, Klöppel G, et al.: Glycoprotein-hormone alpha-chain production by pancreatic endocrine tumors: A specific marker for malignancy. Immunocytochemical analysis of tumors of 155 patients. Cancer 51:277–282, 1983.
47. Graeme-Cook F, Bell DA, Flotte TJ, et al.: Aneuploidy in pancreatic insulinomas does not predict malignancy. Cancer 66:2365–2368, 1990.
48. Lee CS, Charlton IG, Williams RA, et al.: Malignant potential of aneuploid pancreatic endocrine tumors. J Pathol 169:451–456, 1993.
49. Pelosi G, Zamboni G, Doglioni C, et al.: Immunodetection of proliferating cell nuclear antigen assess the growth fraction and predicts malignancy in endocrine tumors. Am J Surg Pathol 16:1215–1225, 1992.
50. Graeme-Cook F, Nardi G, Compton CC: Immunocytochemical staining for human chorionic gonadotrophin subunits does not predict malignancy in insulinomas. Am J Clin Pathol 93:273–276, 1990.
51. Whipple AO, Frantz VK: Adenoma of islet cells with hyperinsulinism: A review. Ann Surg 101:1299–1304, 1935.
52. Grant CS: Gastrointestinal endocrine tumors. Insulinoma. Baillieres Clin Gastroenterol 10:645–671, 1996.
53. Broughan TA, Leslie JD, Soto JM, et al.: Pancreatic islet cell tumors. Surgery 99:671–678, 1986.
54. Mann JR, Rayner PH, Gourevitch A: Insulinoma in childhood. Arch Dis Child 44:435–442, 1969.
55. Rawlinson DG, Christiansen RO: Light and electron microscopic observations on a congenital insulinoma. Cancer 32:1470–1476, 1973.
56. Carney CN: Congenital insulinoma (nesidioblastoma): Ultrastructural evidence for histogenesis from pancreatic ductal epithelium. Arch Pathol Lab Med 100:352–356, 1976.
57. Marrano D, Campione O, Santini D, et al.: Cystic insulinoma: A rare islet cell tumor of the pancreas. Eur J Surg 160:519–522, 1994.
58. Roth J, Klöppel G, Madsen OD: Distribution patterns of proinsulin and insulin in human insulinomas: An immunohistochemical analysis in 76 tumors. Virchows Arch B Cell Pathol Incl Mol Pathol 63:51–61, 1992.
59. Mukai K, Grotting JC, Greider MH, et al.: Retrospective study of 77 pancreatic endocrine tumors using the immunoperoxidase method. Am J Surg Pathol 6:387–399, 1982.
60. Sacchi B, Bani D, Biliotti G: The endocrine pancreas in patients with insulinomas. An immunocytochemical and ultrastructural study of the non-tumoral tissue with morphometrical evaluations. Int J Pancreatol 5:11–28, 1989.
61. Mallinson CN, Bloom SR, Warin AP, et al.: A glucagonoma syndrome. Lancet 2:1–5, 1974.
62. Bloom SR, Polak JM: Glucagonoma syndrome. Am J Med 82(suppl 5B):25–36, 1987.
63. Frankton S, Bloom SR: Gastrointestinal endocrine tumors. Glucagonomas. Baillieres Clin Gastroenterol 10:697–705, 1996.
64. Soga J, Yukuwa Y: Glucagonomas/diabetico-dermatogenic syndrome (DDS): A statistical evaluation of 407 reported cases. J Hepatobiliary Pancreat Surg 5:312–319, 1998.
65. Croughs RJ, Hulsmans HA, Israel DE, et al.: Glucagonoma as a part of the polyglandular syndrome. Am J Med 52:690–698, 1972.
66. Roggli VL, Judge DM, McGavran MD: Duodenal glucagonoma: A case report. Hum Pathol 10:350–353, 1979.
67. Hunstein W, Trumper LH, Dummer R, et al.: Glucagonoma syndrome and bronchial carcinoma. Ann Int Med 109:920–921, 1988.
68. Sarui H, Yoshimoto K, Okumura S, et al.: Cystic glucagonoma with loss of heterozygosity on chromosome 11 in multiple endocrine neoplasia type 1. Clin Endocrinol (Oxf) 46:511–516, 1997.
69. Hamid QA, Bishop AE, Sikri KL, et al.: Immunocytochemical characterization of 10 pancreatic tumors, associated with the glucagonoma syndrome, using antibodies to separate regions of the pro-glucagon molecule and other neuroendocrine markers. Histopathology 10:119–133, 1986.
70. Cavallo-Perin P, De Paoli M, Guiso G, et al.: A combined glucagonoma and VIPoma syndrome. First pathologic and clinical report. Cancer 62:2576–2579, 1988.
71. Bani D, Biliotti G, Sacchi TB: Morphological changes in the human endocrine pancreas induced by chronic excess of endogenous glucagon. Virchows Arch B Cell Pathol Incl Mol Pathol 60:199–206, 1991.
72. Deveney CW, Deveny KS, Way LW: The Zollinger–Ellison syndrome: 23 years later. Ann Surg 188:384–393, 1978.
73. Hirschowitz BI: Zollinger–Ellison syndrome: Pathogenesis, diagnosis and management. Am J Gastroenterol 92[suppl]:445–485, 1997.
74. Wolfe MM, Jensen RT: Zollinger–Ellison syndrome. Current concepts in diagnosis and management. N Engl J Med 317:1200–1209, 1987.
75. Jensen RT: Gastrointestinal endocrine tumors. Gastrinoma. Baillieres Clin Gastroenterol 10:603–643, 1996.

76. Fang M, Ginsberg AL, Glassman L, et al.: Zollinger–Ellison syndrome with diarrhea as the predominant clinical feature. Gastroenterology 76:378–387, 1979.
77. Komorowski RA, Caya JG: Hyperplastic gastropathy: Clinicopathologic correlation. Am J Surg Pathol 15:577–585, 1991.
78. Buchanan KD, Johnson CF, O'Hare M, et al.: Neuroendocrine tumors: A European view. Am J Med 81[suppl 6B]:14–22, 1986.
79. Jacobsen O, Bardram L, Rehfeld JF: The requirement for gastrin measurements. Scand J Clin Lab Invest 46:423–426, 1986.
80. McGuigan JE, Wolfe MM: Secretin injection test in the diagnosis of gastrinoma. Gastroenterology 79:1324–1331, 1980.
81. Eire PF, Rodriguez Pereira C, Barca Rodriguez P, et al.: Uncommon case of gastrinoma in a child. Eur J Pediatr Surg 6:173–174, 1996.
82. Cherner JA, Doppman JL, Norton JA, et al.: Selective venous sampling for gastrin to localize gastrinomas. Ann Intern Med 105:841–847, 1986.
83. Stabile BE, Morrow DJ, Passaro E Jr: The gastrinoma triangle: Operative implications. Am J Surg 147:25–31, 1984.
84. Bardram L: Gastrin in non-neoplastic pancreatic tissue from patients with and without gastrinomas. Scand J Gastroenterol 25:935–943, 1990.
85. Pipeleers-Marichal M, Somers G, Willems G, et al.: Gastrinomas in the duodenums of patients with multiple endocrine neoplasia type 1 and the Zollinger–Ellison syndrome. N Engl J Med 322:723–727, 1990.
86. Donow C, Pipeleers-Marichal M, Schroder S, et al.: Surgical pathology of gastrinoma. Site, size, multicentricity, association with multiple endocrine neoplasia type 1, and malignancy. Cancer 68:1329–1334, 1991.
87. Mignon M, Cadiot G: Diagnostic and therapeutic criteria in patients with Zollinger–Ellison syndrome and multiple endocrine neoplasia type 1. J Intern Med 243:489–494, 1998.
88. Capella C, Riva C, Rindi G, et al.: Histopathology, hormone products and clinicopathologic profile of endocrine tumors of the upper small intestine. A study of 44 cases. Endocr Pathol 2:92–110, 1992.
89. Stamm B, Häcki WH, Klöppel G, et al.: Gastrin-producing tumors and the Zollinger–Ellison syndrome. *In* Dayal Y (ed): Endocrine Pathology of the Gut and Pancreas. Boca Raton, FL: CRC Press, 1991, pp 155–194.
90. Antonioli DA, Dayal Y, Dvorak AM, et al.: Zollinger–Ellison syndrome: Cure by surgical resection of a jejunal gastrinoma containing growth hormone releasing factor. Gastroenterology 92:814–823, 1987.
91. Oberhelman HA Jr: Excisional therapy for ulcerogenic tumors of the duodenum. Long-term results. Arch Surg 104:447–453, 1972.
92. Hoffman JD, Fox PS, Wilson SD: Duodenal-wall tumors and the Zollinger–Ellison syndrome. Arch Surg 107:334–339, 1973.
93. Weber HC, Venzon DY, Lin JT, et al.: Determinants of survival in patients with Zollinger–Ellison syndrome: A prospective long-term study. Gastroenterology 108:1637–1649, 1995.
94. Cherner JA, Jensen RT, Dubois A, et al.: Gastrointestinal dysfunction in systemic mastocytosis: A prospective study. Gastroenterology 95:657–667, 1988.
95. Chey WY, Chang TM, Lee KY, et al.: Ulcerogenic tumor syndrome of the pancreas associated with a non-gastrin acid secretagogue. Ann Surg 210:139–149, 1989.
96. Ganguli PC, Elder JB, Polak JE, et al.: Antral-gastrin cell hyperplasia in peptic ulcer disease. Lancet 1:1288, 1974.
97. Straus E, Gerson CD, Yallow RS: Hypersecretion of gastrin associated with the short bowel syndrome. Gastroenterology 66:175–180, 1974.
98. Sloas DD, Hirschowitz BI, Chey WY: A non-gastrin malignant ampullary tumor causing gastric acid and pepsin hypersecretion. J Clin Gastroenterol 12:573–578, 1990.
99. Vinik AT, Strodel WE, Eckhauser FE, et al.: Somatostatinomas, PPomas, and neurotensinomas. Semin Oncol 14:263–281, 1987.
100. Capella C, Riva C, Rindi G, et al.: Histopathology, hormone products and clinicopathological profile of endocrine tumors of the upper small intestine. Endocr Pathol 2:92–110, 1991.
101. Maki M, Kaneko Y, Ohta Y, et al.: Somatostatinoma of the pancreas associated with von Hippel–Lindau disease. Intern Med 34:661–665, 1995.
102. Ozbakir O, Kelestimur F, Ozturk F, et al.: Carcinoid syndrome due to a malignant somatostatinoma. Postgrad J Med 71:695–698, 1995.
103. Stavri GT, Pritchard GA, Williams EJ, et al.: Somatostatinoma of the pancreas with hypercalcemia. A case report. Eur J Surg Oncol 18:298–300, 1992.
104. Axelrod L, Bush MA, Hirsch HJ, et al.: Malignant somatostatinoma: Clinical features and metabolic studies. J Clin Endocrinol Metabol 52:886–896, 1981.
105. O'Brien TD, Chejfec G, Prinz RA: Clinical features of duodenal somatostatinomas. Surgery 114:1144–1147, 1993.
106. Mao C, Shah A, Hanson DJ, et al.: von Recklinghausen's disease associated with duodenal somatostatinoma: Contrast of duodenal versus pancreatic somatostatinomas. J Surg Oncol 59:67–73, 1995.
107. Dayal Y, Doos WG, O'Brien MJ, et al.: Psammomatous somatostatinomas of the duodenum. Am J Surg Pathol 7:653–665, 1983.
108. Verner JV, Morrison AB: Non-beta islet cell tumors and the syndrome of watery diarrhea, hypokalemia and hypochlorhydria. Clin Gastroenterol 3:595–608, 1974.
109. Matsumoto KK, Peter JB, Schultze RG, et al.: Watery diarrhea and hypokalemia associated with pancreatic islet cell adenoma. Gastroenterology 50:231–242, 1966.
110. Kane MG, O'Dorisio TM, Krejs GJ: Production of secretory diarrhea by intravenous infusion of vasoactive intestinal polypeptide. N Engl J Med 309:1482–1485, 1983.
111. Brenner RW, Sank LI, Kerner MB, et al.: Resection of a vipoma of the pancreas in a 15-year-old girl. Pediatr Surg 21:983–985, 1986.
112. Long RG, Bryant MG, Mitchell SJ, et al.: Clinicopathological study of pancreatic and ganglioneuroblastoma tumors secreting vasoactive intestinal polypeptide (Vipomas). Br Med J 282:1767–1771, 1981.
113. Mekhjian HS, O'Dorisio TM: VIPoma syndrome. Semin Oncol 14:282–291, 1987.
114. Park SK, O'Dorisio MS, O'Dorisio TM: Vasoactive intestinal polypeptide-secreting tumours: Biology and therapy. Baillieres Clin Gastroenterol 10:673–696, 1996.
115. Bloom SR, Christofides ND, Yiangan T, et al.: Peptide histidine isoleucine (PHI). and Verner–Morrison syndrome (abstract). Gut 24:473, 1983.

116. O'Dorisio TM, Mekhjian H, Gaginella TS: Medical therapy of VIPomas. Endocrinol Clin North Am 18:545–556, 1989.
117. Solcia E, Capella C, Riva C, et al.: The morphology and neuroendocrine profile of pancreatic epithelial VIPomas and extrapancreatic VIP producing neurogenic tumors. Ann NY Acad Sci 527:508–517, 1988.
118. Ooi A, Kameya T, Tsumaraia M, et al.: Pancreatic endocrine tumors associated with WDHA syndrome. An immunohistochemical and electron microscopic study. Virchows Arch[A] 405:311–323, 1985.
119. Crowley PF, Slavin JL, Rode J: Massive amyloid deposition in pancreatic VIPoma: A case report. Pathology 28:377–379, 1996.
120. Rood RP, DeLellis RA, Dayal Y, et al.: Pancreatic cholera syndrome due to a vasoactive intestinal polypeptide-producing tumor: Further insights into pathophysiology. Gastroenterology 94:813–818, 1988.
121. Ordonez NG, Balsaver AM, Mackay B: Mucinous islet cell (amphicrene) carcinoma of the pancreas associated with watery diarrhea and hypokalemia syndrome. Hum Pathol 19:1458–1461, 1988.
122. Rosenstein BJ, Engelman K: Diarrhea in a child with a catecholamine secreting ganglioneuroblastoma. J Pediatr 63:217–226, 1963.
123. Quak SH, Prabhakaran K, Kwok R, et al.: Vasoactive intestinal polypeptide secreting tumors in children: A case report with literature review. Aust Pediatr J 24:55–58, 1988.
124. Tischler AS, Dayal Y, Balogh K, et al.: The distribution of immunoreactive chromogranins, S-100 protein and vasoactive intestinal polypeptide in compound tumors of the adrenal medulla. Hum Pathol 18:909–917, 1987.
125. Kimura N, Yamamoto H, Okamoto H, et al.: Multiple-hormone gene expression in ganglioneuroblastoma with watery diarrhea, hypokalemia and achlorhydria syndrome. Cancer 71:2841–2846, 1993.
126. Rescorla FJ, Vane DW, Fitzgerald JF, et al.: Vasoactive intestinal polypeptide-secreting ganglioneuromatosis affecting the entire colon and rectum. J Pediatr Surg 23:635–637, 1988.
127. Debas HT, Mulvihill SJ: Neuroendocrine gut neoplasms. Important lessons from uncommon tumors. Arch Surg 129:965–971, 1994.
128. Noseda A, Fuss M, DeNutte N, et al.: Vipoma syndrome simultaneously occurring with small-cell carcinoma of the lung. Arch Intern Med 149:1223, 1989.
129. Bradley C, Haddock G, Pickard RG, et al.: Metastatic vipoma arising from colonic primary tumor. Eur J Surg Oncol 15:386–389, 1989.
130. Watson KJ, Shulkes A, Smallwood RA, et al.: Watery-diarrhea-hypokalemia-achlorhydria syndrome and carcinoma of the esophagus. Gastroenterology 88:798–803, 1988.
131. Hamilton I, Reis L, Ballimore S, et al.: A renal vipoma. Br Med J 281:1323–1324, 1980.
132. Ayub A, Zafar M, Abdulkareem A, et al.: Primary hepatic vipoma. Am J Gastroenterol 88:958–961, 1993.
133. Lundstet C, Linjawi T, Amin T: Liver VIPoma: Report of two cases and literature review. Abdom Imaging 19:433–437, 1994.
134. Verner JV, Morrison AB: Endocrine pancreatic islet disease with diarrhea. Report of a case due to diffuse hyperplasia of non-beta islet tissue with a review of 54 additional cases. Arch Intern Med 133:492–500, 1974.
135. Pasieka JL, Hershfield N: Pancreatic polypeptide hyperplasia causing watery diarrhea syndrome: A case report. Can J Surg 42:55–58, 1999.
136. Sano T, Asa SL, Kovacs K: Growth hormone releasing-producing tumors: Clinical, biochemical and morphological manifestations. Endocr Rev 9:357–373, 1988.
137. Caplan RH, Koob L, Abellera RM, et al.: Care of acromegaly by operative removal of an islet cell tumor of the pancreas. Am J Med 64:874–882, 1978.
138. Berger G, Trouillas J, Bloch B, et al.: Multihormone carcinoid tumor of the pancreas. Secreting growth hormone-releasing factor as a cause of acromegaly. Cancer 54:2097–2108, 1984.
139. Thorner MO, Frohman LA, Leong DA, et al.: Extrahypothalamic GRF secretion is a rare cause of acromegaly. Plasma GRF in 177 acromegalic patients. J Clin Endocrinol Metab 59:846–849, 1984.
140. Sano T, Yamasaki R, Saito H, et al.: Growth hormone releasing hormone (GHRH) secreting pancreatic tumor in a patient with multiple endocrine neoplasm type I. Am J Surg Pathol 11:810–819, 1987.
141. Rivier J, Spress J, Thorner M, et al.: Characterization of a growth-hormone releasing factor from a human pancreatic islet cell tumor. Nature 300:276–278, 1982.
142. Dayal Y, Lin HD, Tallberg K, et al.: Immunocytochemical demonstration of growth hormone-releasing factor in gastrointestinal and pancreatic endocrine tumors. Am J Clin Pathol 85:13–20, 1986.
143. Clark ES, Carney JA: Pancreatic islet cell tumor associated with Cushing's syndrome. Am J Surg Pathol 8:917–924, 1984.
144. Liddle GW, Givens JR, Nicholson WE, et al.: The ectopic ACTH syndrome. Cancer Res 25:1057–1061, 1965.
145. Maton PN, Gardner JD, Jensen RT: Cushing's syndrome in patients with the Zollinger–Ellison syndrome. N Engl J Med 315:1–5, 1986.
146. Melmed S, Yamashita S, Kovacs K, et al.: Cushing's syndrome due to ectopic proopiomelanocortin gene expression by islet cell carcinoma of the pancreas. Cancer 59:772–778, 1987.
147. Passmore SJ, Berry PJ, Oakhill A: Recurrent pancreatoblastoma with inappropriate adrenocorticotrophic hormone secretion. Arch Dis Child 63:1494–1496, 1988.
148. Corrin B, Gilby ED, Jones NF, et al.: Oat cell carcinoma of the pancreas with ectopic ACTH secretion. Cancer 31:1523–1527, 1973.
149. Gullo L, De Giorgio R, D'Errico A, et al.: Pancreatic exocrine carcinoma producing adrenocorticotrophic hormone. Pancreas 7:172–176, 1992.
150. Mao C, Carter P, Schaeffer P, et al.: Malignant islet cell tumor associated with hypercalcemia. Surgery 117:37–40, 1995.
151. Ratcliffe WA, Bowden SJ, Dunne FP, et al.: Expression and processing of parathyroid hormone-related protein in a pancreatic endocrine cell tumor associated with hypercalcemia. Clin Endocrinol (Oxf) 40:679–686, 1994.
152. Mitlak BH, Hutchison JS, Kaufman SD, et al.: Parathyroid hormone-related peptide mediates hypercalcemia in an islet cell tumor of the pancreas. Horm Metab Res 23:344–346, 1991.
153. Vair DB, Boudreau SF, Reid EL: Pancreatic islet-cell neoplasia, with secretion of a parathormone-like substance and hypercalcemia. Can J Surg 30:108–110, 1987.
154. Miraliakbari BA, Asa SL, Boudreau SF: Parathyroid hormone-like peptide in pancreatic endocrine carcinoma and adenocarcinoma associated with hypocalcemia. Hum Pathol 23:882–887, 1992.

155. Arps H, Dietel M, Schulz A, et al.: Pancreatic endocrine carcinoma with ectopic PTH-production and paraneoplastic hypercalcemia. Virchows Arch [A] 408:497–503, 1986.
156. Heitz PU, Harder F, Haas HG, et al.: Tumor of the pancreas inducing hypercalcemia. Ultrastruct Pathol 13:585–588, 1989.
157. Brayko CM, Doll DC: Squamous cell carcinoma of the pancreas associated with hypercalcemia. Gastroenterology 83:1297–1299, 1982.
158. Monno S, Nagata A, Homma T, et al.: Exocrine pancreatic cancer with humoral hypercalcemia. Am J Gastroenterol 79:128–132, 1984.
159. Feurle GE, Helmstaedter V, Tischbirek K, et al.: A multihormonal tumor of the pancreas producing neurotensin. Dig Dis Sci 26:1125–1133, 1981.
160. Blackburn AM, Bryant MG, Adrian TE, et al.: Pancreatic tumors produce neurotensin. J Clin Endocrinol Metab 52:820–822, 1981.
161. Chiang HC, O'Dorisio TM, Maton PN, et al.: Prospective study of multiple hormone production and symptomatic secondary endocrine tumors in patients with the Zollinger–Ellison syndrome (ZES). Gastroenterology 96:A529, 1989.
162. Alumets J, Sundler F, Falkmer S, et al.: Neurohormonal peptides in endocrine tumors of the pancreas, stomach and upper small intestine: I. An immunohistochemical study of 27 cases. Ultrastruct Pathol 5:55–72, 1983.
163. Mao C, Attar A, Domenico DR, et al.: Carcinoid tumors of the pancreas. Status report based on two cases and review of the world's literature. Int J Pancreatol 23:153–164, 1998.
164. Ordonez NG, Manning JT, Raymond AK: Argentaffin endocrine carcinoma (carcinoid) of the pancreas with concomitant breast metastasis: An immunohistochemical and electron microscopic study. Hum Pathol 16:746–751, 1985.
165. Dollinger MR, Ratner LH, Shamoian CA, et al.: Carcinoid syndrome associated with pancreatic tumors. Arch Intern Med 120:575–580, 1967.
166. Howard JN, Moss NH, Rhoads JE: Collective review: Hyperinsulinism and islet cell tumors of the pancreas. Int Abstr Surg 90:417–455, 1950.
167. Kent RB, van Heerden JA, Weiland LH: Non-functioning islet cell tumors. Ann Surg 193:185–190, 1981.
168. Fink RS, Adrian TE, Margot DH, et al.: Increased plasma pancreatic polypeptide in chronic alcohol abuse. Clin Endocrinol (Oxf) 18:417–421, 1983.
169. Besterman HS, Adrian TE, Mallinson CN, et al.: Gut hormone release after intestinal resection. Gut 23:854–861, 1982.
170. Berger D, Crowther RC, Floyd JC, et al.: Effect of age on fasting plasma levels of pancreatic hormones in man. J Clin Endocrinol Metab 47:1183–1189, 1987.
171. Eckhauser FE, Cheung PS, Vinik AI, et al.: Non-functioning malignant neuroendocrine tumors of the pancreas. Surgery 100:978–988, 1986.
172. Kloppel G, Willemer S, Stamm B, et al.: Pancreatic lesions and hormonal profile of pancreatic tumors in multiple endocrine neoplasia type 1. Cancer 57:1824–1832, 1986.
173. Eriksson B, Oberg K, Skogeid B: Neuroendocrine pancreatic endocrine tumor. Acta Oncol 28:373–377, 1989.
174. La Rosa S, Sessa F, Capella C, et al.: Prognostic criteria in non-functioning pancreatic endocrine tumors. Virchows Arch 429:323–333, 1996.
175. Venkatesh S, Ordonez NG, Ajani J: Islet cell carcinoma of the pancreas. A study of 98 patients. Cancer 65:354–357, 1990.
176. Broughan TA, Leslie JD, Soto JM, et al.: Pancreatic islet cell tumors. Surgery 99:671–678, 1986.
177. Larsson C, Skogseid B, Oberg K, et al.: Multiple endocrine neoplasia maps to chromosome 11 and is lost in insulinoma. Nature 332:85–87, 1988.
178. Bale AE, Norton JA, Wong EL, et al.: Allelic loss of chromosome 11 in hereditary and sporadic tumors related to familial multiple endocrine neoplasia type 1. Cancer Res 51:1154–1157, 1991.
179. Lips CJ, Vasen HF, Lamers CB: Multiple endocrine neoplasia syndromes. CRC Crit Rev Oncol/Hematol 2:117–184, 1984.
180. Oberg K, Skogseid B, Eriksson B: Multiple endocrine neoplasia type 1. Acta Oncol 28:383–387, 1989.
181. Majewski JT, Wilson SD: The MEA-I syndrome: An all or none phenomenon? Surgery 86:475–484, 1979.
182. Stefanini P, Carboni M, Patrassi N, et al.: Beta-islet cell tumors of the pancreas: Results of a study on 1,067 cases. Surgery 75:597–609, 1974.
183. Jensen RT, Gardner JD, Raufman J-P, et al.: Zollinger–Ellison syndrome: Current concepts and management. Ann Intern Med 98:59–75, 1983.
184. O'Connor TP, Wade TP, Sunwoo YC, et al.: Small cell undifferentiated carcinoma of the pancreas. Report of a patient with tumor marker studies. Cancer 70:1514–1519, 1992.
185. Reyes CV, Wang T: Undifferentiated small cell carcinoma of the pancreas: A report of five cases. Cancer 47:2500–2503, 1981.
186. Chetty R, Clark SP, Pitson GA: Primary small cell carcinoma of the pancreas. Pathology 25:240–242, 1993.
187. Hobbs RD, Stewart AF, Ravin ND, et al.: Hypercalcemia in small cell carcinoma of the pancreas. Cancer 53:1552–1554, 1984.
188. Gordon DL, Lo MC, Schwartz MA: Carcinoid of the pancreas. Am J Med 51:412–415, 1971.
189. Ordonez NG, Cleary KR, Mackay B: Small cell undifferentiated carcinoma of the pancreas. Ultrastruct Pathol 21:467–474, 1997.
190. Jaffe R, Hashida Y, Yunis EJ: Pancreatic pathology in hyperinsulinemic hypoglycemia of infancy. Lab Invest 42:356–365, 1980.
191. Rahier J, Goebbels RM, Henquin JC: Cellular composition of the human diabetic pancreas. Diabetologi 24:366–371, 1983.
192. Grube D, Bohn R: The microanatomy of human islets of Langerhans, with special reference to somatostatin (D-) cells. Arch Histol Jpn 46:327–353, 1983.
193. Orci L, Malaisse-Lagae F, Baetens D: Pancreatic-polypeptide rich regions in the human pancreas. Lancet 2:1200–1201, 1978.
194. Bommer G, Friedl U, Heitz PU, et al.: Pancreatic PP cell distribution and hyperplasia. Immunocytochemical distribution in the normal human pancreas, in chronic pancreatitis and pancreatic carcinoma. Virchows Archive [A] 387:319–331, 1980.
195. Sempoux C, Guiot Y, Dubois D, et al.: Pancreatic B-cell proliferation in persistent hyperinsulinemic hypoglycemia of infancy: An immunohistochemical study of 18 cases. Mod Pathol 11:444–449, 1998.
196. Goudswaard WB, Houthoff J, Koudstaal J, et al.: Nesidioblastosis and endocrine hyperplasia of the pancreas: A secondary phenomenon. Hum Pathol 17:46–53, 1986.

197. Dahms BB, Landing BH, Blaskovics M, et al.: Nesidioblastosis and other islet cell abnormalities in hyperinsulinemic hypoglycemia of infancy. Hum Pathol 11:641–649, 1980.
198. Witte DP, Greider MH, DeSchryver-Kecskemeti K, et al.: The juvenile human endocrine pancreas: Normal v idiopathic hyperinsulinemic hypoglycemia. Semin Diagn Pathol 1:30–42, 1984.
199. Sempoux C, Guiot Y, Lefevre A, et al.: Neonatal hyperinsulinemic hypoglycemia: Heterogeneity of the syndrome and keys for differential diagnosis. J Clin Endocrinol Metab 83:1455–1461, 1998.
200. Rahier J, Fält K, Müntefering H, et al.: The basic structural lesion of persistent neonatal hypoglycemia with hyperinsulinism: Deficiency of pancreatic D cells or hyperactivity of B cells? Diabetologia 26:282–289, 1984.
201. Rahier J, Sempoux C, Fournet JC, et al.: Partial or near-total pancreatectomy for persistent neonatal hyperinsulinemic hypoglycemia: The pathologist's role. Histopathology 32:15–19, 1998.
202. de Lonlay-Debeney P, Poggi-Travert F, Fournet J-C, et al.: Clinical features of 52 neonates with hyperinsulinism. N Engl J Med 340:1169–1175, 1999.
203. Ray MB, Zumwalt R: Islet-cell hyperplasia in genetic deficiency of alpha-1-proteinase deficiency. Am J Clin Pathol 85:681–687, 1986.
204. Perry TL: Tyrosinemia associated with hypermethioninemia and islet cell hyperplasia. Can Med Assoc J 97:1067–1075, 1967.
205. Milner RD, Dinsdale F, Wirdnam PK, et al.: Pancreatic endocrine cell fractions in erythroblastosis fetalis. Diabetes 32:313–315, 1983.
206. Rosenberg AM, Haworth JC, Degroot GW, et al.: A case of leprechaunism with severe hyperinsulinemia. Am J Dis Child 134:170–175, 1980.
207. Stefan Y, Bordi C, Grasso S, et al.: Beckwith–Wiedemann syndrome: A quantitative, immunohistochemical study of pancreatic islet cell populations. Diabetologia 28:914–919, 1985.
208. Bani Sacchi T, Bani D, Biliotti G: Nesidioblastosis and islet cell changes related to endogenous hypergastrinemia. Virchows Archiv B Cell Pathol Incl Mol Pathol 48:261–276, 1985.
209. Ghishan FK, Soper RT, Nassif ED, et al.: Chronic diarrhea of infancy: Nonbeta islet cell hyperplasia. Pediatrics 64:46–49, 1979.
210. Pasieka JL, Hershfield N: Pancreatic polypeptide hyperplasia causing watery diarrhea syndrome: A case report. Can J Surg 42:55–58, 1999.
211. Martella EM, Ferraro G, Azzoni C, et al.: Pancreatic-polypeptide cell hyperplasia associated with pancreatic or duodenal gastrinomas. Hum Pathol 28:149–153, 1997.
212. Fong TL, Warner NE, Kumar D: Pancreatic nesidioblastosis in adults. Diabetes Care 12:108–114, 1989.
213. Albers N, Lohr M, Bogner U, et al.: Nesidioblastosis of the pancreas in an adult with persistent hyperinsulinemic hypoglycemia. Am J Clin Pathol 91:336–340, 1989.
214. Kim HK, Shong YK, Han DJ, et al.: Nesidioblastosis in an adult with hyperinsulinemic hypoglycemia. Endocr J 43:163–167, 1996.
215. Klöppel G, Willemer S, Stamm B, et al.: Pancreatic lesions and hormonal profile of pancreatic tumors in multiple endocrine neoplasia type I. An immunocytochemical study of nine patients. Cancer 57:1824–1832, 1986.
216. Pilato FP, D'Adda T, Banchini E, et al.: Nonrandom expression of polypeptide hormones in pancreatic tumors. An immunohistochemical study in a case of multiple islet cell neoplasia. Cancer 61:1815–1820, 1988.
217. Gould VE, Memoli VA, Dardi LE, et al.: Nesidiodysplasia and nesidioblastosis of infancy: Ultrastructural and immunohistochemical analysis of islet cell alterations with and without associated hyperinsulinemic hypoglycemia. Scand J Gastroenterol Suppl 70:129–142, 1981.
218. Gould VE, Memoli VA, Dardi LE, et al.: Nesidiodysplasia and nesidioblastosis of infancy: Structural and functional correlations with the syndrome of hyperinsulinemic hypoglycemia. Pediatr Pathol 1:7–31, 1983.

Chapter

10

GALLBLADDER AND CYSTIC DUCT: DEVELOPMENT, ANATOMY, HISTOLOGY, AND CONGENITAL ANOMALIES

DEVELOPMENT

The gallbladder may first be recognized in the fourth week of fetal life, as a bud developing from the primitive endoderm near the junction of foregut and midgut. This outgrowth, which is opposite the dorsal pancreatic bud, grows into the surrounding mesoderm and becomes the future liver. By a process of elongation and branching, the caudal portion of this hepatic bud forms the gallbladder and cystic duct. By the 5th week of fetal life, when the embryo is approximately 5 mm long, the gallbladder may be recognized as a tubular structure, lined by epithelium. At the 8th week of gestation, the gallbladder and biliary tree has developed a lumen, and by the 18th week, all layers of the gallbladder wall are fully developed.[1] As the fetal gut rotates, the origin of the common bile duct (ampulla of Vater) comes to lie to the left side of the duodenum.

GROSS ANATOMY

The gallbladder is a pear-shaped saccular structure that lies on the undersurface of the right lobe of the liver, where it is partly sunk into a depression on the liver surface. On the inferior aspect of the gallbladder, the surface is covered by serosa that is continuous with the liver capsule. The superior aspect is directly attached by connective tissue to the lower border of the liver. The portions of liver and gallbladder that are in apposition are sometimes referred to as the "bare area," as it is not covered by serosa. Occasionally, however, the attachment to the liver is thinned and elongated, forming a short mesentery, which suspends the gallbladder from the liver.

In an adult, the normal gallbladder measures up to 10 cm in length and 3 to 4 cm in width, with the wall measuring 1 to 2 mm in thickness.[2] Its capacity is usually 40 to 70 mL, but in situations of extreme dilation, this can increase to 100 mL.[3] The organ is divided into the fundus (Fig. 10–1), or blind-ended portion, the central body, and a narrower S-shaped neck that joins the cystic duct. The term *infundibulum* refers to the tapering portion of the body, before it joins the neck. This portion of the gallbladder may be identified by the presence of the cholecystoduodenal ligament, a peritoneal fold that connects the infundibulum to the duodenum. Hartmann's pouch is a small bulge in the wall at the junction of the neck and cystic duct. It is not regarded as a normal anatomic feature and probably occurs as a result of chronic inflammation.[1–4]

The mucosal surface of the first part of the cystic duct, near where it joins the gallbladder, is thrown into a series of grossly visible mucosal folds. These are referred to as Heister's valves and appear to have the function of preventing

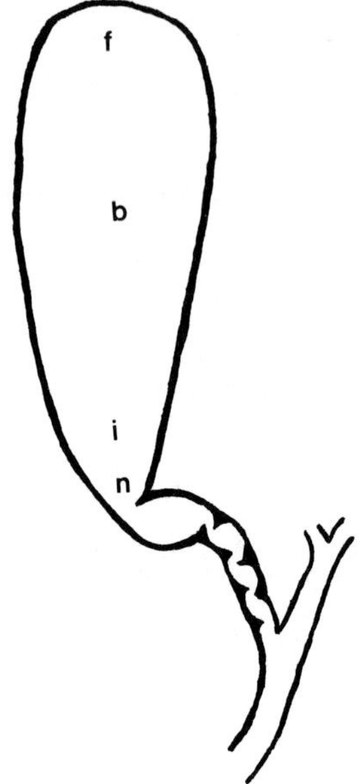

Figure 10–1. Anatomy of the normal gallbladder: f, fundus; b, body; i, infundibulum; n, neck.

collapse of the cystic duct when it is not distended with bile. This permits a more even flow of bile, without extreme gallbladder contractions. These valves have a spiral configuration down the duct.

Blood supply to the gallbladder is normally from the cystic artery, a branch of the right hepatic artery. At the neck of the gallbladder, the artery bifurcates into superficial and deep branches, which supply the free wall and hepatic wall of the gallbladder, respectively. The artery is usually single, although in 14% of individuals, a double cystic artery is present, with the superficial and deep branches arising directly from the right hepatic artery. In a smaller percentage of patients, the cystic artery may arise directly from either the superior mesenteric artery, the common hepatic artery, the left hepatic artery, the celiac artery, or even from the aorta. In the majority of patients, the cystic artery passes to the right of, and posterior to, the common hepatic bile duct. In 30% of patients, however, it originates to the left of the common bile duct, and in 17% of patients, it is anterior to it.[5] The venous drainage of the gallbladder is variable, with some veins communicating with the liver directly and some communicating with the portal vein. Lymphatic drainage from the lateral portion of the gallbladder is to the superior pancreaticoduodenal node. From the medial portion, lymph drains to the cystic node.

FUNCTION

The gallbladder concentrates and stores bile. It also adds mucus, which is released from the surface epithelium and the mucus glands located in the neck. Bile flow into and out of the gallbladder is believed to be the result of pressure gradients caused by selective muscle contraction and relaxation, under neural and hormonal control. About 800 mL to 1 L of bile from the liver enters the gallbladder daily. This is concentrated by a process of active electrolyte transport. Emptying of bile into the duodenum occurs after a fatty meal, when cholecystokinin causes contraction of the gallbladder wall and relaxation of the sphincter of Oddi (located at the ampulla of Vater). Motilin causes contraction of the gallbladder between meals and pancreatic polypeptide secretion results in its relaxation.[6]

HISTOLOGIC APPEARANCES

The wall of the gallbladder is composed of four layers: mucosa, lamina propria, muscularis, and outer connective tissue. The inferior part of the gallbladder is also covered by a serosal membrane that is continuous with the liver capsule. There is no muscularis mucosa or submucosa.

The mucosa consists of a single layer of columnar epithelium that is thrown into a series of branching folds (Fig. 10–2). These folds are barely appreciated by naked eye inspection, as a roughening of the mucosal surface. They are most prominent in an empty gallbladder and least obvious when it is distended. The epithelial nuclei are oval shaped, regular, and basally located, with an even distribution of chromatin and only occasional small nucleoli (Fig. 10–3). The cytoplasm is clear or lightly eosinophilic and contains a mixture of sulfomucin and nonsulfated sialomucin.[7] Occasional columnar cells are present that are narrow with a darkly eosinophilic cytoplasm. These have been called "pencil cells" and probably just represent compressed and contracted columnar cells.[2] Rare basal cells are identified that probably represent the reserve (stem) cells. These are flattened cells with dark elongated nuclei that lie parallel to and just above the basement membrane. A few chromogranin-positive endocrine cells may be present in the surface epithelium of the neck region, but none are normally present in the fundus or body.

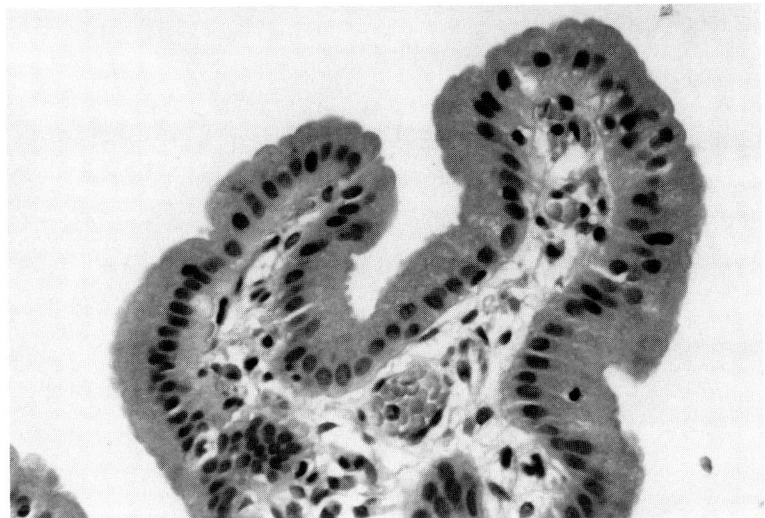

Figure 10–2. Normal pattern of mucosal folds of the gallbladder epithelium.

Mucus-secreting glands are present in the lamina propria and, occasionally, the adventitia of the gallbladder neck.[8] These are tubuloalveolar in type. The epithelium lining closely resembles that of the surface mucosa and is dissimilar to metaplastic antral gastric, or Brunner's glands, which have a bubbly appearing cytoplasm (Fig. 10–4). In common with the surface epithelium, the glandular cells contain sulfated and nonsulfated acid mucin only.

The gallbladder epithelium contains small numbers of T lymphocytes; however, there are normally no Paneth's cells or melanocytes. With immunohistochemical stains, there is staining for α_1-antitrypsin and α_1-antichymotrypsin and some weak positivity for polyclonal carcinoembryonic antigen.

Ultrastructurally,[8,9] the surface columnar epithelial cells have numerous apical microvilli, with filamentous glycocalyx and core rootlets. Within the cytoplasm are abundant mitochondria, Golgi complex, mucus granules, lysosomes, and small amounts of rough endoplasmic reticulum. At the apex of the cells, there are junctional complexes; below these, the cell membranes have complex interdigitations.

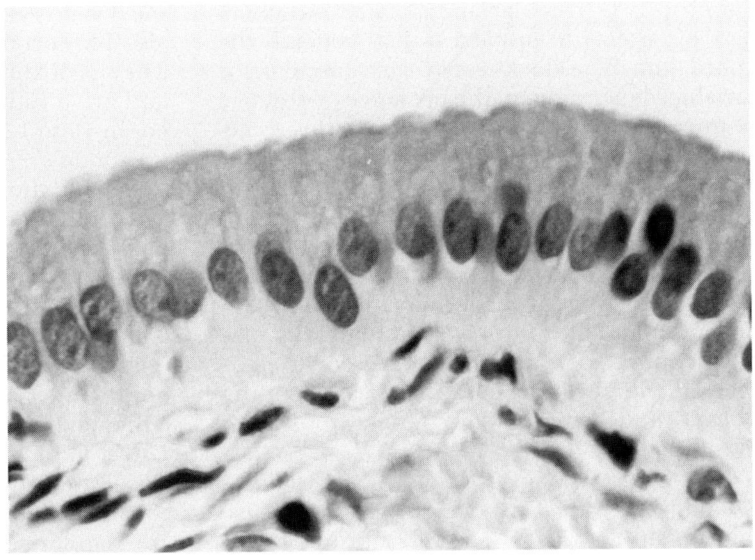

Figure 10–3. Normal columnar epithelium of the gallbladder, with basal regular nuclei and eosinophilic cytoplasm.

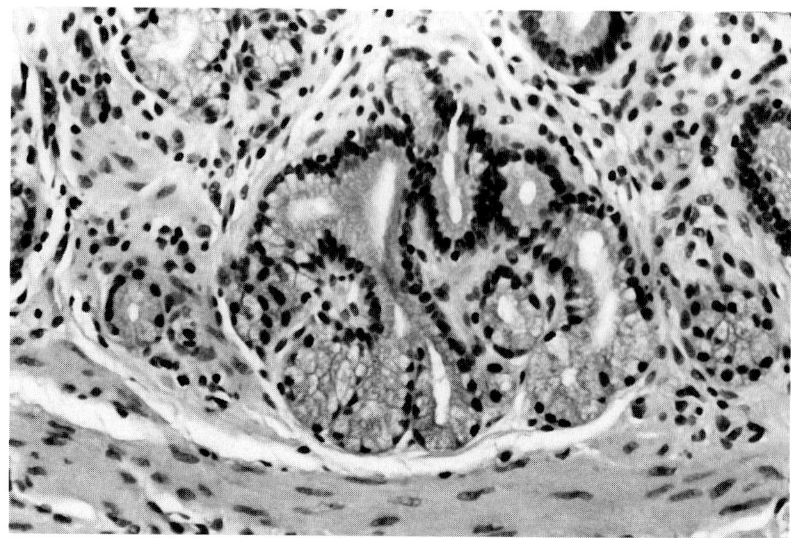

Figure 10–4. Mucus-secreting glands of the lamina propria of the gallbladder.

The lamina propria contains loose connective tissue and small numbers of lymphocytes, macrophages, and plasma cells. Neutrophils are normally absent. It lies between the mucosa and the muscularis and fills up the cores of the mucosal folds. Nerve fibers, small blood vessels, and lymphatics are also present.

The muscularis consists of loosely arranged bundles of smooth muscle, with intervening fibrovascular cores, that may be oriented in a circular, longitudinal, or oblique fashion. Collagen, reticulin, and elastic fibers are also present. There are no separate defined layers, as in the bowel wall. The junction of muscularis and lamina propria is irregular and isolated muscle fibers often extend upward to just beneath the epithelium. The thickness of the muscularis is variable, depending on the presence or absence of muscular contraction, and also varies somewhat in different parts of the gallbladder.

The subserosa, or adventitia, which surrounds the gallbladder, contains variable amounts of fibroelastic and adipose tissue, together with vessels, nerves, and ganglia. Occasional macrophages and lymphocytes may also be present. Collections of ganglion cells may be encountered in up to 90% of resected specimens.[10] The adventitia in the bare area is continuous with the interlobular connective tissue of the liver.

Downgrowths of mucosa (Aschoff–Rokitansky sinuses) may occur, to a minor extent, in up to 42% of otherwise histologically normal gallbladders examined at autopsy.[11] The sinuses may extend into the deep lamina propria, muscularis, or even subserosa. They are lined by histologically normal epithelium and accompanied by an adjacent cuff of lamina propria. Aschoff–Rokitansky sinuses are not found in fetuses, although early outpouchings can be encountered in infants.[12] They are therefore considered to be an acquired abnormality, probably resulting from episodes of overdistension, followed by vigorous contractions.[12]

Luschka's ducts are microscopic accessory bile ducts, typically located in the adventitial connective tissue, between the gallbladder and the liver (Fig. 10–5). Occasionally, they may also be encountered in a subserosal location. They probably represent embryonic remnants and are a rather common finding, being present in 10 to 12% of unselected cholecystectomy specimens.[12,13] Luschka's ducts may communicate with the intrahepatic biliary system and can drain bile after a cholecystectomy. Most are blind-ended, although occasionally they communicate with the lumen of the gallbladder, especially in cases where there is obstructive jaundice.[14] Luschka's ducts are not etiologically related to Aschoff–Rokitansky sinuses and do not connect to them. Histologically, they have a diameter ranging from a few microns, up to 1 to 2 mm. They are lined by epithelium that closely resembles intrahepatic bile ductules and consists of cuboidal epithelium with nuclei that are regular with even chromatin distribution

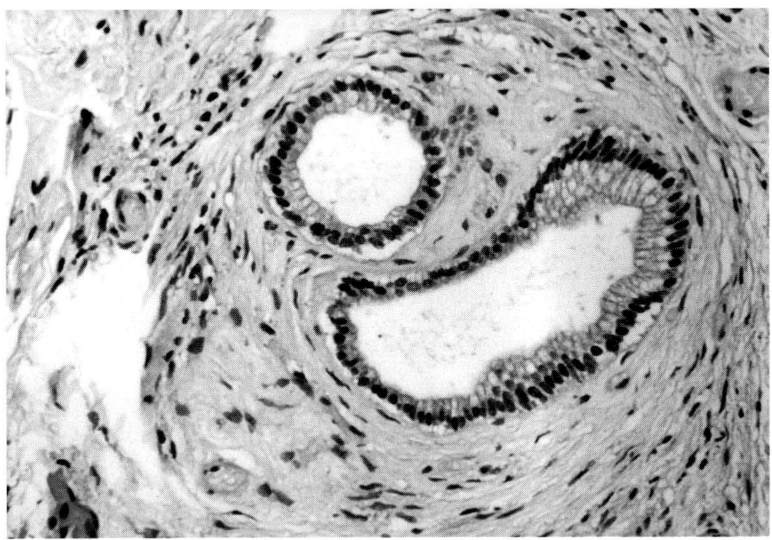

Figure 10–5. Luschka's ducts present in the bare area of the gallbladder. Histologically, they resemble intrahepatic bile ducts but may be surrounded by a ring of connective tissue.

and only small nucleoli. They are surrounded by a ring of connective tissue. The ducts may occur singly or in small groups. Some may be dilated, in which case the lining epithelium can be attenuated.

CONGENITAL ANOMALIES

Agenesis and Hypoplasia

Agenesis of the gallbladder occurs in up to 0.13% of the population and is the result of a failure of the cystic bud to develop.[15–17] Patients with this anomaly fall into one of three broad groups.[18] children with multiple congenital anomalies, asymptomatic adults in whom the abnormality is first discovered at autopsy, and symptomatic adults who have choledocholithiasis.[17,19] In rare instances, patients develop clinical symptoms that mimic cholecystitis but have no abnormality present to explain symptomatology. In the past, patients may have been subjected to surgery for "nonfunctioning" gallbladders that were actually "not present." Surprisingly, ultrasound examination will not always prevent this mistake.[17,19] Considerable confusion may occur at the time of laparoscopic surgery, when the gallbladder is not located at the usual site, and its absence may give rise to concern that there is an ectopic location.[19–21] In instances of gallbladder agenesis, the cystic duct is also almost invariably absent and the undersurface of the liver may not contain the usual depression. There may be poor delineation of the quadrate lobe. Other congenital anomalies that have been associated with agenesis include polycystic kidneys,[22] tracheoesophageal fistula,[22] cardiac abnormalities,[22,23] annular pancreas,[24] the Klippel-Feil syndrome,[25] and gastrointestinal anomalies, including imperforate anus,[26] duodenal atresia,[27] and shortening of the ascending colon.[28] It may also occur in congenital hypoplasia of the right lobe of the liver.[29]

Examples of gallbladder hypoplasia and atrophy are also recorded but are much rarer than agenesis. Two types are described.[30] Congenital hypoplasia, which is also associated with atresia and hypoplasia of the extrahepatic biliary system, results in the gallbladder being reduced to a bulb of fibrous and muscular tissue, attached to the end of the cystic duct. The lumen is extremely narrow, with a central lining of compressed epithelial structures. This type of hypoplasia may be difficult, if not impossible, to distinguish from an acquired inflammatory destruction. Intrauterine-acquired hypoplasia may occur, secondary to inflammation resulting from giant cell hepatitis, cystic fibrosis, or α_1-antitrypsin deficiency. This situation generally results in an intact but miniature gallbladder.[31] Cases have been described in which there is apparent presence of a gallbladder, with absence of the cystic duct. It is difficult to explain this situation embryologically, and it is possible that the "gallbladder" is actually a dilated cystic duct with secondary inflammation and proximal fibrous obliteration of the duct lumen.

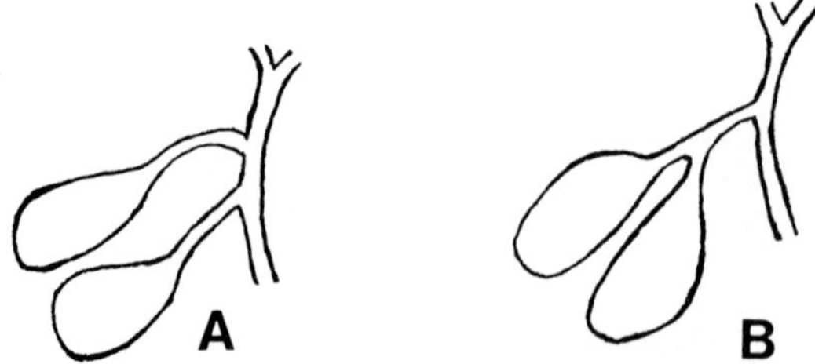

Figure 10–6. Duplication of the gallbladder. *A*, Each gallbladder may have a separate cystic duct draining into the common duct, or *B*, both cystic ducts may fuse to form a common distal portion. (From Weedon D: Pathology of the Gallbladder. New York, Masson Publishing, 1984.)

Duplication and Triplication

Duplication[32,33] of the gallbladder is an uncommon occurrence. These twin gallbladders may be drained by their own separate cystic duct[34] or by one bifid duct that drains both bladders[35] (Fig. 10–6). There are rare examples of cases where one of the cystic ducts drains directly into either the left or right hepatic duct[36,37] or even into the duodenum.[38] Duplication of the gallbladder is also associated with abnormalities of vascular supply, including an anomalous anteriorally displaced right hepatic artery.[39] Twin gallbladders may be quite separate or may be closely apposed within the same sheath of fibrous tissue and peritoneum (Fig. 10–7). Under those circumstances, it may be difficult at surgery to appreciate that the anomaly is in fact present. Closely apposed gallbladders are often affected by the same disease process, whereas with separated gallbladders, one may be diseased and the other normal. Diseases described as involving twin gallbladders include gallstones,[40] cholecystitis,[41] and cholesterolosis.[42] Duplication of the gallbladder and cystic ducts predisposes to chronic cholangitis, which may ultimately lead to cirrhosis.[32]

Rare cases of cystic duct duplication, in the presence of a single gallbladder, have been described. Usually, both ducts enter the gallbladder at separate locations, although occasionally they fuse in a Y formation to form a single common cystic duct. Abnormal insertion of the distal end of the cystic duct may occur and is relatively common. It may enter either the left or, more frequently, the right hepatic duct.[43,44] Of much more relevance to the practicing surgeon, however, is the rather common situation where the cystic duct runs for a distance alongside the common bile duct before being inserted into it. Sometimes, both ducts are surrounded by the same fibrous sheath. If this anatomic situation is not recognized, both ducts may be inadvertently ligated and transected at the time of cholecystectomy.

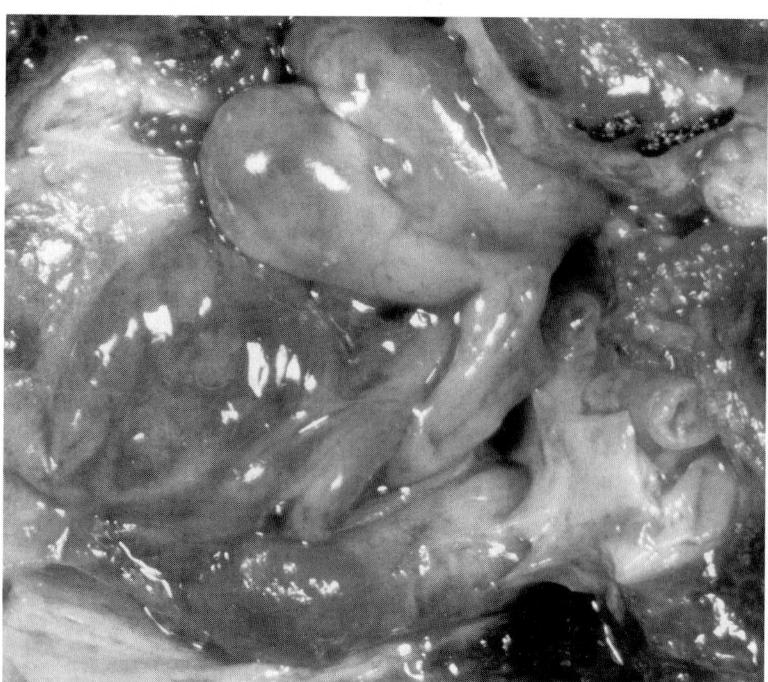

Figure 10–7. Duplication of the gallbladder. In this example, the surrounding common sheath of connective tissue is well demonstrated.

Triplication of the gallbladder is a real anatomic rarity.[45–47] A variety of cystic duct(s) draining the gallbladders has been described (Fig. 10–8). The gallbladders may all be of similar size, or there may be one or more that are vestigial. Cholelithiasis, cholecystitis, or adenocarcinoma may be present.[45]

Malposition

Minor malpositions of the gallbladder, usually of little clinical significance, include an intrahepatic gallbladder[48–52] and a floating gallbladder (one that is suspended from the undersurface of the liver by its own mesentery).[53] Intrahepatic gallbladders rarely cause specific clinical problems, although they are subject to diseases commonly encountered in normally positioned organs. These include cholecystitis,[49] gallstones,[50] and abscess formation.[51] Problems may, however, arise at cholecystectomy, when liver tissue may have to be excised to allow exposure to the gallbladder. In most instances, however, the gallbladder is not deeply buried in the liver. Intrahepatic gallbladders may also cause diagnostic confusion on imaging studies[52] if the possibility of a malposition is not considered.

Floating gallbladder is present in about 5% of individuals and is said to be more common in women.[53] In these circumstances, the elongation of the mesentery produces a risk of torsion and subsequent gangrene. Floating gallbladder has also been associated with hypoplasia of the left lobe of the liver.[54]

Other rare sites of misplaced gallbladders include locations on the left side of the liver,[55–57] suprahepatic area,[58–60] retroperitoneum, falciform ligament,[61] lesser sac, abdominal wall, and transverse orientation. A left-sided gallbladder may naturally occur in individuals with situs inversus.[55,62] In other examples, it appears that the gallbladder is attached to the left lobe of the liver, with the cystic duct either crossing the midline and entering a normally located common hepatic duct from the right side or entering either a left-sided common hepatic duct or the left hepatic duct. These anomalies are often first diagnosed at laparotomy, when it may be observed that the gallbladder is present to the left of the round ligament. This finding has given rise to the speculation that in fact, the primary abnormality is an abnormally placed umbilical vein and that displacement of the gallbladder is secondary.[56,63] In individuals with non–situs inversus–related left-sided gallbladder, there is a very high incidence of abnormal intrahepatic venous drainage.[57]

Suprahepatic gallbladder is a rare condition.[58–60,64] It may arise from entrapment of a gallbladder between the liver and diaphragm, occurring secondary to a long gallbladder mesentery. More commonly, however, it is associated with hypoplasia of the right lobe of the liver. Rarely, even an intrathoracic location has been recorded,[65,66] with associated diaphragmatic defects. These abnormally positioned gallbladders are also subject to the usual complications of inflammation and stone formation,[60] and one example caused a bronchobiliary fistula.[66]

Retropositioned gallbladders are found in the retroperitoneum, behind the liver.[67] At this location, they may give rise to considerable problems in diagnosis and surgical removal, if complications develop. Much rarer examples of malpositioning have been described. These include a gallbladder embedded in the falciform ligament,[61] with the cystic duct and gallbladder vessels present within the ligamentum teres.[64] Gallbladder herniation into the lesser sac has been described, in which the opening of the foramen of Winslow is abnormally large and the gallbladder mesentery is abnormally long.[68] Subcutaneous location in the anterior

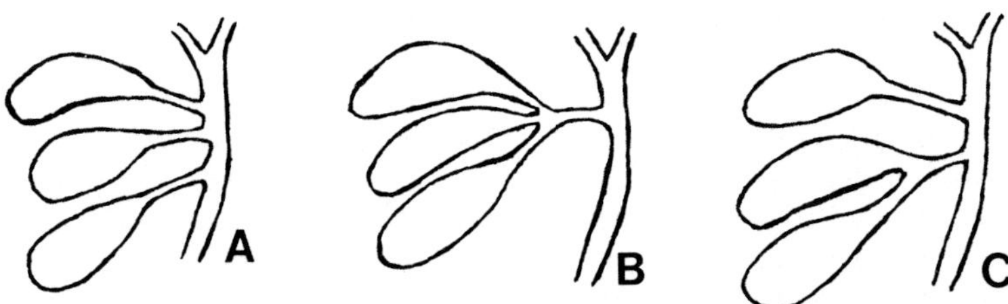

Figure 10–8. Triplication of the gallbladder: The cystic ducts *A,* may each drain separately into the bile duct; *B,* may drain into a distal common cystic duct; or *C,* may be in a composite arrangement. (From Weedon D: Pathology of the Gallbladder. New York, Masson Publishing, 1984.)

abdominal wall, just below the costal margin, has been described, but this case is difficult to explain embryologically, as there was no peritoneal lined hernia sac present.[69] Lastly, a transverse position of a normally located gallbladder has been recorded.[70]

Multiseptate Gallbladder

Multiseptate gallbladder is a congenital anomaly that is readily diagnosed by ultrasound examination.[71,72] It consists of a partitioning of the lumen by thin septa, covered by normal mucosa and consisting of muscle and lamina propria, continuous with the gallbladder wall. These septa may be fenestrated (communicating)[71,73] or noncommunicating.[74,75] The whole gallbladder may be involved, or the anomaly may be confined to the neck region. Patients with this condition tend to present with biliary colic and may or may not have associated gallstones.[71] The abnormality is thought to be the result of incomplete cavitation of the developing solid gallbladder bud. It has been described in association with gallbladder hypoplasia.[76]

Most examples of hourglass gallbladder are acquired as a result of chronic cholecystitis,[77] the single incomplete septum separating the two portions being composed of fibrous tissue or thickened muscle. However, rare congenital forms exist that are a variant of multiseptate gallbladder (uniseptate gallbladder).[78] Cholecystitis, or cholelithiasis, may be found in one or both of the compartments, irrespective of the etiology of the hourglass configuration.

Diverticula and Cysts

Most gallbladder diverticula are also acquired as a result of chronic inflammation and are analogous to diverticula of the colon.[79] The outpouchings are therefore false, or pseudodiverticula, and are lined only by mucosa with an incomplete muscular coat. They may arise as a result of traction from peritoneal adhesions, or erosion of the wall by intraluminal calculi, leading to damage of the muscularis (pulsion diverticula). Strictly speaking, Aschoff–Rokitansky sinuses are examples of pseudodiverticula; however, they are almost invariably microscopic in size and do not become large enough to present as clinical diverticula. Rarely, true congenital diverticula may occur in the gallbladder.[80,81] These probably arise after incomplete cavitation in the developing gallbladder bud. Congenital diverticula may be distinguished from acquired false diverticula, as they contain all four layers of the normal gallbladder in their wall (mucosa, lamina propria, muscularis, and adventitia).

Diverticula vary in size from 0.6 mm to 8 cm in diameter. They may be so large that they impinge on, or even erode, adjacent organs, such as the duodenum. They may contain calculi[81] and even become calcified themselves. In common with choledochal cysts, adenocarcinoma may occasionally complicate gallbladder diverticula.[82]

A variety of gallbladder cysts have been described. Fundal cysts probably represent diverticula, in which the neck has been "pinched off," as a result of ongoing inflammation.[83] Mesothelial cysts arise from the peritoneal covering,[84] and true congenital cysts[85,86] may arise from dilation of Luschka's ducts. These may be lined by a simple columnar epithelium or ciliated epithelium.

Phrygian Cap

The term *phrygian cap* is used to describe an abnormality seen most readily in cholecystograms and at ultrasound examination. It consists of a small mucosal fold, containing disorganized muscle, located toward the distal portion of the fundus.[87] In the laboratory, it is best demonstrated if the gallbladder is inflated with formalin and fixed before sectioning. This anomaly is considered as an anatomic variant, present in up to 6% of gallbladders. It has no specific significance, provided the correct diagnosis is made radiologically, ultrasonographically,[88] or by nuclear scan.[89]

Heterotopia

The presence of heterotopic tissue in the gallbladder has to be distinguished from simple metaplasia. Most examples of metaplasia consist of either gastric surface epithelium with underlying antral type mucus glands, or intestinal mucosa resembling duodenum, which may contain Brunner's glands. On the other hand, the term *heterotopia* implies a mass lesion containing tissue foreign to the site. In the gallbladder, heterotopic tissue may consist of gastric fundic mucosa,[90] liver,[90] pancreas,[91] adrenal,[92] and even thyroid.[93]

Gastric fundic heterotopia may arise secondary to embryonic displacement of cells from the primitive stomach. Examples are usually recorded in gallbladders from patients younger than those presenting with chronic cholecystitis and pyloric metaplasia.[90,94–96] Sessile polypoid islands may be found throughout the gallbladder, although the neck[94] and the fundus[97] are the most common sites. Generally, these polyps are 1 to 2.5 cm in diameter. Microscopically, these heterotopic foci consist of chief cells, parietal cells, and superficial epithelial cells, located either within the mucosa or as a nodule in the lamina propria.[97] There may be adjacent thickening of the muscularis, with Aschoff–Rokitansky sinuses and surface intestinal metaplasia. Gastric fundal heterotopia may be asymptomatic and discovered incidentally[96] or may cause abdominal pain.[95] Rarely, associated peptic ulceration has been recorded.[98]

It is not uncommon for gallbladders to be submitted to the pathology laboratory with small fragments of liver attached to the bare area. This represents normal tissues excised from the undersurface of the liver and does not constitute heterotopia. To qualify as heterotopic, the liver has to be present as a discrete nodule in the gallbladder, separated from the normal liver by a layer of adventitia. It may be present within the wall, or at a subserosal location.[90,99] The nodules may vary in size from 0.5 to 1.5 cm in diameter. Larger masses than this have been described but should probably be regarded as accessory hepatic lobes. Histologically, the liver may be normal or may demonstrate a variety of hepatocellular diseases. Any bile produced may drain via an accessory duct directly into the gallbladder.[100]

Ectopic pancreatic tissue in the wall of the gallbladder is an uncommon finding[91,101] and presents as a nodule, usually $<$1.0 cm in diameter, located within the wall. No site within the gallbladder is particularly favored. Extension to the mucosa may occur, resulting in formation of a sessile polyp,[102] containing ducts draining to the surface the secretions of ectopic exocrine elements. Microscopically, the ectopic tissue is organized into lobules of acini, with intervening ducts and islets. A variety of complicating diseases have been described, including acute pancreatitis, with adjacent fat necrosis.[103] As well as being found within the gallbladder wall, ectopic pancreatic tissue may also be located alongside the common bile duct.[104]

Ectopic adrenal tissue is relatively common in a variety of intra-abdominal locations, but surprisingly, there is only one example described, which occurred in the gallbladder subserosa.[92] This nodule was 3 mm in diameter and not associated with any obvious complication. Adrenal cortex and a small amount of medulla was present.

Ectopic thyroid tissue has also been demonstrated within the gallbladder.[93] How this arises is not clear. The ectopic tissue in the report of Curtis and Sheahan[93] measured only a few millimeters in diameter and did not appear to have any clinical significance.

REFERENCES

1. Albores-Saavedra J, Henson DE: Tumors of the gallbladder and extrahepatic bile ducts. *In*: Atlas of tumor pathology, second series, fascicle 22. Washington, DC: Armed Forces Institute of Pathology, 1986, pp 3–16.
2. Frierson HF: The gross anatomy of the gallbladder, extrahepatic bile ducts, Varterian system and minor papilla. Am J Surg Pathol 13:146–162, 1989.
3. Schoetz DJ, La Morte WW, Wise WE: Gallbladder compliance: A significant physiologic and pathophysiologic concept. Curr Surg 37:204–208, 1980.
4. Hand BH: Anatomy and function of the extrahepatic biliary system. Clin Gastroenterol 2:3–29, 1973.
5. Michels NA: Variational anatomy of the hepatic, cystic and retroduodenal arteries. Arch Surg 66:20–32, 1953.
6. Pomeranz IS, Davison JS, Shaffer EA: In vitro effects of pancreatic polypeptide and motilin on contractility of human gallbladder. Dig Dis Sci 28:539–544, 1983.
7. Laitio M: Morphology and histochemistry of nontumorous gallbladder epithelium. A series of 103 cases. Pathol Res Pract 167:335–345, 1980.
8. Laitio M, Nevalainen T: Gland ultrastructure in the human gallbladder. J Anat 120:105–112, 1975.
9. Evett RD, Higgins JA, Brown AL: The fine structure of normal mucosa in the human gallbladder. Gastroenterology 47:49–60, 1964.
10. Fine G, Raju UB: Paraganglia in the human gallbladder. Arch Pathol Lab Med 104:265–268, 1980.
11. Robertson HE, Ferguson WJ: The diverticula (Luschka's cysts) of the gallbladder. Arch Pathol Lab Med 40:312–333, 1945.
12. Halpert B: Morphological studies on the gallbladder. II. The "true Luschka ducts" and the "Rokitansky–Aschoff sinuses" of the human gallbladder. Bull Johns Hopkins Hosp 41:77–103, 1927.
13. Elfving G: Crypts and ducts in the gallbladder wall. Acta Pathol Microbiol Immunol Scand A 49[suppl 135]:1–45, 1960.
14. Bielby JO: Diverticulosis of the gallbladder. The fundal adenoma. Br J Exp Pathol 48:455–461, 1967.
15: Richards RJ, Taubin H, Wasson D: Agenesis of the gallbladder in symptomatic adults. A case and review of the literature. J Clin Gastroenterol 16:231–233, 1993.
16. Watemberg S, Rahmani H, Avrahami R, et al.: Agenesis of the gallbladder found at laparoscopy for cholecystectomy: An unpleasant surprise. Am J Gastroenterol 90:1020–1021, 1995.

17. Azmat N, Francis KR, Mandava N, et al.: Agenesis of the gallbladder revisited laparoscopically. Am J Gastroenterol 88:1269–1270, 1993.
18. Bennion RS, Thompson JE, Tomkins RK: Agenesis of the gallbladder without extrahepatic biliary atresia. Arch Surg 123:1257–1260, 1988.
19. Serow F, Klin B, Strauss S, et al.: False positive ultrasonography in agenesis of the gallbladder: A pitfall in the laparoscopic cholecystectomy approach. Surg Laparosc Endosc 3:144–146, 1993.
20. Raule M, Bagni M, Marioni M, et al.: Agenesis of the gallbladder in adults: a diagnostic problem. Br J Surg 81:676, 1994.
21. Cabajo Caballero MA, Martin del Olmo JC, Blanco Alvarez JI, et al.: Gallbladder and cystic duct absence. An infrequent malformation in laparoscopic surgery. Surg Endosc 11:483–484, 1997.
22. Gerwig WH, Countryman LK, Gomez AC: Congenital absence of the gallbladder and cystic duct. Report of six cases. Ann Surg 153:113–125, 1961.
23. Schlossman RE, Tartell M, Weisbach MS, et al.: Agenesis of the gallbladder associated with mitral annulus prolapse. A possibly unreported entity. NY State J Med 82:1249–1251, 1982.
24. Martinoli S, Schmitt HE, Allgower M: [An unusual triad: Gallbladder agenesis, annular pancreas and portal anomaly]. Helv Chir Acta 46:767–770, 1980.
25. Gajic SI. Gallbladder agenesis in a patient with Klippel–Feil syndrome. Arch Pathol Lab Med 105:682–683, 1981.
26. Turkel SB, Swanson V, Chandrosoma P: Malformations associated with congenital absence of the gallbladder. J Med Genet 20:445–449, 1983.
27. Coughlin JP, Rector FE, Klein MD: Agenesis of the gallbladder in duodenal atresia: Two case reports. J Pediatr Surg 27:1304, 1992.
28. Reid DA: Congenital absence of gallbladder associated with a high caecum and absence of ascending colon. Br Med J 2:1154–1155, 1959.
29. Kakitsubata Y, Kakitsubata S, Watanabe K: Gallbladder abnormalities associated with hypoplasia of the right lobe of the liver. Radiat Med 15:71–74, 1997.
30. Stolkind E: Congenital abnormalities of the gallbladder and extrahepatic ducts. Br J Child Dis 36:295–307, 1939.
31. Orava S, Leiviska T: Hypoplasia and aplasia of the gallbladder, a report of two cases. Acta Chir Scand 138:420–424, 1972.
32. Granot E, Deckelbaum RJ, Gordon R, et al.: Duplication of the gallbladder associated with childhood obstructive biliary disease and biliary cirrhosis. Gastroenterology 85:946–950, 1983.
33. Gigot J, Van Beers B, Goncette L, et al.: Laparoscopic treatment of gallbladder duplication. A plea for the removal of both gallbladders. Surg Endosc 11:475–482, 1997.
34. Harlaftis N, Gray SW, Skandalakis JE: Multiple gallbladders. Surg Gynecol Obstet 145:928–934, 1977.
35. Ingegno AP, D'Albora JB: Double gallbladder. Roentgenographic demonstration of a case of the "Y" type; classification of accessory gallbladder. Am J Roentgenol 61:671–676, 1949.
36. Ritchie AWS, Crucioli V: Double gallbladder with cholecystocolic fistula. A case report. Br J Surg 67:145–146, 1980.
37. Gorecki PJ, Andrei VE, Musacchio T, et al.: Double gallbladder originating from left hepatic duct: A case report and review of the literature. JSLS 2:337–339, 1998.
38. Hurst JM, Mayo RA: Unsuspected latent paring of the cystic primordium. South Med J 73:950–951, 1980.
39. Udelsman R, Sugarbaker PH: Congenital duplication of the gallbladder associated with an anomalous right hepatic artery. Am J Surg 149:812–815, 1985.
40. Chouhan AL, Chouhan S, Chouhan MK: Duplication of gallbladder associated with cholelithiasis: Sonographic detection. J Clin Ultrasound 23:556–557, 1995.
41. Moore TC, Hurley AG: Congenital duplication of the gallbladder. Review of the literature and report of an unusual symptomatic case. Surgery 35:283–289, 1954.
42. Oldfield MC, Wright CJE: Double gallbladder. Report of a case. Br J Surg 38:116–117, 1950.
43. Watson JF: Anomalous cystic and common bile ducts associated with cholecystitis. Am J Surg 118:459–462, 1969.
44. Kobak MW, Bettman RB: Anomalous insertion of the right hepatic duct into the cystic duct. Ann Surg 129:528–532, 1949.
45. Roeder WJ, Mersheimer WL, Kazarian KK: Triplication of the gallbladder with cholecystitis, cholelithiasis and papillary adenocarcinoma. Am J Surg 121:746–748, 1971.
46. Kurtzweg FT, Cole PA: Triplication of the gallbladder, review of the literature and report of a case. Am Surg 45:410–412, 1979.
47. Foster DR: Triple gallbladder. Br J Radiol 54:817–818, 1981.
48. Wysong CB, Gorten RJ: Intrahepatic gallbladder. South Med J 73:825–826, 1980.
49. Schmahman JD, Dent DM, Mervis B, et al.: Cholecystitis in an intrahepatic gallbladder. A case report. S Afr Med J 62:1042–1043, 1982.
50. Lusink C, Sali A: Intrahepatic gallbladder and obstructive jaundice. Med J Aust 142:53–54, 1985.
51. Bakalakos EA, Melvin WS, Kirkpatrick R: Liver abscess secondary to intrahepatic perforation of the gallbladder, presenting as a liver mass. Am J Gastroenterol 91:1644–1646, 1996.
52. Velchick MG, Noel AW: False positive liver scan due to intrahepatic gallbladder detection. Clin Nuc Med 12:50–52, 1987.
53. Anon: Wandering gallbladder. Br Med J 2:193, 1975.
54. Maeda N, Horie Y, Shiota G, et al.: Hypoplasia of the left hepatic lobe associated with floating gallbladder: Report of a case. Hepatogastroenterology 45:1100–1103, 1998.
55. Mayo CW, Rice RG: Situs inversus totalis. A statistical review of data on 76 cases with special reference to disease of the biliary tract. Arch Surg 58:724–730, 1949.
56. Nagai M, Kubota K, Kawasaki S, et al.: Are left-sided gallbladders really located on the left side? Ann Surg 225:274–280, 1997.
57. Ogawa T, Ohwada S, Ikeya T, et al.: Left-sided gallbladder with anomalies of the intrahepatic portal vein and anomalous junction of the pancreatobiliary ductal system: A case report. Hepatogastroenterology 42:645–649, 1995.
58. Faintuch J, Machado MC, Raia AA: Suprahepatic gallbladder with hypoplasia of the right lobe of the liver. Arch Surg 115:658–659, 1980.
59. Shen BS, Lin XZ, Chen CY, et al.: Suprahepatic gallbladder and right lobe anomaly of the liver in patients with biliary cancer. Dig Dis Sci 40:2411–2416, 1995.

60. Sato N, Matoba N, Fujii T, et al.: Suprahepatic gallbladder associated with cholelithiasis. Am J Gastroenterol 92:1388–1389, 1997.
61. Nelson PA, Schmitz RL, Perutsea S: Anomalous position of the gallbladder within the falciform ligament. Arch Surg 66:679–681, 1953.
62. Southam JA: Left sided gallbladder: Calculous cholecystitis with situs inversus. Ann Surg 182:135–137, 1975.
63. Fujita N, Shirai Y, Kawaguchi H, et al.: Left-sided gallbladder on the basis of a right-sided round ligament. Hepatogastroenterology 45:1482–1484, 1998.
64. Naganuma S, Ishida H, Konno K, et al.: Sonographic findings of anomalous position of gallbladder. Abdom Imaging 23:67–72, 1998.
65. Organ CH, Hayes DF: Supradiaphragmatic right lobe of liver and gallbladder. Arch Surg 115:989–990, 1980.
66. Allison MC, Milkins S, Burroughs AK, et al.: Bronchobiliary fistula due to acute cholecystitis in a suprahepatic gallbladder. Postgrad Med J 63:291–294, 1987.
67. Hsu KL, Cheng YF, Ko SF: Hypoplastic right hepatic lobe with retrohepatic gallbladder complicated by hepatolithiasis and liver abscess: A case report. Hepatogastroenterol 44:803–807, 1997.
68. Norkar BB, Whelan JG, Crech JL: Herniation of the gallbladder through the foramen of Winslow. Dig Dis Sci 25:228–232, 1980.
69. Bullard RW: Subcutaneous or extraperitoneal gallbladder. JAMA 129:949, 1945.
70. Burke J: An anomaly in the position of the gallbladder. JAMA 177:508–509, 1961.
71. Naritomi G, Kimura H, Konomi H, et al.: Multiseptate gallbladder as a cause of biliary pain. Am J Gastroenterol 89:1891–1892, 1994.
72. Hahm KB, Yim DS, Kang JK, et al.: Cholangiographic appearance of multiseptate gallbladder: Case report and a review of the literature. J Gastroenterol 29:665–668, 1994.
73. Okuda K, Nakajima M, Nakayama M, et al.: Multiseptate gallbladder. Report of a case with a review of the literature. Acta Hepatogastroenterol 26:70–75, 1979.
74. Tan CEL, Howard ER, Driver M, et al.: Non-communicating multiseptate gallbladder and choledochal cyst: A case report and review of publications. Gut 34:853–856, 1993.
75. Paciorek ML, Lockner D, Daly C, et al.: A unique presentation of multiseptate gallbladder. Dig Dis Sci 42:2519–2523, 1997.
76. Jena PK, Hardie RA, Hobsley M: Multiseptate hypoplastic gallbladder. Br J Surg 64:192–193, 1977.
77. Halpert RD, Bedi DG, Tirman PJ, et al.: Segmental adenomyosis of the gallbladder. A radiologic, sonographic and pathologic correlation. Am Surg 55:570–572, 1989.
78. St-Vil D, Luks FI, Hancock BJ, et al.: Diaphragm of the gallbladder: A case report. J Pediatr Surg 27:1301–1303, 1992.
79. Kramer AJ, Bregman A, Zeddies CA, et al.: Gallbladder diverticulum: A case report and review of the literature. Am Surg 64:298–301, 1998.
80. Allison JG: Cholecystocele: A congenital anomaly of the gallbladder. Arch Surg 113:994–997, 1978.
81. Kassner EG, Klotz DH: Cholecystitis and calculi in a diverticulum of the gallbladder. J Pediatr Surg 10:967–968, 1975.
82. Chin NW, Chapman I: Carcinoma in a true diverticulum of the gallbladder. Am J Gastroenterol 83:667–669, 1988.
83. Sworn MJ, Gay P: A fundal cyst of the gallbladder. An unusual abdominal mass. Med J Aust 2:307–308, 1975.
84. Hoffman CJ, Hales ED, Malachowski ME, et al.: Mesothelial cyst of the gallbladder. J Clin Ultrasound 17:50–52, 1989.
85. Jacobs E, Ardichvilli D, D'Avanzo E, et al.: Cyst of the gallbladder. Dig Dis Sci 36:1796–1802, 1991.
86. Kakitsubata Y, Kakitsubata S, Marutsuka K, et al.: Epithelial cyst of the gallbladder demonstrated by ultrasonography: A case report. Radiat Med 13:309–310, 1995.
87. Ober WB, Wharton RN: On the "Phrygian Cap." N Engl J Med 255:571–572, 1956.
88. Edell S: A comparison of the "phrygian cap" deformity with bistable and gray scale ultrasound. J Clin Ultrasound 6:34–35, 1978.
89. Smergel EM, Maurer AH: Phrygian cap simulating a mass lesion in hepatic scintigraphy. Clin Nucl Med 9:131–133, 1984.
90. Boyle L, Gallivan MV, Chun B, et al.: Heterotopia of gastric mucosa and liver involving the gallbladder. Report of two cases with literature review. Arch Pathol Lab Med 116:138–142, 1992.
91. Mutschman PN: Aberrant pancreatic tissue in the gallbladder wall. Am J Surg 72:282–283, 1946.
92. Busuttil A: Ectopic adrenal within the gallbladder wall. J Pathol 113:231–233, 1974.
93. Curtis LE, Sheahan DG: Heterotopic tissues in the gallbladder. Arch Pathol 88:677–683, 1969.
94. Lamont N, Winthrop AL, Cole FM, et al.: Heterotopic gastric mucosa in the gallbladder: A cause of chronic abdominal pain in a child. J Pediatr Surg 26:1293–1295, 1991.
95. Vallera DU, Dawson PJ, Path FR: Gastric heterotopia in the gallbladder. Case report and review of the literature. Path Res Pract 188:49–52, 1992.
96. Uchiyama S, Imai S, Suzuki T, et al.: Heterotopic gastric mucosa of the gallbladder. J Gastroenterol 30:543–546, 1995.
97. Yamamoto M, Murakami H, Ito M, et al.: Ectopic gastric mucosa of the gallbladder: Comparison with metaplastic polyp of the gallbladder. Am J Gastroenterol 84:1423–1426, 1989.
98. Larsen EH, Diederich PJ, Sorensen FB: Peptic ulcer of the gallbladder: A case report. Acta Chir Scand 151:575–576, 1985.
99. Tejada E, Danielson C: Ectopic or heterotopic liver (choristoma) associated with the gallbladder. Arch Pathol Lab Med 113:950–952, 1989.
100. Ashby EC: Accessory liver lobe attached to the gallbladder. Br J Surg 56:311–312, 1969.
101. Ben-Baruch D, Sandbank Y, Wolloch Y: Heterotopic pancreatic tissue in the gallbladder. Acta Chir Scand 152:557–558, 1986.
102. Kondi-Paphiti A, Antoniou AG, Kotsis T, et al.: Aberrant pancreas in the gallbladder wall. Eur Radiol 7:1064–1066, 1997.
103. Qizilbash AH: Acute pancreatitis occurring in heterotopic pancreatic tissue in the gallbladder. Can J Surg 19:413–414, 1976.
104. Pearson S: Aberrant pancreas. Arch Surg 63:168–184, 1951.

Chapter

11

GALLSTONES, CHOLECYSTITIS, AND REACTIVE CHANGES IN THE GALLBLADDER MUCOSA

CHOLELITHIASIS

The prevalence of gallstones is quite variable in different parts of the world, but in all groups studied they are more common in women. In the United States, they are present in about 10% of the general population.[1] In Europe, the prevalence is similar, with about 10% to 20% of women between the ages of 30 and 50 years and 15% to 40% of women older than 50 affected.[2] Higher rates are recorded in Latin American women,[3,4] with lower rates for women in Asia,[4,5] for women in sub-Saharan Africa,[6] and for black women living in the United States.[7]

Gallstones are quite uncommon in children, although gallstone incidence increases with age. The sex differences in prevalence are most marked among young adults but lessen with age, so that in those older than 60 years, the male-to-female ratio narrows to 1:2. Familial and socioeconomic factors associated with a higher prevalence include obesity,[8] increase in parity,[9] rapid dieting,[10] and low economic status.[8,11] The influence of these factors appears, however, to be relatively minor.

Medical conditions found to be strongly associated with an increased tendency to develop gallstones include hypertriglyceridemia,[12] Crohn's disease,[13] and total parenteral nutrition (TPN).[14] Triglyceride levels generally correlate with total body weight and so the influence of obesity may be mediated in this way. Crohn's disease probably causes stone formation, by depleting bile salts, which may be malabsorbed by a diseased terminal ileum. Patients on TPN are prone to develop biliary sludge, a precursor to stone formation. The reasons for sludge formation are not completely understood. Diabetes mellitus and hypercholesterolemia have only a weak correlation with stone formation. The individuals most at risk seem to be those who are obese, and develop hyperinsulinemia.[15] Drug therapies associated with gallstone formation include estrogen replacement therapy,[16] oral contraceptives,[9] and blood cholesterol–reducing agents, such as clofibrate.[17] Recent trends, however, have lowered the amount of estrogen prescribed for replacement therapy and also the amount present in oral contraceptives. This appears to have had an effect of reducing the risk of gallstone formation.[8,18]

Gallstones are of two major types and are classified according to their chemical composition. The vast majority of stones encountered in North America, especially among Hispanic Americans,[4] are cholesterol stones, which by definition contain > 75% cholesterol, with smaller amounts of calcium bilirubinate. Cholesterol gallstones are also extremely common in Native Americans in both North and South America.[19] The epidemiology of gallstone disease in these populations is consistent with the hypothesis that dominant lithogenic genes are present. Occasional examples, sometimes referred to as pure cholesterol stones, contain > 90% cholesterol. Pure cholesterol stones account for < 10% of all biliary calculi. Most of the remaining stones are pigment stones, consisting predominately of calcium bilirubinate, with smaller amounts (< 25%) of cholesterol. Two major subtypes are described: black pigment stones, which contain calcium bilirubinate, calcium phosphate, and calcium carbonate, and brown pigment stones, which contain calcium bilirubinate, calcium palmitate, and cholesterol. Both types of pigment stones have a glycoprotein matrix.

In gallstone disease, anywhere from one to several thousand calculi may be present. In up to one third of patients, culture of bile may reveal evidence of bacteria. However, when stones are present in the extracystic ducts, the prevalence of infection rises to 75%. The prevalence of chronic cholecystitis in patients with gallstones is variable and depends on criteria used for the diagnosis of inflammation. Nevertheless, there are many patients with cholecystolithiasis unaccompanied by cholecystitis and even more patients in whom the degree of inflammation is trivial. This strongly suggests, therefore, that in North America at least, most examples of cholecystitis occur as a complication of gallstones and are not an initiating factor. An exception to this statement is found in the case of brown pigment stones, which are rare in North America but which are strongly associated with ascending cholangitis and biliary inflammation.

The pathogenesis of cholesterol stones now appears to be firmly established and requires that bile, supersaturated with cholesterol, be secreted by the liver.[20,21] This can occur because of either an increased secretion of cholesterol or a reduced secretion of water, bile salts, and phospholipids. As it is secreted by the liver, bile contains aggregates of cholesterol and phospholipids. These are termed *vesicles*. Stabilization and solubilization of vesicles is achieved by their structural arrangement, which places hydrophilic radicals on the outside of the vesicle and hydrophobic elements on the inside. Bile salts do not play a role in vesicle formation but do have the ability to dissolve portions of vesicles and form smaller aggregates termed *micelles*. Micelles represent solubilized bile and vesicles represent cholesterol in a metastable (supersaturated) form. A variety of agents and complex reactions contribute to the stability of vesicles, but when these mechanisms break down, vesicles start to aggregate, forming crystals, and ultimately, cholesterol precipitation occurs.[22] Crystal formation is also a highly complex process and governed by a variety of influences. Because the presence of supersaturated bile within the gallbladder is a rather common occurrence, these factors are key in determining whether an individual is a stone former. The gallbladder also appears to play a key role in gallstone formation. As well as storing bile, the gallbladder concentrates it, especially at night, or during periods of fasting. This results in a higher cholesterol–to–bile salt ratio and the conversion of small unilaminar vesicles to larger, unstable, multilaminar forms. Nucleation and precipitation may be enhanced by mucin present within the gallbladder. During prolonged periods of fasting, a layer of mucus present within the gallbladder may contain multilamellar vesicles and microcrystals, recognizable by ultrasound examination as biliary sludge, a probable precursor of stone formation.[23]

The typical mixed cholesterol stones are generally multiple and rarely measure more than 2.0 cm in diameter. They are commonly multifaceted and have a smooth contour (Fig. 11–1). The cut surface reveals a laminated configuration, with alternating layers having a variegated appearance, depending on how much pigment is present (Fig. 11–2). In contrast, pure cholesterol stones are larger, usually between 2 and 4 cm in diameter. They are round or ovoid in appearance and the cut surface shows a radial arrangement of crystals. Pigment either is absent, or is present only in scanty amounts.

Experimental studies of cholesterol stone formation have used the prairie dog,[24] or its close relative, the ground squirrel.[25] Within 12 hours of intake of a cholesterol-enriched diet, the cholesterol saturation index within gallbladder bile increases. Within 18 hours, a layer of mucus forms on the surface of the gallbladder mucosa, and at 24 hours, the mucus is noted, by scanning electron microscopic examination, to contain small crystals.[25] This formation of crystals corresponds to a further increase in cholesterol within bile and a drop in the concentration of bile salts. After 2 weeks of this lithogenic diet, a progressive aggregation of cholesterol crystals is observed. After 10 weeks of feeding, the first visible stones of up to 1 mm in diameter are observed, and after 20 weeks of feeding, these calculi have increased to 2 mm in size.[25] The importance of minute crystal formation and the presence of a mucus layer are emphasized as critical initiating events. Inhibition of mucus

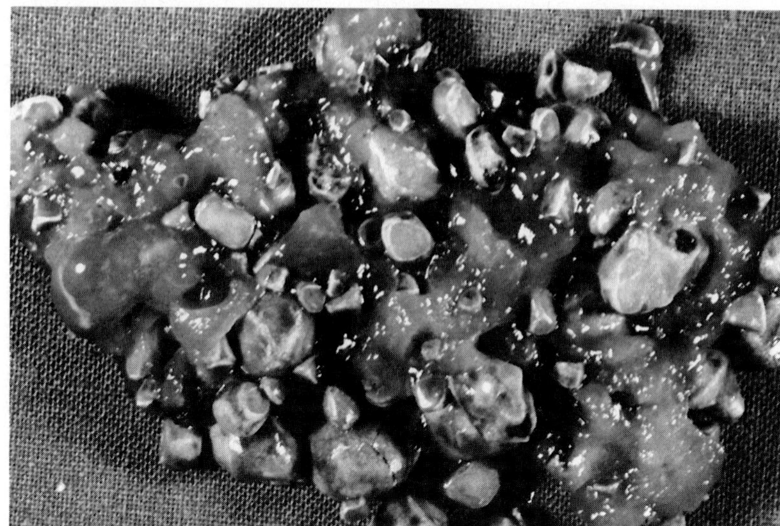

Figure 11–1. Multiple-smooth surfaced, faceted cholesterol stones in mucoid gallbladder contents.

formation—for example, by administration of aspirin—prevents this crystal formation.[24,26] In humans, an additional factor, impaired gallbladder contractility, may also be significant.[27]

Pigment stones comprise only a minority of gallstones—approximately 10% to 25%—in North America, but they are much more common in Asian populations.[28] The sex incidence is approximately equal. Black stones contain calcium bilirubinate and calcium carbonate and may be radiopaque (50%). They are most commonly found in the elderly and in individuals with hemolytic disorders, cirrhosis, and sclerosing cholangitis.[29] Grossly, they are present as multiple 2- to 5-mm shiny, irregular, multifaceted calculi. The pathogenesis appears to be an increase in bile concentration of unconjugated bilirubin, which combines with calcium to produce calcium bilirubinate. This process may also be influenced by changes in concentration of bile salts, lecithin, or ionized calcium.

Brown stones are found in the setting of biliary stasis and ascending infection, especially due to *Escherichia coli.* They, not uncommonly, complicate Oriental cholangiohepatitis and may be located within the common bile duct and intrahepatic ducts, as well as within the gallbladder.[30] It appears that the bacterial organisms have the ability to elaborate phospholipase A, which can break down phospholipids to form lysolecithin and free fatty acids. These generate free bile acids from bile salts and cause the precipitation of unconjugated bilirubin and fatty acids as calcium bilirubinate, calcium palmitate, and calcium stearate. In this process,

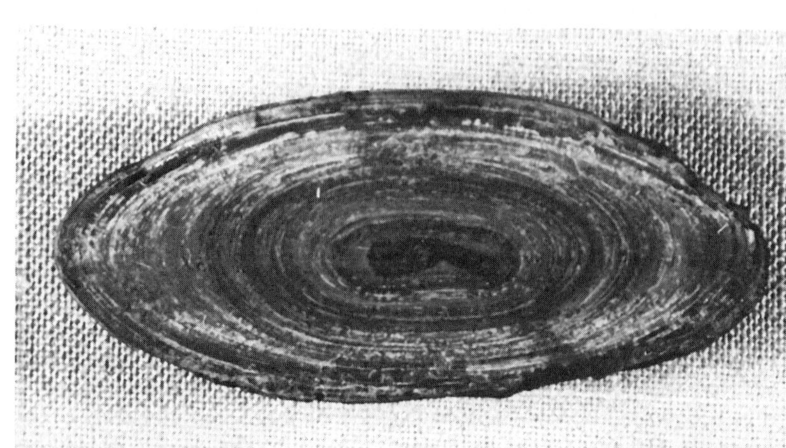

Figure 11–2. Cut surface of a cholesterol stone showing a typical laminated configuration.

bilirubin that was previously conjugated may become unconjugated. Brown stones are similar in size and configuration to black stones but have a softer texture and a flaky appearance. In southeast Asia, it is not uncommon to find that brown stones contain remnants of parasites or their eggs.

The vast majority of gallstones are clinically silent.[31,32] Many, but not all, tend to remain so over time. However, patients with gallstones who do present with symptoms are likely to have recurrent episodes if cholecystectomy is not performed. When symptoms do develop, they usually consist of right upper quadrant pain, flatulence, and intolerance of fatty food. The characteristics of the pain are highly variable and it is not always colicky in type. Conversely, occasional patients with typical biliary colic are not demonstrated to have gallstones. The risk of entirely asymptomatic individuals with gallstones subsequently developing symptoms is controversial. Estimates range from 31% for developing biliary pain after 2 years[32] to 10% for developing symptoms after 5 years and 18% for developing symptoms after 15 years.[31] In another study of 298 patients who presented with mild or nonspecific complaints, recurrence was at a rate of 6% per year for the first 5 years but declined to 2% per year after 15 years. However, the incidence of severe events was < 1% per year.[33] Complications of gallstones include acute and chronic cholecystitis, choledocholithiasis, acute pancreatitis, and gallbladder cancer. Details of these relationships are provided in other chapters. A search for groups of asymptomatic individuals with a higher risk of developing complications has not been rewarding. At least in North America, where gallbladder cancer is rare, routine cholecystectomy for asymptomatic gallstones to prevent cancer does not seem justified.

Gallstones have occasionally been described in children[34] and even neonates.[35] Calculi may also occur in the fetal gallbladder and frequently undergo spontaneous resolution, with no apparent residual biliary tract disease.[36] Many childhood gallstones are pigment stones that arise as a result of hemolytic anemia. Generally, it is considered that gallstones in children are less likely to impact and cause jaundice than are those occurring in adults.[34]

UNUSUAL TYPES OF GALLSTONES

Unusual clinical types of gallstones include disappearing gallstones, intramural gallstones, floating gallstones, and gas-containing stones. Although the topic of disappearing gallstones is interesting, such gallstones are a rarely observed phenomenon.[37,38] Possible reasons for disappearance include spontaneous passage via the common bile duct,[39] spontaneous passage via a cholecystoenteric fistula, and spontaneous dissolution. Undoubtably, all mechanisms may be operative. Spontaneous dissolution has been linked to dieting[37] and hormonal factors occurring during pregnancy.[40]

Intramural gallstones[41,42] may arise when stones become adherent to the gallbladder wall, causing ulceration and eventually erosion into the muscularis. This mechanism may result in part of the stone being embedded in the wall and part of it being exposed to the lumen. When gallstones are found wholly within the gallbladder wall, they have probably been formed in preexistent diverticula, or Aschoff–Rokitansky sinuses.

Many gallstones float, as can easily be demonstrated in the surgical pathology cutting room or autopsy suite. Undoubtably, this is usually a result of their high cholesterol content.[43,44] However, this may also occur when bile develops a high specific gravity, either secondary to the use of certain radiologic contrast media or as a result of fasting and bile concentration.[45] The term *floating gallstone* is of radiologic interest only and does not signify specific clinical or pathologic features.[46]

Gallstones containing gas are not uncommon, accounting for 22% in the largest reported series.[46] The volume of gas can be up to 0.5 mL per stone,[47] and gas is frequently present within triradiate fissures. The gas appears to be predominately nitrogen, with smaller amounts of carbon dioxide and traces of oxygen.[48] It has been hypothesized that the gas forms as a result of bacterial action, but this has not been confirmed.[49] The presence of gas within calculi makes them much more susceptible to the effects of ultrasonic lithotripsy.[50]

CHOLESTEROLOSIS

Cholesterolosis of the gallbladder represents the accumulation of neutral lipid, particularly cholesterol esters and triglycerides, within macrophages of the lamina propria. The condition may be diffuse or patchy. Four different patterns of gross involvement have been described: a diffuse granular type, accounting for up to 80% of cases; cholesterol polyposis, accounting for 10% of cases; diffuse granular cholesterolosis plus cholesterol polyps; and a localized granular type.[51] The granular forms are grossly characterized by the presence of numerous yellowish spots or thin streaks < 1 mm in diameter on the mucosal surface (Fig. 11–3). Where the localized form is present, the changes may be limited to the gallbladder neck or midportion. Only rarely is the fundus involved in isolation. Interestingly, cholesterolosis does not extend outside of the gallbladder to involve the cystic duct. When cholesterolosis is present, the bile tends to have an increased viscosity, giving it a tarry consistency. Detached masses of foam cells, termed *lipoidic corpuscles,* may be present as yellowish flecks suspended within the bile. The coexistence of gallstones and cholesterolosis is well recognized[52] and appears to be more frequent in surgically resected gallbladders than in autopsy cases. Many associated stones are solitary (30%) and, not surprisingly, are of the cholesterol type. The wall of the gallbladder is usually of normal thickness, except in cases of cholesterolosis associated with stones, where it may have additional changes of chronic cholecystitis. When cholesterolosis is in the form of seedlike accumulations and the background mucosa is red, this appearance has been likened to that of a strawberry.

Microscopically, the cholesterol deposits are in the form of ill-circumscribed collections of foamy histiocytes in the lamina propria at the base of the mucosa, often extending upward to involve mucosal folds, which may themselves appear hypoplastic.[53] Downward extension to the muscularis may occur but is rare. The histiocyte nuclei are usually small and have inconspicuous nucleoli (Fig. 11–4). These deposits are generally not associated with other types of inflammation and giant cells are absent. In a small number of patients, however, lipofuscin is present, both within the histiocytes and the adjacent gallbladder epithelium. This can be recognized as a brownish, granular pigment that is weakly periodic acid–Schiff (PAS) positive and is probably related to bile leakage into the mucosa. The fat within the histiocytes is optically clear but may be stained on frozen sections with techniques, such as oil red O. The clear spaces within histiocytes are PAS negative, indicating an absence of mucus. Adjacent to the stromal collections of foam cells, there may be prominent venular dilation, with minor degrees of fibrosis, particularly at the tips of the mucosal folds. Rarely, foam cells are encountered within the lumen of these vessels. Weak associations appear to exist among cholesterolosis, gallbladder neural hyperplasia, and adenomyosis.[54]

Ultrastructural changes, seen in the gallbladder of individuals with cholesterolosis, have been extensively studied.[55–57] One of the earliest lesions described is the presence of lipid droplets within the cytoplasm of superficial epithelial cells. These cells also contain numerous well-developed mitochondria and smooth endoplasmic reticulum. Inserted between the epithelial cells are macrophages with protruded processes, containing the same organelle arrangement as the epithelial cells. With progression of the lesion, macrophages come to lie freely in the lamina propria. As they become foam cells, they accumulate lipid droplets. It has been postulated that free cholesterol is absorbed by epithelial cells and becomes esteri-

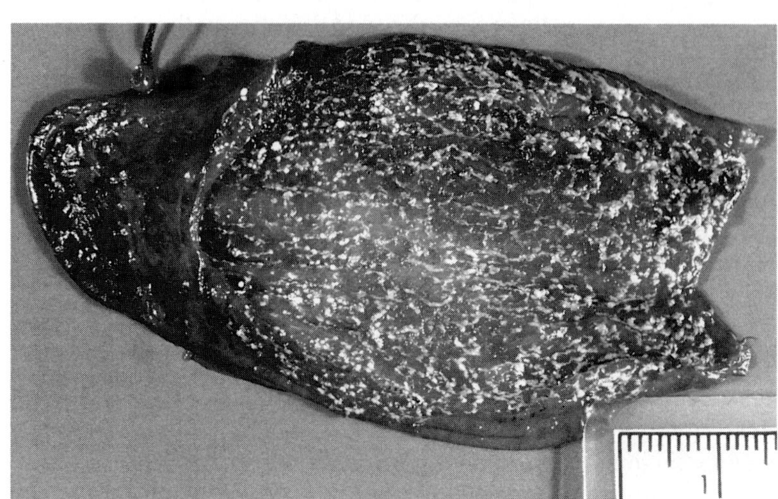

Figure 11–3. Cholesterolosis of the gallbladder. Note the cream-colored mucosal flecks.

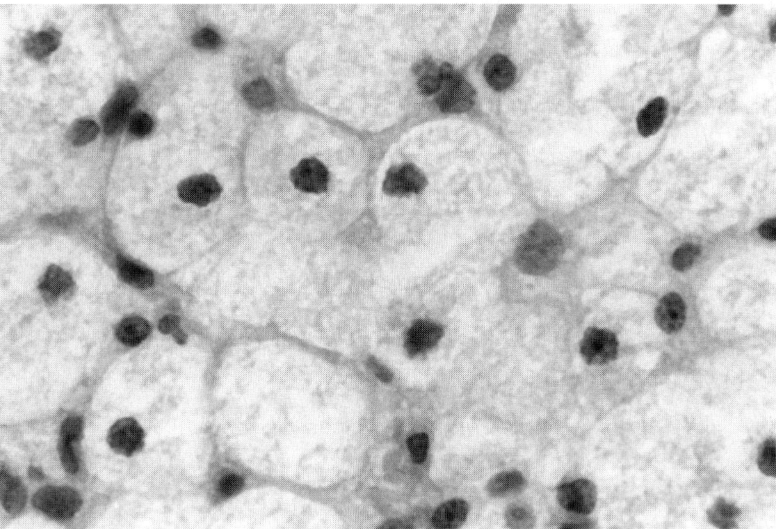

Figure 11–4. Microscopically, cholesterolosis consists of foamy histiocytes containing neutral lipid.

fied in the endoplasmic reticulum, where it is initially stored as lipid droplets. Later, these droplets are released into the interstitium, where they are phagocytosed and stored by macrophages. Accumulation of foam cells may occur as the macrophages become too distended and rigid to pass through the endothelium of lymphatics.[57] The pathogenetic factors underlying the formation of cholesterolosis are less well understood. The traditional point of view[58] is that in cholesterolosis, the gallbladder mucosa contains a marked excess of triglycerides, with significant elevation of esterified sterols and free methyl sterols. This suggests that free sterols can be transferred from bile to the gallbladder mucosa and that altered hepatic cholesterol synthesis is a major factor in the development of cholesterolosis. More recent results[59] suggest that patients with cholesterolosis have normal hepatic cholesterol formation and esterification but that their bile has a sevenfold increase in the level of esterified cholesterol and that the level of esterification correlates with bile saturation by cholesterol. Deposition of cholesterol, therefore, appears to occur after mucosal absorption from supersaturated luminal bile.[60] It is clear, however, that high plasma cholesterol levels do not correlate with gallbladder cholesterolosis.[61]

Cholesterolosis may be encountered in adult patients of any age, although it appears to be most frequent in the fifth and sixth decades of life. There is a marked female predominance.[52] Cholesterolosis may be asymptomatic and discovered incidentally. However, it has also been associated with postprandial distress, abdominal pain, and even jaundice. These symptoms, which are often of several years' duration, are relieved by cholecystectomy. Cholesterolosis is associated with obesity and diabetes mellitus but does not appear to be related to coronary artery disease.[52]

CHOLECYSTITIS

Acute Cholecystitis

Acute cholecystitis is a distinct clinical syndrome, characterized by right upper quadrant pain, nausea, vomiting, fever, and mild jaundice. A clinical distinction is made between acute cholecystitis accompanied by gallstones and acalculous cholecystitis (see following section). Typically, acute calculous cholecystitis begins with an abrupt onset of abdominal pain that is clinically similar to biliary colic. The pain may be continuous, although it can wax and wane in intensity. Initially, pain is experienced in the epigastrium before it later localizes to the right upper quadrant. The pain is accompanied by abdominal tenderness, with nausea and vomiting. A low-grade fever is common, but symptoms do vary, and particularly in the elderly, they may be milder and nonspecific. Jaundice is present in between 20% and 40% of patients.[62,63] Generally, the degree of jaundice is mild and high levels of serum bilirubin should raise the suspicion that calculi have become impacted in the common bile duct. In approxi-

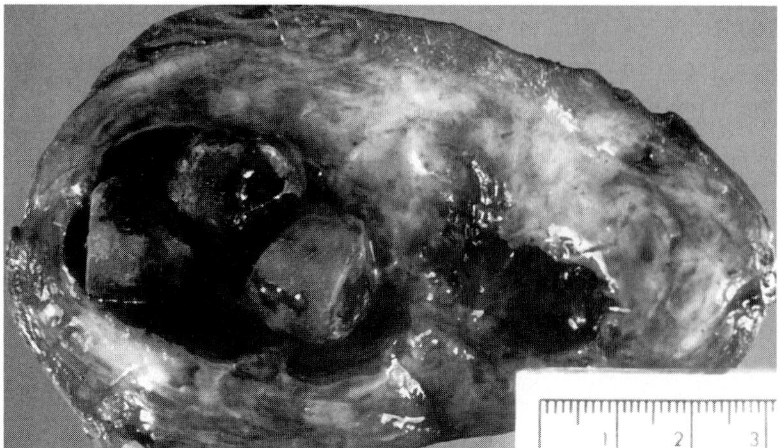

Figure 11–5. Gangrenous acute calculous cholecystitis with blackening of the wall due to gross hemorrhagic discoloration.

mately 50% of patients, the symptoms resolve without the need for surgery. In the remainder, cholecystectomy is required or complications may ensue, particularly if bacterial infection occurs. Patients with complications often have a high fever. Pus may accumulate within the gallbladder(empyema), or there may be gallbladder rupture, with formation of a subhepatic abscess.

The diagnosis of acute calculous cholecystitis is made clinically and is aided by ultrasound examination. In 30% of patients, an enlarged gallbladder is clinically palpable. Ultrasound examination can demonstrate the presence and location of gallstones and also whether there is thickening of the gallbladder wall. The finding of gallstones within the cystic duct or impacted in the neck of the gallbladder is considered highly significant.[64]

The exact mechanism by which gallstones produce acute cholecystitis remains unknown, although there is a strong correlation with stone impaction. It is postulated that the primary event is damage to the mucosal surface, leading to release of inflammatory mediators. Lecithin, a normal constituent of bile, may be converted into lysolecithin by the action of phospholipase A, a constituent of biliary epithelium.[65] Lysolecithin appears to have the ability to elevate prostaglandin production and start the inflammatory cascade.[66]

The gross pathologic findings in acute cholecystitis consist of a dilated gallbladder, covered by a serosal membrane that frequently may be hemorrhagic. Occasionally, adhesions form to adjacent organs and prominent serosal vessels are common. In more extreme examples, the gallbladder surface is blackened and necrotic (so-called gangrenous cholecystitis)[67] (Fig. 11–5). The wall is almost invariably thickened, sometimes up to 2 cm (Fig. 11–6). This is due to a combination of edema and inflammatory exudation. Secondary infection is present in approximately 50% of patients. If anaerobic gas-forming organisms are present, this may result in the formation of small bubbles within the

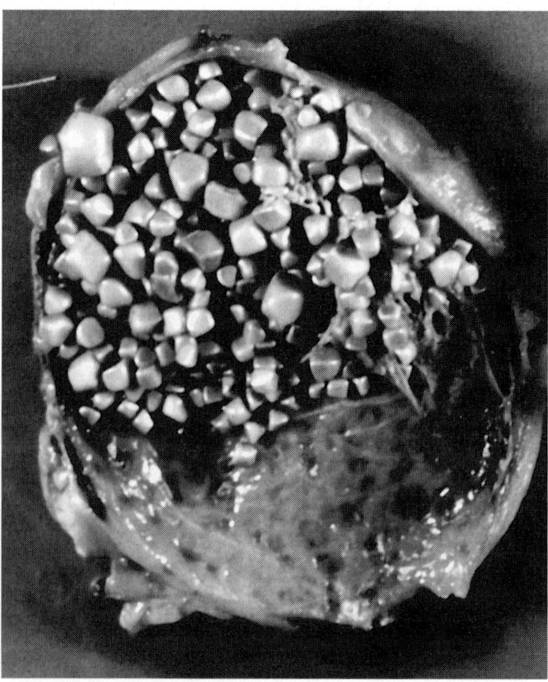

Figure 11–6. Acute calculous cholecystitis. Note the mural thickening and mucosal ulceration.

tissues (emphysematous cholecystitis).[68] Examination of the mucosa reveals diffuse reddening, with multiple ulcers or sometimes global ulceration, with a covering of mucopus. The gallbladder lumen contains a mixture of bile, mucus, pus, and hemorrhagic material. Stones of any type are present, often impacted in Hartmann's pouch or within the cystic duct itself (15% of patients).

Microscopic appearances of acute cholecystitis vary, according to the severity and duration of the disease. In the milder, early forms, the gallbladder wall and mucosa may simply be edematous and congested (Fig. 11–7). Later, a variable degree of transmural, acute inflammatory exudation develops. More severe acute cholecystitis is characterized by hemorrhage into the wall, with widespread ulceration. Microabscesses may be present, and in extreme examples, the wall of the gallbladder is necrotic. Near total mucosal denudation may be present, with surviving islands of mucosa displaying conspicuous regenerative atypia. If cholecystectomy is delayed longer than 7 days after the onset of symptoms, evidence of chronic inflammation and healing by fibrosis may be present. These include infiltration by lymphocytes, plasma cells, and hemosiderin-containing macrophages. Small numbers of eosinophils may be noted during the phase of resolution, but a diagnosis of eosinophilic cholecystitis should not be entertained unless eosinophils are abundant and are present in sheets. Resolution of acute cholecystitis occurs gradually, with organization and fibrosis. This may require 2 to 3 months to be fully developed.

The pathologic diagnosis of acute cholecystitis is somewhat controversial, and considerable discrepancy may exist between the surgeon's opinion and the final diagnosis of pathology.[69] Several reasons have been advanced to explain this discrepancy.[70] These include a reluctance on the part of pathologists to diagnose acute inflammation, where zero or few neutrophils are present in the gallbladder wall, and a tendency to diagnose only chronic cholecystitis in examples where acute and chronic inflammation coexist. Unlike acute appendicitis, the wall of the gallbladder in acute cholecystitis is not usually extensively infiltrated by large numbers of neutrophils. This is because the initiating agent is chemical rather than bacterial.[71] Because an intraoperative diagnosis of acute cholecystitis is probably correct, it is recommended that to prevent pathologic underdiagnosis, attention be paid to other findings in acute cholecystitis, particularly submucosal edema congestion and mucosal ulceration. Although ulcers can occur in chronic cholecystitis, they are not common, particularly if they are extensive.

Acalculous Cholecystitis

Acalculous cholecystitis accounts for just 5% to 10% of all cases of acute cholecystitis.[72–74] It is most common in people over 65 years of age, particularly men (the male-to-female ratio is

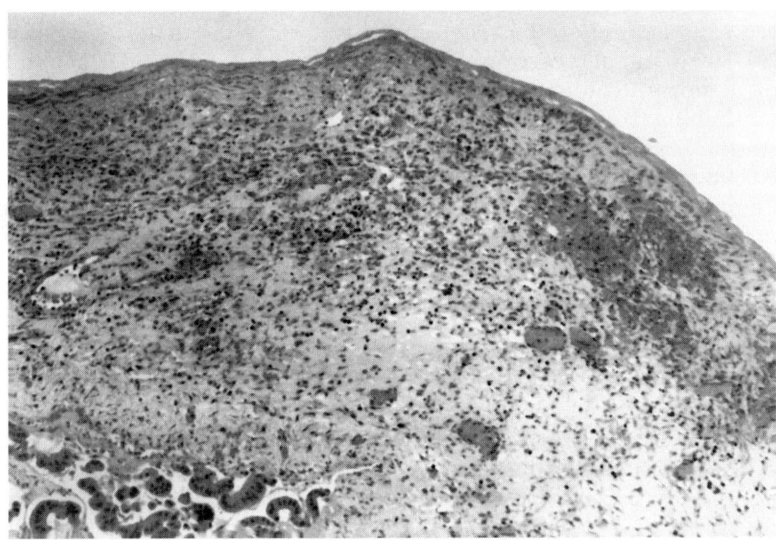

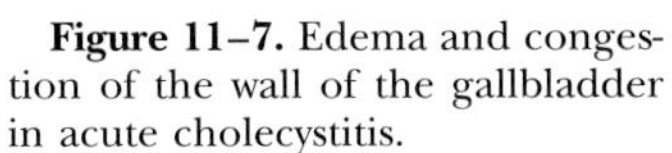
Figure 11–7. Edema and congestion of the wall of the gallbladder in acute cholecystitis.

2:1). The clinical symptoms are often nonspecific and a high index of suspicion is necessary. Early radiologic evaluation is recommended.[73] There are a variety of precipitating factors, including fasting, immobility, and hemodynamic instability.[73,74] Many patients have suffered trauma,[75,76] burns,[77] or sepsis.[78–80] The disease may also complicate major surgery[81] or severe medical conditions, such as acute leukemia[82] or systemic lupus erythematosus.[83] In some instances, it may have an infectious origin. Causative organisms include *Salmonella typhi,*[79] *Clostridia,*[80] *Vibrio cholerae,*[84–86] *Legionella,*[87] *Campylobacter jejuni,*[88] *Haemophilus segnis,*[89] *H. parainfluenzae,*[90] and *leptospira.*[91] Acute acalculous cholecystitis may also be drug induced[92] and can occur, for unknown reasons, in bone marrow transplant recipients.[93] Associated diseases that may be provoking factors include alcoholism,[94] diabetes mellitus, advanced malignancy, or generalized vasculitis.[95] Acute acalculous cholecystitis generally has a more fulminant clinical course than does acute cholecystitis with gallstones and a mortality that approaches 40%.[73] By the time the diagnosis is established, more than half of the patients have already developed complications, such as gangrene, perforation, or empyema.

The pathogenetic mechanism underlying acute acalculous cholecystitis is probably mucosal ischemia. This may be triggered by release of activated factor XII.[96] Ischemia renders the gallbladder mucosa vulnerable to injury from bile acids, which exert a detergent effect, breaking down tissues within the gallbladder wall. Superinfection by gram-negative bacteria and anaerobes (bowel flora) is common and further exacerbates the damage, although in most cases, it is considered a secondary event.[97]

Grossly and microscopically, the appearances of acute acalculous cholecystitis are indistinguishable from acute cholecystitis without stones,[98] except that the degree of inflammation is generally more severe. Gangrene may be identified in up to 40% of patients, and there may be abscess formation, perforation, empyema, or emphysematous cholecystitis.[99]

Emphysematous Cholecystitis

Emphysematous cholecystitis is a variant of acute cholecystitis in which the wall or lumen of the gallbladder contains gas. Gas may also be present within the cystic duct and bile ducts.[100–102] Typically, it complicates acalculous cholecystitis but can occasionally occur in acute cholecystitis with calculi. The immediate cause is infection by gas-forming bacteria, usually *Clostridium perfringens,*[100] although other organisms, such as *E. coli, Klebsiella,* or anaerobic streptococci may also be responsible.

In most instances, the correct diagnosis is suggested by imaging studies. These include plain abdominal radiographs, ultrasound, and computed tomography scan. Of these, ultrasound is the most useful, as it may detect small amounts of gas not readily identified on plain radiographs. A variety of characteristics have been described on ultrasound,[103] including the presence of champagne-like bubbles (effervescent gallbladder).[104]

Patients with this condition are usually elderly men, many of whom have diabetes mellitus.[100] The symptom onset is generally abrupt, with upper abdominal pain, either epigastric or right sided in distribution, accompanied by nausea and vomiting. The patients are febrile, with increasing fever, as the illness progresses. Distinction from simple acalculous cholecystitis may be difficult, although high fevers are very suggestive of an infectious cholecystitis. Treatment is with high-dose antibiotics and general supportive measures, followed by cholecystectomy. Despite optimum treatment, mortality remains high, in the region of 15% overall.[100]

At gross inspection, the gallbladder is distended, with gangrenous areas of the wall. Perforation is noted in 13% of patients.[100] The omentum may be adherent to the serosal surface and there may be adjacent localized pockets of pus. A foul-smelling odor emanates from the tissues. On opening the gallbladder, it is found to contain variable quantities of purulent material. Slough, consisting of a mixture of necrotic mucosa, pus, and fibrin, covers the wall and may even produce a mucosal cast. The wall of the gallbladder is friable, with visible gas bubbles or evidence of crepitus on palpation. The wall is generally grossly discolored and is often obviously necrotic. Microscopically, the appearances are somewhat variable, ranging from full-thickness infarction to a dense transmural neutrophil infiltrate. Fibrin thrombi are commonly encountered within vessels. Gas bubbles, present within the wall, may be difficult to recognize as such, because they tend not to be surrounded by neutrophils and may easily be confused with foci of edema. Stains for organisms, particularly Gram stains, are usually highly informative. The presence of gram-positive bacilli is highly suggestive of infection by clostridial species.

The exact clinical and pathologic mechanism permitting the development of emphysematous cholecystitis, have yet to be elucidated. They are, in all likelihood, similar to those causing simple acalculous cholecystitis. Most probably, there is an underlying vascular cause, resulting from either a primary obliterative endarteritis or interference in the vascular supply from blockage of the cystic duct. The organisms are derived from the bowel and may reach the gallbladder from lymphatic spread. Gas is probably initially generated within the gallbladder lumen and may enter the wall via breaches in the mucosal lining of the Aschoff–Rokitansky sinuses.

PERFORATION OF THE GALLBLADDER

Clinically, perforations of the gallbladder have been divided into acute cases (20%), subacute cases (35%), and chronic cases (45%). These categories relate to the speed of symptom onset, which may vary from the rapid development of a severe illness to a gradual progression of mild disease. They correspond approximately to situations of free perforation localized perforation, and cholecystenteric fistula. However, classification according to underlying cause is probably more logical, and a wide variety of causes are recognized.[105]

Perforation occurs acutely in approximately 10% of patients with acute calculous cholecystitis. It also complicates acute acalculous cholecystitis[106] and emphysematous cholecystitis,[100] when the wall of the gallbladder becomes necrotic. Acute perforation may also result from gallbladder ischemia and infarction secondary to vascular diseases of the gallbladder or to torsion. Usually, these individuals have a free perforation with peritonitis and are severely ill.

Acute gallbladder perforation is occasionally a complication of gallbladder trauma. This can occur after blunt injury to the abdominal wall[107,108] or injury occurring at the time of gallstone lithotripsy.[109] If recognized early, these perforations should be treated by immediate cholecystectomy. However, small leaks can become walled off by chronic inflammation and fibrous tissue and may be managed by initial conservative therapy, followed by elective cholecystectomy.

The most subtle form of perforation is one that results in the formation of a fistula from the gallbladder into an adjacent organ. The duodenum is the organ most commonly involved, but fistulas may also extend into the colon and, rarely, into the stomach, jejunum, thorax, and kidney. Occasionally, a fistula may extend from the gallbladder to other parts of the biliary system, such as the liver or common bile duct. In the majority of instances, gallbladder fistulas are the result of gallstones eroding through the wall. These cases are discussed fully in the section on fistulas later in this chapter.

EMPYEMA

Empyema of the gallbladder is defined as a gallbladder with obstructed cystic duct that contains frank pus. This distinguishes it from mucocele and simple acute cholecystitis.[110] Extensive surveys[111,112] have identified empyemas in between 2.4% and 11% of all patients undergoing cholecystectomy at major medical centers in both Europe and the United States. Empyema may be present in up to 40% of patients given an initial clinical diagnosis of acute cholecystitis.[112] The average age range of patients is 63 to 71 years.

Of particular importance is the fact that in many instances, empyema may be clinically unrecognized because the clinical findings are inconsistent.[110] Most patients have right hypochondrial pain, but less than half have significant pyrexia.[111] In 11 of 34 cases of acute cholecystitis in the series reported by Fry et al.,[112] the correct diagnosis was not made preoperatively. The clinical significance of this missed diagnosis is great, as the mortality of empyema is high (15% to 25% of patients).

Empyema is one outcome in the natural history of acute cholecystitis of both the calculous and acalculous variety. Organisms cultured from the pus include *E. coli* and *Klebsiella*.[112] The excised specimen generally shows a distended gallbladder, with a thickened wall, although there may be areas of gangrene and even perforation. In acute disease, the mucosa is extensively ulcerated with hemorrhage, neutrophil infiltration, and edema in the wall. Necrosis of the wall is present in examples accompanied by perforation. Empyema can, however, show more chronic changes, in which the mucosa is focally replaced by granulation tissue and the wall shows early fibrotic changes, with a relative absence of both acute and chronic inflammatory cells.

GALLBLADDER HYDROPS AND MUCOCELE

Hydrops and mucocele of the gallbladder are basically the same condition, with the exception that in hydrops, the gallbladder contains a watery fluid and in mucocele, it contains mucus. The term *mucocele* refers to reactive inflammatory conditions only and specifically excludes primary neoplastic conditions of the gallbladder, such as cystadenoma, where mucus overproduction may also occur.

Hydrops and mucoceles in adults are the result of an obstruction of the cystic duct, generally secondary to an impacted calculus. Other causes include fibrosis, kinking of the cystic duct, and external compression of the duct from, for example, a cirrhotic liver nodule.[113] Obstruction, leading to hydrops or mucocele, may also result from low-grade neoplasms, such as cystic duct carcinoma[114] and granular cell tumor.[115] Generally, these abnormalities do not spontaneously resolve and cholecystectomy is required for relief of symptoms.

In the pediatric age group, however, hydrops is commonly a reversible condition that occurs secondary to infections or inflammatory diseases. These include Kawasaki syndrome (mucocutaneous lymph node syndrome),[116,117] Epstein–Barr virus infection,[118] Henoch–Schönlein syndrome,[119] typhoid fever,[120] scarlet fever,[121] familial Mediterranean fever,[122] and leptospirosis.[122] Irreversible causes of childhood mucoceles include atresia of the cystic duct[123] and cystic fibrosis.[124]

Symptoms and physical signs of hydrops and mucoceles are similar in both adults and children. They include vomiting and the presence of a right-sided upper abdominal mass. Pain and tenderness may be present and, particularly in children, may be misdiagnosed as appendicitis or intussusception. A hugely enlarged gallbladder may produce pressure symptoms, with obstruction of adjacent bowel, particularly the duodenum.[125]

The gross appearances of hydrops and mucocele can be striking. It is not uncommon for adult specimens to weigh 2 kg, contain 1.5 L of fluid, and measure 15 cm in length. Opening the specimen reveals material that varies from thin, watery bile-stained fluid to viscid mucus. At these extremes, it is easy to determine whether the term *hydrops* or *mucocele* is more appropriate. In many instances, however, the fluid is thin and cloudy but slightly mucous to the touch, so that choice of one term or another is arbitrary. In adults, a calculus is almost invariably found impacted at the gallbladder outlet. Other stones may be present, floating free in the contained fluid. In adults, the gallbladder wall tends to be thickened, with partial fibrous replacement of the muscularis. In children, the wall is usually attenuated and may transilluminate. The lining of the gallbladder is a single layer of rather flattened epithelium and inflammation is typically scanty. In children, attention should be paid to the cystic duct, with careful gross and microscopic observation to determine the cause of stenosis or obliteration and whether there is any congenital anomaly that may be identified.

CHRONIC CHOLECYSTITIS

Chronic cholecystitis is the most common gallbladder disease, and in > 95% of cases, it is associated with cholelithiasis. Its epidemiology and clinical presentation is therefore very similar to that of gallstones. Specifically, it is three times more common in women than in men, tends to affect individuals in their forties and fifties, and is usually manifest clinically as episodes of biliary colic. However, many patients are entirely asymptomatic and their condition is diagnosed only when cholecystectomy is performed, because calculi have been discovered incidentally on abdominal ultrasound examination. The small number of patients with acalculous chronic cholecystitis may also experience right upper quadrant pain, presumably due to gallbladder dysmotility. It is assumed that the chronic inflammation is a result of longstanding irritation from bile salts and calculi and not vice versa. In about one third of patients, bile cultures are positive, usually for *E. coli,* presumably representing the residuum of a prior attack of acute cholecystitis.[126] Subclassification of chronic cholecystitis into those cases with evidence of a prior attack of acute cholecystitis and those without does not seem to serve any useful clinical purpose. This distinction may, however, explain the marked histologic differences seen in various gallbladders removed for "gallbladder pain." It is interesting to note that with the use of polymerase chain reaction technology, *Helicobacter* species DNA has been recovered from bile or resected gallbladder tissue of some individuals with cholecystitis.[127] Sequencing has revealed evidence of *H. bilis, H. pullorum* and *Flexispira rappini.* It remains to be seen whether the presence of these

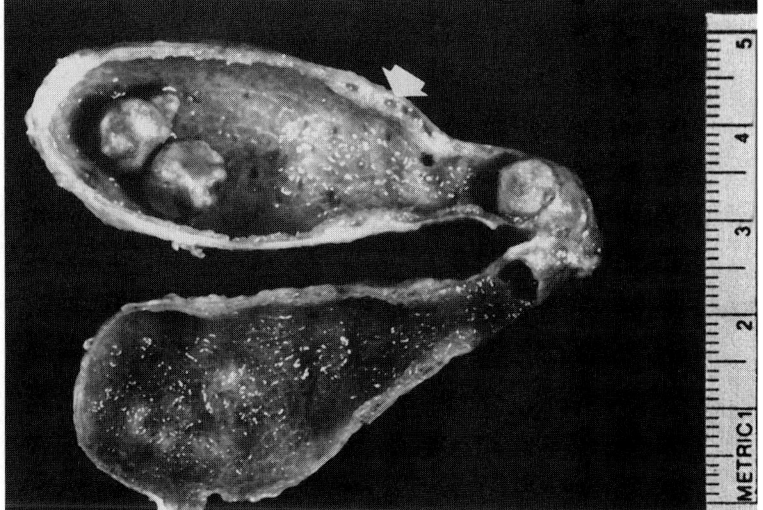

Figure 11–8. Chronic cholecystitis. Note the thickening of the wall with Aschoff–Rokitansky sinus formation (*arrow*). A stone is impacted in Hartmann's pouch.

organisms is as significant in the gallbladder as it is in the stomach.

A wide variety of gross and microscopic findings may be encountered in chronic cholecystitis, depending on the duration and severity of the disease. In the majority of instances, the gallbladder may appear virtually normal grossly, with only minor degrees of thickening of the wall and serosal scarring. With progressive disease, the wall of the gallbladder becomes thickened and Aschoff–Rokitansky sinuses form (Fig. 11–8). More severe and prolonged disease produces a shrunken gallbladder, with marked fibrous thickening of the wall and dense serosal scarring, with resulting adhesions to adjacent organs. The mucosa may appear flattened or granular in appearance and may show regenerative-type polypoid proliferation or superficial ulcers.

Microscopically, the typical features of chronic cholecystitis include a relatively scanty inflammatory infiltrate, mainly confined to the lamina propria. This includes lymphocytes, plasma cells, and smaller numbers of acute inflammatory cells, including occasional eosinophils (Fig. 11–9). The mucosa may be flattened, metaplastic, or regenerative. The muscularis may be thickened and apparently hypertrophic

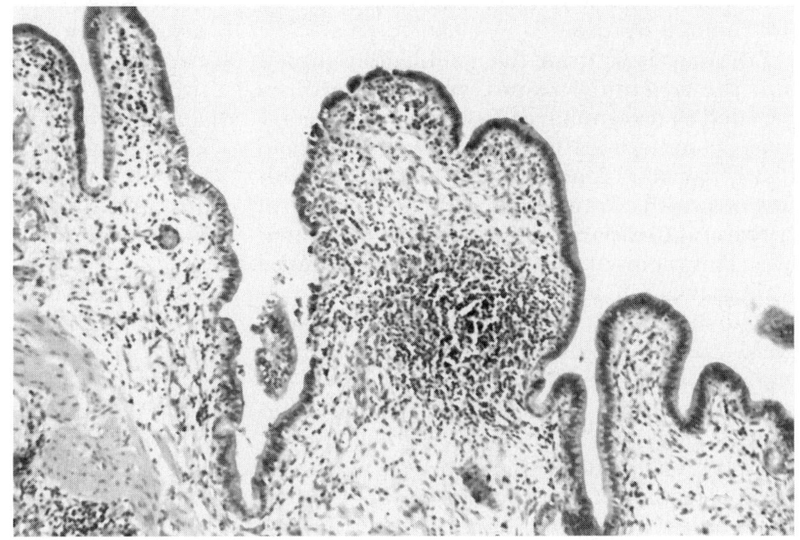

Figure 11–9. The mucosa in chronic cholecystitis with a mixture of acute and chronic inflammatory cells.

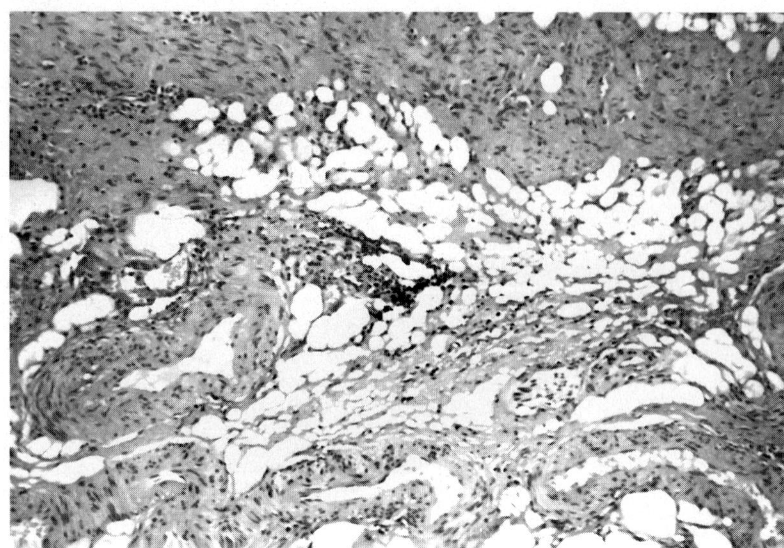

Figure 11–10. Adventitial scarring of the gallbladder mucosa in chronic cholecystitis.

but in the milder forms of disease is not scarred. However, the adventitia (subserosal layer) is frequently densely thickened, with diffuse scarring (Fig. 11–10). Scattered chronic inflammatory cells may also be located in this layer. It is recommended that chronic cholecystitis be diagnosed only when the gallbladder is obviously inflamed. It is perfectly possible to encounter normal gallbladders containing symptomatic calculi; therefore, it is not necessary to manufacture a diagnosis of cholecystitis to retrospectively justify cholecystectomy. More severe disease is associated with greater numbers of inflammatory cells and more dense and more extensive fibrosis. In some patients, dense lamina propria fibrosis is associated with neuronal hyperplasia and small vessels may show obliterative luminal fibrosis.

Bile may leak from the gallbladder lumen into the adventitial tissues, where it becomes ingested by macrophages. Collections of macrophages, sometimes termed *cholegranulomatous cholecystitis,* may contain foamy histiocytes, with fine brownish cytoplasmic granules, cholesterol crystals, and variable amounts of extravasated bile. This pigment within macrophages may be a mixture of bile and ceroid (lipofuschin). The ceroid stains positively with diastase/PAS and Ziehl–Neelson stains.[128] Large numbers of cholegranulomas, present within the wall of the gallbladder, have been termed *xanthogranulomatous cholecystitis.*

Aschoff–Rokitansky sinuses are an almost invariable feature of moderate and severe degrees of chronic cholecystitis. They consist of irregular herniations of mucosa into the muscularis (Fig. 11–11), sometimes extending out to the subserosa (Fig. 11–12). They are thus analogous to acquired colonic diverticula. Accompanying the mucosa is a coat of normal lamina propria. The lining of the sinuses may consist of inflamed or uninflamed epithelium and may occasionally be ulcerated. Regenerative cytologic changes may be present within sinuses, on occasion giving rise to confusion with very well differentiated infiltrating carcinoma. Occasionally, gallbladders are encountered in which there is true dysplasia in the surface epithelium that also extends down to involve epithelium within sinuses. This, too, can be difficult to distinguish from an infiltrating carcinoma. The most useful microscopic feature in differentiating sinuses from invasive carcinoma is the presence of a thin layer of lamina propria, which surrounds the mucosa of Aschoff–Rokitansky sinuses but is not present around the glands of infiltrating carcinomas.

Follicular Cholecystitis

Follicular cholecystitis is a minor variant of the usual type of chronic cholecystitis in which large numbers of mucosal lymphoid follicles with hyperplastic germinal centers are present.[129] Occasionally, the follicles may be so large and numerous as to give rise to polyp formation. For this diagnosis to be appropriate, many follicles should be present. Small numbers of scattered follicles are encountered in approxi-

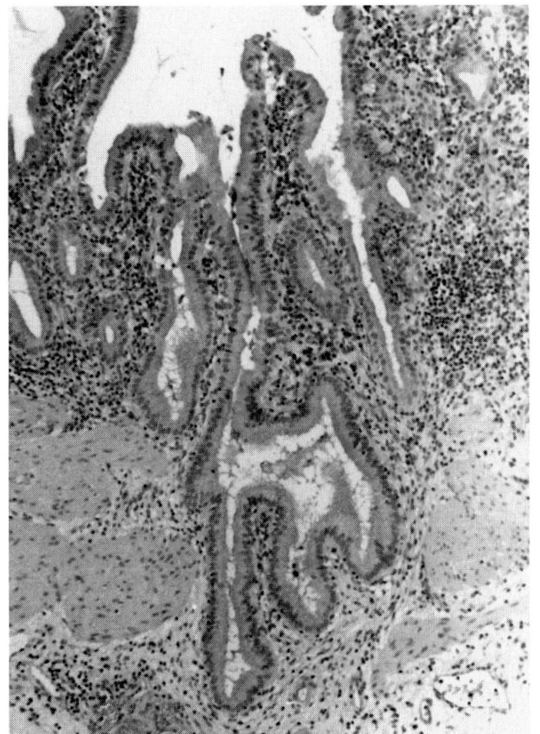

Figure 11–11. Aschoff–Rokitansky sinus in a gallbladder with chronic cholecystitis.

mately 5% of examples of otherwise unremarkable chronic cholecystitis. These cases should not be labeled follicular cholecystitis. Under this rigid criterion for diagnosis, follicular cholecystitis is present in only 0.08% of cholecystectomy specimens.[129] Usually, the diagnosis is clear-cut, as follicular proliferation dominates the histologic picture (Fig. 11–13). Follicular cholecystitis has no specific clinical picture that can be used to distinguish it preoperatively from the usual type of chronic cholecystitis.

Follicular cholecystitis was originally described in typhoid fever[129] but is now recognized as occurring in other infections, especially those due to gram-negative organisms.[130] It has also been described in sclerosing cholangitis.[131] Gross inspection of the mucosa may reveal either normal findings or a granular appearance with flattened nodules 1 to 3 mm in diameter. Calculi may or may not be present. On microscopic examination, the follicles are seen to be located mainly in the lamina propria, where they widen and flatten the normal mucosa folds. They have the typical appearance of reactive follicles, with sharply defined germinal centers, containing tingible body macrophages and mitotic figures.

Porcelain Gallbladder

Porcelain gallbladder is another complication of long-standing chronic cholecystitis. It consists of multiple areas of dystrophic calcification, located predominately within the muscle and lamina propria, so that on palpation and gross inspection, the organ has an eggshell-like appearance. Gentle pressure may result in cracking of the sheets of calcification.

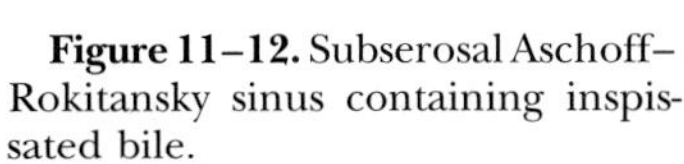

Figure 11–12. Subserosal Aschoff–Rokitansky sinus containing inspissated bile.

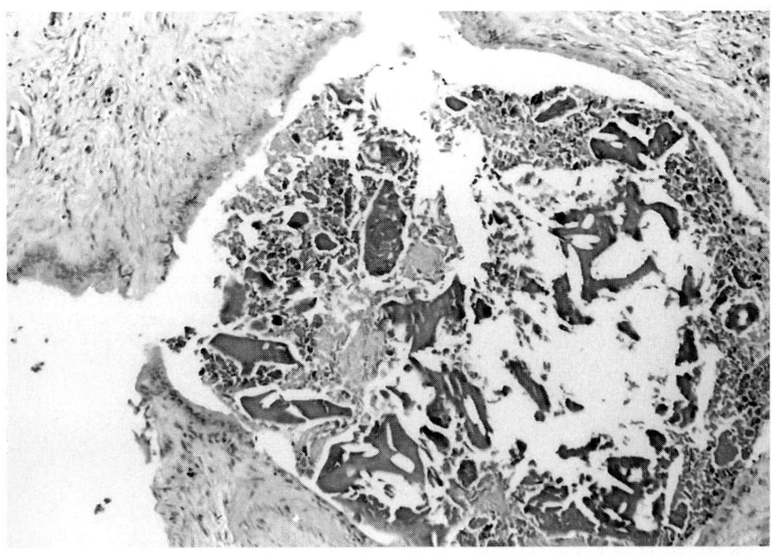

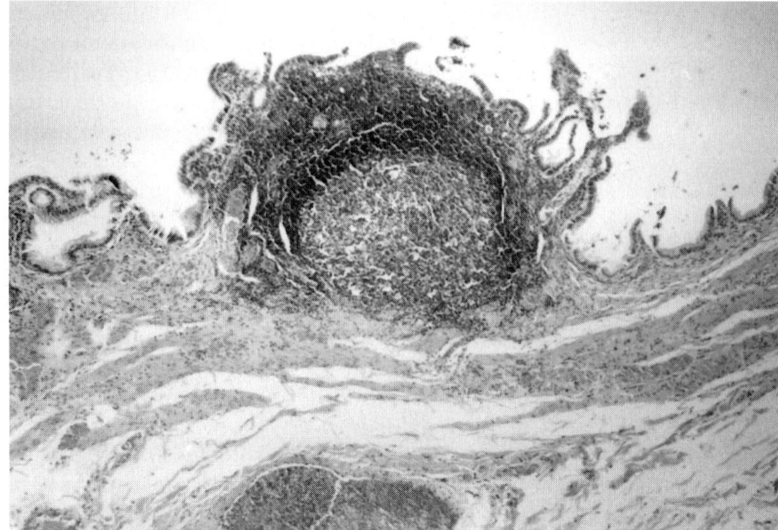

Figure 11–13. Follicular cholecystitis demonstrating a lymphoid follicle containing a germinal center.

Porcelain gallbladder is a rare condition and is present in 0.6% to 0.8% of all cholecystectomy specimens. Patients' mean age of disease onset is 54 years, and the condition is five times more common in women than in men.[132] One case has been described in a 10-year-old child.[133] Diagnosis is often made preoperatively on plain abdominal x-rays by identifying thin, curvilinear calcifications in the right upper quadrant of the abdomen.[134,135] Ultrasound examination produces a variety of characteristic appearances[136,137] and may identify "complete" and "incomplete" patterns of calcification.[137] The cause of the condition is unknown; intramural hemorrhage, local alterations in calcium metabolism, irritation by gallstones, and chronic infection have all been postulated, but there is little confirmatory evidence. The deposited mineral is mainly calcium phosphate, with smaller amounts of calcium carbonate.

On gross inspection, the gallbladder is generally shrunken and has a thick, fibrous wall containing calcium deposits (Fig. 11–14). The calcification may be eggshell thin or, rarely, so thick that a saw is required to produce tissue blocks for decalcification. The lumen of the gallbladder generally contains either multiple calculi or a thick sludge focally adherent to the mucosal surface.

Histologic examination confirms the presence of mural fibrosis and calcification associated with variable but usually sparse amounts

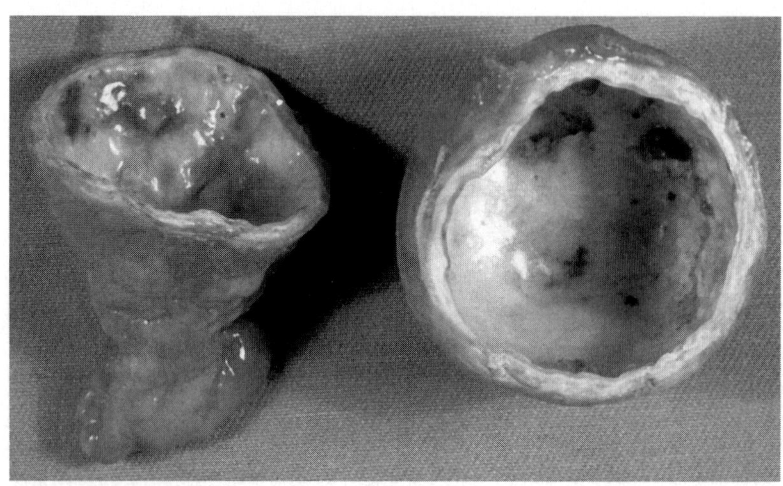

Figure 11–14. Porcelain gallbladder. Note the thickening and rigidity of the wall with deposition of whitish calcified material.

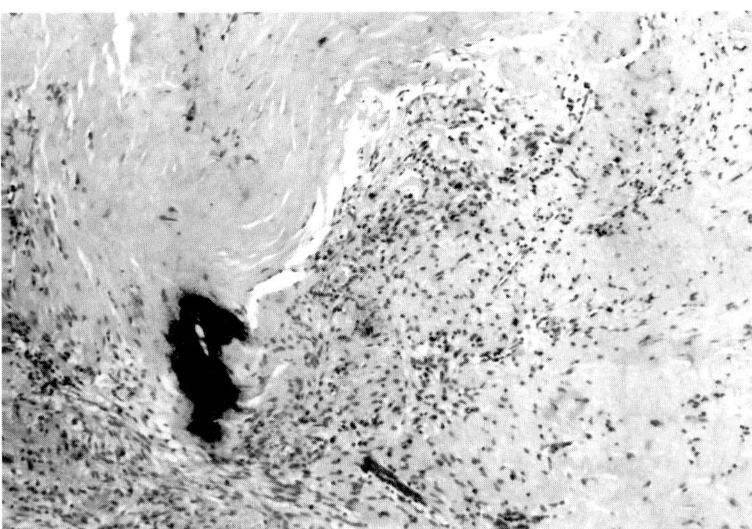

Figure 11–15. Porcelain gallbladder with calcification in dense mural fibrous tissue.

of chronic inflammation (Fig. 11–15). Two patterns of calcification are described: a more common "complete" type, in which the muscularis shows broad bands of calcification, and a rarer "incomplete," or focal type, in which there are localized calcium deposits within the mucosa.[137,138] Metaplastic bone formation is generally absent. The mucosal surface may be ulcerated or may have residual epithelium sometimes showing antral or squamous metaplasia.

Porcelain gallbladders have been associated with the subsequent development of carcinoma. In some series, the risk is estimated to be as high as 20%,[134] but this may be somewhat exaggerated because of a case selection bias. The risk is reported to be higher with "incomplete" calcification.[137] Most commonly, the tumors are poorly differentiated adenocarcinomas, but squamous cell carcinomas have also been reported.[139]

The term *limy bile* has been applied to a situation in which the gallbladder contents consist of creamy or yellowish green–colored material, with a doughy consistency. The bile contains precipitated calcium salts, which are opaque on plain x-ray, giving rise to an appearance resembling that of a normal cholecystogram.[140,141] Once the gallbladder is opened in the laboratory, the majority of the bile will drain away, although there may be a residuum adherent to the mucosal surface. The gallbladder itself shows chronic cholecystitis, and in some instances, there may be mural calcification also. The pathogenesis of the condition is obscure but may be related to cystic duct obstruction, followed by a pH change in the bile. In some, but not all, cases, an impacted gallstone is present. The presence of limy bile does not appear to have any clinical significance, and it may undergo spontaneous resolution, probably as a result of drainage of the abnormal bile down the cystic duct.[142]

Adenomyomatosis and Adenomyoma

Both adenomyomatosis and adenomyoma are regarded as a complication of cholelithiasis and cholecystitis. They are considered to represent simply exaggerated forms of Aschoff–Rokitansky sinus formation. Adenomyoma is a localized form of adenomyomatosis, and both are usually discovered incidentally by radiologic examination or when an excised gallbladder is received in the laboratory.

Aschoff–Rokitansky sinuses are acquired structures consisting of outpouchings of the gallbladder mucosa into the wall. They are thus analogous to acquired colonic diverticula. Their prevalence increases with age and they are present, to a greater or lesser extent, in approximately 90% of routine cholecystectomy specimens performed for cholecystolithiasis.[143] Many authors have concluded that they arise as a "blowout" phenomenon, secondary to raised intraluminal pressures. In support of this suggestion is the fact that they tend to occur at points of weakness in the gallbladder wall at the site of penetrating blood vessels.[144] The raised pressure is thought to occur during episodes of biliary colic. Aschoff–Rokitansky sinuses in an excised gallbladder are usually accompanied by chronic cholecystitis; nevertheless, both conditions may occur by themselves. In a series of 125 cholecystectomy specimens studied by Elfving,[143] Aschoff–Rokitansky sinuses were present in 86.4%. In 9.6%, the lamina propria alone was involved; in 46.4%, they extended into the muscularis; and in a further 30.4%, they penetrated the muscularis to involve the adventitia. Elfving observed that the more deeply penetrating sinuses tended to be associated with extensive cholecystitis. The lining of sinuses is similar to the normal surface mucosa, although it can become inflamed and display metaplastic changes.

In generalized adenomyomatosis, the whole of the gallbladder wall is thickened, sometimes up to 10 mm.[145,146] Mucosal proliferation results in extensive Aschoff–Rokitansky sinus formation with branching sinuses and cyst formation. The muscularis is hypertrophied and possibly hyperplastic. Prominent mucosal folds are present on the mucosal surface. The sinuses are generally larger than usual and may contain inspissated bile. The point at which florid Aschoff–Rokitansky sinus formation becomes adenomyomatosis is not precisely defined (Fig. 11–16).

Adenomyomatosis, when specifically looked for in cholecystectomy specimens, occurs in 1% to 7% of specimens.[147,148] However, these figures include cases of both segmental and generalized adenomyomatosis. Generalized adenomyomatosis is considerably less frequent, with a possible prevalence of 0.05% in unselected cholecystectomy specimens. Adenomyosis is three times more common in women than it is in men. Most instances occur in adults, although there are small numbers of examples occurring in the pediatric age group.[149,150]

Segmental adenomyomatosis has a variety of configurations, depending on its localization. It is characterized by a thickened band or segment of the gallbladder wall, within which it grossly and microscopically resembles the generalized form. Four subtypes have been distinguished[151] (Fig. 11–17): (a) a proximal subtype, in which thickening extends from the cystic duct to the middle of the gallbladder and in which the proximal gallbladder is often dilated; (b) a distal subtype, which is the mirror image of subtype a, where the distal half of the gallbladder is affected; (c) a middle segmental subtype—the rarest—in which the central portion of the gallbladder is involved with normal distal and proximal portions and which may produce an hourglass or dumbbell distortion of the gallbladder; (d) miscellanous forms—subtypes a, b, and c can occur as mixed or irregular forms—grouped together. The most common association is a combination of subtypes b and c. Although the four are described as distinct subtypes,[151] it is clear that all are really part of the same disease spectrum. This subdivision, therefore, is useful only for descriptive purposes.

Localized adenomyosis is a tumorlike nodule whose usual location is at the fundus of the gallbladder.[152,153] At this location, the term *adenomyoma* is generally used to describe the lesion, although there is widespread recognition that it is nonneoplastic in nature. Rarely, adenomyomas have been described in the gallbladder neck,[153] extrahepatic bile ducts, and the sphincter of Oddi.[154] Most commonly, adenomyomas are spherical or hemispherical nodules, measuring 1 to 2 cm in diameter (Fig. 11–18). Occasionally, they may be polypoid and can be confused radiologically with gallbladder cancer. This occurs most frequently when there is abundant associated inflammation.[155] Grossly, ade-

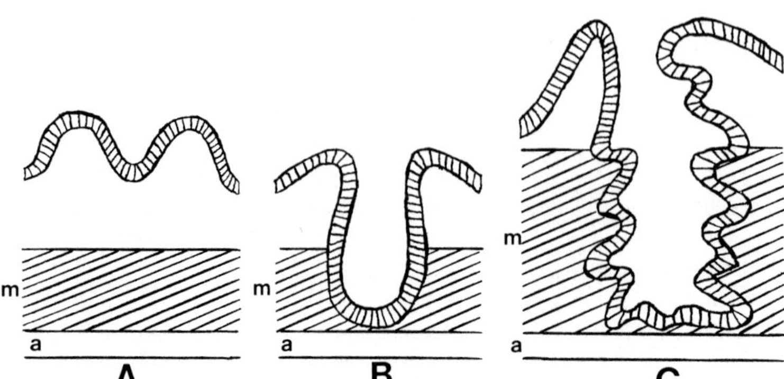

Figure 11–16. Sinus formation in the gallbladder: *A,* normal gallbladder; *B,* Aschoff–Rokitansky sinus formation; *C,* adenomyosis. (From Bilhartz LE: *In* Sleisenger MK, Fordtran JS (eds): Gastrointestinal Disease, 5th ed. Philadelphia: WB Saunders, 1993, pp 1858–1868.)

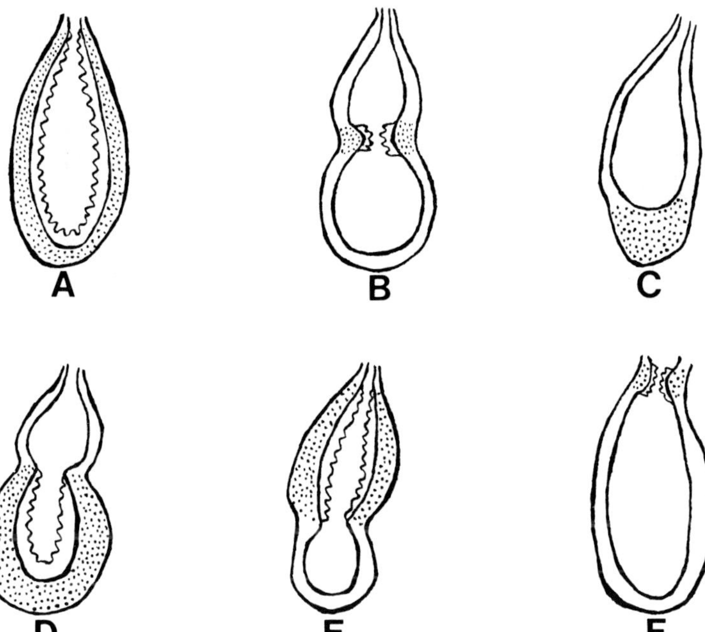

Figure 11–17. Adenomyomatosis of the gallbladder: *A,* generalized type; *B,* middle segmental involvement; *C,* adenomyoma; *D,* distal segmental involvement; *E,* proximal segmental involvement; *F,* localized neck. (From Weedon D. Pathology of the Gallbladder. New York: Masson Publishing, 1984, pp 185–194.)

nomyomas are firm, pale gray lesions with umbilication on the mucosal surface. The cut surface may demonstrate small cystic structures (Fig. 11–19). Microscopically, the cysts have a complex branching structure and may contain inspissated bile or even small calculi.

The traditional viewpoint is that adenomyosis in either focal segmental or generalized forms is not a preneoplastic condition.[156] However, recent reports have cast some doubt on this opinion. A study by Ootani et al.[157] examined 3,197 cholecystectomy specimens and found adenomyosis in 279 (8.8%). Overall, cancer was present in 12 of 188 patients with segmental adenomyosis (6.4%). In all 12 examples, the carcinoma was located in the distal gallbladder and the adenomyosis involved either the distal gallbladder also or a segment in the middle of the gallbladder. In gallbladders without adenomyosis, cancer was found in 3.1%. No cancers were present in 9 patients with generalized adenomyosis or in 82 patients with fundal adenomyoma. Furthermore, several authors have recently described an association between adenomyosis and anomalous union of the pancreaticobiliary duct (AUPBD).[158–160] AUPBD (see

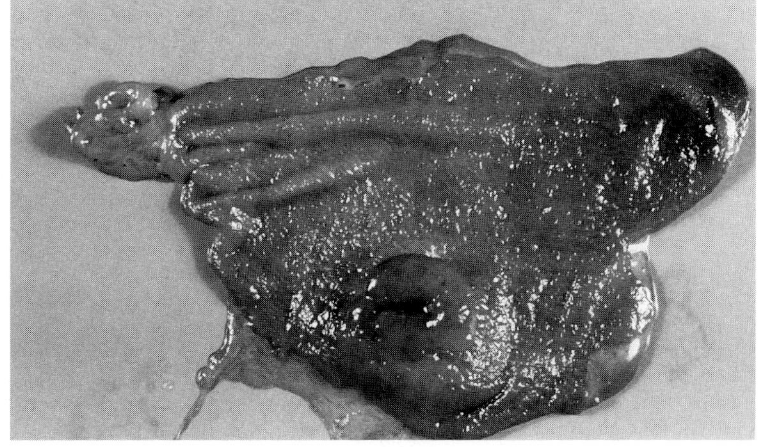

Figure 11–18. Adenomyoma of the fundus of the gallbladder. Note the central umbilication.

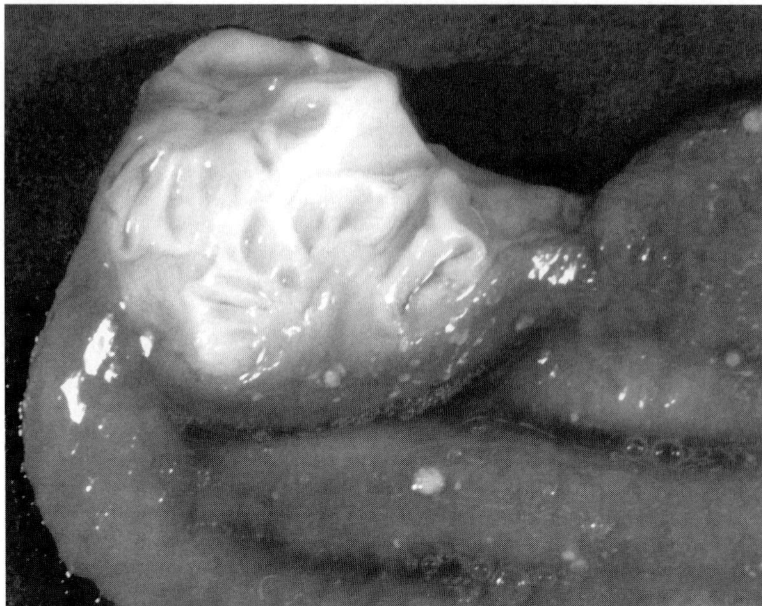

Figure 11–19. Cut surface of a gallbladder adenomyoma displaying dilated Aschoff–Rokitansky sinuses.

Chapters 13 and 14) is a congenital anomaly occurring at the lower end of the common bile duct at its junction with the main pancreatic duct. The anomaly permits reflux of pancreatic secretions up the bile duct and into the gallbladder. The presence of AUPBD has a statistical association with gallbladder cancer. What is not clear is whether it is adenomyosis or another mucosal change (hyperplasia) that represents the premalignant lesion.

Xanthogranulomatous Cholecystitis

Xanthogranulomatous cholecystitis, another variant of chronic cholecystitis, involves proliferation of foamy macrophages so florid that tumorlike masses, or diffuse infiltrative plaques,[161] can be detected by naked-eye examination of the gallbladder.[162,163] Xanthogranulomatous cholecystitis may also be diagnosed by preoperative ultrasound examination of the gallbladder.[164,165] The gallbladder wall is thickened (3 to 20 mm) and contains nodules varying in size from 6 to 12 mm (mean, 10.5 mm) in diameter.[164] These nodules may be echogenic, isoechoic, or hypoechoic.

The masses usually have an intramural location but occasionally may produce sessile nodules, partly covered by mucosa. The lesions, which may be multiple, appear yellowish, creamy colored, or light brown and are ill circumscribed, with a softish consistency (Fig. 11–20). They may measure up to 3.0 cm in diameter. Microscopically, the lesions may contain, as well as foamy histiocytes, a variety of other inflammatory cells, including lymphocytes and giant cells reacting to foreign material, particularly cholesterol crystals (Fig. 11–21). Typically, the foam cells contain lightly pigmented lipofuscin (ceroid) granules. Pools of extravasated bile pigment may also be seen. With time, organization occurs and fibroblastic proliferation may predominate. Rarely, with superimposed *E. coli* infection, the histiocytes may contain Michaelis–Gutmann bodies and fulfill the morphologic criteria for malacoplakia.[166] Fine-needle aspiration cytology demonstrates abundant histiocytes, foam cells, and multinucleate giant cells, with a background of pink granular debris and lymphocytes.[167]

The majority of examples of xanthogranulomatous cholecystitis are associated with gallstones. The reaction seems to be initiated by rupture of an Aschoff–Rokitansky sinus, with liberation of bile into the gallbladder wall. The foam cells are macrophage derived and are invariably immunopositive for KP1, HAM56, CD11b, and CD68. The accompanying lymphocytes are predominately T cells, with a CD4 and CD8 phenotype. These findings indicate a delayed hypersensitivity reaction of cell-mediated immunity.[168]

Xanthogranulomatous cholecystitis has been reported in 4.2%[168] and 8.9%[169] of unselected

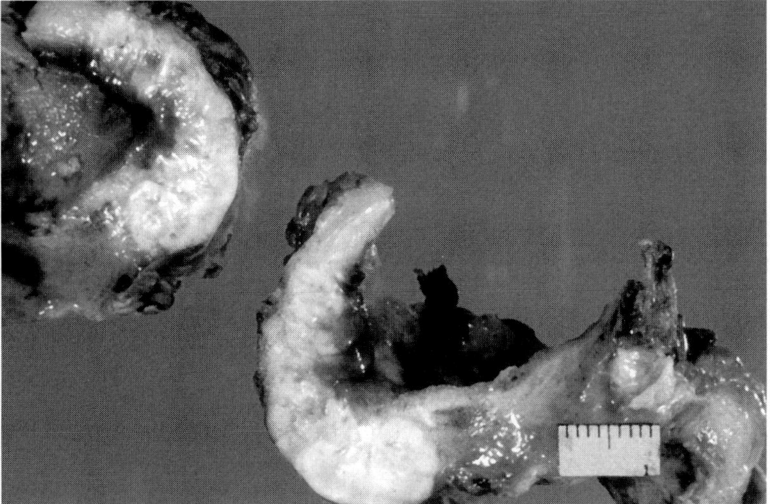

Figure 11–20. Gallbladder with plaquelike thickening of the wall due to xanthogranulomatous cholecystitis.

cholecystectomy specimens. Although cases have been identified in association with gallbladder carcinoma,[169] this is usually considered to be a chance association. Some examples of xanthogranulomatous cholecystitis may have elevated serum CA 19-9 without carcinoma being present.[170]

Eosinophilic Cholecystitis

Eosinophilic cholecystitis should be diagnosed only when there is a massive infiltration of the gallbladder wall by sheets of eosinophils. These may occur as a pure population or mixed with other inflammatory cells, especially lymphocytes. Smaller numbers of eosinophils are not uncommonly encountered in the healing phases of acute and chronic cholecystitis and do not, therefore, fulfill the criteria for this diagnosis.[171] As rigidly defined, therefore, eosinophilic cholecystitis is an uncommon condition (6.4% of cholecystectomy specimens), although up to 22% of gallbladders removed at cholecystectomy may contain some eosinophil infiltration.[171]

Eosinophilic cholecystitis probably represents a group of disorders, rather than a single

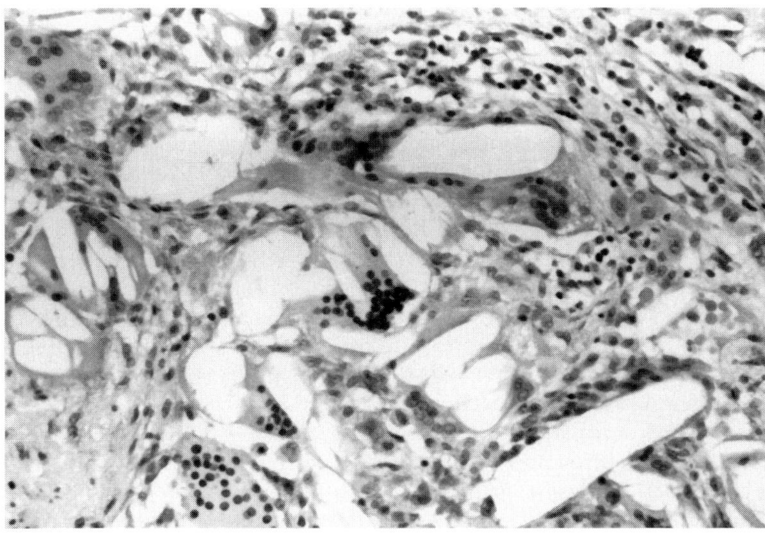

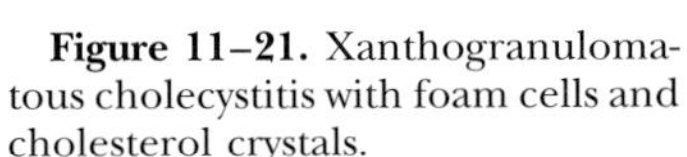

Figure 11–21. Xanthogranulomatous cholecystitis with foam cells and cholesterol crystals.

condition. Several clinical groups are recognized,[172] including

- A group of patients with peripheral eosinophilia who have evidence of asthma or other allergic symptoms. In extreme examples, these individuals may have a hypereosinophilic syndrome with myocardial damage and an eosinophilic pericarditis.
- Patients with peripheral eosinophilia who also have evidence of eosinophil infiltration of other organs within the gastrointestinal tract (eosinophilic gastroenteritis)
- Patients with parasitic disease of the liver and biliary tract
- Individuals with known drug hypersensitivity
- Patients with eosinophilia restricted to the gallbladder, where it represents a form of primary cholecystitis. Here, tissue eosinophilia, rather than the more usual types of inflammatory exudation, is predominant.

Eosinophilia confined to the gallbladder falls into two subtypes. One group consists of male patients who present with subacute left upper abdominal pain and obstructive jaundice due to edema and mural inflammation of the gallbladder and bile duct. Gallstones are not present.[173,174] A second group consists of female patients who present with abdominal pain but without clinical evidence of biliary obstruction. Paradoxically, these women all have cholecystolithiasis.[175,176]

The hypereosinophilic syndrome[177] is a rare condition characterized by an extreme degree of blood eosinophilia (often in the range of 50,000 to 100,000/μL) with corresponding tissue eosinophilia. Multiple organs are involved and death may result from myocardial fibrosis and congestive heart failure. Tissue damage is caused by release of toxic substances from eosinophil granules.[178] Cases have been recognized in which gallbladder disease was a major manifestation of the condition.[178,179]

Eosinophilic gastroenteritis may also affect the gallbladder.[180] Some of these patients, particularly children, may have a food allergy, but in adults, the cause is often unknown. Parasites that have been reported as causing eosinophilic cholecystitis include echinococcus (hydatid cysts).[181] We have seen minor degrees of eosinophilia associated with degenerating ova of schistosomiasis, but infestation by *Opisthorchis* (*Clonorchis*) *sinensis* causes a neutrophilic cholangitis. Little information is available about the relationship between drugs and eosinophilic cholecystitis. A single case report documents the association in a patient taking cephalosporin.[179]

CHOLECYSTITIS AND INFLAMMATORY BOWEL DISEASE

Sclerosing cholangitis is a complication of idiopathic inflammatory bowel disease, either ulcerative colitis or Crohn's disease.[182] However, as the name suggests, the condition generally affects the extra- and intrahepatic bile ducts and spares the gallbladder. One study that formally compared gallbladders of patients with primary sclerosing cholangitis (PSC) to gallbladders of patients with the usual type of chronic cholecystitis found few differences,[183] although as might be expected with an "autoimmune" disease, PSC cholecystitis contained a dense lymphocytic infiltrate with relatively fewer macrophages present.

A more recent study[184] specifically comparing PSC gallbladders with those from other diseases demonstrated a unique type of PSC cholecystitis. This was acalculous, with a diffuse chronic inflammatory infiltrate, especially in the lamina propria, which was rich in plasma cells (lymphoplasmacytic acalculous cholecystitis). It was present in 55% of PSC gallbladders studied. Control gallbladders did not show extensive plasma cell infiltration.

Crohn's disease has rarely been described as involving the gallbladder.[185] The pattern of involvement is similar to that encountered in the bowel, with panmural inflammation, characterized by lymphoid aggregates, fibrosis, and discrete noncaseating granulomas.

UNUSUAL TYPES OF GALLBLADDER INFECTION

Most infections of the gallbladder are bacterial and produce the clinical and pathologic picture of acute or chronic cholecystitis.[78,97,126] Gut flora are the typical causative organisms, especially *E. coli*. However, a variety of unusual and some exotic infections have been described. These include bacteria, viruses, fungi, and parasites (Table 11–1).

Typhoid Fever

Typhoid fever classically localizes to the gallbladder after the third week of infection, where

Table 11–1. Infections of the Gallbladder

Bacteria
Escherichia coli
Klebsiella
Clostridium perfringens
Salmonella
Campylobacter jejuni
Vibrio cholerae
Brucella abortus
Legionella
Haemophilus segnis
Leptospira
Mycobacterium tuberculosis
Mycobacterium leprae
Mycobacterium avium-intracellulare
Treponema pallidum
Actinomyces israelii
Fungi
Candida species
Cryptococcus neoformans
Torulopsis glabrata
Viruses
Epstein–Barr virus
Hepatitis A
Cytomegalovirus
Protozoa
Giardia lamblia
Trypanosoma cruzei
Leishmania donovani
Entamoeba histolytica
Isospora belli
Cryptosporidia
Enterocytozoon bieneusi
Encephalitozoon intestinalis
Pneumocystis carinii

it becomes a source of residual organisms.[79] In many instances, no gallbladder symptoms are produced and the individual becomes a "carrier." However, when organisms do localize to the gallbladder, they may result in an episode of acute cholecystitis.[79] This episode can happen as early as 3 weeks after acquisition of the disease or may develop many years later.[186] The gallbladder becomes distended, with areas of hemorrhage and necrosis. Perforation is common, but if this does not occur, an empyema may develop. Chronic typhoid cholecystitis may resemble the usual appearance of chronic cholecystitis and gallstones may be present.[187] Impaction of gallstones can result in hydrops formation.[120] Some authors[129] have emphasized the association of *S. typhi* with chronic follicular cholecystitis. Other salmonella organisms that may colonize the gallbladder and biliary tract include *S. paratyphi,*[188] *S. virchow,*[189] *S. javiana,*[190] *S. heidelberg,*[191] *S. indiana,*[192] and *S. oranienberg.*[193] Persistence of infection may be facilitated by morphologic abnormalities in the biliary tract, such as gallstones[187] and Caroli's syndrome.[191] For many years, it has been recognized that chronic typhoid cholecystitis predisposes to the development of gallbladder carcinoma.[188,194,195] The precise risk of carcinoma varies between different studies, which have surveyed diverse populations. In Bolivia, the odds ratio (OR) for carcinoma development was 12.7 (confidence interval [CI], 1.5 to 598),[188] whereas in Scotland,[188] the risk was greater (OR, 167; CI, 54 to 389). A study from northern India[195] also showed a higher prevalence of bile culture positivity for *Salmonella* among patients with gallbladder cancer than among matched controls.

Cholera

For many years, it has been recognized that individuals with cholera may develop disease in the gallbladder as well as in the small intestine.[84] Typically, the patients live in Third World countries,[85] although visitors to those countries may become infected and import the disease when they return home.[86] Both O1 toxin–positive and Ol-negative types have been recovered.[85,86] Infections with *V. cholerae* produce no specific pathology and the gallbladder resembles the usual type of acute acalculous cholecystitis. In common with cholera, the gallbladder may also become infected in cases of diarrhea due to *C. jejuni.*[88] These, too, resemble typical acute cholecystitis, although some gallbladders may contain calculi and otherwise appear as typical chronic cholecystitis.[196] Other organisms recovered from the gallbladder include *H. segnis,*[89] *Legionella,*[87] *Brucella,*[197] and *Leptospira.*[91,198,199] Infections of the gallbladder by anaerobic gas forming organisms have been discussed in the section on emphysematous cholecystitis.

Tuberculosis

Tuberculosis of the gallbladder is exceedingly rare, particularly in westernized countries. It is also relatively uncommon in Third World countries, where tuberculous pulmonary infection is more prevalent.[200–204] This infrequency of gallbladder tuberculosis may be a result of the inhibitory effect of bile on growth of the organism. When infection does occur, it may be present as an isolated finding, as a component of miliary tuberculosis, or in association with tuberculous peritonitis. It seems probable that in most instances, spread of infection occurs via the bloodstream, although in instances of tuberculous peritonitis, dissemination could reach the gallbladder via lymphatics. Gallbladder tuberculosis may occur at any age, although the majority of patients are older than 40 years. Women are more commonly affected than men. Symptomatology is quite nonspecific and consists of vague upper abdominal discomfort and pain, sometimes related to food. Jaundice is unusual. Examination of the excised gallbladder generally reveals a shrunken fibrotic organ with a thickened wall and numerous dense serosal adhesions. The wall is grayish in color and small tubercles may be visible on the serosa. The lumen may contain pus, which may be liquid or may have the classical caseous appearance. Gallstones may or may not be present and the mucosa is generally extensively ulcerated. On microscopic examination, widespread or even confluent granuloma formation is seen, with central caseous necrosis. Ziehl–Neelson staining may identify acid-/alcohol-fast bacteria. Nonspecific chronic inflammation and fibrosis often entirely replace the muscularis. Complications of gallbladder tuberculosis include free perforation, localized perforation,[204] and fistula formation.[205] Fistulas may form between the gallbladder and the common bile duct, or the duodenum. There are no reported examples of carcinoma complicating gallbladder tuberculosis, although there is one instance of an association with papillomatosis.[203]

Leprosy

Leprosy rarely affects the gastrointestinal tract.[206,207] There is only one report[207] providing details of the morphologic appearances. In this case, the gallbladder was edematous and had focal areas of hemorrhage, producing a gross "mosaic" pattern. Microscopically, the changes had a lepromatous, rather than tuberculoid, pattern. Areas of necrosis and nonspecific inflammation were noted and Fite's stain showed organisms within macrophages and endothelial cells.

Syphilis

No recent descriptions exist of syphilis involving the gallbladder. Older reports mention that in tertiary syphilis, gummas may form within the wall of the gallbladder or in adjacent structures, such as the liver, where they may indent the gallbladder.

Actinomycosis

Actinomycosis of the gallbladder is a rare condition. Most reports describe an inflammatory mass in the region of the gallbladder that may also involve the common bile duct;[208–210] however, there are reports of cases that clinically mimicked acute[211] and chronic[212] cholecystitis. At laparotomy, the gallbladder is usually thick walled and inflamed. It may contain pus in which yellow flecks are identified. These are collections of organisms, the so-called sulfur granules. Inflammatory tissue may surround the gallbladder and involve the undersurface of the liver, and rarely, this mass may contain multiple sinuses. Gallstones may or may not be present. Histologically, the mucosa is generally extensively ulcerated and replaced by chronically inflamed granulation tissue containing microabscesses. The bacterial colonies are present within the microabscesses. The granules consist of a mass of filamentous organisms that are deeply hematoxophilic on routine sections and are also gram positive. One case has been reported in which actinomycosis was associated with adenocarcinoma.[213] This is regarded as a chance occurrence.

Fungal Infections

Fungi are infrequently the cause of cholecystitis, although *Candida* species are by far the organisms most commonly isolated. The majority of patients are either debilitated or immunosuppressed,[214–216] but in some individuals, infection occurs secondary to endoscopic retrograde cholangiopancreatography (ERCP)[217] or after placement of a stent.[216] In debilitated patients, infection of the gallbladder occurs against a background of infection at multiple other sites, with or without candidemia. In almost all the cases described, candidal infection produced the clinical and pathologic picture of acute cholecystitis. Cystic duct obstruction, as a result of inflammation and edema, is common, and external drainage of this can be a lifesaving procedure. Histologic examination of tissues reveals a nonspecific picture of acute inflammation, with purulent exudate in which hyphae and spores of *Candida* may be identified. In one instance, a xanthogranulomatous reaction was encountered.[218]

Other fungi causing gallbladder disease have been described in individual case reports. Cryptococcal infection is generally part of disseminated disease in patients with acquired immunodeficiency syndrome (AIDS).[219,220] The gallbladder involvement is incidental to life-threatening involvement at other locations. *Torulopsis glabrata* has been isolated from the gallbladder of an individual with adult-onset diabetes mellitus.[221] Granulomatous inflammation was identified on histologic examination and the patient made a complete recovery. Obstructive jaundice may occur when fungal organisms cause an inflammatory lymphadenitis of nodes within the porta hepatis. This has been described with coccidiomycosis[222] and blastomycosis.[223]

Viral Infections

Viral infections of the gallbladder are extremely rare in immunocompetent patients. They have been described in children with Epstein–Barr virus infections, who may develop cholecystitis with hydrops formation.[118] Ultrasound examination of the gallbladder in these cases may show marked thickening of the wall up to 1 cm.[224,225] There are rare cases of hepatitis A cholecystitis.[226,227] In immunosuppressed patients, cytomegalovirus (CMV) infection of the gallbladder is relatively common and frequently occurs in association with protozoal infection.

Protozoal Infections

Protozoal infections of the gallbladder are also most conveniently divided into those cases occurring in immunocompetent patients and those occurring in immunosuppressed individuals. In the former category, infections are rare but may include *Giardia lamblia*,[228–230] *Trypanosoma cruzei*,[231,232] *Leishmania*,[233] and *Entamoeba histolytica*.[234,235] Giardial infection of the small bowel may result in symptoms that mimic cholecystitis. Cases have been described in which giardial cysts and trophozoites have been recovered from bile that has either been aspirated from the gallbladder or harvested from the duodenal papilla.[229] The organism has also been found in mucosal scrapings from individuals with chronic cholecystitis and ulceration.[228] South American trypanosomiasis (Chagas' disease) has a chronic phase in which organisms may localize to destroy ganglion cells throughout the gastrointestinal tract. Typically, the esophagus is affected and becomes dilated and aperistaltic.[232] Rarely, similar changes may be encountered in the biliary system, resulting in dilation of both the gallbladder and bile ducts.[231] This abnormality, which can be demonstrated radiographically, does not seem to be symptomatic. In visceral leishmaniasis (kala-azar), cholecystitis may be present as part of other systemic manifestations but is rarely a prominent feature.[233] Amebiasis of the gallbladder may occur in two forms. Most commonly, an amebic abscess of the liver ruptures into the gallbladder.[234] The gallbladder becomes filled with necrotic material containing sparse numbers of inflammatory cells. The trophozoite form of the amebae are usually readily identified, if they are specifically looked for. In a single-case report,[235] primary amebiasis of the gallbladder is described in which there was no liver abscess. The gallbladder was distended and contained bile-stained mucus. Marked acute and chronic inflammatory changes, along with desquamation of the mucosa, were noted microscopically.

In immunosuppressed patients, viral and protozoal infections of the gallbladder frequently coexist. Most patients have AIDS, but infection may also rarely occur in immunosuppression from other causes. CMV[236–242] may occur in association with coccidian protozoa[237,240,242–244] or microsporidia.[242,245–248] Coccidian parasites include *Cryptosporidia*[240,242,243] and *Isospora belli*.[242,244] Microsporidia include the species *Enterocytozoon bieneusi*[240,245] and *Encephalitozoon* (*Septata*) *intestinalis*.[242,246,248] Additional rarely described organisms encountered in the gallbladders of AIDS patients include *Pneumocystis carinii*[242] and *Mycobacterium avium-intracellulare*.[247] The presence of one of these organisms, or a combination of them, in the biliary system may give rise to the clinical syndrome of AIDS cholangiopathy,[245,249,250] also referred to as AIDS-associated sclerosing cholangitis.[251] This consists of cholestasis, right upper quadrant pain, low-grade fever, and biliary tract dilation. Sometimes there is accompanying stenosis at the ampulla of Vater. The dilation of the biliary system may be simple or may take the form of dilated segments, with intervening stenotic segments. The gallbladder is typically dilated and histologically presents as an acute acalculous cholecystitis. The mucosa may be extensively ulcerated and replaced by granulation tissue. CMV inclusions are most numerous within endothelial cells

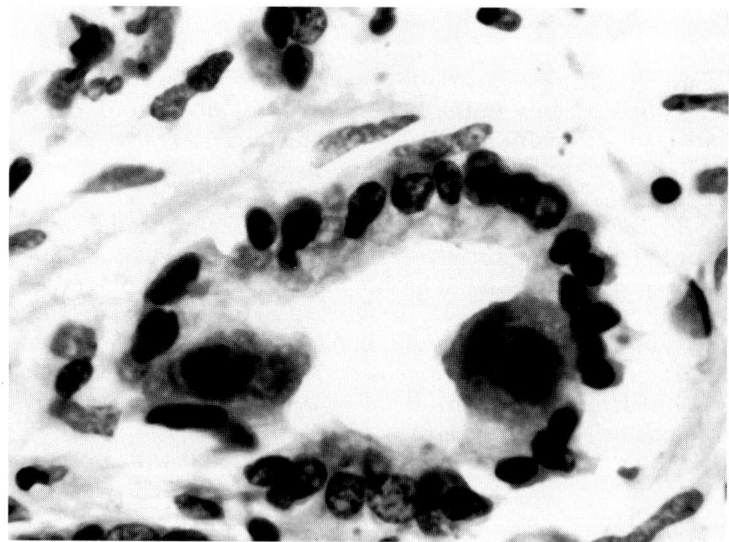

Figure 11–22. Typical cytomegalovirus inclusions from the gallbladder of a person with acquired immunodeficiency syndrome. Note the presence of intranuclear and cytoplasmic inclusions.

present in the granulation tissue but may also be encountered in any surviving epithelial cells. The intranuclear inclusions are round or oval with a smooth outline and are surrounded by a clear halo, separating them from the nuclear membrane, which is enhanced by chromatin condensation. They are generally eosinophilic in routine sections (Fig. 11–22). Cytoplasmic inclusions may also be recognized. These are present as multiple granular basophilic structures. They are PAS positive.

Cryptosporidia in the gallbladder appear, by light microscopy, to be attached to the surface of epithelial cells (Fig. 11–23). However, by electron microscopy, they are seen to be intracellular but extracytoplasmic—that is, they are attached to the inner aspect of the cell membrane. They measure 2 to 2.5 μm in diameter (approximately half the size of a lymphocyte) and are basophilic or amphophilic on routine staining. Giemsa is the most useful special stain, where they appear dark blue.

I. belli may be found within parasitophorous vacuoles in the cytoplasm of the gallbladder epithelial cells. At high-power microscopic examination, several stages in the life cycle may be identified (schizonts, merozoites, and macro- and microgametocytes). Although routine stains are perfectly adequate for identifying the presence of parasitophorous vacuoles, better vi-

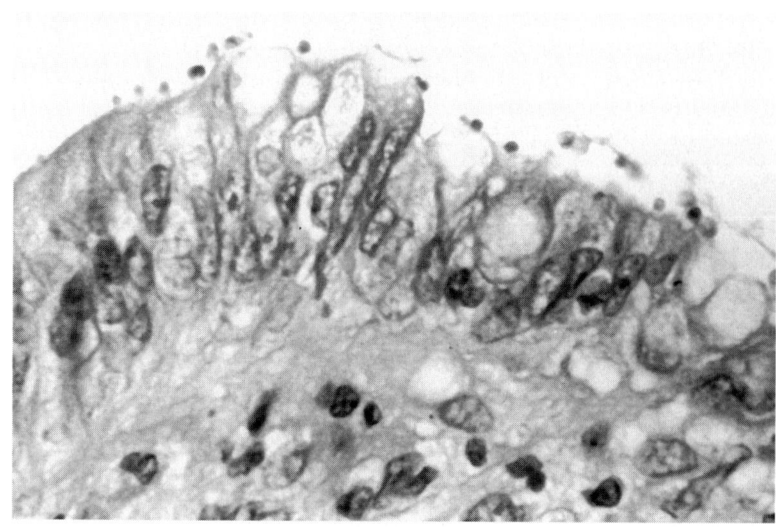

Figure 11–23. *Cryptosporidia* attached to the mucosal surface of the gallbladder.

sualization may be obtained using either Giemsa, trichrome, or PAS stains. Different stages of the life cycle are best appreciated by using plastic sections stained with toluidine blue.[252]

The microsporidia *Enterocytozoon bieneusi* and *Encephalitozoon septata* are also found within parasitophorous vacuoles in the epithelial cell cytoplasm. The vacuoles are relatively easily recognized on routine sections, but speciation requires considerable experience and reference should be made to specialized texts for the details. One basic distinction, however, is that *Encephalitozoon septata* occurs within separated parasitiphorous vacuoles resembling honeycombs, whereas *Enterocytozoon bieneusi* is found within a single vacuole.[253]

Parasitic Infections

A variety of helminths (worms) may cause disease of the gallbladder. However, in the majority of cases, it is the bile ducts that are primarily affected. These are discussed in Chapter 15 on bile duct inflammation. The gallbladder may, however, be involved in patients with schistosomiasis (*Bilharzia*). Gallstones may complicate cholecystitis; characterized by a fibrocalcific reaction in the gallbladder wall.[254,255]

VASCULITIS

Almost any form of vasculitis can involve the gallbladder; however, none are common. They are listed in Table 11–2.

Polyarteritis nodosa may be encountered as a manifestation of generalized disease or as a monoarterial form, isolated to the gallbladder.[256–261] The disease may present clinically as an acute acalculous cholecystitis or may be discovered incidentally in gallbladders removed for cholelithiasis. At surgery, the gallbladder wall is often thickened and edematous. On histologic examination alone, there is no way of distinguishing the two forms, so the surgeon should be advised that the arteritis may simply be an incidental finding or may herald the later onset of a widespread and severe disease. Systemic involvement may occur up to 1 year after the initial diagnosis at cholecystectomy. The histologic hallmark of polyarteritis is the finding of fibrinoid necrosis, involving medium-size arteries (Fig. 11–24). This may be accompanied by a mixed acute and chronic inflammatory infiltrate. In some cases, eosinophil infiltration can occur. This should be distinguished from eosinophilic cholecystitis, which may display perivascular inflammation but lacks fibrinoid necrosis. The necrosis initially involves the media, with destruction of the elastic laminae and smooth muscle. In larger vessels, only a segment of the wall may be affected (Fig. 11–25), so that when fibrous healing occurs, a beadlike (nodose) aneurysm may form. In the acute phase, endothelial damage may result in thrombosis. The wall of the arteries may be so necrotic that rupture and intra-abdominal hemorrhage occurs. If healing takes place, focal scarring of the vessel wall may be a precursor to formation of the typical beaded aneurysm. Small foci of infarction may be seen in the wall and the mucosa may show focal ulceration.

Churg–Strauss syndrome may affect the gallbladder as part of a systemic disease but is rarely isolated to that organ.[261–264] It consists of a disease resembling polyarteritis nodosa but accompanied by asthma, pulmonary infiltrates, and eosinophilia. Histologically, it is characterized by a necrotizing granulomatous vasculitis, resembling Wegener's granulomatosis. Within the gallbladder, it presents as an acute acalculous cholecystitis, with small (2- to 10-mm) nodules in the wall. These represent foci of granulomatous vasculitis, with surrounding tissue inflammation, in which eosinophils can be prominent. The diagnosis of Churg–Strauss syndrome cannot be made by histologic examination alone; it requires correlation with clinical and other laboratory findings.

Rheumatoid vasculitis affecting the gallbladder is rare.[265,266] In most described cases, the individuals have severe arthritis, low serum complement levels, and high levels of circulating immune complexes. Necrotizing vasculitis, resembling polyarteritis nodosa, is the most common histologic finding, but it is also possi-

Table 11–2. Types of Vasculitis Involving the Gallbladder

Polyarteritis nodosa
Localized
Generalized
Allergic granulomatosis (Churg–Strauss syndrome)
Rheumatoid vasculitis
Systemic lupus erythematosus
Henoch–Schönlein purpura
Mixed connective-tissue disease
Wegener's granulomatosis

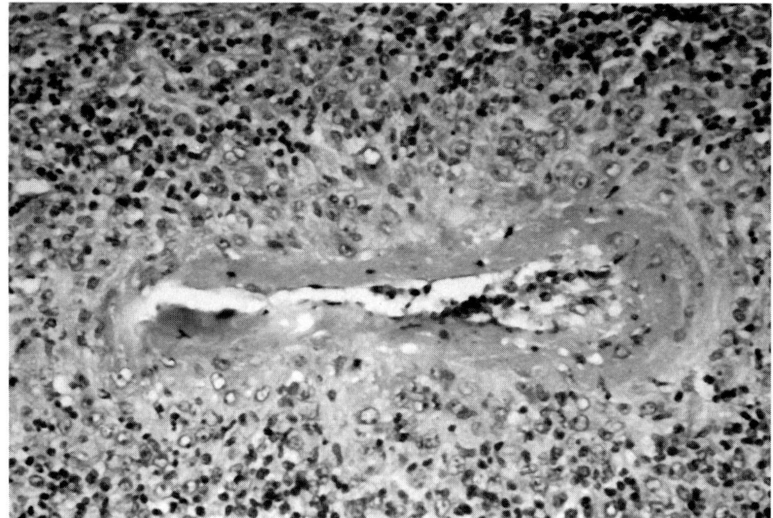

Figure 11–24. Polyarteritis in the wall of the gallbladder. This is characterized by fibrinoid necrosis with destruction of the media and elastic laminae.

ble to encounter a small vessel vasculitis.[261] Lupus erythematous affects the gastrointestinal tract in 10% to 64% of patients. Gallbladder involvement is less common but does occur[267,268] and, again, tends to be present in individuals with severe systemic disease. Inflammation typically involves small vessels, including venules. A similar small-vessel vasculitis has also been described in the gallbladder as a complication of mixed connective-tissue disease.[269]

Henoch-Schönlein syndrome consists of palpable cutaneous purpura, arthritis, and abdominal pain. Typically, it affects children, who develop an intestinal vasculitis with rectal bleeding. Surprisingly, gallbladder involvement is rare.[270,271] In one described patient, the gallbladder was edematous, with submucosal hemorrhage and bleeding manifest clinically as hemobilia. Microscopic examination revealed small-vessel leucocytoclastic vasculitis. In other reports, the patient developed hydrops of the gallbladder.[119,271] Wegener's granulomatosis is a systemic vasculitis, with a classical clinical triad of sinusitis and pulmonary and renal involvement. Rarely, the gastrointestinal tract, including the gallbladder, can be affected.[272] The histologic appearances are typically those of a necrotizing vasculitis, with "geographic" areas

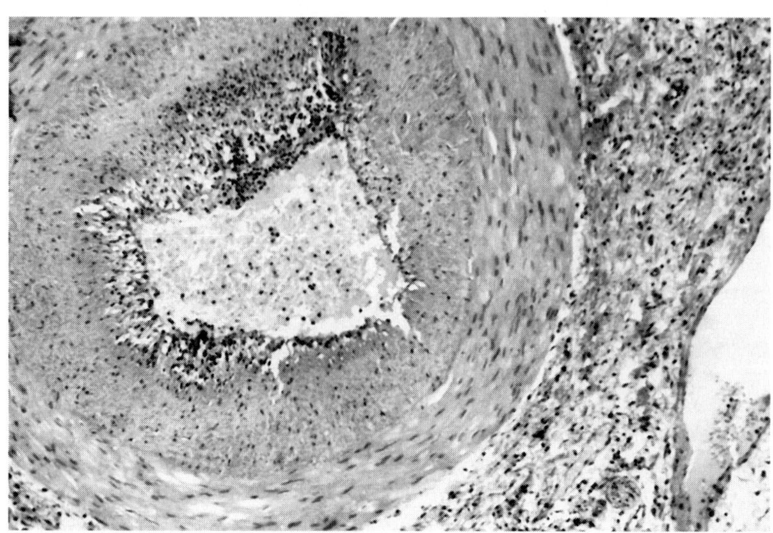

Figure 11–25. The main cystic artery involved by polyarteritis nodosa. Note the segmental inflammation.

of necrosis (i.e., the outline of the necrotic tissue is completely irregular).

ISCHEMIA AND INFARCTION

Vascular insufficiency is an uncommon cause of gallbladder disease. A variety of underlying causes exist (Table 11–3). Much of the literature on this subject is confusing and contradictory, as causes may overlap and it is sometimes difficult to be sure which is a primary and which is a secondary complication.

Vasculitis has already been discussed. Vascular occlusive disease may involve arteries or veins and may occur at the level of the cystic vessels or, more proximally, in the celiac or hepatic vessels. Varying degrees of ischemic damage to the gallbladder have been described, either partial or complete. The term *gangrenous cholecystitis* has been applied to global infarction. In some cases, this is secondary to severe acalculous cholecystitis,[77,273] whereas in other cases it has a primary ischemic cause.[274]

A large number of causes of arterial insufficiency leading to gallbladder ischemia have been described. Older literature tended to emphasize primary thrombosis,[275,276] atherosclerotic emboli,[277] and compression of vessels by neoplasms growing in the porta hepatis. More recent reports have emphasized exotic causes of ischemia. These include transcatheter arterial embolization in patients undergoing treatment for malignant hepatic neoplasms,[278,279] surgical mishaps,[280] penetrating duodenal ulcer injuring the cystic artery,[281] cocaine abuse,[282] and antiphospholipid syndrome.[283] Arterial occlusion may also occur in cases of torsion (volvulus). This list is by no means exhaustive.

Table 11–3. Causes of Gallbladder Infarction

Arterial occlusion
Thrombosis
Emboli
Vasculitis
Tumor compression
Surgical damage
Volvulus
Hypertension
Venous occlusion
Thrombosis
Tumor compression
Inflammation
Acute acalculous cholecystitis
Acute calculous cholecystitis
Trauma
Radiotherapy

Some authors have pointed out that severe hypertension without vascular occlusion or thrombosis may also result in gallbladder infarction.[284] It must be presumed that spasm of vessels is responsible for the damage in these cases, the best documented example of which occurred in a man with malignant hypertension.[284]

In a series of 43 cholecystectomies performed for ischemic damage to the gallbladder, full-thickness infarction of the wall was observed in 27 (63%) and mucosal necrosis with partial muscularis necrosis in the remaining 16 (37%).[274] Grossly, it was possible to divide the cholecystectomy specimens into those with a thickened wall (35) and those with an attenuated wall (8). All 35 gallbladders with a thickened wall had gallstones and the ischemia was considered to arise from local thrombosis occurring within the wall of the gallbladder. These 35 cases consisted of all 16 cases with lesser degrees of infarction plus 19 of the 27 cases with more extensive infarction. In the remaining 8 cases of extensive infarction, the gallbladder was dilated and ischemic changes were thought to have arisen as a result of extramural vascular insufficiency. These gallbladders did not contain calculi.

Histologic changes in infarcted gallbladders mimic those of infarction in other organs. The mucosa may be partly or completely eroded, with granulation tissue at the base of any ulcers. Surviving mucosa is often flattened and atrophic. The lamina propria is edematous and hemorrhagic. Varying degrees of infarction and early fibrosis may be found in the muscularis. Chronic ischemic cholecystitis analogous to chronic ischemic colitis does not appear to have been described. This probably reflects the fact that even minor degrees of gallbladder ischemia are symptomatic and likely to result in a cholecystectomy when the disease is in an acute stage.

TORSION AND VOLVULUS

The terms *torsion* and *volvulus* are regarded as synonymous in reference to the gallbladder. Torsion occurs when the gallbladder either has a long mesentery supporting it on the undersurface of the liver or has no mesentery at all and is attached to the porta hepatis only by a pedicle consisting of the cystic duct, vein, and artery. In most instances, the underlying abnormality is congenital, but it may be acquired in rare circumstances when there is fibrosis, atrophy, and retraction of the liver, resulting in a lengthening of the existing peritoneal attachment of the gallbladder.

Torsion occurs when the gallbladder twists on its long axis. Twisting exceeding 180° is often referred to as complete torsion and almost invariably results in compromise of the blood supply. Lesser degrees of twisting are termed incomplete torsion. Rotation may occur in a clockwise or anticlockwise direction.

Factors precipitating torsion are poorly defined. A majority of cases have been described in elderly women;[285] torsion in these women may occur as a result of atrophy of intra-abdominal fat,[286] kyphoscoliosis (leading to a stooping posture),[287] and to the presence of gallstones, which may cause increased weight of the gallbladder.[288] The possibility that stones in the gallbladder are a precipitating factor is supported by the finding that calculi are present in 50% of gallbladders with torsion but in only 5% of control gallbladders.[288]

Symptoms of torsion are usually hard to distinguish from those of biliary colic and acute cholecystitis.[289] In minor degrees of torsion, there may be brief episodes of epigastric or right hypochondrial pain that subsides as the torsion resolves spontaneously. In more severe cases, there is constant abdominal pain and a firm, tender mass may be identified on abdominal examination. The diagnosis is generally made only by laparotomy[290] or laparoscopy.[291] Radiologic evaluation may be normal,[291] but ultrasound examination can reveal a thickened, multilayered gallbladder wall.[292]

Gross and histologic examination of resected gallbladders that have undergone torsion show features of infarction. The lumen contains fresh or altered blood and blood-stained bile. Calculi are present in 50% of cases and may or may not be impacted into the cystic duct. The mucosal surface is also hemorrhagic and the wall, together with mesentery distal to the torsion, is hemorrhagic and edematous. Microscopic examination reveals infarction of varying degree. In early cases, only the mucosa will be necrotic, but in long-standing torsion there may be a panmural infarction, with only "ghost" outlines of original tissue architecture.

Rare examples of torsion have been described in which only the distal portion of the gallbladder, particularly the fundus, is affected.[293] This arises when the proximal portion of the gallbladder is firmly anchored to the undersurface of the liver but the distal portion has a long mesentery.

TRAUMA

Traumatic damage to the gallbladder is rare. When present, it is generally accompanied by damage to the liver and other major abdominal organs.[294,295] Conventionally, injuries are divided into penetrating and blunt. In most series, penetrating injuries are the most common,[296,297] generally resulting from gunshots or stab wounds. Blunt trauma results from motor vehicle accidents, falls, or kicks.[298–300] In one series, the overall mortality associated with gallbladder injury was 16%.[295] However, this was largely because of associated hepatic (50%) and pancreatic (17%) damage. Isolated gallbladder injury occurred in only 8% of cases.

A variety of gallbladder injuries may follow trauma. Contusions are probably the least significant of these, although they are among the most common. Often, they will not become apparent until laparotomy, because of the presence of other more severe injuries. In published reports on series[298,299] of blunt trauma, they accounted for between 45% and 68% of gallbladder injuries. Gross examination of resected specimens will show areas of hemorrhage into the wall, associated with edema. The lamina propria is generally most severely affected, although there may be mucosal disruption and small amounts of intraluminal bleeding. Large hematomas may cause pressure on the muscularis, leading to necrosis and subsequent rupture. If immediate cholecystectomy is not performed, the hematomas will organize with an initial inflammatory response and later focal fibrosis and hemosiderin deposition.

Avulsion of the gallbladder is the second most commonly encountered injury in blunt trauma, accounting for between 45% and 32% of cases.[298,299] Varying degrees of avulsion may be recognized. Occasionally, the gallbladder may become totally detached from both the liver and biliary tract and float free within the abdomen. Partial avulsions may detach the gallbladder from the undersurface of the liver, leaving it still connected to the bile duct. In both types of avulsion, there can be considerable bleeding into the peritoneal cavity and sometimes this may originate from a damaged cystic artery.

Rarer types of injury due to blunt trauma include lacerations that may or may not be accompanied by rupture.[301] Injuries of this type are most common in normal gallbladders, which are thin walled, in contrast to gallbladders thickened by chronic cholecystitis. The other main predisposing factor to this type of injury is the recent ingestion of alcohol. This seems to work in two ways: first, by causing sphincteric constriction, resulting in gallbladder distension, and second, by relaxing musculature in the anterior abdominal wall, thus producing less resistance to a blow. Children also seem prone to traumatic rupture, presumably because they tend to have normal gallbladders and less well developed abdominal musculature.[294,300,302] Free perforation of the gallbladder will result in leakage of bile into the peritoneal cavity. Provided the bile is sterile, this is well tolerated, but the presence of infected bile results in a high mortality.

It has recently become recognized that gallbladder trauma may occasionally result in acute acalculous cholecystitis.[303–306] Postulated causes of this include bile stasis, ischemia, infection, factor XII activation, and the Schwarzman reaction.[306] The trauma may not necessarily occur in the gallbladder region and may be relatively minor—for example, trauma occurring after elective surgery.[305] It has been recognized as occurring in 0.5% of patients after injury or severe burns,[304] commonly after an interval of 2 to 3 weeks. The mortality is high, up to 80% in one series.[303] At cholecystectomy, the gallbladder is generally distended and contains viscid bile. Acute inflammation leads to focal necrosis of the wall and subsequent perforation.

FISTULAS

Fistulas involving the gallbladder are quite uncommon. Most reports are of single cases, or small groups of cases, so that general conclusions are hard to draw. In one of the larger series involving 33 cases, fistulas represented 1.9% of all patients treated for biliary tract disease over a 12-year period.[307] This is in accordance with older estimates.

Various causes have been identified (Table 11–4). The vast majority (> 90%) occur in individuals with gallstones and chronic cholecystitis. Not surprisingly, therefore, the male-to-female ratio is 1 : 1.5, with an age range at occurrence of 43 to 85 years and an average age of 63 to 70 years.[307,308] It is supposed that fistulas arise as a result of pericystic inflammation and fibrosis, with tethering of adjacent viscera to the gallbladder peritoneum. Calculi become attached to the gallbladder mucosal surface, with initial mucosal erosion and then lodging of a stone in the base of an ulcer. With the action of repeated gallbladder contractions, the stone is driven first into the gallbladder wall, then out into the pericystic fibrous tissue, and ultimately into and through the wall of an adjacent organ.

Table 11–4. Causes of Gallbladder Fistula

Causes
Gallstones
Peptic ulcers
Trauma
Crohn's disease
Tuberculosis
Malignant neoplasm
Congenital

Rarer causes of fistula formation include penetrating gastric and duodenal peptic ulcers,[309] trauma,[310] Crohn's disease,[311] and tuberculosis.[312] Malignant fistulas also fall into this group of rarely occurring causes. Although the primary neoplasm is usually present within the gallbladder,[307,313] it can also be found in the colon, stomach, or pancreas. Congenital fistulas of the biliary tract generally involve the bile ducts but not the gallbladder.

Fistulas from the gallbladder may communicate with a variety of other organs. The most commonly occurring fistula leads to the duodenum,[308,310,314–316] colon,[317,318] and stomach.[319,320] Exceptionally, fistulas may join the gallbladder to the skin,[321–324] thoracic cavity,[325,326] bronchus,[327,328] and umbilicus.[329] The term *Mirizzi syndrome* is applied to a situation in which a calculus impacts in the neck of the gallbladder and erodes through the wall toward either the hepatic duct or common bile duct, initially causing external compression but eventually a fistula.[330,331]

Patients with cholecystoduodenal fistulas generally have a history of chronic cholecystitis, which is sometimes accompanied by episodes of jaundice. A preoperative diagnosis may be made by ERCP or by the finding of pneumobilia. Not uncommonly, the distal opening of the fistula is close to the gastric pylorus and may even straddle it, producing a cholecystoduodenogastric fistula. Complications are rare but include bleeding after erosion of the cystic artery[332] and carcinoma of the gallbladder.[333]

Cholecystocolonic fistulas usually join the gallbladder fundus to the hepatic flexure of the colon. Symptoms are generally nonspecific and usually cannot be distinguished from those of the underlying cholecystitis and gallstone disease. Occasionally, however, they can be specifically related to the abnormal anatomy and include an ascending infection, leading to cholangitis[308] or hepatic abscess formation.[319] Some patients also develop diarrhea,[308] related to drainage of bile acids into the colon, and malabsorption, secondary to the lack of bile salts in the small bowel.[334] Because of the large diameter of the colon, it is unusual for obstruction to result from gallstones, although hemorrhage after erosion of medium-size arteries has been reported.[335]

Cholecystogastric fistulas may occur on their own[320] or as part of a more complex fistula that links gallbladder, stomach, and colon.[319] Although gallstones are the most commonly encountered cause, on rare occasions penetrating peptic ulcer[309] or even gastric carcinomas[336] are responsible. Occasionally, gallstones may enter the stomach, where they obstruct the pylorus or are even vomited up. Pyloric or duodenal bulb obstruction, due to the presence of gallstones, is known as *Bouveret's syndrome.*[337,338] The syndrome mimics pyloric obstruction due to other causes and is characterized by intractable vomiting and abdominal pain. In cases of choledochogastric fistula, the gallbladder is commonly shrunken, fibrotic, and firmly attached to the undersurface of the liver. The gastric end of the fistula usually terminates in the pylorus.

Cholecystocutaneous fistulas were formerly quite common but are now rarely seen. This is probably a reflection of improved surgical management of cholelithiasis, which was formerly the most common cause. Empyema of the gallbladder often precedes spontaneous fistula formation, and a fistulous tract may be formed after gallbladder rupture. The cutaneous opening of the fistula is most commonly in the right upper quadrant of the abdomen, but abscess tracking along the falciform ligament can lead to an opening in the region of the umbilicus.[329] Biliary cutaneous fistulas may complicate biliary surgery, in which case the skin openings may be related to surgical incisions or scars.[321] Cutaneous fistulas to the skin usually discharge a mixture of bile, gallstones, mucus, pus, and necrotic debris.

Fistulas to the pleural cavity and bronchus are most commonly associated with a misplaced gallbladder,[326,328] which may be present on the superior ventral surface of the liver. Fistulas to the pleural cavity present with fever, tachypnea, and septic shock.[325,326] Radiologic examination commonly reveals a pleural effusion with underlying pulmonary consolidation, and thoracentesis yields bile-stained fluid, in which gallstones may be present.[325] Fistulas to the bronchus may present clinically with biloptysis and severe bronchospasm.[327,328,339] Because bile is capable of provoking extreme degrees of irritation, continuous drainage of the gallbladder contents into the bronchial tree is capable of causing respiratory failure, secondary to a chemical pneumonitis. In common with fistulas draining to the skin, fistulas to the thoracic cavity are often precipitated by acute cholecystitis, with empyema and gallbladder rupture.

Mirizzi syndrome is of considerable interest to surgeons because of the high possibility of damage to the common bile duct that may occur at the time of cholecystectomy if it is not correctly identified.[330,331,340–343] Four types of abnormality are recognized. In type I, a gallstone has eroded to a position alongside the bile duct and is causing external compression. In type II, a cholecystobiliary fistula is present, with erosion of up to one third of the circumference of the bile duct. In type III lesions, the bile duct erosion has destroyed two thirds of the bile duct circumference, and in type IV lesions, the duct is completely destroyed.[330] More recent publications have devised different classification schemes.[344,345] These are not clearly superior to the scheme quoted here. For the purposes of pathologic examination, it is, however, clearly important to distinguish cases of Mirizzi syndrome, with or without structural damage to the common bile duct. In a study of 17,395 individuals undergoing surgery for benign biliary tract disease, 210 (1.3%) had Mirizzi syndrome. Of these, 11% had type I lesions, 41% had type II lesions, 44% had type III lesions, and 4% had type IV lesions.[330] Typical clinical presentations include pain (100% of cases), jaundice (100%), and fever, secondary to cholangitis (71%).[341] At surgery, the gallbladder is often small and contracted. No predisposing conditions are known and the patient's medical history is generally typical of uncomplicated cholecystitis and gallstones.[343]

GALLSTONE ILEUS

The syndrome of gallstone ileus occurs when a biliary calculus erodes out of the gallbladder and passes into the bowel, causing obstruction.[346–348] This accounts for 25% of nonstrangulated small bowel obstruction in patients older than 65 years of age, or 2% of obstruction from all causes.[348] In a series of 74 patients of all ages, there were 55 females (74%) and 19 males (26%) with a mean age of 64.8 years[347] and an age range of 13 to 97 years.[348] The reported incidence of gallstone ileus occurring in persons with biliary-enteric fistulas varies from 9% to 72%.[349–350]

Gallstones entering the gastrointestinal tract may spontaneously pass out with feces or they may, in rare instances, be vomited up. Depending on the size of the gallstone, they may, however, create an obstruction. This may be acute or intermittent, as the gallstone passes with difficulty down the bowel. It has been stated that approximately 10% of gallstones passing into the gastrointestinal tract actually cause obstruction.[351] The size of gallstone required for obstruction to occur is generally considered to be > 2.5 to 3.0 cm in diameter,[352] although obviously this will vary in different individuals. The average size of recovered obstructing calculi is between 3.5 and 4.5 cm.[346]

Most gallstones will impact in the terminal ileum (60.5%), with a further 16.1% arresting in the jejunum.[348] This appears to be because this area is the narrowest part of the bowel. Conditions causing small bowel stricture formation, such as Crohn's disease, will render a patient liable to obstruction when relatively small stones fail to pass.[353] Kinking of the bowel, secondary to peritoneal adhesions, may cause a similar problem. Gallstones impacting in the colon are a relatively rare problem, accounting for only 4% of cases of gallstone ileus.[348] The sigmoid colon (the narrowest segment of the large bowel) is the site most commonly involved. Additional sigmoid luminal narrowing may occur in individuals affected with diverticular disease.[354,355] Smaller numbers of stones may become lodged in the rectum as they fail to pass the anal sphincter. These may require manual removal.

As mentioned, gallstone ileus is predominately a disease of elderly women. Many of the patients are in poor general health, with additional medical problems, such as hypertension, cerebrovascular disease, diabetes mellitus, and ischemic heart disease.[346] These factors make for a high surgical risk and have given rise to discussion in surgical circles as to whether initial treatment should consist simply of stone removal (enterolithotomy) or whether stone removal should be combined with cholecystectomy and excision of the fistula. Reported mortality for enterolithotomy alone is 11.7% and for enterolithotomy combined with biliary surgery is 16.9%.[348] Recurrence of gallstone-induced bowel obstruction in patients undergoing enterolithotomy alone is estimated at 6.0%.[348] However, cholecystectomy does not entirely prevent this complication, as more than one stone may have migrated into the bowel prior to surgery.[356] Morbidity after surgery occurs as a result of wound infection (32%); biliary disease, such as cholangitis and cholecystitis (15%); or intraoperative complications (10%).[348]

In gallstone ileus, the bowel at the time of surgery is dilated proximal to the impaction and collapsed distal to it. Pressure of the stone on the mucosa may cause superficial ulceration or, occasionally, deep ulceration and infarction of the bowel wall. Examination of an excised or recovered stone is important, as the presence of facets will suggest that other calculi may be present, either within the gallbladder or more proximally in the bowel. Chemical analysis of excised gallstones is probably advisable to confirm the presence of bilirubin and cholesterol. Occasionally, gallstones within the gastrointestinal tract may be confused with enteroliths, which also appear as brownish circular objects. Enteroliths would not be expected to be found in association with a biliary fistula.

Upper gastrointestinal obstruction may occur when calculi pass via a biliary fistula to lodge in either the gastric pylorus or duodenal bulb (Bouveret's syndrome). Stones at these locations account, respectively, for 14.2% and 3.5% of all cases of gallstone ileus. The clinical features have already been discussed.

HYPERPLASIA AND METAPLASIA

Mucosal hyperplasia in cholecystectomy specimens has been reported in 1%[357] to 21%[358] of cases. This difference is probably explained by variability in the definition of hyperplasia and in the interpretation of minor degrees of abnormality. Minor degrees of hyperplasia seem to have no clinical significance, so it is hardly worth expending a great deal of effort in defining precisely the cutoff between normal and hyperplastic mucosa. More florid examples of hyperplasia are easier to diagnose, although at present it is uncertain whether they, too, have any clinical significance. Many authors consider it doubtful that hyperplasia is a precursor to

Table 11–5. Proposed Classification of Proliferative Lesions of the Gallbladder

Nonneoplastic
Hyperplasia
Inflammatory/regenerative
Metaplasia
Noninvasive neoplastic
Adenoma
Dysplasia (low grade or high grade)
Invasive neoplasm
Adenocarcinoma

dysplasia and carcinoma;[54,358,359] however, others believe that there is a hyperplasia–dysplasia–carcinoma sequence.[360–363] It is appropriate, however, to clearly distinguish among hyperplasia, metaplasia, and dysplasia, as the literature is replete with confusing terms, such as *villous hyperplasia, papillomatosis, adenomatous hyperplasia, adenomyomatous hyperplasia,* and *atypical hyperplasia.* It is recommended that these now be dropped in favor of simple and clear nomenclature, as outlined below.

It is suggested that the terminology used to describe proliferative lesions of the gallbladder should be simplified and brought into line with those currently proposed for similar lesions of the gastrointestinal tract.[364] Only three classes of lesions are proposed (Table 11–5): nonneoplastic lesions, noninvasive neoplastic lesions, and invasive neoplasms. Neoplastic lesions are fully described in the chapter on gallbladder tumors. Noninvasive neoplasms may be subdivided into adenomas (circumscribed lesions not associated with underlying inflammation) and dysplasia (generally flat or sessile lesions, often associated with underlying inflammation). Dysplasia may be high grade and low grade. High-grade dysplasia incorporates carcinoma in situ. Nonneoplastic lesions may be hyperplastic, metaplastic, or reactive (showing nuclear changes secondary to inflammation) or may contain a combination of types. Occasionally, reactive hyperplastic lesions can be difficult to distinguish from adenoma or dysplasia, in which case the term *indefinite for dysplasia* may be used (Fig. 11–26). Where possible, proliferative lesions should be assigned to one of these categories. In the bowel, this assignment has highly significant prognostic differences. In the gallbladder, the exact nature of the epithelial proliferation is less significant for an individual patient because in the overwhelming majority of patients, the organ has already been removed.

Hyperplasia of the gallbladder mucosa may be primary[357,365] or secondary.[358] Most cases are secondary and are the result of mucosal irritation from gallstones or cholesterolosis. Secondary hyperplasia is also described in metachromatic leukodystrophy.[366] The changes tend to be patchy and are difficult to identify grossly, although velvety reddish patches may be present. Primary hyperplasia may be identifiable as small papillary projections and tends to be more widespread. It may even extend into the cystic

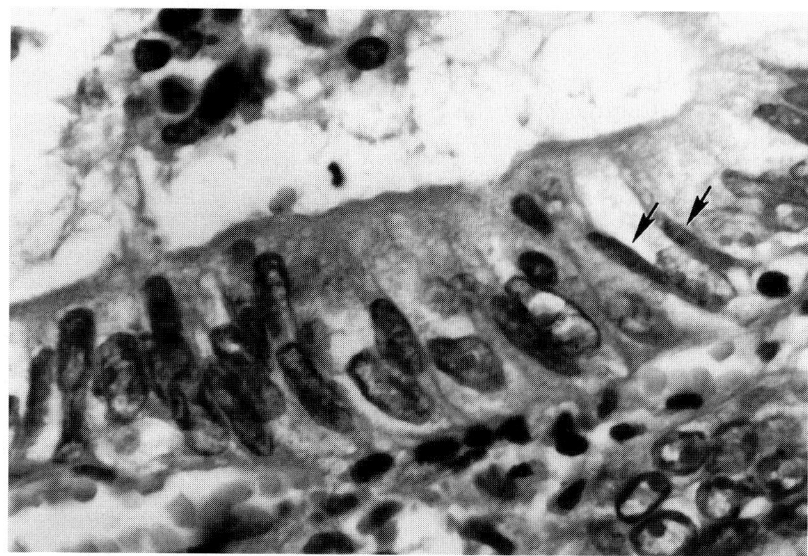

Figure 11–26. Gallbladder mucosa indefinite for dysplasia. Pencil cells are present (*arrows*).

and bile ducts.[365] Primary hyperplasia may rarely occur in association with adenomyomatosis, a combination confusingly termed *adenomyomatous hyperplasia*.[367] In this combination, florid forms of adenomyosis are accompanied by a villous hyperplasia of the lining of Aschoff–Rokitansky sinuses. Mucus gland metaplasia may also be present. Adenomyomatous hyperplasia may also rarely demonstrate hyperplastic Aschoff–Rokitansky sinuses, which extend alongside nerves, thus mimicking an invasive carcinoma.[367]

Microscopically, two types of hyperplasia have been described: villous and spongioid.[358,368] The spongioid type probably represents an artifact in which a complex villous hyperplasia is tangentially sectioned (Fig. 11–27). Villous hyperplasia is characterized by a profound thickening of the mucosa. The folds are taller than normal and closer together. The covering mucosa is usually similar to normal and consists of tall columnar cells with regular basally located nuclei and containing occasional subnuclear clear vacuoles (Fig. 11–28). Occasional "pencil cells" may be encountered. Rarely, the epithelium covering the hyperplastic folds may show low-grade nuclear crowding and pseudostratification, generally accompanied by minor inflammatory changes. In simple hyperplasia, Paneth's cells, endocrine cells, and metaplastic goblet cells are not encountered. Inflammation of the lamina propria may be present but in most cases is not a prominent feature. Localized villous hyperplasia overlaps with, and is probably a precursor to, a hyperplastic polyp.

Hyperplasia is a relatively common finding if cholecystectomy specimens are extensively sectioned, but it is doubtful if this has much significance for the typical North American patient suffering from gallstones. Work from Japan, however, has suggested that, in certain circumstances, hyperplasia may be a precursor or marker lesion for the subsequent development of gallbladder carcinoma.[360–363] Kimura et al.[369] studied patients with an anomalous arrangement of the pancreaticobiliary duct (AAPBD), also known as anomalous union of the pancreaticobiliary duct, or AUPBD,[160–162] and found a 24.6% incidence of gallbladder carcinoma. AAPBD consisted of a junction of the common bile duct and pancreatic duct of Wirsung anatomically outside of the duodenal wall and therefore beyond the influence of the sphincter of Oddi. It seems probable that individuals with this anatomic arrangement have regurgitation and stagnation of pancreatic secretions into the gallbladder. Because of the risk of subsequent carcinoma development, Tokiwa and Iwai examined gallbladders prophylactically removed from 34 children with AAPBD.[362] They found villous hyperplasia without metaplasia or dysplasia in 50% of gallbladders. These changes were not present in control subjects. The morphologic changes were identical to those described above as occurring in elderly North American adults. Furthermore, individuals with hyperplasia had a higher mucosal proliferative index than normal (as measured by the presence of silver-staining nucleolar organizing regions). This work was

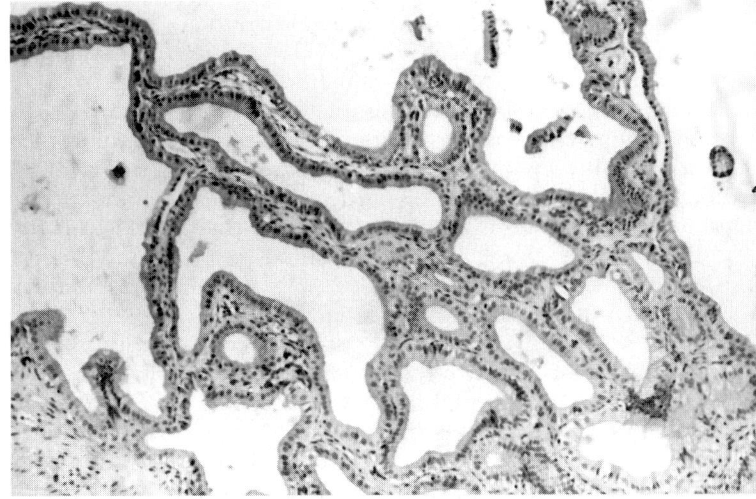

Figure 11–27. Spongioid hyperplasia of the gallbladder mucosa. This probably represents a combination of hyperplasia and tangential sectioning.

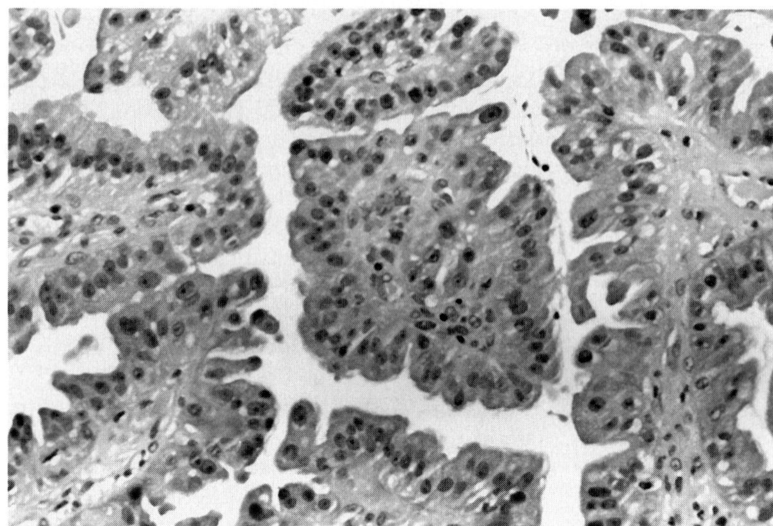

Figure 11–28. Villous hyperplasia of gallbladder mucosa.

confirmed and expanded by Tanno et al.,[363] who examined gallbladders from adults with AAPBD. They found hyperplasia was present in 63% of patients with the anomaly. Florid hyperplasia was present in 37% of patients and was found more frequently in those older than 35 years. Interestingly, 2 of 9 patients (22%) with florid hyperplasia also had K-*ras* mutations, although none had morphologically identifiable dysplasia. These authors point out that hyperplasia, particularly florid hyperplasia, was significantly more common in individuals with AAPBD who did not also have dilation of the common bile duct and in whom stasis of refluxed pancreatic secretions apparently occurred in the gallbladder, not the bile duct. This finding suggests that pancreatic juice reflux may be a cause of gallbladder cancer and that villous hyperplasia is either a marker or precursor lesion for cancer.

Metaplastic changes in the gallbladder may or may not be associated with simple hyperplasia. They may be present as incidental findings, identified only on histologic examination, or they may be polypoid.[368] Polypoid metaplastic lesions are discussed in Chapter 12 and consist of three major types: gastric, intestinal, and squamous.

Nonpolypoid gastric metaplasia produces changes resembling the normal antral mucosa and is characterized by alterations within the surface epithelium as well as by the presence of mucus-secreting glands in the lamina propria.[361,370–372] Mucus gland (pseudopyloric) metaplasia is the most commonly encountered change and may be found in up to 85% of cholecystectomy specimens, if they are thoroughly sampled. Mucus-secreting glands, usually aggregated as small lobules, develop either diffusely or, more commonly, as small nodules within the lamina propria. Larger nodules may actually appear as grossly recognizable sessile polyps. Superficially, these metaplastic glands closely resemble normal gastric antral (pyloric) glands, with rounded or flattened, basally oriented nuclei and a bubbly appearing superficial cytoplasm (Fig. 11–29). Subtle differences from pyloric glands do, however, exist in the secretory products. The mucus produced is mainly neutral in type but can contain small amounts of both sialomucin and sulfated mucin.[372] In addition, pepsinogens I and II and concanavalin A may be detected immunohistochemically.[373] Lysozyme may also be found in antral metaplasia.[373]

Surface epithelial gastric metaplasia is less common than mucus gland metaplasia. Morphologically, the metaplastic cells are somewhat taller than normal gallbladder surface epithelium and contain increased quantities of mucus (Fig. 11–30). This is predominately neutral mucin (PAS positive, alcian blue negative), in contrast to the normal finding of acid mucin within epithelial cells. The finding of gastric mucosa, with glands containing chief and parietal cells (i.e., fundic glands), is usually considered an example of heterotopia rather than of metaplasia.[374]

Intestinal metaplasia is also common in inflammatory conditions of the gallbladder.[349–351]

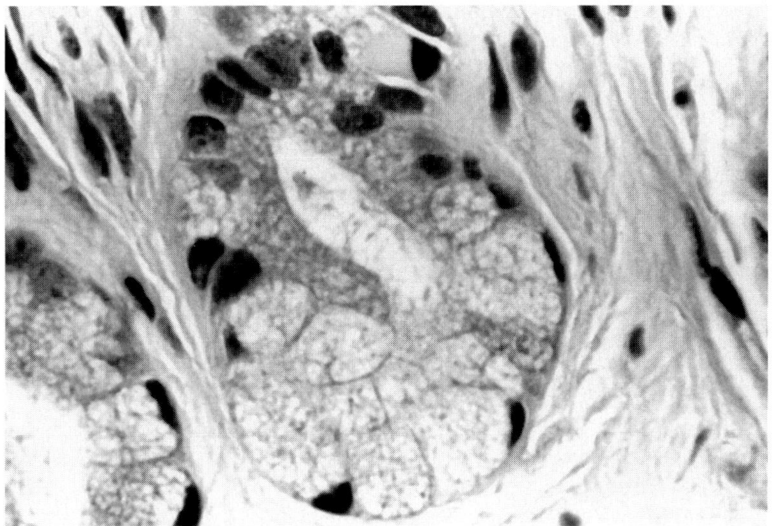

Figure 11–29. Metaplastic pyloric-type glands.

Its frequency increases with age and it is more common in women. It is found usually in association with gastric metaplasia.[375] The presence of goblet cells is the most frequent manifestation, although absorptive cells may occur, along with rarer Paneth's cells and endocrine cells[376] (Fig. 11–31). The goblet cells contain sialomucin, just like the normal small bowel goblet cells.[377] Endocrine cells are found in approximately 16% of routine cholecystectomy specimens. They may be located within metaplastic mucus glands or in the surface epithelium.[377,378] Eighty percent of endocrine cells are serotonin producing. The remainder secrete somatostatin, cholecystokinin, gastrin, or pancreatic polypeptide.[377] Paneth cells in metaplastic gallbladder mucosa tend to have somewhat finer granules than those in normal small intestine. They may be found singly, or in groups, usually within metaplastic mucus glands but also within the surface epithelium.[376] The frequency of metaplastic Paneth's cells in routine cholecystectomy specimens is quoted as 14% in men and 25% in women.[376] Goblet cell metaplasia is most commonly encountered in the superficial epithelium, as either single cells or small groups of cells. Typically, the tip of the mucosal folds is the area most commonly affected. Its prevalence has been stated as 34% in men and 56% in women.[376]

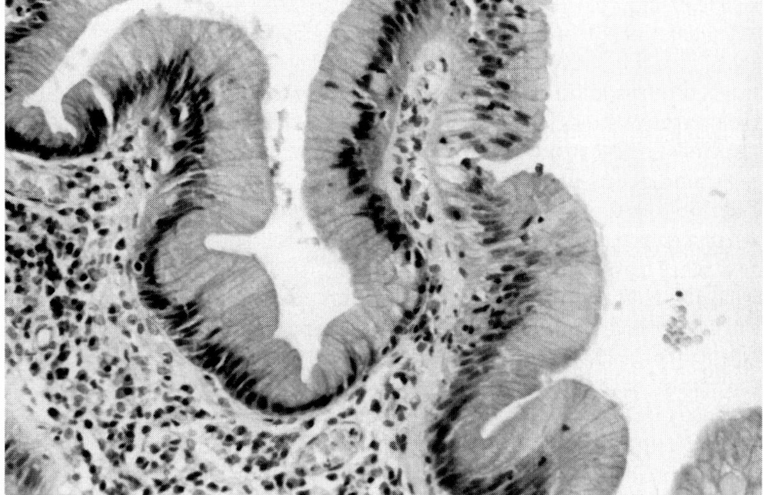

Figure 11–30. Gastric metaplasia in surface epithelium.

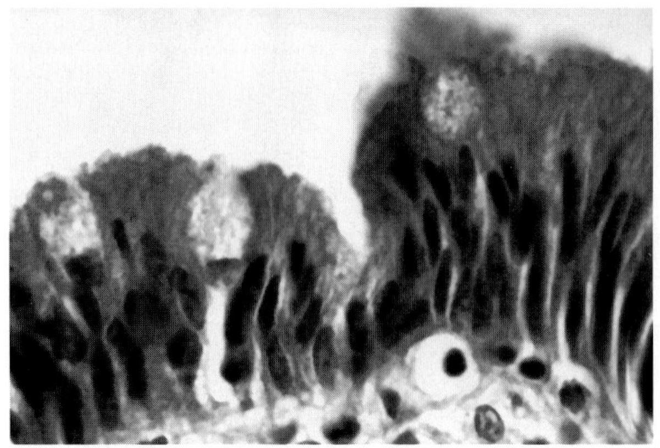

Figure 11–31. Intestinal metaplasia of the gallbladder.

Intestinal metaplasia of the gallbladder is regarded as more significant than pyloric metaplasia in the development of carcinoma.[361,374,379–382] This is not surprising, in view of the evidence that distal (intestinal) carcinomas of the stomach are also thought to arise from intestinal metaplasia. In a study of 162 resected gallbladders from Chile, Duarte et al.[361] found dysplasia in 16% and intestinal metaplasia in 58%. Significantly, however, dysplasia was present in 23% of gallbladders that also had metaplasia but in only 0.06% of gallbladders with no metaplasia. These rather high prevalence rates for dysplasia and metaplasia are not unexpected in Chile, which experiences an extremely high prevalence of gallstones and where carcinoma of the gallbladder is a leading cause of death, especially among women. In contrast, a series of 277 cholecystectomy specimens examined by Dowling and Kelly[381] from Canada, a country with a low incidence of gallbladder cancer, found intestinal metaplasia in 30 cases (11%) but only 1 example of dysplasia (0.36%). This single case of dysplasia also occurred in association with metaplasia. However, in a parallel study of 15 gallbladders containing carcinoma, these authors found intestinal metaplasia adjacent to the tumor in 53% of cases.[381] Furthermore, foci of dysplasia were present within metaplastic epithelium in 67% of cases but were found in nonmetaplastic epithelium in only 13% of cases. These findings support an intestinal metaplasia–dysplasia–carcinoma sequence.[382] However, for an individual patient in whom metaplasia or dysplasia is present in a cholecystectomy specimen, there appears to be little significance, as changes in the gallbladder do not appear to be predictive for subsequent bile duct carcinoma.

Squamous metaplasia of the gallbladder is a rare lesion. It has been associated with porcelain gallbladder[383] and may be present adjacent to primary squamous cell carcinoma.[384] Some authors have presumed that it arises secondary to chronic inflammation and cholelithiasis; however, there must be other, unknown factors involved, given the frequency of gallstones and the rarity of squamous metaplasia. Like squamous metaplasia occurring at other sites in the gastrointestinal tract, it is presumed that in the gallbladder, it arises from reserve cells normally present in small numbers within the epithelium.

REFERENCES

1. Moser AJ, Abedin MZ, Roslyn JJ: The pathogenesis of gallstone formation. Adv Surg 26:357–386, 1993.
2. Rhomberg HP, Judmair G, Lochs A: How common are gallstones? Br Med J 289:1002, 1984.
3. Diehl AK: Epidemiology of gallbladder cancer: A synthesis of recent data. J Natnl Cancer Inst 65:1209–1214, 1980.
4. Maurer KR, Everhart JE, Ezzati TM, et al.: Prevalence of gallstone disease in Hispanic populations in the United States. Gastroenterology 96:487–492, 1989.
5. Kono S, Kochi S, Ohyama S, et al.: Gallstones, serum lipids and glucose intolerance among male officials of self-defence forces in Japan. Dig Dis Sci 33:839–844, 1988.
6. Adedeji A, Akande B, Olmuide F: The changing pattern of cholelithiasis in Lagos. Scand J Gastroenterol 21:63–66, 1986.
7. Sichieri R, Everhart JE, Roth HP: Low incidence of hospitalization with gallbladder disease among blacks in the United States. Am J Epidemiol 131:826–835, 1990.
8. Layde PM, Vessey MP, Yeates D: Risk factors for gallbladder disease: A cohort study of young women attending family planning clinics. J Epidemiol Community Health 36:274–278, 1982.

9. Scragg RK, McMichael AJ, Seamark RF: Oral contraceptives, pregnancy and endogenous oestrogen in gallstone disease—a case-control study. Br Med J 288:1795–1799, 1984.
10. Liddle R, Goldstein RB, Saxon J: Gallstone formation during weight-reduction dieting. Arch Intern Med 149:1750–1753, 1989.
11. Diehl AK, Rosenthal M, Hazuda HP, et al.: Socioeconomic status and the prevalence of clinical gallbladder disease. J Chronic Dis 38:1019–1026, 1985.
12. Rome Group for Epidemiology and Prevention of Cholelithiasis (GREPCO): The epidemiology of gallstone disease in Rome, Italy. Part II. Factors associated with the disease. Hepatology 8:907–913, 1988.
13. Whorwell PJ, Hawkins R, Dewbury K, et al.: Ultrasound survey of gallstones and other hepatobiliary disorders in patients with Crohn's disease. Dig Dis Sci 29:930–933, 1984.
14. Roslyn JJ, Pitt HA, Mann LL, et al.: Gallstone disease in patients on long-term parenteral nutrition. Gastroenterology 84:148–154, 1983.
15. Haffner SM, Diehl AK, Mitchell BD, et al.: Increased clinical prevalence of gallbladder disease in subjects with non-insulin dependent diabetes mellitus. Am J Epidemiol 132:327–335, 1990.
16. Petitti DB, Sidney S, Perlman JA: Increased risk of cholecystectomy in users of supplemental estrogen. Gastroenterology 94:91–95, 1988.
17. Coronary Drug Project Research Group: Gallbladder disease as a side effect of drugs influencing lipid metabolism. Experience in the Coronary Drug Project. N Engl J Med 296:1185–1190, 1977.
18. Royal College of General Practitioners Oral Contraceptive Study: Oral contraceptives and gallbladder disease. Lancet 2:957–959, 1982.
19. Miquel JF, Covarrubias C, Villaroel L, et al.: Genetic epidemiology of cholesterol cholelithiasis among Chilean Hispanics, Amerindians and Maoris. Gastroenterology 115:937–946, 1998.
20. Donovan JM, Carey MC: Physical-chemical basis of gallstone formation. Gastroenterol Clin North Am 20:47–66, 1991.
21. Paumgartner G, Sauerbruch T: Gallstones: Pathogenesis. Lancet 338:1117–1121, 1991.
22. Holzbach RT, Busch N: Nucleation and growth of cholesterol crystals. Kinetic determinants in supersaturated native bile. Gastroenterol Clin North Am 20:67–84, 1991.
23. Carey MC, Cahalane MJ: Whither biliary sludge? Gastroenterology 95:508–523, 1988.
24. Lee SP, La Mont JT, Carey MC: Role of gallstone mucin hypersecretion in the evolution of cholesterol gallstones: Studies in the prairie dog. J Clin Invest 67:1712–1723, 1981.
25. MacPherson BR, Pemsingh RS, Scott GW: Experimental cholelithiasis in the ground squirrel. Lab Invest 56:138–145, 1987.
26. Lee SP, Carey MC, La Mont JT: Aspirin prevention of cholesterol gallstone formation in the prairie dog. Science 211:1429–1431, 1981.
27. Portincasa P, van de Meeberg P, van Erpecum KJ, et al.: An update on the pathogenesis and treatment of cholesterol gallstones. Scand J Gastroenterol 223(Suppl):60–69, 1997.
28. Trotman BW: Pigment gallstone disease. Gastroenterol Clin North Am 20:111–126, 1991.
29. Crowther RS, Soloway RD: Pigment gallstone pathogenesis: From man to molecules. Semin Liver Dis 10:171–180, 1990.
30. Nakanuma Y, Yamaguchi K, Ohta G, et al.: Pathologic features of hepatolithiasis in Japan. Hum Pathol 19:1181–1186, 1988.
31. Gracie WA, Ransohoff DF: The innocent gallstone is not a myth. N Engl J Med 307:798–800, 1982.
32. Thistle JL, Cleary PA, Lachim AM, et al.: The natural history of cholelithiasis: The National Cooperative gallstone study. Ann Intern Med 101:171–175, 1984.
33. Friedman GD, Raviola CA, Fireman B: Prognosis of gallstones with mild or no symptoms. 25 year follow-up in a health maintenance organization. J Clin Epidemiol 42:127–136, 1989.
34. Hawkins PE, Graham FB, Holliday P: Gallbladder disease in children. Am J Surg 111:741–744, 1996.
35. Azabe K, Handa N: Infant cholelithiasis: Report of a case. Surg Today 27:71–75, 1997.
36. Stringer MD, Lim P, Cave M, et al.: Fetal gallstones. J Pediatr Surg 31:1589–1591, 1996.
37. Hansson K, Lundh G, Ramberg L: Spontaneous and total disappearance of stones from the gallbladder. Acta Chir Scand 127:176–180, 1964.
38. Grey R: Disappearing gallstones: Report of two cases. Br J Surg 61:101–103, 1974.
39. Damiscelli B, Livraghi T: Disappearing gallstones: 5 more cases point to the mechanism. Diagn Imaging 50:17–19, 1981.
40. Miller MC: Spontaneous disappearance of gallstones. Gastroenterology 31:588–591, 1956.
41. Iwamura K, Ueno F: Laparoscopic finding of the gallbladder in a case of intramural gallstones. Gastroenterol Jpn 13:442–446, 1978.
42. Mizuno T, Masaoka A, Honda K, et al.: Intramural giant gallstone: Report of a rare case. Am J Gastroenterol 82:454–456, 1987.
43. Dolgin SM, Schwartz JS, Kressel HY, et al.: Identification of patients with cholesterol or pigment gallstones by discriminant analysis of radiographic features. N Engl J Med 304:808–811, 1981.
44. Malet PF, Baker J, Kahn MJ, et al.: Gallstone composition in relation to buoyancy at oral cholecystography. Radiology 177:167–169, 1990.
45. Yeh HC, Goodman J, Rabinowitz JG: Floating gallstones in bile without added contrast media. AJR 146:49–50, 1986.
46. Rominger CJ, Lockwood DW: Floating gallbladder calculi. Their incidence in a review of 1000 cholecystograms. Am J Surg 106:89–93, 1963.
47. Hinkel CL: Fissures in biliary calculi: further observations. AJR 91:979–987, 1954.
48. Kommerell B, Wolpers C: Gashaltige Gallensteine. Fortschr Geb Rontgenstr Nuklearmed ErgamZungsband 58:156–174, 1938.
49. Akerlund A: Über transparente Gashaltige spaltbildringen in Gallensteinen und ihre diagnostische Bedentung. Acta Radiol 19:215–229, 1938.
50. Vakil N, Everbach EC: Gas in gallstones: Quantitative determinations and possible effects on fragmentation by shockwaves. Gastroenterology 101:1628–1634, 1991.
51. Salmenkivi K: Cholesterolosis of the gallbladder. A clinical study based on 269 cholecystectomies. Acta Chir Scand 128(Suppl 324):1–93, 1964.
52. Feldman M, Feldman M, Jr: Cholesterolosis of the gallbladder: An autopsy study of 165 cases. Gastroenterology 27:641, 1954.
53. Elfving G, Palma A, Teir H: Cholesterolosis and mucosal hyperplasia of the gallbladder. Ann Chir Gynaec Fenn 57:28–30, 1968.

54. Jutras JA, Longtin JM, Lévesque HP: Hyperplastic cholecystoses. Am J Roentgenol 83:795–827, 1960.
55. Myllarniemi H, Nickels JI: Observations by scanning electron microscopy of normal and pathological human gallbladder epithelium. Acta Pathol Microbiol Scand [A] 85:42–48, 1977.
56. Hopwood D, Kouroumalis E, Milne G, et al.: Cholecystitis: A fine structural analysis. J Pathol 130:1–13, 1980.
57. Satoh H, Koga A: Fine structure of cholesterolosis in the human gallbladder and the mechanism of lipid accumulation. Microsc Res Tech 39:14–21, 1997.
58. Tilvis RS, Aro J, Strandberg TE, et al.: Lipid composition of bile and gallbladder mucosa in patients with acalculous cholesterolosis. Gastroenterology 82:607–615, 1982.
59. Sahlin S, Stahlberg D, Einarson K: Cholesterol metabolism in liver and gallbladder mucosa of patients with cholesterolosis. Hepatology 21:1269–1275, 1995.
60. Ross PE, Butt AN, Gallacher C: Cholesterol absorption by the gallbladder. J Clin Pathol 43:572–575, 1990.
61. Mendez-Sanchez N, Tanimoto MA, Cobos E, et al.: Cholesterolosis is not associated with high cholesterol levels in patients with and without gallstone disease. J Clin Gastroenterol 25:518–521, 1997.
62. Edlund G, Kempi V, van der Linde W: Jaundice in acute cholecystitis without common duct stones. Acta Chir Scand 149:597–601, 1983.
63. Edlund G, Ljungdahl M: Acute cholecystitis in the elderly. Am J Surg 159:414–416, 1990.
64. Laing FC: Ultrasonography of the acute abdomen. Radiol Clin North Am 30:389–404, 1992.
65. Sjodahl R: On the development of primary acute cholecystitis. Scand J Gastroenterol 18:577–479, 1983.
66. Kaminski DL, Daneshmand H, Dean P, et al.: Prostanoids and leukotrienes in experimental feline cholecystitis. Hepatology 11:1003–1009, 1990.
67. Glenn F, Becker CG: Acute acalculous cholecystitis: An interesting entity. Ann Surg 195:131–136, 1982.
68. Lee BY, Morilla CV: Acute emphysematous cholecystitis: A case report and review of the literature. NY State Med J 92:406–407, 1992.
69. Fitzgibbons RJ Jr, Tseng A, Wang H, et al.: Acute cholecystitis. Does the clinical course correlate with the pathological diagnosis? Surg Endosc 10:1180–1184, 1996.
70. Weedon D: Pathology of the gallbladder. New York: Masson Publishing, 1984, p 92.
71. Strasberg M: Cholelithiasis and acute cholecystitis. Baillieres Clin Gastroenterol 11:643–661, 1997.
72. Babb RR: Acute acalculous cholecystitis: A review. J Clin Gastroenterol 15:238–241, 1992.
73. Kalliafas S, Ziegler DW, Flancbaum L, et al.: Acute acalculous cholecystitis: Incidence, risk factors, diagnosis and outcome. Am Surg 64:471–478, 1998.
74. Barie PS, Fischer E: Acute acalculous cholecystitis. J Am Coll Surg 180:232–244, 1995.
75. Raunest J, Imhof M, Rauen U, et al.: Acute cholecystitis a complication in severely injured intensive care patients. J Trauma 32:433–440, 1992.
76. Lindberg EF, Grinnan GLB, Smith L: Acalculous cholecystitis in Vietnam casualties. Ann Surg 171:152–157, 1970.
77. Munster AM, Brown JR: Acalculous cholecystitis. Am J Surg 113:730–734, 1967.
78. Kuo CH, Changchien CS, Chen JJ, et al.: Septic acute cholecystitis. Scand J Gastroenterol 30:272–275, 1995.
79. Avalos ME, Cerulli MA, Lee RS: Acalculous acute cholecystitis due to *Salmonella typhi*. Dig Dis Sci 37:1772–1775, 1992.
80. Sagar PM, Wedgewood KR, Benson EA: Clostridial cholecystitis—the need for early recognition and treatment. Br J Clin Pract 44:752, 1990.
81. Simic O, Strathausen S, Hess W, et al.: Incidence and prognosis of abdominal complications after cardiopulmonary bypass. Cardiovasc Surg 7:419–424, 1999.
82. Buyukasik Y, Kosar A, Demiroglu H, et al.: Acalculous acute cholecystitis in leukemia. J Clin Gastroenterol 27:146–148, 1998.
83. Kamimura T, Mimori A, Takeda A, et al.: Acute acalculous cholecystitis in systemic lupus erythematosus: A case report and review of the literature. Lupus 7:361–363, 1998.
84. Gomez NA, Leon CJ, Gutierrez J: Acute acalculous cholecystitis due to *Vibrio cholerae*. Surg Endosc 9:730–732, 1995.
85. Asnis DS, Golub R, Bresciani A: *Vibrio cholerae* 01 isolated in the gallbladder of a patient presenting with cholecystitis. Am J Gastroenterol 91:2241–2242, 1996.
86. West BC, Silberman R, Otterson WN: Acalculous cholecystitis and septicemia caused by non-01 *Vibrio cholerae:* First reported case and review of biliary infections with *Vibrio cholerae*. Diagn Microbiol Infect Dis 30:187–191, 1998.
87. Earle KA, Hoffbrand BI: Acalculous cholecystitis complicating Legionnaire's disease. Br J Clin Pract 44:783, 1990.
88. Laudau Z, Agmon NL, Argas D, et al.: Acute cholecystitis caused by *Campylobacter jejuni*. Isr J Med Sci 31:696–697, 1995.
89: Carson HJ, Rezmer S, Belli J: *Hemophilus segnis* cholecystitis: A case report and literature review. J Infect 35:85–86, 1997.
90. Alvarez M, Potel C, Rey L, et al.: Biliary tract infection caused by *Haemophilus parainfluenzae*. Scand J Infect Dis 31:212–213, 1999.
91. Vilaichone RK, Mahachai V, Wilde H: Acute acalculous cholecystitis in leptospirosis. J Clin Gastroenterol 29:280–283, 1999.
92. Kuttah L, Weber F, Cregar RJ, et al.: Acute cholecystitis after autologous bone marrow transplantation for acute myeloid leukemia. Ann Oncol 6:302–304, 1995.
93. Jardines LA, O'Donnell MR, Johnson DL, et al.: Acalculous cholecystitis in bone marrow transplant recipients. Cancer 71:354–358, 1993.
94. Howard RJ: Acute acalculous cholecystitis. Am J Surg 141:194–198, 1981.
95. Imai H, Nakamoto Y, Nakajima Y, et al.: Allergic granulomatosis and angiitis (Churg-Strauss syndrome) presenting as acute acalculous cholecystitis. J Rheumatol 17:247–249, 1990.
96. Becker CG, Dubin T, Glenn F: Induction of acute cholecystitis by activation of factor XII. J Exp Med 151:81–90, 1980.
97. Claesson BE: Microflora of the biliary tree and liver. Dig Dis Sci 4:93–118, 1986.
98. Glenn F: Acute acalculous cholecystitis. Ann Surg 189:458–465, 1979.
99. Ong CL, Wong TH, Rauff A: Acute gallbladder perforation—a dilemma in early diagnosis. Gut 32:956–958, 1991.
100. Mentzer RM, Golden GT, Chandler JG, et al.: A comparative appraisal of emphysematous cholecystitis. Am J Surg 129:10–15, 1975.
101. Lorenz RW, Steffen HM: Emphysematous cholecystitis, diagnostic problems and differential diagnosis of gallbladder gas accumulations. Hepatogastroenterology 37(Suppl 2):103–106, 1990.

102. Gill KS, Chapman AH, Weston MJ: The changing face of emphysematous cholecystitis. Br J Radiol 70:986–991, 1997.
103. Bloom RA, Libson E, Lebensart PD, et al.: The ultrasound spectrum of emphysematous cholecystitis. J Clin Ultrasound 17:251–256, 1989.
104. Wu CS, Yao WJ, Hsiao CH: Effervescent gallbladder: Sonographic findings in emphysematous cholecystitis. J Clin Ultrasound 26:272–275, 1998.
105. Tsai CJ, Wu CS: Risk factors for perforation of the gallbladder. A combined hospital study in a Chinese population. Scand J Gastroenterol 26:1027–1034, 1991.
106. Madl C, Grimm G, Mallek R, et al.: Diagnosis of gallbladder perforation in acute acalculous cholecystitis in critically ill patients. Intensive Care Med 18:245–246, 1992.
107. Gottesman L, Marks RA, Khoury PT, et al.: Diagnosis of isolated perforation of the gallbladder following blunt trauma using sonography and CT Scan. J Trauma 24:280–281, 1984.
108. Greenwald G, Stine RJ, Larson RE: Perforation of the gallbladder following blunt abdominal trauma. Ann Emerg Med 16:452–454, 1987.
109. Janowitz P, Janowitz A, Schumaher KA, et al.: Occult gallbladder perforation: An unusual complication of gallstone lithotripsy. Hepatogastroenterology 39:43–46, 1992.
110. Anonymous: Empyema of the gallbladder—a forgotten disease. Lancet 1:606, 1984.
111. Thornton JR, Heaton KW, Espiner HJ, et al.: Empyema of the gallbladder—reappraisal of a neglected disease. Gut 24:1183–1185, 1983.
112. Fry DE, Cox RA, Harbrecht PJ: Empyema of the gallbladder: A complication in the natural history of acute cholecystitis. Am J Surg 141:366–369, 1981.
113. Lam RC, Neher DA, Starke JC: Hydrops of the gallbladder in cirrhosis of the liver. Mil Med 121:98–100, 1957.
114. Pack GT, Teng PK: Carcinoma of the cystic duct leading to hydrops of the gallbladder. JAMA 203:175–176, 1968.
115. Reul GJ Jr, Rubio PA, Berkman NL: Granular cell myoblastoma of the cystic duct. A case associated with hydrops of the gallbladder. Am J Surg 129:583–584, 1975.
116. Meade RH 3rd, Brandt L: Manifestations of Kawasaki disease in New England outbreak of 1980. J Pediatr 100:558–562, 1982.
117. Wheeler RA, Najmaldin AS, Soubra M, et al.: Surgical presentation of Kawasaki disease (mucocutaneous lymph node syndrome). Br J Surg 77:1273–1274, 1990.
118. Dinulos J, Mitchell DK, Egerton J, et al.: Hydrops of the gallbladder associated with EB virus infection: A report of two cases and a review of the literature. Pediatr Infect Dis J 14:163–164, 1995.
119. McCrindle BW, Wood RA, Nussbaum AR: Henoch-Schönlein syndrome. Unusual manifestations with hydrops of the gallbladder. Clin Pediatrics 27:254–256, 1988.
120. Cohen EK, Stringer DA, Smith CR, et al.: Hydrops of the gallbladder in typhoid fever as demonstrated by sonography. J Clin Ultrasound 14:633–635, 1986.
121. Strauss RG: Scarlet fever with hydrops of the gallbladder. Pediatrics 44:741–745, 1969.
122. Slovis TL, Hight DW, Philippart AI, et al.: Sonography in the diagnosis and management of hydrops of the gallbladder in children with the mucocutaneous lymph node syndrome. Pediatrics 65:789–794, 1980.
123. Schrumpf JO, Handmaher H: Hydrops of the gallbladder in a premature neonate. Am J Dis Child 136:172–173, 1982.
124. Williams RJ: Acquired mucocele of the gallbladder in childhood. Br Med J 1:1047, 1958.
125. Bailey MJ: Duodenal obstruction by a mucocele of the gallbladder. Br J Clin Pract 34:296–298, 1980.
126. Bergan T, Dobling I, Liavag I: Bacterial isolates in cholecystitis and cholelithiasis. Scand J Gastroenterol 14:625–631, 1979.
127. Fox JG, Dewhirst FE, Shen Z, et al.: Hepatic *Helicobacter* species identified in bile and gallbladder tissue from Chileans with chronic cholecystitis. Gastroenterology 114:755–763, 1998.
128. Amazon K, Rywlin AM: Ceroid granulomas of the gallbladder. Am J Clin Pathol 73:123–127, 1980.
129. Estrada RL, Brown NM, James CE: Chronic follicular cholecystitis. Radiologic, pathologic and surgical aspects. Br J Surg 48:205–209, 1960.
130. Hatae Y, Kikuchi M: Lymph follicular cholecystitis. Acta Pathol Jpn 29:67–72, 1979.
131. Thorpe MEC, Scheuer PJ, Sherlock S: Primary sclerosing cholangitis, the biliary tree and ulcerative colitis. Gut 8:435–448, 1967.
132. Cornell CM, Clarke R: Vicarious calcification involving the gallbladder. Ann Surg 149:267–272, 1959.
133. Casteel HB, Williamson SL, Golladay ES, et al.: Porcelain gallbladder in a child: A case report and review. J Pediatr Surg 25:1302–1303, 1990.
134. Ashur H, Siegal B, Oland Y, et al.: Calcified gallbladder (porcelain gallbladder). Arch Surg 113:594–596, 1978.
135. Weiner PL, Lawson TL: Porcelain gallbladder. Am J Gastroenterol 64:224–227, 1975.
136. Kane RA, Jacobs R, Katz J, et al.: Porcelain gallbladder: Ultrasound and CT appearance. Radiology 152:137–141, 1984.
137. Shimizu M, Miura J, Tanaka T, et al.: Porcelain gallbladder: Relation between its type by ultrasound and incidence of cancer. J Clin Gastroenterol 11:471–476, 1989.
138. Oschner SF, Carrera GM: Calcification of the gallbladder ("Porcelain Gallbladder"). Am J Roentgenol 89:847–853, 1963.
139. Polk HC Jr: Carcinoma and the calcified gallbladder. Gastroenterology 50:582–585, 1966.
140. Vitella L, Stubbs A, Purser S, et al.: Limy "milky" bile without apparent gallbladder obstruction by a gallstone. Aust N Z J Surg 57:405–408, 1987.
141. Fowler CL, Soriano H, Ferry GD, et al.: Limy bile syndrome. J Pediatr Surg 28:1568–1569, 1993.
142. Nomura F, Suzuki Y, Suzuki K, et al.: Spontaneous disappearance of limy bile: Report of a case and review of the literature. Am J Gastroenterol 79:884–888, 1984.
143. Elfving G: Crypts and ducts in the gallbladder wall. Acta Pathol et Microbiol Scand [A] 49(suppl 135):1–45, 1960.
144. Halpert B: Significance of the Rokitansky–Aschoff sinuses. Am J Gastroenterol 36:534–539, 1961.
145. Ram MD, Midha D: Adenomyomatosis of the gallbladder. Surgery 78:224–229, 1975.
146. Meguid MM, Aun F, Bradford ML: Adenomyomatosis of the gallbladder. Am J Surg 147:260–262, 1984.
147. Shepard VD, Walters W, Dockerty MB: Benign neoplasms of the gallbladder. Arch Surg 45:1–18, 1942.
148. Bricker DL, Halpert B: Adenomyoma of the gallbladder. Surgery 53:615–620, 1963.

149. Fenkel LD, Javitt NB, McSherry CK: Cholecystadenoma and the use of cholecystokinin. J Pediatr 79:468–470, 1971.
150. Albert D, Callea F, Camoni G, et al.: Adenomyosis of the gallbladder in childhood. J Pediatr Surg 33:1411–1412, 1998.
151. Aguirre JR, Boher RO, Guraieb S: Hyperplastic cholecystoses, a new contribution to the unitarian theory. Am J Roentgenol 107:1–13, 1969.
152. Young TE: So-called adenomyoma of the gallbladder. Am J Clin Pathol 31:423–427, 1959.
153. Arbab AA, Brashfield R: Benign tumors of the gallbladder. Surgery 61:535–540, 1967.
154. Burhaus R, Myers RT: Benign neoplasms of the extrahepatic biliary ducts. Am Surg 37:161–166, 1971.
155. Sasatomi E, Miyazaki K, Mori M, et al.: Polypoid adenomyoma of the gallbladder. J Gastroenterol 32:704–707, 1997.
156. Aldridge MC, Gruffaz F, Castaing D: Adenomyomatosis of the gallbladder. A premalignant lesion. Surgery 109:107–110, 1991.
157. Ootani T, Shirai Y, Tsukada K, et al.: Relationship between gallbladder carcinoma and the segmental type of adenomyomatosis of the gallbladder. Cancer 69:2647–2652, 1992.
158. Kainuma O, Asano T, Nakagoliri T, et al.: A case of gallbladder adenomyomatosis with pancreaticobiliary maljunction and an anomaly of the cystic duct joined the common channel. Am J Gastroenterol 93:1156–1158, 1998.
159. Chang LY, Wang HP, Wu MS, et al.: Anomalous pancreaticobiliary ductal union—an etiologic association of gallbladder cancer and adenomyomatosis. Hepatogastroenterology 45:2016–2109, 1998.
160. Tanno S, Obara T, Maguchi H, et al.: An association between anomalous pancreaticobiliary ductal union and adenomyomatosis of the gallbladder. J Gastroenterol Hepatol 13:175–180, 1998.
161. Fligiel S, Lewin KJ: Xanthogranulomatous cholecystitis. Case report and review of the literature. Arch Pathol Lab Med 106:302–304, 1982.
162. Goodman ZD, Ishak KG: Xanthogranulomatous cholecystitis. Am J Surg Pathol 5:653–659, 1981.
163. Roberts KM, Parson MA: Xanthogranulomatous cholecystitis: Clinicopathological study of 13 cases. J Clin Pathol 40:412–417, 1987.
164. Kim PN, Ha HK, Kim YH, et al.: US findings in xanthogranulomatous cholecystitis. Clin Radiol 53:290–292, 1998.
165. Muguruma N, Okamura S, Okahisa T, et al.: Endoscopic sonography in the diagnosis of xanthogranulomatous cholecystitis. J Clin Ultrasound 27:347–350, 1999.
166. Charpentier P, Prade M, Bognel C, et al.: Malakoplakia of the gallbladder. Hum Pathol 14:827–828, 1983.
167. Shukla S, Krishnani N, Jain M, et al.: Xanthogranulomatous cholecystitis. Fine needle aspiration cytology in 17 cases. Acta Cytol 41:413–418, 1997.
168. Nakashiro H, Haraoka S, Fujiwara K, et al.: Xanthogranulomatous cholecystitis. Cell composition and possible pathogenetic role of cell-mediated immunity. Pathol Res Pract 191:1078–1086, 1995.
169. Dixit VK, Prakash A, Gupta A, et al.: Xanthogranulomatous cholecystitis. Dig Dis Sci 43:940–942, 1998.
170. Adachi Y, Iso Y, Moriyama M, et al.: Increased serum CA 19-9 in patients with xanthogranulomatous cholecystitis. Hepatogastroenterology 45:77–80, 1998.
171. Dabbs DJ: Eosinophilic and lymphoeosinophilic cholecystitis. Am J Surg Pathol 17:497–501, 1993.
172. Rosengart TK, Rotterdam H, Ranson H: Eosinophilic cholangitis: A self-limited cause of extrahepatic biliary obstruction. Am J Gastroenterology 85:582–585, 1990.
173. Leegaard M: Eosinophilic cholecystitis. Acta Chir Scand 146:295–296, 1980.
174. Butler TW, Feintuch TA, Caine WP: Eosinophilic cholangitis, lymphadenopathy and peripheral eosinophilia. A case report. Am J Gastroenterol 80:572–574, 1985.
175. Fox H, Mainwaring AR: Eosinophilic infiltration of the gallbladder. Gastroenterology 63:1049–1052, 1972.
176. Kerstein MD, Sheahan DG, Gudjonsson B, et al.: Eosinophilic cholecystitis. Am J Gastroenterol 66:349–352, 1976.
177. Fauci AS, Harley JB, Roberts WC, et al.: The idiopathic hyper-eosinophilic syndrome: Clinical, physiologic and therapeutic considerations. Ann Intern Med 97:78–92, 1978.
178. Tajima K, Katagiri T: Deposits of eosinophil granule proteins in eosinophilic cholecystitis and eosinophilic colitis associated with the hyper-eosinophilic syndrome. Dig Dis Sci 41:282–288, 1996.
179. Felman RH, Sutherland DB, Conklin JL, et al.: Eosinophilic cholecystitis, appendiceal inflammation, pericarditis and cephalosporin-associated eosinophilia. Dig Dis Sci 39:418–422, 1994.
180. Steffer RM, Wyllie R, Petras RE, et al.: The spectrum of eosinophilic gastroenteritis. Report of six pediatric cases and review of the literature. Clin Pediatrics 30:404–411, 1991.
181. Russell CO, Dowling JP, Marshall RD: Acute eosinophilic cholecystitis associated with hepatic echinococcosis. Gastroenterology 77:758–760, 1979.
182. Balan V, LaRusso NF: Hepatobiliary disease in inflammatory bowel disease. Gastroenterol Clin North Am 24:647–669, 1995.
183. Jeffrey GP, Reed WD, Carrello S, et al.: Histological and immunohistochemical study of the gallbladder lesion in primary sclerosing cholangitis. Gut 32:424–429, 1991.
184. Jesserun J, Bilio-Solis A, Manivel JC: Diffuse lymphoplasmacytic acalculous cholecystitis: A distinctive form of chronic cholecystitis associated with primary sclerosing cholangitis. Hum Pathol 29:512–517, 1998.
185. McClure J, Banerjee SS, Schofield PS: Crohn's disease of the gallbladder. J Clin Pathol 37:516–518, 1984.
186. Axelrod L, Munster AM, O'Brien TF: Typhoid cholecystitis and gallbladder carcinoma after an interval of 67 years. JAMA 217:83, 1971.
187. Lai CW, Chan RC, Cheng AF, et al.: Common bile duct stones: A cause of chronic salmonellosis. Am J Gastroenterol 87:1198–1199, 1992.
188. Caygill CP, Hill MJ, Braddick M, et al.: Cancer mortality in typhoid and paratyphoid carriers. Lancet 343:83–84, 1994.
189. Beiler HA, Kuntz C, Eckstein TM, et al.: Cholecystolithiasis and infection of the biliary tract with *Salmonella virchow*—a very rare case in early childhood. Eur J Ped Surg 5:369–371, 1995.
190. Lee JG, McLeod ME, Meyers WC, et al.: Successful laparoscopic management of perforated gallbladder associated with *Salmonella javiana* infection. N Carol Med J 53:594–595, 1992.
191. Waldram R, Vahrman J, Williams R: *Salmonella heidelberg* infection in Caroli's syndrome. Gastroenterology 68:151–153, 1995.

192. Campbell CW, Eckman MR: Acute acalculous cholecystitis caused by *Salmonella indiana.* JAMA 233:815, 1975.
193. Bonta JA, Lovinggood CG: Acute cholecystitis in childhood: Report of a case. Surgery 31:309–311, 1952.
194. Strom BL, Soloway RD, Rios–Dalenz JL, et al.: Risk factors for gallbladder cancer. An international case control study. Cancer 76:1745–1756, 1995.
195. Nath G, Singh H, Shukla VK: Chronic typhoid carriage and carcinoma of the gallbladder. Eur J Cancer Prev 6:557–559, 1997.
196. Darling WM, Peel RN, Skirrow MB, et al.: Campylobacter cholecystitis. Lancet I:1302, 1979.
197. Morris SJ, Greewald RA, Turner RL, et al.: *Brucella*-induced cholecystitis. Am J Gastroenterol 71:481–484, 1979.
198. Barton LL, Escobedo MB, Keating JP, et al.: Leptospirosis with acalculous cholecystitis. Am J Dis Child 126:350–351, 1973.
199. Wong ML, Kaplan S, Dunkle LM, et al.: Leptospirosis: A childhood disease. J Pediatr 90:532–537, 1977.
200. Bergdahl L, Boquist L: Tuberculosis of the gallbladder. Br J Surg 59:289–292, 1972.
201. Misgar MS, Kariholu PL, Bhat DN, et al.: Tuberculosis of the gallbladder. J Indian Med Assoc 74:196–197, 1980.
202. Ahmad MN, Zargar HU, Shahdad NA, et al.: Tuberculosis of gallbladder. J Postgrad Med 29:258–260, 1983.
203. Nakajo S, Yamamoto M, Urushihara T, et al.: Diffuse papillomatosis of the gallbladder complicated by tuberculosis. Acta Pathol Jpn 38:1473–1480, 1988.
204. Hahn ST, Park SH, Shin WS, et al.: Gallbladder tuberculosis with perforation and intrahepatic biloma. J Clin Gastroenterol 20:84–86, 1995.
205. Al Nakib B, Jacob GS, Al Liddawi H, et al.: Choledochoduodenal fistula due to tuberculosis. Endoscopy 14:64–65, 1982.
206. Bernard JC, Vazquez CA: Visceral lesions in lepromatous leprosy. Study of sixty necropsies. Int J Lepr Other Mycobact Dis 41:94–101, 1973.
207. Taylor CE: Leprosy of the large intestine and gallbladder. Case report and review of the literature. Trans R Soc Trop Med Hyg 39:125–132, 1945.
208. Brewer JH, Allen MJ: Actinomycosis of the gallbladder with liver abscess. South Med J 73:1070–1072, 1980.
209. Smithers BM, Wall DR, Weedon D: Actinomycosis of the gallbladder. Aust N Z J Surg 53:587–588, 1983.
210. Hadley DA, Porschen RK, Juler GL: Actinomycosis of the common bile duct presenting as chronic cholecystitis. Surgery 90:117–119, 1981.
211. Freland C, Massoubre B, Horeau JM, et al.: Actinomycosis of the gallbladder due to *Actinomyces naeslundi.* J Infect 15:251–257, 1987.
212. Arora B, Punia RS, Arora DR: Actinomycotic cholecystitis. Ind J Gastroenterol 16:68, 1997.
213. Merle-Melet M, Mory F, Stempfel B, et al.: *Actinomyces naeslundi,* acute cholecystitis and carcinoma of the gallbladder. Am J Gastroenterol 90:1530–1531, 1995.
214. Irani M, Truong LD: Candidiasis of the extrahepatic biliary tract. Arch Pathol Lab Med 110:1087–1090, 1986.
215. Hiatt JR, Kobayashi MR, Doty JE, et al.: Acalculous candida cholecystitis: A complication of critical surgical illness. Am Surg 57:825–829, 1991.
216. Diebel LN, Raafat AM, Dulchavsky SA, et al.: Gallbladder and biliary tract candidiasis. Surgery 120:760–764, 1996.
217. Takano H, Yoshikawa T, Nishida K, et al.: Candida cholecystitis as an unusual complication of endoscopic retrograde cholangiography. Endoscopy 28:790–791, 1996.
218. Brown H, Talamini M, Westra WH: Xanthogranulomatous cholecystitis due to invasive *Candida albicans* in a patient with AIDS. Clin Infect Dis 22:186–187, 1996.
219. Washington K, Gottfried MR, Wilson ML: Gastrointestinal cryptococcosis. Mod Pathol 4:707–711, 1991.
220. Flum DR, Steinberg SD, Sarkis AY, et al.: Role of cholecystectomy in acquired immunodeficiency syndrome. J Am Coll Surg 184:233–239, 1997.
221. Warren GH, Marsh S: Granulomatous *Torulopsis glabrata* cholecystitis in a diabetic. Am J Clin Pathol 78:406–410, 1982.
222. Rothman PE, Graw RG Jr, Harris JC Jr, et al.: Coccidiodomycosis—possible fomite transmission. Am J Dis Child 118:792–801, 1969.
223. Chaib E, deOliveira CM, Prado PS, et al.: Obstructive jaundice caused by blastomycosis of the lymph nodes around the common bile duct. Arq Gastroenterol 25:198–202, 1988.
224. O'Donovan N, Fitzgerald E: Gallbladder wall thickening in infectious mononucleosis: An ominous sign. Postgrad J Med 72:299–300, 1996.
225. Sainsbury R, Smith PK, Le Quesne G, et al.: Gallbladder wall thickening with infectious mononucleosis hepatitis in an immunosuppressed adolescent. J Pediatr Gastroenterol Nutr 19:123–125,1994.
226. Mourani S, Dobbs SM, Genta RM, et al.: Hepatitis A virus-associated cholecystitis. Ann Int Med 120:398–400, 1994.
227. Klar A, Branski D, Nadjari M, et al.: Gallbladder and pancreatic involvement in hepatitis A. J Clin Gastroenterol 27:143–145, 1998.
228. McGowan JM, Nussbaum CC, Burroughs EW: Cholecystitis due to *Giardia lamblia* in a left sided gallbladder. Ann Surg 128:1032–1037, 1948.
229. Petersen H: Giardiasis (lambliasis). Scand J Gastroenterol 7(suppl 14):1–44, 1972.
230. Soto JM, Dreiling DA: *Giardia lamblia.* A case presentation of chronic cholecystitis and duodenitis. Am J Gastroenterol 67:265–269, 1977.
231. Köberle F: Enteromegaly and cardiomegaly in Chagas disease. Gut 4:399–405, 1963.
232. Pinotti HW, Felix VN, Zilberstein B, et al.: Surgical complications of Chagas' disease: Megaesophagus, achalasia of the pylorus and cholelithiasis. World J Surg 15:198–204, 1991.
233. Fahal AH, el Hag IA, el Hassan AM, et al.: Leishmanial cholecystitis and colitis in a patient with visceral leishmaniasis. Trans Soc Trop Med Hyg 89:284, 1995.
234. Powell SJ, Sutton JB, Lautre G: Hemobilia in amebic liver abscess. S Afr Med J 47:1555–1557, 1973.
235. Hashim M: Pathological lesions of the gallbladder associated with ulcerations and bilharziasis of the intestines. J Egypt Med Assoc 14:461–475, 1931.
236. Kavin H, Jonas RB, Chowdhury L, et al.: Acalculous cholecystitis and cytomegalovirus infection in the acquired immunodeficiency syndrome. Ann Intern Med 104:53–54, 1986.
237. Blumberg RS, Kelsey P, Perrone T, et al.: Cytomegalovirus and cryptosporidium-associated acalculous gangrenous cholecystitis. Am J Med 76:1118–1123, 1984.
238. Adolph MD, Bass SN, Lee SK, et al.: Cytomegaloviral acalculous cholecystitis in acquired immunodeficiency patients. Am Surg 59:679–684, 1993.

239. Agha FP, Nostrant TT, Abrams GD, et al.: Cytomegalovirus cholecystitis in a homosexual man with acquired immunodeficiency syndrome. Am J Gastroenterol 81:1068–1072, 1986.
240. Hinnant K, Schwartz A, Rotterdam H, et al.: Cytomegaloviral and cryptosporidial cholecystitis in two patients with AIDS. Am J Surg Pathol 113:57–60, 1989.
241. Bigio EH, Haque AK: Disseminated cytomegalovirus infection presenting with acalculous cholecystitis and acute pancreatitis. Arch Pathol Lab Med 113:1287–1289, 1989.
242. French AL, Beaudet LM, Benator DA, et al.: Cholecystectomy in patients with AIDS: Clinicopathologic correlations in 106 cases. Clin Infect Dis 21:852–858, 1995.
243. Boige N, Bellaiche M, Cornet D, et al.: Hydrops-like cholecystitis due to cryptosporidiosis in an HIV-infected child. J Ped Gastroenterol Nutr 26:219–221, 1998.
244. Benator DA, French AL, Beandet LM, et al.: *Isospora belli* infection associated with acalculous cholecystitis in a patient with AIDS. Ann Intern Med 121:663–664, 1994.
245. Pol S, Romana CA, Richard S, et al.: Microsporidia infection in patients with the human immunodeficiency virus and unexplained cholangitis: N Engl J Med 328:95–99, 1993.
246. Knapp PE, Saltzman JR, Fairchild P: Acalculous cholecystitis associated with microsporidial infection in a patient with AIDS. Clin Infect Dis 22:195–196, 1996.
247. Orenstein JM, Dieterich DT, Kotler DP: Systemic dissemination by a newly recognized intestinal microsporidia species in AIDS. AIDS 6:1143–1150, 1992.
248. Liberman E, Yen TS: Foamy macrophages in acquired immunodeficiency syndrome cholangiopathy with *Encephalitozoon intestinalis.* Arch Pathol Lab Med 121:985–988, 1997.
249. Bouche H, Housset C, Dumont JL, et al.: AIDS related cholangitis: Diagnostic features and course in 15 patients. J Hepatol 17:34–39, 1993.
250. Benhamen Y, Caumes E, Gerosa Y, et al.: AIDS related cholangiopathy: Critical analysis and prospective series of 26 patients. Dig Dis Sci 38:1113–1118, 1993.
251. Forbes A, Blanshard C, Gazzard B: Natural history of AIDS related sclerosing cholangitis: A study of 20 cases. Gut 34:116–121, 1993.
252. Orenstein JM: Isosporiasis. *In:* Connor DH, Chandler FW, Schwartz DA, Manz HJ, Lack EE (eds): Pathology of Infectious Diseases. Vol. II. Stamford, CT: Appleton & Lange, pp 1185–1190, 1997.
253. Orenstein JM: Microsporidiosis. *In:* Connor DH, Chandler FW, Schwartz DA, Manz HJ, Lack EE (eds): Pathology of Infectious Diseases. Vol. II. Stamford, CT: Appleton & Lange, pp 1223–1240, 1997.
254. al-Saleem T, al-Janabi T: Schistosomal cholecystitis: Report of six cases. Ann Roy Coll Surg Engl 71:366–367, 1989.
255. Bakhotmah MA: Gallbladder bilharzias. HPB Surg 9:175–177, 1996.
256. LiVolsi VA, Perzin KH, Porter M: Polyarteritis of the gallbladder presenting as acute cholecystitis. Gastroenterology 65:115–123, 1973.
257. Chen KTK: Gallbladder vasculitis. J Clin Gastroenterol 11:537–540, 1989.
258. Nohr M, Lanstsen J, Falk E: Isolated necrotizing arteritis of the gallbladder. Case report. Acta Chir Scand 155:485–487, 1989.
259. Parangi S, Oz MC, Blume RS, et al.: Hepatobiliary complications of polyarteritis nodosa. Arch Surg 126:909–912, 1991.
260. Ito M, Sano K, Inaba M, et al.: Localized necrotizing arteritis. A report of two cases involving the gallbladder and pancreas. Arch Pathol Lab Med 115:780–783, 1991.
261. Burke AP, Sobin LH, Virmani R: Localized vasculitis of the gastrointestinal tract. Am J Surg Pathol 19:338–349, 1995.
262. Lasser A, Ghofrany S: Necrotizing granulomatous vasculitis (allergic granulomatosis) of the gallbladder. Gastroenterology 71:660–662, 1976.
263. Imai H, Nakamoto Y, Nakajima Y, et al.: Allergic granulomatosis and angiitis (Churg–Strauss syndrome) presenting as acute acalculous cholecystitis. J Rheumatol 17:247–249, 1990.
264. Ohwada S, Yanagisawa A, Joshita T, et al.: Necrotizing granulomatous vasculitis of transverse colon and gallbladder. Hepatogastroenterology 44:1090–1094, 1997.
265. Fayemi AO, Ali M, Barun EV: Necrotizing vasculitis of the gallbladder and the appendix. Similarity in the morphology of rheumatoid arthritis and polyarteritis nodosa. Am J Gastroenterol 67:608–612, 1977.
266. Fernandez-Nebro A, Valdivielso P, Sanchez-Carrillo JJ, et al.: Localized rheumatoid vasculitis presenting as acute alithiasic cholecystitis. Am J Med 91:90–92, 1991.
267. Swanepoel CR, Floyd A, Allison H, et al.: Acute acalculous cholecystitis complicating systemic lupus erythematosus: Case report and review. Br Med J 286:251–252, 1983.
268. Newbold KM, Allum WH, Downing R, et al.: Vasculitis of the gallbladder in rheumatoid arthritis and systemic lupus erythematosus. Clin Rheumatol 6:287–289, 1987.
269. Kuipers EJ, van Leeuwen MA, Nikkels PG, et al.: Hemobilia due to vasculitis of the gallbladder in a patient with mixed connective tissue disease. J Rheumatol 18:617–618, 1991.
270. Kumon Y, Hisatake K, Chikamori M, et al.: A case of vasculitic cholecystitis associated with Schönlein-Henoch purpura in an adult. Gastroenterol Jpn 23:68–72, 1988.
271. Choong CK, Beasley SW: Intra-abdominal manifestations of Henoch-Schönlein purpura. J Pediatr Child Health 34:405–409, 1998.
272. Fauci AS, Haynes BF, Katz P, et al.: Wegener's granulomatosis: Prospective clinical and therapeutic experience with 85 patients for 21 years. Ann Intern Med 98:76–85, 1983.
273. Hallendorf LC, Dockerty MB, Waugh JM: Gangrenous cholecystitis and infarction of the gallbladder. Surg Clin North Am 28:979–998, 1948.
274. Matz LR, Lawrence-Brown MMD: Ischemic cholecystitis and infarction of the gallbladder. Aust N Z J Surg 52:466–471, 1982.
275. Sjodahl R, Wetterfors J: Acute cholecystitis with an occluding thrombus of the cystic artery. Acta Chir Scand 140:77–81, 1974.
276. Loughran CF, Thirn CR: Gallbladder infarction: A radiographic mimic of emphysematous cholecystitis. Eur J Radiol 5:109–110, 1985.
277. Henrich WL, Huehnegerth RJ, Rosch J, et al.: Gallbladder and liver infarction occurring as a complication of acute bacterial endocarditis. Gastroenterology 68:1602–1607, 1975.

278. Kuroda C, Iwasaki M, Tanaka T, et al.: Gallbladder infarction following hepatic transcatheter arterial embolization. Angiographic study. Radiology 149:85–89, 1983.
279. Takayasu K, Moriyama N, Muramatsu Y, et al.: Gallbladder infarction after hepatic artery embolisation. AJR 144:135–138, 1985.
280. Kitigawa T, Iriyama K: Hepatic infarction as a complication of gastric cancer surgery: Report of four cases. Surg Today 28:542–546, 1998.
281. Ford GA, Simpson AH, Gear MW, et al.: Duodenal ulceration into the cystic artery. Postgrad Med J 66:144–146, 1990.
282. Boutros HH, Pantler S, Chakrabarti S: Cocaine-induced ischemic colitis with small vessel thrombosis of colon and gallbladder. J Clin Gastroenterol 24:49–53, 1997.
283. Dessailloud R, Papo T, Vaneecloo S, et al.: Acalculous ischemic gallbladder necrosis in the catastrophic antiphospholipid syndrome. Arthritis Rheum 41:1318–1320, 1998.
284. Rosen Y, Chen C: Infarction of the gallbladder: A complication of hypertension. Case report. Am J Gastroenterol 67:249–252, 1977.
285. Steiber AC, Bauer JJ: Volvulus of the gallbladder. Am J Gastroenterol 78:96–98, 1983.
286. Kazmann HA, Guthorn PJ: Volvulus of the gallbladder. Am J Surg 85:580–581, 1953.
287. Mouzas GL: Torsion of the gallbladder in a kyphoscoliotic patient. Postgrad Med J 36:686–687, 1960.
288. Bothra R: Torsion of the gall-bladder in the aged. Br J Surg 60:359–360, 1973.
289. Loksen A, Wilson BW, Sherman R: Torsion of the gallbladder: A case report and review of the literature. Am Surg 63:975–978, 1997.
290. McDonald PH, Pace RF: Volvulus of the gallbladder: A case report. Can J Surg 33:282–283, 1990.
291. Nguyen T, Geraci A, Bauer JJ: Laparoscopic cholecystectomy for gallbladder volvulus. Surg Endosc 9:519–521, 1995.
292. Hamdi M, Blondiau JV, Algaba R, et al.: Gallbladder volvulus: A case report. Could the ultrasound be the key of the early diagnosis. Acta Chir Belg 96:41–43, 1996.
293. Merriman TE, Houghton G, Ventura R: Torsion of the fundus of the gallbladder. Aust N Z J Surg 63:821–822, 1993.
294. Schachter P, Czerniak A, Shemesh E, et al.: Isolated gallbladder rupture due to blunt abdominal trauma. HPB Surgery 1:359–362, 1989.
295. Burgess P, Fulton RL: Gallbladder and extrahepatic injury following abdominal trauma. Injury 23:413–414, 1992.
296. McNabney WK, Rudek R, Pemberton LB: The significance of gallbladder trauma. J Emerg Med 8:277–280, 1990.
297. Hills MW, Richardson AJ, Tait N: Non–iatrogenic trauma to the extrahepatic biliary tract. Aust N Z J Surg 63:190–194, 1993.
298. Soderstrom CA, Maekawa K, Du Priest RW Jr, et al.: Gallbladder injuries resulting from blunt abdominal trauma: An experience and review. Ann Surg 193:60–66, 1981.
299. Wiener I, Watson LC, Wolma FJ: Perforation of the gallbladder due to blunt abdominal trauma. Arch Surg 117:805–807, 1982.
300. Sharma O: Blunt gallbladder injuries: Presentation of twenty-two cases with review of the literature. J Trauma 39:576–580, 1995.
301. Spigos DG, Tan WS, Larson G, et al.: Diagnosis of traumatic rupture of the gallbladder. Am J Surg 141:731–735, 1981.
302. Yadav K, Pathak IC: Biliary peritonitis following blunt abdominal trauma in children. Report of a case. Am J Gastroenterol 72:444–447, 1979.
303. Du Priest RW Jr, Khaneja SC, Cowley RA: Acute cholecystitis complicating trauma. Ann Surg 189:84–89, 1979.
304. Rice J, Williams HC, Flint LM, et al.: Post-traumatic acalculous cholecystitis. South Med J 73:14–17, 1980.
305. Herlin P, Ericsson M, Holmin T, et al.: Acute acalculus cholecystitis following trauma. Br J Surg 69:475–476, 1982.
306. Okada Y, Tanabe R, Mukaida M: Post-traumatic acute cholecystitis. Relationship to the initial trauma. Am J Forensic Med Pathol 8:164–168, 1987.
307. Yamashita H, Chijiiwa K, Ogawa Y, et al.: The internal biliary fistula—reappraisal of incidence, type, diagnosis and management of 33 consecutive cases. HPB Surgery 10:143–147, 1997.
308. Hession PR, Rawlinson J, Hall JR, et al.: The clinical and radiologic features of cholecystocolic fistulae. Br J Radiol 69:804–809, 1996.
309. Marshall SF, Polk RC: Spontaneous internal biliary fistulas. Surg Clin North Am 38:679–691, 1958.
310. Griffith CD, Saunders JH: Cholecystoduodenocolic fistula following abdominal trauma. Br J Surg 69:99–100, 1982.
311. Porter JM, Muller DC, Silver D: Spontaneous biliary-enteric fistulas. Surgery 68:597–601, 1970.
312. Al Nakib B, Jacob GS, Al Liddawi H, et al.: Choledochoduodenal fistula due to tuberculosis. Endoscopy 14:64–65, 1982.
313. Khaira HS, Awad RW, Thompson AK: Squamous carcinoma of the gallbladder presenting with biliary-colic fistula, 1982. Eur J Surg Oncol 21:581–582, 1995.
314. Pangan JC, Estrada R, Rosales R: Cholecystoduodenocolic fistula with recurrent gallstone ileus. Arch Surg 119:1201–1203, 1984.
315. Byard RW, Thorner PS, Cutz E, et al.: Xanthogranulomatous cholecystitis and cholecystoduodenal fistula associated with total parenteral nutrition in a six year old child. Pathology 22:239–241, 1990.
316. Van Landingham SB, Broders CW: Gallstone ileus. Surg Clin North Am 62:241–247, 1982.
317. Slasky BS, Campbell WL: Cholecystosigmoid fistula. Am J Gastroenterol 78:276–279, 1983.
318. Gibbons CP, Ross B: Cholecystoduodenocolic fistula and gallstone ileus. Postgrad Med J 60:698–699, 1984.
319. Hakim M, Boyd R, Stricoff R, et al.: Cholecystogastrocolic fistula with intrahepatic abscess: A rare complication of biliary stone disease. Am Surg 63:472–474, 1997.
320. Nessler E, Stoss F, Walser J: The cholecystogastric fistula. Surg Endosc 5:46–47, 1991.
321. Abril A, Ulfohn A: Spontaneous cholecystocutaneous fistula. South Med J 77:1192–1193, 1984.
322. Hakaim AG, Vogt DP: Spontaneous cholecystocutaneous fistulas. Clev Clin Q 53:363–365, 1986.
323. Gibson TC, Howat JM: Cholecystocutaneous fistula. Br J Clin Pract 41:980–982, 1987.
324. Birch BR, Cox SJ: Spontaneous external biliary fistula uncomplicated by gallstones. Postgrad Med J 67:391–392, 1991.
325. Cunningham LW, Grobman M, Paz HL, et al.: Cholecystopleural fistula with cholelithiasis presenting as a right pleural effusion. Chest 97:751–752, 1990.

326. Delco F, Domenighetti G, Kauzlaric D, et al.: Spontaneous bilithorax (thoracobilia) following cholecystopleural fistula presenting as an acute respiratory insufficiency. Chest 106:961–963, 1994.
327. Genell SN, Fork FT, Jiborn H: Bronchobiliary fistula in chronic pancreatitis. Case report. Acta Chir Scand 153:473–475, 1987.
328. Allison MC, Milkins S, Burroughs AK, et al.: Bronchobiliary fistula due to acute cholecystitis in a suprahepatic gallbladder. Postgrad J Med 63:291–294, 1987.
329. Davies CJ, Fontaine CJ: Spontaneous cholecystoumbilical fistula. Br J Radiol 57:1034–1036, 1984.
330. Csendes A, Diaz JC, Burdiles P, et al.: Mirizzi syndrome and cholecystobiliary fistula: A unifying classification. Br J Surg 76:1139–1143, 1989.
331. Mishra MC, Vashishtha S, Tandon R: Biliobiliary fistula: Preoperative diagnosis and management implications. Surgery 108:835–839, 1990.
332. Schenken JR, Adamson JR: Fatal gastrointestinal tract hemorrhage: A complication of ulcerative cholecystitis, cholelithiasis and cholecystoduodenal fistula. Am J Clin Pathol 53:423–424, 1970.
333. Berliner SD, Burson LC: One-stage repair for cholecyst-duodenal fistula and gallstone ileus. Arch Surg 90:313–316, 1965.
334. Rau WS, Matern S, Gerok W, et al.: Spontaneous cholecystocolonic fistula. A model situation for bile acid diarrhea and fatty acid diarrhea as a consequence of disturbed enterohepatic circulation of bile acids. Hepatogastroenterology 27:231–237, 1980.
335. Kaplan BJ: Massive lower gastrointestinal hemorrhage from cholecystocolic fistula. Dis Colon Rectum 10:191–196, 1966.
336. Dowse JLA: Spontaneous internal biliary fistulae. Gut 5:429–436, 1964.
337. Nielsen SM, Nielsen PT: Gastric retention caused by gallstones (Bouveret's syndrome). Acta Chir Scand 149:207–208, 1983.
338. Ah-Chong K, Leong YP: Gastric outlet obstruction due to gallstones (Bouveret syndrome). Postgrad Med J 63:909–910, 1987.
339. Collie DA, Redhead DN, Garden OJ: Cholecystobronchocolic fistula: A late complication of biliary sepsis. Case report of diagnosis and management. HPB Surgery 7:319–326, 1994.
340. Yip AW, Chow WC, Chan J, et al.: Mirizzi syndrome with cholecystodochal fistula: Preoperative diagnosis and management. Surgery 111:335–338, 1992.
341. Ibrarullah M, Saxena R, Sikora SS, et al.: Mirizzi's syndrome: Identification and management strategy. Aust N Z J Surg 63:802–806, 1993.
342. Curet MJ, Rosendale DE, Congilosi S: Mirizzi syndrome in a Native American population. Am J Surg 168:616–621, 1994.
343. Tanaka N, Nobori M, Furuya T, et al.: Evolution of Mirizzi syndrome with biliobiliary fistula. J Gastroenterol 30:117–121, 1995.
344. Nagakawa T, Ohta T, Kayahara M, et al.: A new classification of Mirizzi syndrome from diagnostic and therapeutic viewpoints. Hepatogastroenterology 44:63–67, 1997.
345. Dorrance HR, Lingam MK, Hair A, et al.: Acquired abnormalities of the biliary tract from chronic gallstone disease. J Am Coll Surg 189:269–273, 1999.
346. Moss JF, Bloom AD, Mesleh GF, et al.: Gallstone ileus. Am Surg 52:424–428, 1987.
347. Schutte H, Bastias J, Csendes A, et al.: Gallstone ileus. Hepatogastroenterology 39:562–565, 1992.
348. Reisner RM, Cohen JR: Gallstone ileus: A review of 1001 reported cases. Am Surg 60:441–446, 1994.
349. Re Mine WH: Biliary-enteric fistulas: Natural history and management. Adv Surg 7:69–94, 1973.
350. Levowitz BS: Spontaneous internal biliary fistulas. Ann Surg 154:241–251, 1961.
351. Raiford TS: Intestinal obstruction due to gallstones (gallstone ileus). Ann Surg 153:830–838, 1961.
352. MacKenney RP: The management of gallstone ileus. J Coll Surg Edinb 21:292–295, 1976.
353. Senofsky GM, Stabile BE: Gallstone ileus associated with Crohn's disease. Surgery 108:114–117, 1990.
354. Milsom JW, Mackerrigan JM: Gallstone obstruction of the colon. Report of two cases and review of management. Dis Colon Rectum 28:367–370, 1985.
355. Garcia-Lopez S, Sebastian JJ, Uribarrena R, et al.: Successful endoscopic relief of large bowel obstruction in a case of sigmoid colon gallstone ileus. J Clin Gastroenterol 24:291–292, 1997.
356. Davies JB, Sedman PC, Benson EA: Gallstone ileus—beware the second silent stone. Postgrad Med J 72:300–301, 1996.
357. Yamamoto M, Nakajo S, Ito M, et al.: Primary mucosal hyperplasia of the gallbladder. Acta Pathol Jpn 38:393–398, 1988.
358. Elfving G, Silvonen E, Teir H: Mucosal hyperplasia of the gallbladder in cases of cholecystolithiasis. Acta Chir Scand 77:384–388, 1969.
359. Christensen AH, Ishak KG: Benign tumors and pseudotumors of the gallbladder. Report of 180 cases. Arch Pathol 90:423–432, 1970.
360. Yamamoto M, Nakajo S, Tahara E: Histological classification of epithelial polypoid lesions of the gallbladder. Arch Pathol Jpn 38:181–192, 1988.
361. Duarte I, Llanos O, Domke H, et al.: Metaplasia and precursor lesions of gallbladder carcinoma. Frequency, distribution and probability of detection in routine histologic samples. Cancer 72:1878–1884, 1993.
362. Tokiwa K, Iwai N: Early mucosal changes of the gallbladder in patients with anomalous arrangement of the pancreatobiliary duct. Gastroenterology 110: 1614–1618, 1996.
363. Tanno S, Obara T, Fujii T, et al.: Proliferative potential and k-*ras* mutation in epithelial hyperplasia of the gallbladder in patients with anomalous pancreatobiliary duct union. Cancer 83:267–275, 1998.
364. Lewin KJ: Nomenclature problems of gastrointestinal epithelial neoplasia. Am J Surg Pathol 22:1043–1047, 1998.
365. Albores-Saavedra J, Defortuna SM, Smothermon WE,: Primary papillary hyperplasia of the gallbladder and cystic and common bile ducts. Hum Pathol 21:228–231, 1990.
366. Oak S, Rao S, Karmankar S, et al.: Papillomatosis of the gallbladder in metachromatic leukodystrophy. Pediatr Surg Int 12:424–425, 1997.
367. Albores–Saavedra J, Henson DE: Adenomyomatous hyperplasia of the gallbladder with perineural invasion. Arch Pathol Lab Med 119:1173–1176, 1995.
368. Albores-Saavedra J, Vardaman CJ, Vuitch F: Nonneoplastic polypoid lesions and adenomas of the gallbladder. Pathol Annu 28(part I):145–177, 1993.
369. Kimura K, Ohto M, Saisho H, et al.: Association of gallbladder carcinoma and anomalous pancreatobiliary duct union. Gastroenterology 89:1258–1265, 1985.
370. Sato H, Mizushima M, Ito J, et al.: Sessile adenoma of the gallbladder. Re-appraisal of its importance as

a precancerous lesion. Arch Pathol Lab Med 109:65–69, 1985.

371. Yamaguchi K, Enjoji M: Gallbladder polyps. Inflammatory hyperplastic and neoplastic types. Surg Pathol 1:203–213, 1988.
372. Tatematsu M, Furihata C, Miki K, et al.: Complete and incomplete pyloric gland metaplasia of human gallbladder. Acta Pathol Jpn 37:39–46, 1987.
373. Aroni K, Kittas C, Papadimitriou CS, et al.: An immunohistochemical study of the distribution of lysozyme, al-antitrypsin and al-antichymotrypsin in the normal and pathological gallbladder. Virchows Arch [A] Pathol Anat Histopathol 403:281–289, 1984.
374. Boyle L, Gallivan MV, Chun B, et al.: Heterotopia of gastric mucosa and liver involving the gallbladder. Report of two cases with literature review. Arch Pathol Lab Med 116:138–142, 1992.
375. Yamamoto M, Nagako S, Tahara E: Endocrine cells and lysozyme immunoreactivity in the gallbladder. Arch Pathol Lab Med 110:920–927, 1986.
376. Albores-Saavedra J, Nadji M, Henson DE, et al.: Intestinal metaplasia of the gallbladder: A morphologic and immunohistochemical study. Hum Pathol 17:614–620, 1986.
377. Kozuka S, Hachisuka K: Incidence by age and sex of intestinal metaplasia of the gallbladder. Hum Pathol 15:779–784, 1984.
378. Tsutsumi Y, Nagura H, Osamura Y, et al.: Histochemical studies of metaplastic lesions in the human gallbladder. Arch Pathol Lab Med 108:917–921, 1984.
379. Laitio M: Histogenesis of epithelial neoplasms of the human gallbladder. I. Dysplasia. Path Res Pract 178:51–56, 1983.
380. Kozuka S, Kurashina M, Tsubone M, et al.: Significance of intestinal metaplasia for the evolution of cancer in the biliary tract. Cancer 54:2277–2285, 1984.
381. Dowling GP, Kelly JK: The histogenesis of adenocarcinoma of the gallbladder. Cancer 58:1702–1708, 1986.
382. Yamagiwa H, Tomiyama H: Intestinal metaplasia-dysplasia-carcinoma sequence of the gallbladder. Acta Pathol Jpn 36:989–997, 1986.
383. Cornell CM, Clarke R: Vicarious calcification involving the gallbladder. Arch Surg 149:267–272, 1959.
384. Hanada M, Shimizu H, Takami M: Squamous cell carcinoma of the gallbladder associated with squamous metaplasia and adenocarcinoma in situ of the mucosal columnar epithelium. Acta Pathol Jpn 36:1879–1886, 1986.

Chapter

12

NONNEOPLASTIC POLYPS OF THE GALLBLADDER

Gallbladder polyps may be neoplastic or nonneoplastic.

The true frequency of gallbladder polyps is not known. Benign gallbladder neoplasms are considered to be rarities, with a quoted frequency of 0.4% to 0.5% in cholecystectomy specimens.[1,2] Our experience is that nonneoplastic polyps are considerably more common than this and may be present in between 2.5% to 10% of surgically resected gallbladders. This higher figure is also confirmed by several studies using modern imaging techniques,[3–6] with ultrasound examination and enhanced computed tomography being particularly useful for identifying small polyps.[7–9] Sensitive imaging methods may, however, detect gallstones or biliary sludge adherent to the gallbladder wall and erroneously interpret this finding as evidence of a mucosal polyp. The majority of gallbladder polyps are therefore not neoplasms and instead represent reactive or inflammatory conditions (Table 12–1). In typical cases, the histologic distinction between hyperplastic, mucus gland, and inflammatory polyps is clear-cut. However, overlapping forms exist, suggesting that at least in some instances, they have a common origin: chronic inflammation and irritation. Gallbladder polyps are more common in individuals with diabetes mellitus.[4]

The clinical management of gallbladder polyps, discovered incidentally by imaging studies, presents some problems,[10–16] even though the majority are benign and do not increase in size when followed over a period of time.[5,6,16] In studies from Japan,[12,17] it has been shown that neoplastic polyps tend to be solitary and large. Ninety-four percent of benign polyps are < 10 mm in diameter, whereas 88% of malignant polyps exceeded this size.[12] Ninety-seven percent of cholesterol polyps measure < 10 mm in diameter.[17] Multiple polyps are more likely to be benign than they are to be malignant. However, when fewer than three polyps are present in the gallbladder, the incidence of neoplasia is 37%, even in polyps measuring between 5 and 10 mm in diameter.[18] The currently recommended treatment is that polyps > 10 mm in diameter should be excised by elective cholecystectomy. Polyps smaller than this may also be treated by cholecystectomy if the patient has symptoms sufficient to justify the procedure; otherwise, they may be safely followed by sequential ultrasound examination and excised only if they continue to grow.[18]

CHOLESTEROL POLYPS

Cholesterol polyps are generally small lesions measuring < 1.0 cm in diameter.[7,8,17,19] They account for between 50% and 60% of all gallbladder polyps.[7,10,11] Grossly, they have a branched multilobular appearance, have a narrow base, and are yellowish cream in color. They are often multiple, with a median number of 8, but up to 30 are present in some gallbladders.[18] In 20% of patients, they are solitary lesions. Cholesterol polyps may occur in a localized area of cholesterolosis, and in about 5% of patients, there is diffuse cholesterolosis.[19]

Microscopically, there is a central solid core with a coarse papillary surface configuration

Table 12–1. Nonneoplastic Polyps of the Gallbladder

Cholesterol polyp
Hyperplastic polyp
Metaplastic polyp
Inflammatory polyp
Lymphoid polyp
Mucus gland polyp
Hamartoma

(Fig. 12–1). The papillae tend to be simple, without the complex branching pattern typical of benign epithelial neoplasms. The core and stroma of the papillae contain large numbers of foamy macrophages (Fig. 12–2). Other inflammatory cells are generally absent. The polyps are covered by histologically unremarkable biliary type epithelium, which may be attenuated, so that it is cuboidal rather than columnar. Generally, ulceration of the surface does not occur.

Cholesterol polyps have a weak connection with the presence of gallbladder calculi, especially cholesterol calculi, but there is no known malignant potential. Curiously, for such small and apparently incidental lesions, there is an association with the presence of right upper quadrant pain, which may vary in duration from several months to several years.[19] Occasional examples have been recorded in which cholesterol polyps have become detached from the gallbladder mucosa and impacted in the distal bile duct, causing obstructive jaundice.[20]

HYPERPLASTIC/METAPLASTIC POLYPS

Hyperplastic polyps are the second most common type of gallbladder polyp, accounting for approximately 20% of cases. The vast majority of polyps occur secondary to cholecystitis or cholelithiasis. However, rarely, they may occur in association with chronic ulcerative colitis[21,22] or metachromatic leukodystrophy.[23,24] The term *localized papillary hyperplasia* may also be used to describe these polyps, but the older name, *adenomatous hyperplasia,*[19] should be avoided, as it serves to confuse what is essentially a reactive lesion with a benign neoplasm. Most examples of gallbladder mucosal hyperplasia are diffuse and nonpolypoid, recognizable grossly by the velvety appearance they give to the mucosa. These are discussed in the section on reactive lesions of the gallbladder (Hyperplasia and Metaplasia) in Chapter 11. Hyperplastic polyps, which appear polypoid to the naked eye, are

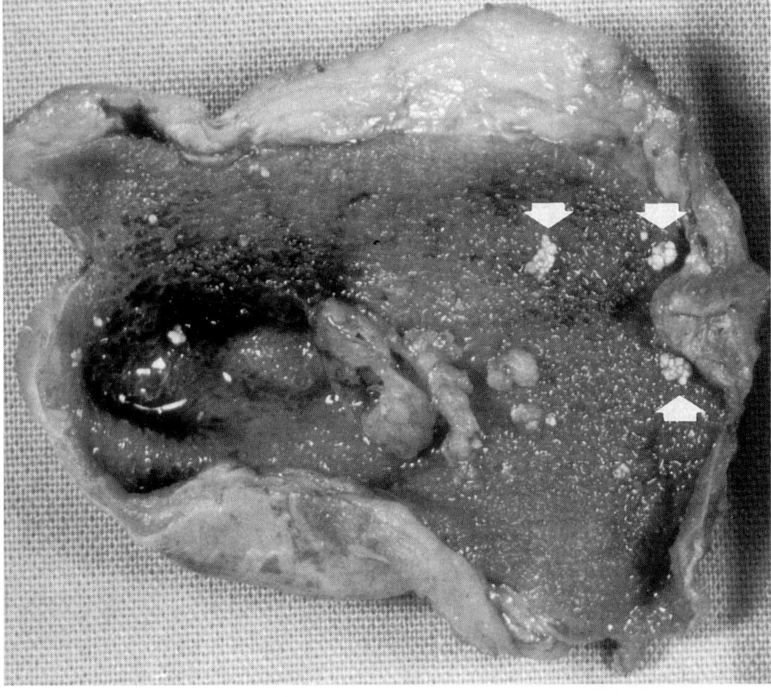

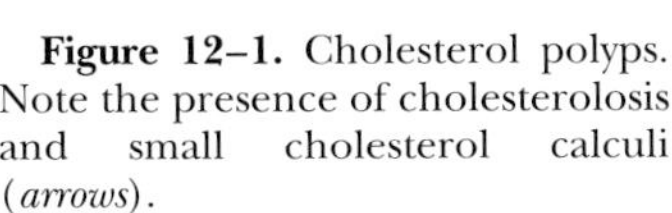

Figure 12–1. Cholesterol polyps. Note the presence of cholesterolosis and small cholesterol calculi (*arrows*).

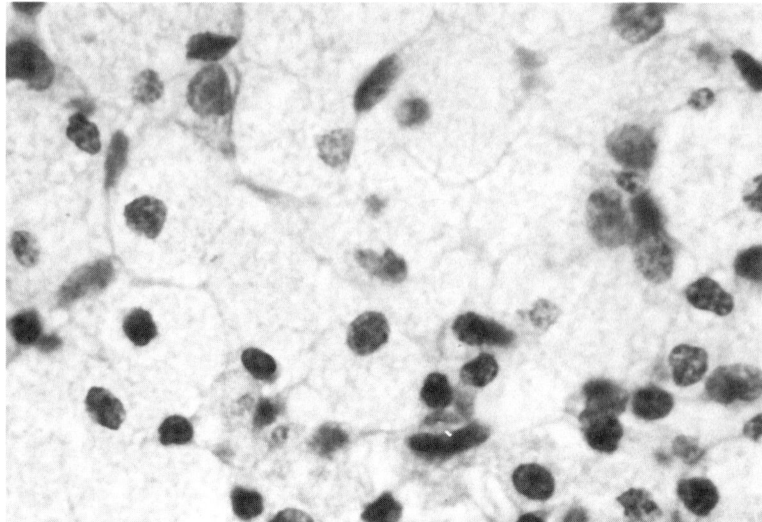

Figure 12–2. Macrophages with expanded clear cytoplasm present within the core of a cholesterol polyp.

regarded as a localized, more florid variant of diffuse mucosal hyperplasia.

Hyperplastic polyps are small, usually measuring < 5 mm in diameter, although rare larger lesions are encountered.[25] They may be multiple and either sessile or pedunculated in gross configuration. Microscopically, they consist of prominent hyperplastic mucosal folds and papillae, covered by mucosa resembling normal gallbladder epithelium[21] (Fig. 12–3). Metaplastic changes are common, and in many cases, there is no clear-cut separation between hyperplastic and metaplastic polyps, with many mixed forms present. These terms should therefore be regarded as clinically equivalent. Metaplasia may consist of gastric-type surface mucosa, intestinal mucosa with goblet cells, and occasionally glands, resembling gastric pyloric mucus-secreting glands. There may also be Paneth's cells and endocrine cells present as part of intestinal metaplasia. Gallbladder metaplasia is also discussed more fully in Chapter 11.

It is not uncommon for hyperplastic/metaplastic polyps to show focal inflammation, especially toward the surface. Generally, this takes the form on nonspecific chronic inflammation, consisting predominately of lymphocytes but with smaller numbers of plasma cells, histio-

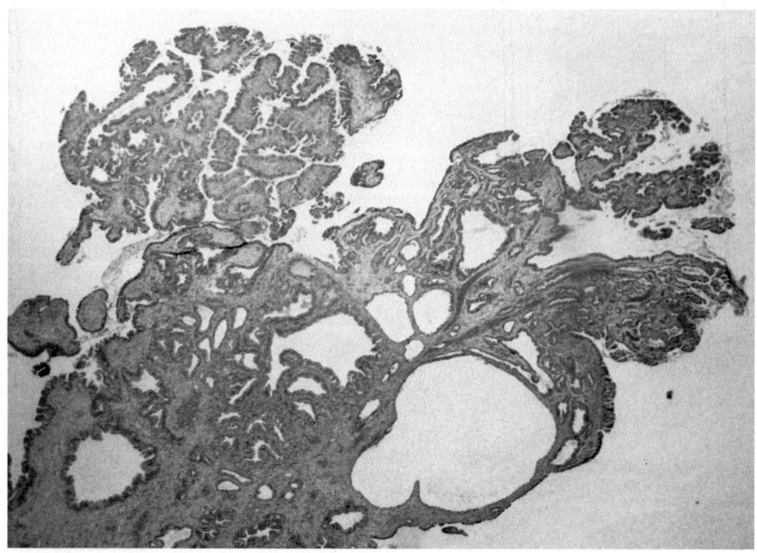

Figure 12–3. Hyperplastic polyp with mucosal folds covered by normal-appearing biliary epithelium. There is a minor inflammatory component.

cytes, eosinophils, and neutrophils. This may be accompanied by reactive epithelial changes that can be confused with dysplasia, leading to an erroneous diagnosis of adenoma. The histopathologic features useful in separating gallbladder adenomas from reactive changes are similar to those used in other areas of the gastrointestinal tract—for example, the stomach. Adenomas of the gallbladder closely resemble colonic adenomas. The whole polyp shows a similar degree of dysplasia, with the epithelium being composed of hyperchromatic cigar-shaped nuclei, demonstrating loss of polarity. As a general rule, adenomas are not inflamed or are only lightly inflamed. Reactive changes in hyperplastic polyps are focal and almost invariably accompanied by inflammation. The nuclei are enlarged and vesicular and occasionally may be pseudostratified or crowded (Fig. 12–4).

Papillary hyperplasia may also occur as an isolated finding (primary hyperplasia).[26] In the cases described, there was widespread villous hyperplasia, which formed either multiple small projections or single broad-based lesions. In some of these cases, there was extensive adenomyosis (Aschoff–Rokitansky sinus formation) and the surface hyperplasia was similar to the hyperplastic epithelium lining sinuses. Histologically, primary hyperplasia shows similarity of the covering epithelium to normal gallbladder epithelium, with the addition of minor inflammatory and metaplastic changes. As mentioned previously, hyperplastic polyps show the same range of appearances that may be identified in hyperplastic nonpolypoid mucosa.

There is some controversy as to whether hyperplastic polyps should be regarded as a precursor of dysplasia and gallbladder carcinoma. At present, it seems that cases in which the association does occur are rare. In these instances, the gallbladder is also inflamed and contains calculi.[21] It seems possible, therefore, that in the majority of cases any association is purely incidental.

INFLAMMATORY POLYPS

There are various types of inflammatory polyps that may occur in the gallbladder; all arise basically as a result of prior, usually repeated episodes of cholecystitis. The two major varieties are granulation tissue polyps and fibrous polyps,[27] however, these are not pure entities and have many overlapping features.

Inflammatory polyps may measure up to 1.5 cm in diameter, with fibrous polyps generally being larger than the granulation tissue polyps. Approximately half the polyps are solitary, and in the remaining examples, between two and five polyps are present.[19] Grossly, both types appear as firm, reddish gray lesions.[11] The polyps have a broad base and a leaflike configuration.

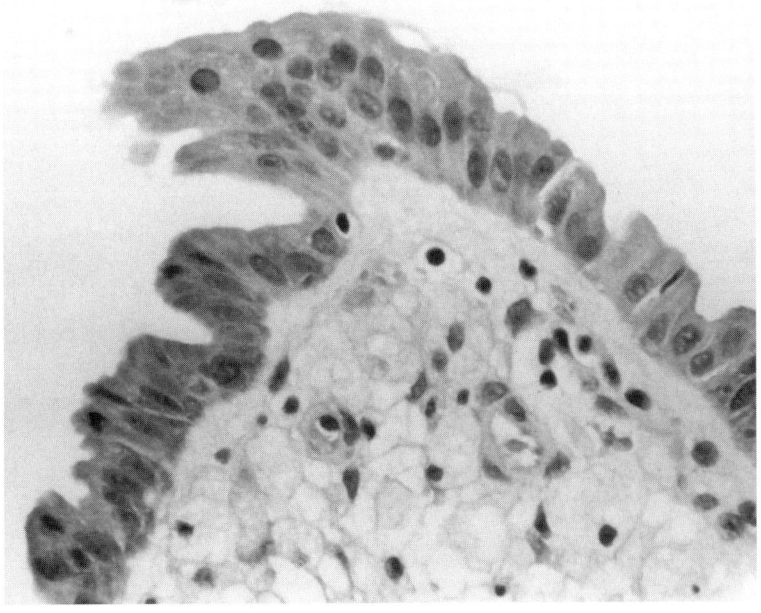

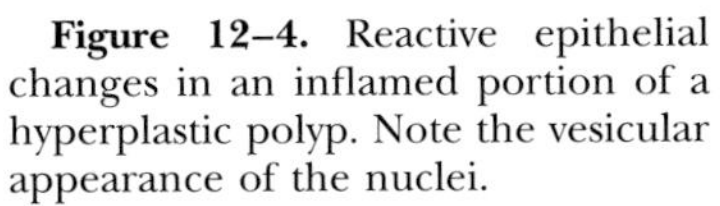

Figure 12–4. Reactive epithelial changes in an inflamed portion of a hyperplastic polyp. Note the vesicular appearance of the nuclei.

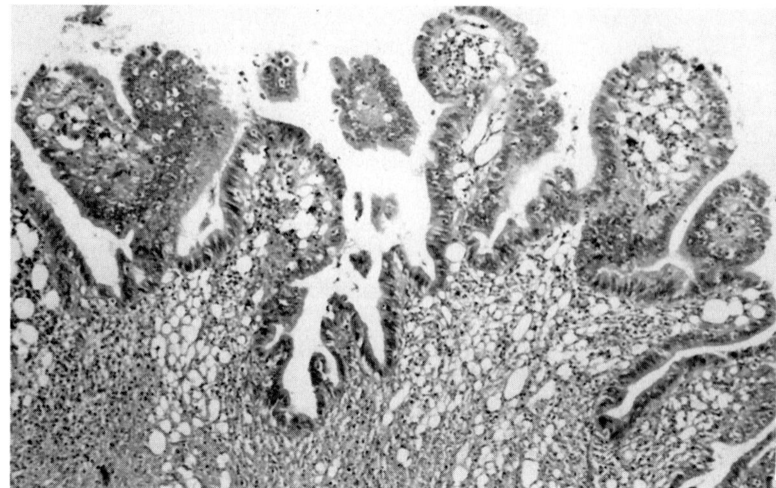

Figure 12–5. Granulation tissue polyp.

They are often denuded of mucosa on the surface. The granulation tissue polyps consist of proliferating vascular channels, with a varying admixture of acute and chronic inflammatory cells.[21] There may be stromal hemorrhage (Fig. 12–5). In fibrous polyps, the stroma contains trapped and distorted glandlike structures, representing invaginations of the surface epithelium. These are surrounded by an edematous fibrous stroma, containing smaller numbers of inflammatory cells, usually lymphocytes (Fig. 12–6). Care must be taken not to confuse focal epithelial atypia occurring in inflamed areas with dysplasia. (See Hyperplastic/Metaplastic Polyps, above.)

LYMPHOID POLYPS

Focal lymphoid hyperplasia with the gallbladder may rarely become polypoid. Each polyp is seldom > 5 mm in diameter, and, not uncommonly, the lesions are multiple (up to 20 polyps). The polyps typically occur in women between the ages of 52 and 80 years (mean age, 65 years).[21] Histologically, these polyps are iden-

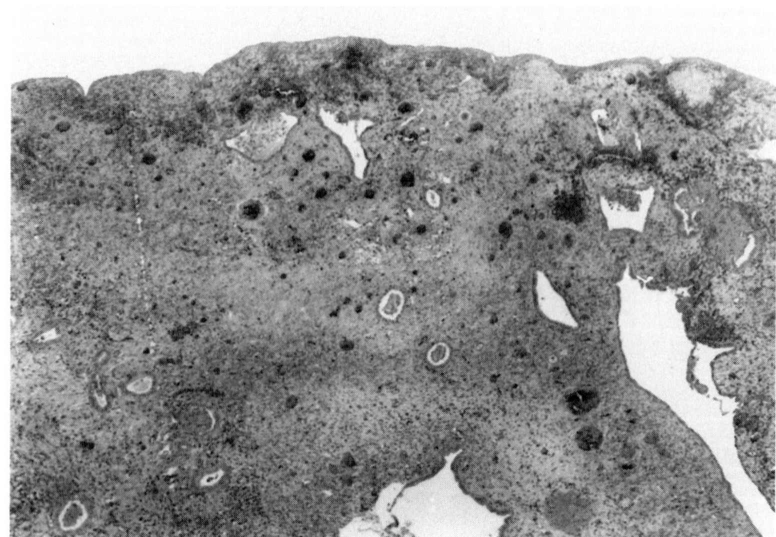

Figure 12–6. Fibrous area of inflammatory polyp with an edematous stroma and entrapped invaginations of the surface epithelium.

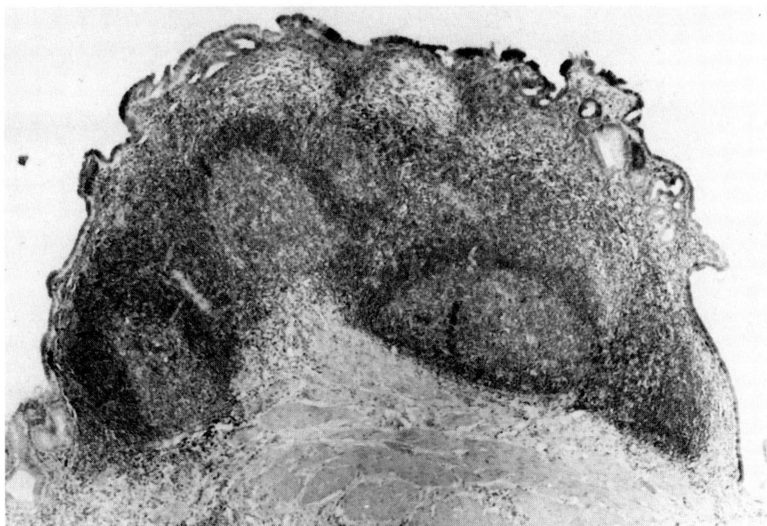

Figure 12–7. Lymphoid polyp of the gallbladder, with prominent germinal centers.

tical to prominent Peyer's patches or to lymphoid polyps of the rectum.[28] They are covered by normal but attenuated biliary epithelium and have a stroma consisting of mature lymphocytes, with reactive germinal centers (Fig. 12–7). At the lower border of the polyp, lymphocytes may spill over to involve the muscularis of the gallbladder.[21,27,29] Distinction from well-differentiated malignant lymphoma is not usually a problem, because the germinal centers are well defined and contain tingible body macrophages. Malignant lymphoma of the gallbladder is usually large cell in type and is advanced at the time of diagnosis. It presents as a large mass and widespread lymphoid infiltration. In problem cases, special techniques will demonstrate polyclonality in benign lymphoid polyps.

Most often, lymphoid polyposis is associated with chronic cholecystitis and gallstones; however, the more florid examples of polyposis may have an associated biliary tract infection, especially with *Klebsiella pneumoniae,*[21] *Escherichia coli,*[21] or *Salmonella typhi.*[30] Lymphoid hyperplasia of the gallbladder has also been described in association with hypogammaglobulinemia and lymphoid hyperplasia of the small bowel.[31]

MUCUS GLAND (PSEUDOPYLORIC GLAND) POLYPS

Mucus glands are normally present in the submucosa of the gallbladder, predominately in the neck region, and histologically resemble Brunner's glands of the duodenum. They may undergo enlargement and form sessile nodules, usually measuring ≤ 5 mm in diameter. They may be multiple. Mucus gland polyps have many similarities to hyperplastic polyps, except that they consist of hyperplastic glands rather than hyperplastic surface epithelium. They are sessile, with a smooth, rounded surface (Fig. 12–8). Most authorities believe that these polyps occur as a result of hyperplasia,[21] although others think they may be examples of benign neoplasia[27,32] or heterotopia.[33]

The hyperplastic mucus glands have a resemblance to gastric antral and Brunner's glands and are lined by tall, columnar, mucin-producing cells with basal nuclei. However, unlike antral glands, the cytoplasm is clear rather than bubbly in appearance. Occasional endocrine cells may also be present.[21] Nuclear atypia is not usually encountered, unless there is superimposed chronic inflammation. The nodules show poor demarcation at their base and merge with the surrounding nonhyperplastic tissues.

HAMARTOMATOUS POLYPS

Hamartomatous polyps may be found in the gallbladder in both Peutz–Jeghers syndrome[34–36] and Cowden's disease.[37] Histologically, the lesions are similar to hyperplastic polyps but may also contain foci of gastric pyloric gland metaplasia.[35] In one patient with Peutz–Jeghers syndrome, polyps in the gallbladder were associated with an adenocarcinoma.[35]

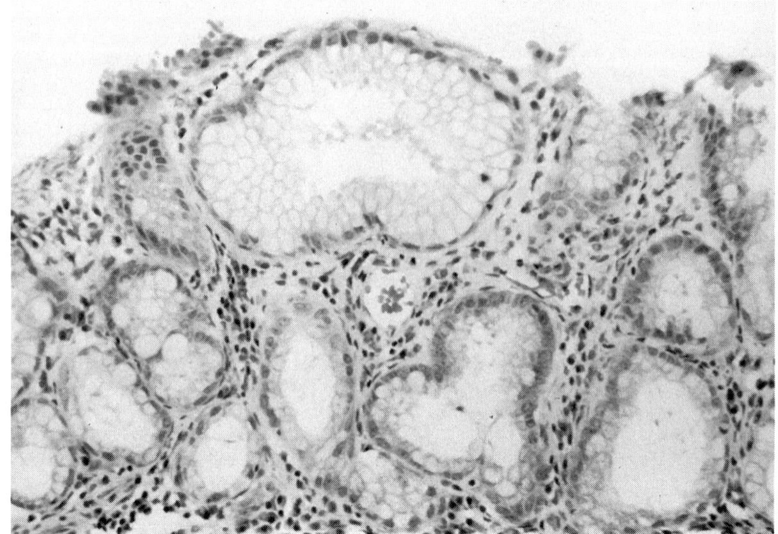

Figure 12–8. Mucus gland polyp with a rounded surface contour containing hyperplastic mucus glands.

REFERENCES

1. Kane CF, Brown CH, Hoerr SO: Papilloma of the gallbladder. Report of eight cases. Am J Surg 83:161–164, 1952.
2. Albores-Saavedra J, Henson DE: Tumors of the gallbladder and extrahepatic bile ducts. *In:* Atlas of tumor pathology, second series, fascicle 22. Washington, DC: Armed Forces Institute of Pathology, 1986, pp 17–27.
3. Shinchi K, Kono S, Honjo S, et al.: Epidemiology of gallbladder polyps: An ultrasonographic study of male self-defence officials in Japan. Scan J Gastroenterol 29:7–10, 1994.
4. Chen CY, Lu CL, Chang FY, et al.: Risk factors for gallbladder polyps in the Chinese population. Am J Gastroenterol 92:2066–2068, 1997.
5. Collett JA, Allan RB, Chisholm RJ, et al.: Gallbladder polyps: Prospective study. J Ultrasound Med 17:207–211, 1998.
6. Moriguchi H, Tazawa J, Hayashi Y, et al.: Natural history of polypoid lesions of the gallbladder. Gut 39:860–862, 1996.
7. Ruhe AH, Zachman JP, Mulder BD, et al.: Cholesterol polyps of the gallbladder. Ultrasound demonstration. J Clin Ultrasound 7:386–388, 1979.
8. Price RJ, Stewart ET, Foley D, et al.: Sonography of polypoid cholesterolosis. AJR 139:1197–1198, 1982.
9. Furukawa H, Takayasu K, Mukai K, et al.: CT evaluation of small polypoid lesions of the gallbladder. Hepatogastroenterology 42:800–810, 1995.
10. Nugent FW, Meissner WA, Hoelscher FE: The significance of gallbladder polyps. JAMA 178:426–428, 1961.
11. Selzer DW, Dockerty MB, Stauffer MH, et al.: Papillomas (so-called) in the non-calculous gallbladder. Am J Surg 103:472–476, 1962.
12. Koga A, Watanabe K, Fukuyama T, et al.: Diagnosis and operative indications for polypoid lesions of the gallbladder. Arch Surg 123:26–29, 1988.
13. Kubota K, Bandai Y, Noie T, et al.: How should polypoid lesions of the gallbladder be treated in the era of laparoscopic cholecystectomy? Surgery 117:481–487, 1995.
14. Mangel AW: Management of gallbladder polyps. South Med J 90:481–483, 1997.
15. Toda K, Souda S, Yoshikawa Y, et al.: Significance of laparoscopic excisional biopsy for polypoid lesions of the gallbladder. Surg Laparosc Endosc 5:267–271, 1995.
16. Moriguchi H, Tazawa J, Hayashi Y, et al.: Natural history of polypoid lesions in the gallbladder. Gut 39:860–862, 1996.
17. Shinkai H, Kimura W, Muto T: Surgical indication for small polypoid lesions of the gallbladder. Am J Surg 175:114–117, 1998.
18. Bilhartz LE: Acute acalculous cholecystitis, adenomyomatosis, cholesterolosis and polyps of the gallbladder. *In* Sleisenger MH, Fordtran JS (eds): Gastrointestinal Disease: Pathophysiology, Diagnosis, Management, 5th ed. Philadelphia: WB Saunders, 1993, pp 1858–1868.
19. Christensen AH, Ishak KG: Benign tumors and pseudotumors of the gallbladder. Arch Pathol 90:423–432, 1970.
20. Takii Y, Shirai Y, Kanehara H, et al.: Obstructive jaundice caused by a cholesterol polyp of the gallbladder: Report of a case. Surg Today 24:1104–1106, 1994.
21. Albores-Saavedra J, Vardaman CJ, Vuitch F: Nonneoplastic polypoid lesions and adenomas of the gallbladder. Pathol Annu 28(part 1):145–177, 1993.
22. Almagro UA: Diffuse papillomatosis of the gallbladder. Am J Gastroenterol 80:274–278, 1985.
23. Warfel KA, Hull MT: Villous papilloma of the gallbladder associated with leukodystrophy. Hum Pathol 15:1192–1194, 1984.
24. Dische MR: Metachromatic leukodystrophic polyposis of the gallbladder. J Pathol 97:388–390, 1969.
25. Kubota K, Bandai Y, Araki Y, et al.: Giant hyperplastic polyp of the gallbladder: A case report. J Clin Ultrasound 24:203–206, 1996.
26. Albores-Saavedra J, Defortuna SM, Smotherson WE: Primary papillary hyperplasia of the gallbladder and cystic and common bile ducts. Hum Pathol 21:228–231, 1990.
27. Yamaguchi K, Enjoji M: Gallbladder polyps. Inflammatory, hyperplastic and neoplastic types. Surg Pathol 1:203–213, 1988.

28. Ranchod M, Lewin KJ, Dorfman RF: Lymphoid hyperplasia of the gastrointestinal tract. A study of 26 cases and a review of the literature. Am J Surg Pathol 2:383–400, 1978.
29. Estrada RL, Brown NM, James CE: Chronic follicular cholecystitis. Radiological, pathological and surgical aspects. Br J Surg 48:205–209, 1960.
30. Mallory TB, Lawson GM: Chronic typhoid cholecystitis. Am J Pathol 7:71–76, 1931.
31. Sauerbrie E, Castelli M: Hypogammaglobulinemia and nodular lymphoid hyperplasia of the gut. J Can Assoc Radiol 30:62–63, 1979.
32. Kushima R, Remmele W, Stolte M, et al.: Pyloric gland type adenoma of the gallbladder with squamoid spindle cell metaplasia. Pathol Res Prac 192:963–969, 1996.
33. Boyle L, Gallivan MV, Chun B, et al.: Heterotopia of gastric mucosa and liver involving the gallbladder. Report of two cases and review of the literature. Arch Pathol Lab Med 116:138–142, 1992.
34. Foster DR, Foster DB: Gall-bladder polyps in Peutz–Jeghers syndrome. Postgrad J Med 56:373–376, 1980.
35. Wada K, Tanaka M, Yamaguchi K, et al.: Carcinoma and polyps of the gallbladder associated with Peutz–Jeghers syndrome. Dig Dis Sci 32:943–946, 1987.
36. Guzman P, Roa I, Villaseca M, et al.: Peritoneal pseudomyxoma in a child with a gallbladder Peutz–Jeghers-like hamartomatous polyp: A case report. J Pediatr Surg 33:1320–1322, 1998.
37. Marra G, Armelao F, Vecchio FM, et al.: Cowden's disease with extensive gastrointestinal polyposis. J Clin Gastroenterol 18:42–47, 1994.

Chapter

13

NEOPLASMS OF THE GALLBLADDER

Table 13–1 shows the World Health Organization (WHO) classification of neoplasms of the gallbladder.[1]

ADENOMA

Adenoma is defined by the WHO monograph as "a benign neoplasm of glandular epithelium which is typically polypoid and well-demarcated."[1] The term *adenoma* implies the presence of glandular dysplasia within the lesion. In the past, a clear distinction between adenoma and nonpolypoid epithelial dysplasia in the gallbladder has not been drawn, as both lesions consist of dysplastic epithelium. Furthermore, some authors have used the terms *adenoma* and *dysplasia* interchangeably or have used one term and excluded the other. This blurring of terminology is understandable, as there is morphologic overlap between adenoma and nonpolypoid dysplasia. However, by convention, an adenoma is polypoid, is well demarcated, and arises in normal mucosa, whereas nonpolypoid dysplasia is poorly demarcated, is flat, and arises in chronically diseased mucosa in association with gastric or intestinal metaplasia. Yamamoto et al. have, however, described two types of adenoma, one derived from normal gallbladder epithelium and the other derived from and containing metaplastic epithelium.[2]

Adenomas are usually solitary but may be multiple in nearly one third of cases.[3] Most adenomas are sporadic, but a minority have been reported in patients with familial adenomatous polyposis or Peutz–Jeghers syndrome.[4,5] Adenomas are rare; the largest reported series is 51 cases from the Armed Forces Institute of Pathology.[3] Early articles have referred to it as "papilloma," meaning papillary adenoma.[6] Eleven adenomas of the gallbladder that were found in 5,200 surgical biliary tract cases comprised 7 villous adenomas, 2 pedunculated adenomas, and 2 examples of diffuse papillomatosis.[7]

Symptoms associated with adenoma include pain in the right upper quadrant of the abdomen, nausea, and vomiting.[3] However, it is doubtful whether these symptoms can be attributed to the adenoma, as in many instances, it is discovered incidentally in a gallbladder removed for cholecystitis or cholelithiasis.[6,7] In the largest reported series, 60% of gallbladders showed significant cholecystitis and 33% contained calculi.[3] An adenoma responsible for massive fecal chloride loss has been reported.[8]

Grossly, adenomas are usually < 2 cm in diameter, papillary or lobulated in configuration, and red to tan in color (Fig. 13–1). Microscopically, they show three growth patterns—tubular, villous (or papillary), and tubulovillous. Individual cells closely resemble those of colonic adenomas. The nuclei are crowded and cigar shaped. They are basally located, although some loss of polarity may be seen. Cytoplasmic mucus vacuoles are generally absent. In most tumors, only low-grade dysplasia is encountered: The nuclei occupy ≤ 50% of the cell volume and are regular in outline, with an even distribution of chromatin. "Metaplastic adenomas" may show goblet cells, Paneth's cells, en-

Table 13–1. Epithelial Tumors of Gallbladder and Extrahepatic Bile Ducts (World Health Organization Classification)

Benign
Adenoma
Cystadenoma
Papillomatosis (adenomatosis)
Dysplasia and carcinoma in situ
Malignant
Carcinoma in situ
Adenocarcinoma not otherwise specified
Papillary adenocarcinoma
Adenocarcinoma, intestinal type
Mucinous adenocarcinoma
Clear cell adenocarcinoma
Signet ring cell adenocarcinoma
Adenosquamous carcinoma
Squamous cell carcinoma
Small cell carcinoma (oat cell carcinoma)
Undifferentiated carcinoma
Endocrine tumors
Carcinoid tumor
Mixed carcinoid-adenocarcinoma
Paraganglioma

From Albores-Saavedra J, Henson DE, Sobin LH: Histological Typing of Tumors of the Gallbladder and Extrahepatic Bile Ducts, 2nd ed. Berlin: Springer-Verlag, 1991, pp 7–21.

docrine cells, and, rarely, squamoid morules.[3,9,10] Most of the endocrine cells contain serotonin. Extensive squamous metaplasia has been described in some adenomas.[11] Adenomas give rise to only a minority of gallbladder cancers, dysplasia being a more common precancerous lesion. Molecular studies confirm this histologic impression and show that adenomas lack the molecular abnormalities that are found in dysplasia, carcinoma in situ, and invasive carcinoma of the gallbladder.[12] Conversely, some adenomas show K-*ras* mutations, which are rare in gallbladder carcinomas.[12]

The distinction of adenoma from hyperplastic (or metaplastic polyp) is not always clear-cut.[13] Adenomas typically show glandular proliferation in a back-to-back pattern with minimal intervening stroma, variable cellular pleomorphism, and nuclear hyperchromasia.[2] Hyperplastic polyps lack dysplasia, typically showing mild crowding of glands, sometimes with glandular dilation and either normal gallbladder epithelium or metaplastic epithelium.[7,13–16]

The differential diagnosis of adenoma also includes gastric heterotopia, which may present as a polyp or intramural nodule. This may be identified by recognizing the presence of gastric fundic mucosa with chief cells and parietal cells. Table 13–2 compares the features of ectopic gastric mucosa and metaplastic polyp. Pyloric type mucosal nodules may also grossly mimic an adenoma.[16] Pancreatic or thyroid heterotopia rarely coexists with gastric heterotopia.[16]

PAPILLOMATOSIS

The WHO monograph definition of papillomatosis is "a clinicopathological condition characterized by multiple recurring papillary adenomas that may involve extensive areas of the extrahepatic bile ducts and even extend into the gallbladder and intrahepatic bile ducts."[1] This tumor is the pathologic equivalent of the papillary mucinous neoplasm of the pancreas. Rarely, it is confined to the gallbladder, but in most examples there is involvement of the intra- and extrahepatic bile ducts (see Chapter 16). The tumor extensively involves the mucosal surface, as soft gray-white to tan friable cauliflower-like masses. Microscopically, the

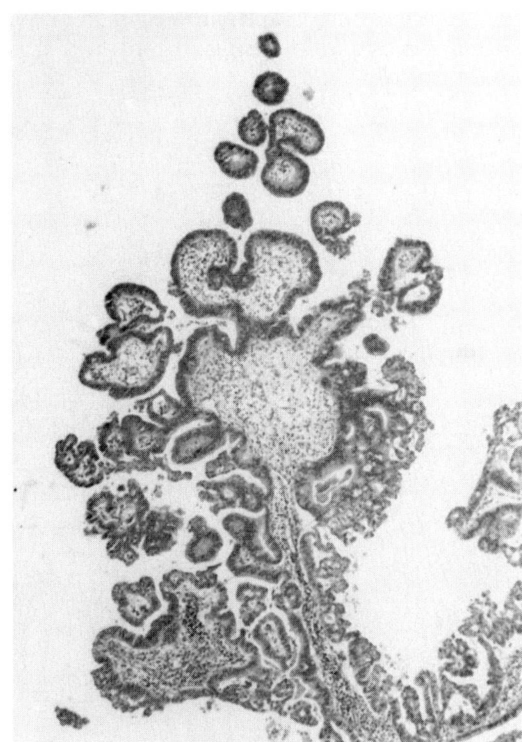

Figure 13–1. Papillary adenoma of the gallbladder.

Table 13–2. Comparison of Ectopic Gastric Mucosa and Metaplastic Polyp

	Ectopic Gastric Mucosa	Metaplastic Polyp
Sex	No difference	Male < female
Age	Younger (31.3 y)	Older (60.7)
Stone	Less common (28.6%)	More common (77.8%)
Macroscopic	Polyp or intramural mass	Polyp
Microscopic		
Fundic gland	Present	Absent
Mucous gland	Present	Present
Paneth cell	Absent	Present (22.2%)
Goblet cell	Absent	Present (44.4%)
Metaplasia nearby	Absent	Present (66.7%)

From Yamamoto M, Murakami H, Ito M, et al: Ectopic gastric mucosa of the gallbladder: Comparison with metaplastic polyp of the gallbladder. Am J Gastroenterol 84:1423–1426, 1989.

polyps are villous or tubulovillous adenomas (Figs. 13–2, 13–3). High-grade dysplasia is often present, making the distinction from papillary carcinoma difficult and indicating a greater proclivity to progress to cancer than ordinary adenoma. Most examples occur sporadically; however, a case of diffuse papillomatosis of the gallbladder was described in a man with primary sclerosing cholangitis and ulcerative colitis.[17] In this clinical setting, papillomatosis can be regarded as a dysplasia arising in chronically inflamed mucosa.

MUCINOUS CYSTIC NEOPLASM (CYSTADENOMA AND CYSTADENOCARCINOMA)

Mucinous cystic neoplasm of the gallbladder is the pathologic counterpart of the mucinous cystic neoplasm of the pancreas[18] (see Chapter 8). It is defined by the WHO expert panel as "a multiloculated thin-walled tumour that contains mucinous or serous fluid. The locules are lined by a single layer of cuboidal or columnar cells that stain for mucin."[1] The epithelium of

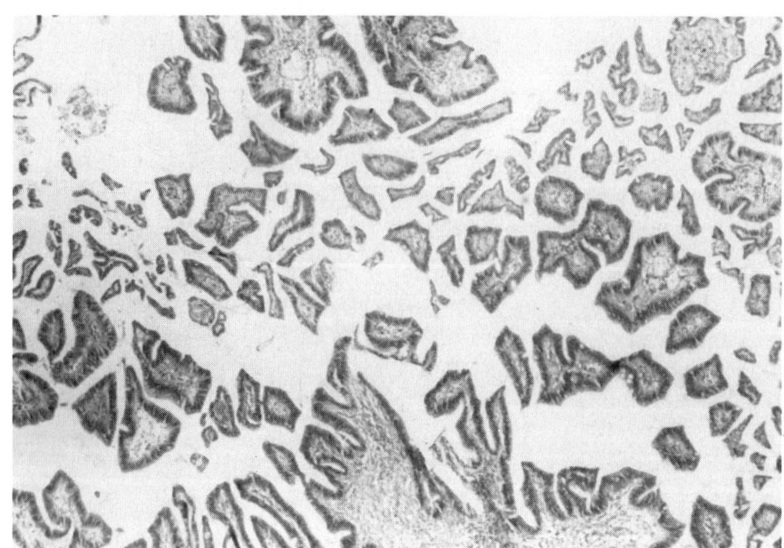

Figure 13–2. Papillomatosis of the gallbladder. Note the multiple complex branching fronds.

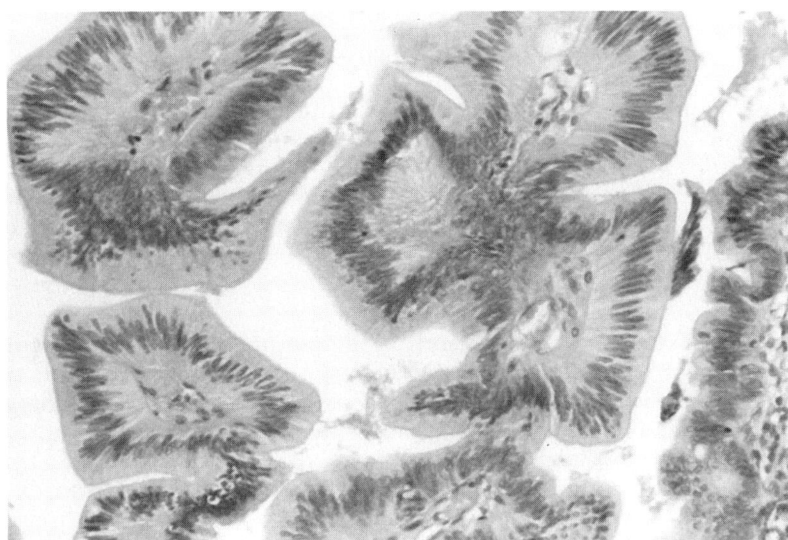

Figure 13–3. Papillomatosis of the gallbladder. Note the close resemblance of the epithelium to a villous adenoma of the colon.

the cystadenomas is simple columnar in type, resembling bile duct or gastric foveolar epithelium. Typically, small numbers of endocrine cells are present. The stroma is composed of cellular connective tissue that resembles ovarian stroma.[18,19] Malignant transformation has been described in about 25% of cases, although mainly in cysts located in liver.[20] This tumor is a great rarity in gallbladder. In the largest reported series, only two cases involved gallbladder, one of which was malignant.[20] Mucinous cystic neoplasms are also rare in extrahepatic bile ducts but are well characterized in liver. They range in size from 2.5 to 30 cm. Most patients are middle-aged women, and almost all cases occurring in women have the distinctive ovarian-like stroma. Most cases in men lack the ovarian-like stroma.

Borderline mucinous cystic tumors are characterized by proliferating epithelium, growing as complex papillary folds. The epithelium shows increased dysplasia and is multilayered. Malignant mucinous tumors show high-grade dysplasia, with irregular epithelial proliferation and stromal invasion.

OTHER BENIGN MUCOSAL TUMORLIKE LESIONS

A villous mucosal lesion of nonadenomatous type due to mucosal infiltration by metachromatic leukodystrophy has been described at autopsy in a child aged 27 months.[21] A tumor similar to mixed salivary tumor has also been reported in the gallbladder.[22] Its histogenesis is unclear.

DYSPLASIA AND CARCINOMA IN SITU

Dysplasia is an epithelial abnormality that is identifiably on the morphologic pathway to cancer and is at increased risk of becoming cancer, when compared to normal epithelium. It is not usually detectable by the naked eye, and when it does form a mass, it may be mistaken for an adenoma. Dysplasia arises in mucosa that is previously diseased. In the gallbladder, it may be associated with anomalous union of the pancreaticobiliary duct (AUPBD) and regurgitation of pancreatic juice into the gallbladder.[23] Dysplasia is seen adjacent to carcinomas in two thirds of patients and is considered the precursor of carcinoma.[24–27] The reported incidence of dysplasia in excised gallbladders is 0.4% in Canada,[26] 2.2% in Japan (where cases were extensively sampled),[27] 5% in Australia,[28] 33.8% in Finland (9.9% moderate or severe),[24] and 48% in Mexico (where the incidence of carcinoma of the gallbladder is very high).[25] These widely divergent figures reflect different rates of cholecystectomy, different extent of sampling, different risk of gallbladder carcinoma, and elastic diagnostic criteria. The size of the areas of dysplasia found in these studies was generally very small.

Dysplasia may be grossly flat, elevated, nodular or villous, unifocal or multifocal. The morphologic features of dysplasia are cellular crowding, pseudostratification, nuclear atypia (enlargement and hyperchromatism), loss of cellular or nuclear polarity, cellular and nuclear pleomorphism, increased mitosis, and absence of features of regeneration[25,26] (Fig. 13–4). It can extend down Aschoff–Rokitansky sinuses and raise a suspicion of invasion. However, the absence of stromal desmoplasia is an important diagnostic point against carcinoma. The background to dysplasia is usually metaplasia of pyloric gland or intestinal type, and the dysplastic epithelium itself often shows metaplastic features, such as goblet cells or Paneth's cells, or contains antigens appropriate to stomach or intestine but not to gallbladder.[29–32]

Squamous cell dysplasia and squamous cell carcinoma in situ have been found beside invasive squamous cell carcinomas of the gallbladder.

THE DYSPLASIA–CARCINOMA SEQUENCE

In the gallbladder, the dysplasia–carcinoma sequence is the main histogenetic pathway to gallbladder cancer and is far more common than the adenoma–carcinoma sequence. Many authors have not drawn a distinction between adenoma and dysplasia in the gallbladder: Some have used the word *adenoma* to describe any polypoid dysplasia; others use it for all dysplasias; some use the word *dysplasia* to describe only a flat lesion, not visible to the naked eye. Dysplasia-associated masses may be recognized in the gallbladder, just as they are in the colon. The crucial distinction between a dysplastic mass and an adenoma is that dysplasia is a more widespread lesion and occurs in flat mucosa, alongside the mass, as well as at other locations within the gallbladder.

In a study of 1,605 cholecystectomies, all dysplasias were described as adenomas and these comprised 11 benign adenomas (interpreted as meaning low-grade dysplasia), 7 adenomas with malignant change (interpreted here as meaning high-grade dysplasia or carcinomas in situ), and 79 invasive carcinomas.[33] All the low-grade lesions were ≤ 12 mm in diameter (average, 5.5 mm), whereas the high-grade lesions were ≥ 12 mm in diameter. The average age of patients with low-grade dysplasia was 50.5 years; with high-grade dysplasia, 58.3 years; and with invasive carcinoma, 64.8 years.[33] This age differential with increasing dysplasia provides an indication of time scale in the dysplasia–carcinoma sequence. All high-grade dysplasias were associated with lesser degrees of dysplasia and there was an increase in size of the lesion with increase in dysplasia. A residue of dysplasia was found in 19% of the invasive carcinomas.[33] Unfortunately, this study did not document the presence or absence of mucosal metaplasia.

Dysplasia or carcinoma in situ is not grossly different from chronic cholecystitis and it can be difficult to distinguish from regenerative atypia microscopically.[34] Dysplasia arises from the surface epithelium adjacent to or overlying metaplastic antral-type glands and less often in-

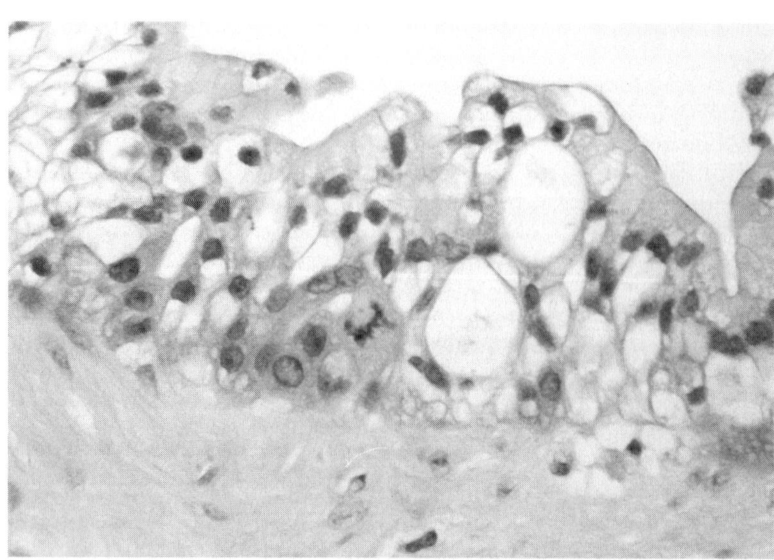

Figure 13–4. Hyperplasia and low-grade dysplasia of the gallbladder mucosa. Note that the epithelium is thickened and disorganized and contains an atypical mitosis.

volves the mucosal infoldings.[24,34,35] Carcinoma in situ was present with follicular cholecystitis in 4 of 18 patients (22%) in one series, although none of these was demonstrated to have chronic infection.[34]

Black found dysplasia in the mucosa surrounding 45 of 48 carcinomas.[35] Two of the three remaining carcinomas were confined to a polyp that resembled a colonic adenoma.[35] He called dysplasia "atypical adenomatous hyperplasia" and described a spectrum of epithelial abnormalities from "adenomatous change to adenomatous hyperplasia with extreme atypia to frank carcinoma in situ."[36] Many of these foci of epithelial abnormality were multicentric.[36] The designation of carcinoma in situ by Black and colleagues was sometimes based on cytologic and architectural features, but sometimes only on similarity to frankly invasive glands.[36] In his discussion, Black mentioned that frank carcinomas outnumbered atypical hyperplasia in cholecystectomy specimens by at least 10:1, a figure that mirrors the great excess of carcinomas over dysplasias in the Japanese series.[33] Laitio, by contrast, found dysplasia in 24 of 71 sequential cholecystectomies (33.8%) performed at a mean patient age of 56.5 years.[24] This extraordinarily high rate of dysplasia in routinely resected gallbladders, in relatively young Europeans, suggests a loose definition of dysplasia; Laitio's categories of low-grade and moderate-grade dysplasia might have been better termed *reactive* or *indeterminate.* These discrepancies among experts indicate how imprecise our criteria are. At present, it is recommended that terminology and identification of dysplasia be based on criteria used in describing similar lesions in the colon, stomach, and esophagus (negative for dysplasia; indefinite for dysplasia, low-grade dysplasia, high-grade dysplasia, and infiltrating carcinoma). Molecular biology may ultimately clarify the field. Regenerative atypia is the main condition that must be distinguished from dysplasia and generally consists of a heterogeneous cell population, which contrasts with the relatively monotonous cells that comprise dysplasia and carcinoma in situ.[34]

In practice, if dysplasia is recognized or suspected, the pathologist should reexamine the gallbladder and submit extra blocks from the suspicious area, or the entire organ, in order not to miss a carcinoma. The excision margin of the cystic duct should be examined to determine whether dysplasia reaches the margin. If dysplasia involves the deeper glands of adenomyomatosis or of Aschoff–Rokitansky sinuses, the distinction from well-differentiated carcinoma can be difficult. The following criteria may be helpful in this distinction: (1) Aschoff–Rokitansky sinuses tend to have a smoothly rounded contour, whereas carcinomas have an irregular or branching contour. (2) Aschoff–Rokitansky sinuses carry with them a thin coating of lamina propria, whereas carcinomas either have a fibroblastic stroma or cut directly across muscle fibers, with no intervening stroma. (3) Carcinomas may show neural invasion, whereas Aschoff–Rokitansky sinuses usually do not.

THE METAPLASIA–DYSPLASIA SEQUENCE

Metaplasia is a response to mucosal damage and regeneration. The causes include gallstones, cholecystitis, ulceration, and reflux of pancreatic juice (in patients with AUPBD). The main forms of metaplasia in the gallbladder are intestinal type and antral type.[37,38] The intestinal type is characterized mainly by goblet cells, but endocrine cells and Paneth's cells may also be present.[38–40] Endocrine cells in areas of goblet cell metaplasia may be immunoreactive for gastrin, somatostatin, pancreatic polypeptide, or motilin.[41] Gastric antral (pseudopyloric) metaplasia is characterized by antral-type glands that contain sulfated mucin, may contain endocrine cells and lysozme, and may be associated with foci of gastric foveolar-type mucosa on the surface.[38] Gastric body–type metaplasia is rare.[42] All forms of metaplasia increase steadily with age and are more frequent in female than in male patients under the age of 70 years.[39,43] In Chilean patients with gallstones whose gallbladders were completely blocked for histologic sectioning, antral metaplasia was found in 95.1%, intestinal metaplasia in 58.1%, hyperplasia in 46.9%, dysplasia in 16%, and carcinoma in situ in 2.5%. Significant associations of intestinal metaplasia with hyperplasia, intestinal metaplasia with dysplasia, and hyperplasia with dysplasia were found.[43] Laitio found dysplasia in 24 of 71 sequential patients undergoing cholecystectomy (33.8%) in a significant association with metaplasia and colocated with it in 58.3% of patients.[24] In a complementary article, Laitio[42] examined the mucosa adjacent to infiltrating carcinomas and found metaplasia in 92% of patients, mainly of antral type (78.4%), a figure close to the 73.3% incidence that Yamagiwa found in gallbladders without dysplasia or stone but lower than the 89.2% incidence in gallbladders with stones.[27] Yamamoto diagnosed metaplasia by silver staining for endocrine cells and immunostaining for lysozyme, mucus cells, and Paneth's cells and found one or more metaplastic markers in 82% of carcinomas of gallbladder. The frequency of metaplastic changes did not increase with size of the tumor, suggesting that metaplasia was not secondary to tumor.[16]

Cumulatively, the work of these authors makes a case for a pathway to carcinoma through metaplasia and dysplasia in the context of gallstones, at least in countries where carcinoma of the gallbladder is common.[24,26,27,33,43] Intestinal and gastric antigens are present in metaplasia of the gallbladder mucosa.[29–32] Carcinoembryonic antigen (CEA) is present in the apical regions of the normal gallbladder epithelial cells and within the cytoplasm in carcinomas.[25] Mucin in the carcinomas is mainly nonsulfated acid mucin (as in metaplasia), not normal sulfated gallbladder mucin.

MUCOSAL HYPERPLASIA

Primary and secondary forms of mucosal hyperplasia of the gallbladder, in the sense of increased mucosal height and elongation of the mucosal folds, have been described by Elfving and colleagues.[44–47] The secondary type occurs in association with stones, cholesterolosis, adenomyomatosis, and metachromatic leukodystrophy. Primary hyperplasia, affecting the entire mucosa, was seen in 9% of patients undergoing cholecystectomy in Finland. The patients included children who presented with upper abdominal pain that often radiated to the back or shoulder.[45] Most had symptomatic relief after cholecystectomy. At that time (the late 1960s), it was not recognized that AUPBD can result in reflux of pancreatic juice into the biliary tree and endoscopic retrograde cholangiopancreatography was not available, so we cannot tell what proportion of these patients had this congenital anomaly. Hyperplasia consists of enlargement or elongation of the mucosal folds. Two patterns of hyperplasia are recognized: villous and spongioid[48,49] (see Chapter 11). In a series from Japan, metaplasia accompanied hyperplasia in two thirds of patients.[49] In some patients, dysplasia was also present.[48]

The normal gallbladder mucosa measures 0.3 to 0.6 mm in height, and hyperplasia, defined as a height > 0.6 mm, is present in 41% of gallbladders accompanied by AUPBD.[49] Hyperplasia has been divided into two grades, low grade and high grade, defined, respectively, as mucosal architecture with three or fewer branchings and with more than three branchings.[50] The "adenomatous hyperplasia" described by Christensen and Ishak, may also represent this form of hyperplasia, as they described it as papillary or villous or forming a glandular spongelike network.[3] Only 6 of their 18 patients had gallstones. The hyperplasia was focal in 7 and diffuse in 11. The papillary hyperplasia illustrated by Hultén et al. might have been of this type, too.[7]

All patients with cholesterolosis have mucosal hyperplasia, comprising lengthening of the folds and increased mucosal height. Elfving and colleagues suggested that hyperplasia preceded the cholesterolosis.[46,51] In addition to diffuse hyperplasia, epithelial changes in reaction to cholelithiasis consist of increased epithelial turnover, increased numbers of mucin cells, foci of atrophy, ulcers, regenerative change that includes multilayering of the nuclei and hyperchromatism, and metaplasia.[47]

The term *hyperplasia* was used in a different sense by Albores-Saavedra et al., who described it as "pseudostratification of the epithelium, nuclear crowding, taller than normal columnar cells with or without increased mucin production, and occasional normal mitotic figures."[52] Used in this sense, hyperplasia has been found in 83% of gallbladders in Mexico City[52] and in 46.9% of gallbladders with cholelithiasis in Chile.[43] *Atypical hyperplasia* has been defined as hyperplasia with "some loss of architecture and disorganization of the epithelium, as well as nuclear atypia" and appears to be synonymous with *dysplasia*[52] and with the term *atypical adenomatous hyperplasia* used by Black.[35] Because of a lack of uniform terminology and definitions, it is difficult to evaluate the relevance of hyperplasia as a precursor of carcinoma of the gallbladder in North America.

CARCINOMA OF THE GALLBLADDER

Carcinoma of the gallbladder is a tumor of the elderly that varies widely in incidence with ethnicity and affects women more than men in a ratio about 3:1 (2.7:1 in the largest U.S. study).[53] It is twice as common as carcinoma of the extrahepatic bile ducts. In the United

States, 5,000 new carcinomas of the gallbladder are diagnosed annually.

The clinical presentation is with right upper quadrant abdominal pain (70%), jaundice (50%), and weight loss,[54–56] but in many patients, the tumors are found incidentally at cholecystectomy for cholecystitis and stones. Other symptoms include ascites,[57] fever,[58] duodenal obstruction,[57] anemia, and melena secondary to duodenal invasion. An abdominal mass is palpable in 50% of patients. Occasionally, patients present with perforation of the gallbladder, local abscess, or fistula.[59]

The Surveillance, Epidemiology, and End Results (SEER) Program of the National Cancer Institute, which covers about 9.6% of the population of the United States, found that the average age of men with gallbladder cancer is 71 years (range, 22 to 103 years) and of women is 72.7 years (range, 26 to 99 years).[53] Overall, one third of patients are younger than 70 and two thirds are older.

Molecular Changes in Gallbladder Cancer

The principal changes described to date comprise gene mutations of p53 and p16[INK4]/*CDKN2a* and loss of heterozygosity at the loci for p53 (17p, 92%), *CDKN2a* (9p21, 50%), 8p21 (44%), and DCC (18q, 35%).[60–62] These mutations and chromosomal alterations are found in dysplasias and carcinomas in situ, accompanying invasive gallbladder carcinomas, and also in adjacent normal-appearing mucosa.[62] In early carcinoma of the gallbladder, defined as tumor that has not invaded muscle coat, the *ras* p21 oncogene is overexpressed in 92%, *myc* in 69%, *erb*-B2 in 69%, epidermal growth factor in 46%, and transforming growth factor in 62% in contrast to cholecystitis, where the corresponding figures are significantly lower. Thus, *ras* p21 may play as important a role in initiation of gallbladder cancer as it does in colorectal cancer and pancreatic cancer.[63]

Risk Factors for Development of Cancer of the Gallbladder

Gallstone disease is the main risk factor (Table 13–3) for carcinoma and numerous studies have shown a strong correlation between the presence of gallstones and gallbladder cancer.[35,64–67] In most series, at least 70% of patients with cancer have gallstones and the percentage of patients stated not to have stones ranges from 3.4% to 17%.[35] Gallstones grow at a rate of about 2 mm in diameter per year. With time, the proportion of small stones decreases and the proportion of large stones increases. There is a strong correlation between gallstone size and gallbladder cancer.[68] Those races and peoples who are prone to cholelithiasis and who develop gallstones early in life are also prone to carcinoma of the gallbladder. These include aboriginals in the United States, Mexico, Chile, and Bolivia, in whom cancer of the gallbladder is the leading cause of cancer mortality in women. These ethnic groups produce highly lithogenic bile. Carcinoma of the gallbladder is far more common in Native Americans than in blacks or whites. The rate among Native American women is 21 per 100,000, compared with 1.4 per 100,000 among white women. Of Native Americans with carcinoma of the gallbladder who could be evaluated, 93% had gallstones.[35] Gallstones are found in 73% of Pima Indian women between the ages of 25 and 34 years.[69] Other studies have shown similar rates in the Chippewa, Sioux, Arapaho, and Shoshone nations.[35] In Chile, the crude mortality rate from biliary cancer was 9.9 in 1988 and the age-adjusted mortality was 13.3, among the highest in the world.[43] Almost 90% of these were primary gallbladder cancers.[70] In Bolivia, the risk of gallbladder cancer is different in various racial groups: People who speak Aymara have a far higher risk than that of those who speak Quechua.[71] Carcinoma of the gallbladder is increased among the Maori in New Zealand.[72] The incidence in Japan is higher than in white Americans but less than in Native Americans.

Lowenfels and colleagues studied the relationship between gallstones and gallbladder cancer in three racial groups—whites, blacks, and Southwestern Native Americans. For non–Native Americans, the relative risk estimate was 4.4; for the Native Americans, it was 20.9. These

Table 13–3. Risk Factors for Carcinoma of the Gallbladder

Gallstones
Pancreatobiliary maljunction
Typhoid carriers
Helicobacter species
Adenomyomatosis
Polyposis coli
Primary sclerosing cholangitis

authors estimate that the proportion of gallbladder cancer attributable to gallstones (population attributable risk) is 30% for blacks, 50% for whites, and 90% for Native Americans.[72] Silent gallstones in middle-aged whites and blacks are associated with a low risk of gallbladder cancer estimated at not more than 0.5% in 20 years,[72] but for young North American aboriginal women with silent gallstones, the ultimate risk of gallbladder cancer may be as high as 4% to 5%,[72] and for these people, cholecystectomy may be warranted as a prophylactic procedure. Thus, the duration of gallstone disease is likely an important factor, producing a higher incidence of the disease in peoples who routinely develop gallstones in adolescence. The association of female sex with gallbladder cancer is a reflection of the female predominance of gallstones. Obesity and a high-carbohydrate diet are also associated with gallstones. Constipation is another risk factor, as it promotes gallstone formation.[73] The pathway from normal mucosa to cancer in patients with gallstones likely involves mucosal abrasion or ulceration, regeneration, metaplasia, and dysplasia. This sequence may potentiate other carcinogenic influences, such as chronic infection as typified by chronic typhoid (see below) or, possibly, *Helicobacter* infections. Whether AUPBD potentiates the effect of stones is uncertain as yet.

Pancreaticobiliary Maljunction

Pancreaticobiliary maljunction, or AUPBD, in which the common bile duct joins the pancreatic duct outside the duodenal wall, means that the sphincter of Oddi is distal to the junction of the ducts and consequently the pancreatic secretions can reflux through the biliary system and into the gallbladder. This anomaly has been recognized as a causative factor for choledochal cyst and dilation of the bile ducts since 1973.[74] Since then, it has been observed that carcinoma of the biliary tract and gallbladder frequently develops in patients with AUPBD, with or without dilation of the common bile duct.[75] In the largest Japanese series reported to date, 17 (35%) of 48 patients with AUPBD were given a diagnosis of gallbladder cancer,[76] and other studies found AUPBD in association with 12% to 24% of gallbladder cancers, an association that strongly supports a causative relationship.[77–79] In a review of 569 patients with AUPBD, dilation of the extrahepatic bile duct was present in 84% of patients and no dilation was found in 14%.[80] The undilated type of AUPBD is associated more strongly with gallbladder carcinoma than is the dilated type,[76,81] and cancer in the undilated type presents at a more advanced stage.[76] Possibly, where dilation of the ducts is present, this acts as a reservoir for the refluxed pancreatic secretions, which do not enter the gallbladder. Therefore, prophylactic cholecystectomy is recommended for patients with undilated-type AUPBD.[79,81] This anomaly may also predispose to pancreatitis and pancreatic duct neoplasms.[82]

How does carcinoma arise? In patients with AUPBD, the gallbladder becomes a repository for pancreatic secretions, as evidenced by high pancreatic amylase levels in the gallbladder bile. Anomalous union results in mucosal hyperplasia of the gallbladder as an early and characteristic change, both in children and in adults.[49,50,83,84] In children with maljunction, hyperplasia was found in 50% of 28 patients,[83] and in adults with maljunction, the incidence of hyperplasia has been reported to range from 38.5% to 87%. Metaplasia is associated with the hyperplasia in two thirds of patients,[49] but not at a rate significantly different from that of controls without maljunction.[50] It is likely that the pancreatic juice causes repetitive exfoliation and regeneration and that the increased proliferation predisposes to an increased rate of random mutations. Experimental exposure of the biliary tree to pancreatic juice results in epithelial damage and accelerated cell turnover, conditions known to favor neoplasia.[50,84,85] A comparison between 6 patients with stage I gallbladder cancer with AUPBD and 20 without showed an equal incidence of p53 mutations (67%) but a higher incidence of K-*ras* mutation in patients with AUPBD than without (50% versus 6%).[84] Tanno et al. showed that K-*ras* mutations were mainly associated with high-grade hyperplasia, which they defined as "mucosal architecture of more than three branchings."[50]

The majority of patients with cancer of the gallbladder secondary to AUPBD have advanced disease at diagnosis, permitting curative surgery in only 20%.[76,81] Long-term survivors are few. The incidence of gallstones is very low in these patients.[81]

Typhoid and Paratyphoid Carriers

In typhoid carriers, the gallbladder is the principal seat of the persistent infection because the presence of stones protects the organisms from elimination. Only cholecystectomy and removal of stones will clear the bile of bacteria. There is a weak association between hepatobiliary cancer and the typhoid carrier state. In the Typhoid Carrier Registry of the New York City Department of Health, 5.7% of deaths among the 471 carriers were due to hepatobiliary cancers, compared to < 1% of controls (p = < 0.001).[86] By contrast, 15.5% of carriers and 14% of controls died because of other neoplasms. An interesting finding was that most of the excess deaths were from carcinoma of the gallbladder in male carriers, who had a death rate of 5.5% from gallbladder cancer.[87] A British study confirmed that chronic typhoid and paratyphoid carriers have a great increase in relative risk for gallbladder cancer, with a lesser increase in risk for cancer of pancreas, colorectum, and lung and all neoplasms.[88] Other supporting evidence is the finding of an odds ratio of 12.7 for a history of physician-diagnosed typhoid in Latin American patients with gallbladder cancer, compared with controls,[71] and from India, where a significantly higher number of patients with gallbladder cancer had *Salmonella typhi* or *S. paratyphi-A* in bile than did controls with cholelithiasis or without.[89] Chronic follicular cholecystitis occurs in some of these patients, with a lymphoplasmacytic infiltrate and lymphoid follicle formation.[90]

Helicobacter *Infection*

Preliminary evidence has recently emerged that *Helicobacter* species may infect the gallbladder and perhaps play a role in the high rate of cancer of the gallbladder in Chilean women.[91] There are many strains of *Helicobacter* that infect the bile ducts and gallbladders of animals, and it was hypothesized that similar strains might infect humans. Studies in Chilean patients undergoing cholecystectomy for chronic cholecystitis detected *Helicobacter* DNA in the gallbladder contents or wall by polymerase chain reaction analysis, but the organisms could not be cultured from the bile samples (which had been frozen without cryoprotection). Thirteen of 23 bile samples and 9 of 23 gallbladder tissues were positive for *Helicobacter* DNA using *Helicobacter*-specific 16S ribosomal RNA primers. Eight sequences were subjected to phylogenetic analysis and five represented strains of *H. bilis,* two were strains of *Flexispira rappini,* and one was a strain of *H. pullorum.* The study did not report the morphology of the cholecystitis; it will be interesting to see whether these organisms are responsible for follicular cholecystitis. The authors cite references to the isolation of *F. Rappini, H. pullorum,* and *H. canis* from patients with diarrhea and of *H. cinaedi* and *H. fennelliae* from homosexual men with proctitis, which indicates that these species can infect humans.[91]

Adenomyomatosis

Adenomyomatosis comprises surface epithelial hyperplasia with muscle coat hypertrophy and protrusion of mucosal diverticula through the wall. Though typically benign, adenomyomatosis is considered by some to be a potentially important factor in cancer causation, being associated with 11.4% of cancers in one series.[92] There are eight recorded cases of cancer arising directly in adenomyomatosis, sometimes connected with mucinous metaplasia or with villous adenoma similar to the type that arises in the appendix.[93] Perineural "invasion" can occur in adenomyomatosis, but should not be mistaken for adenocarcinoma, as the glands have bland cytologic features.[94]

Adenomas and Polyps

Adenomas are described above and precede only a minority of cancers. A polyp of the gallbladder that is > 1 cm in diameter, is solitary, and is found in a patient older than 60 years should arouse suspicion of carcinoma.[95] A few cases of gallbladder cancer have been described with polyposis coli, but not enough to be regarded as more than a chance association.[96]

Primary Sclerosing Cholangitis

Carcinoma of the bile ducts and gallbladder are increasingly recognized as complications of primary sclerosing cholangitis (PSC),[97–103]), although PSC accounts for only a small number of cases of carcinoma of the gallbladder.[97] It appears that the inflammatory change in PSC extends through the entire biliary tree and into the gallbladder.[102] Diffuse papillomatosis of the gallbladder has been described with PSC.[17] There is a significant positive association between cigarette smoking and hepatobiliary carcinoma in patients with PSC.[97]

Histologic Types of Carcinoma of the Gallbladder

The WHO classification of malignant epithelial tumors of the gallbladder is listed in Table 13–1.[1]

Table 13–4. Histologic Types of Gallbladder Carcinoma, SEER Program, 1977–1986

Tumor Type	No. of Patients	% of Total	Mean Age (Yr)	2-Year Survival Rate	Median Survival (Mo)
Adenocarcinoma NOS	1,970	75.8	72.1	0.14	4
Carcinoma NOS	200	7.6	74.5	0.06	2
Papillary	151	5.8	71.9	0.47	20
Mucinous	125	4.8	71.4	0.12	4
Adenosquam	95	3.6	71.8	0.08	3
Squamous	45	1.7	69.6	0.09	4
Oat cell	13	0.5	67	0	2

Key: NOS, not otherwise specified; SEER, Surveillance, Epidemiology, and End Results (National Cancer Institute).
From Hensen DE, Albores-Saavedra J, Corle D: Carcinoma of the gallbladder. Histologic types, stage of disease, grade, and survival data. Cancer 70:1493–1497, 1992.

Adenocarcinoma not otherwise specified (NOS) is a gland-forming tumor that often contains mucin (Table 13–4). It varies from well differentiated (Fig. 13–5) to poorly differentiated, most tumors being moderately differentiated[53] (Table 13–5, Fig. 13–6). Most carcinomas are of this type (Table 13–4). The glands are tubular and of medium size, closely packed, or separated by desmoplasia. The epithelium is columnar or cuboidal and sometimes flattened. The nuclei vary from regular to pleomorphic and from pale and vesicular to hyperchromatic. Cytoplasm is usually moderate in quantity, eosinophilic or amphophilic, or pale. Focally, the tumor may form cords or sheets of tumor cells. Mucins are present in variable amounts, both intracytoplasmic and luminal. Alcian blue–positive mucin is mainly luminal. CEA is present at the juxtaluminal cytoplasm.[104] Inflammatory cells may infiltrate the tumor. Clear-cell foci have a reticular or cribriform pattern or form solid sheets and resemble fetal gut. The cytoplasm is rich in glycogen.

Papillary adenocarcinoma is composed of villous structures, lined by cuboidal or columnar cells that often contain mucin (Fig. 13–7). Goblet cells, Paneth's cells, or endocrine cells are sometimes present. These tumors often have a large intraluminal component of exophytic growth, similar to a villous adenoma of the colon (Fig. 13–8). The invasive component is often superficial at presentation and the prognosis is then better than the average. The invasive component may be desmoplastic and less differentiated than the villous component, which is merely carcinoma in situ in many instances. The carcinomas may dedifferentiate as they invade and the superficial components show more intestinal differentiation than do the deeper components.

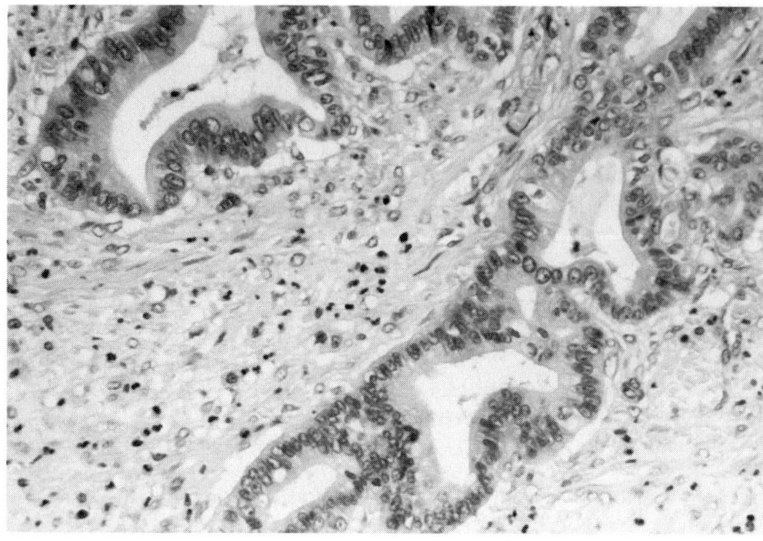

Figure 13–5. Well-differentiated adenocarcinoma not otherwise specified.

Table 13–5. Relation Between Histologic Grade of Adenocarcinoma NOS and Survival, SEER Program

Grade	No. of Patients	% of Cases	Median Survival (Mo)	2-Year Survival Rate
1	265	20.5	7	0.3
2	443	34.2	6	0.14
3	594	42.4	4	0.08
4	38	2.9	3	0.07

Key: NOS, not otherwise specified; SEER, Surveillance, Epidemiology, and End Results (National Cancer Institute).

From Henson DE, Albores-Saavedra J, Corle D: Carcinoma of the gallbladder. Histologic types, stage of disease, grade, and survival data. Cancer 70:1493–1497, 1992. Copyright © 1992 American Cancer Society. Reprinted by permission of Wiley-Liss, Inc., a subsidiary of John Wiley & Sons, Inc.

Intestinal-type adenocarcinoma is composed of cells of intestinal type, particularly goblet cells, colonic-type epithelium, and even Paneth's cells and endocrine cells. Two types of intestinal pattern are described by Albores-Saavedra and colleagues. The first type includes a predominance of goblet cells (Fig. 13–9) and absorptive columnar cells, and the second resembles colonic adenocarcinoma[105] (Fig. 13–10). A major feature in two thirds of colonic-type tumors is the presence of many glands, lined by benign-appearing columnar epithelium, in which the nuclei are bland and ovoid or elongated. Endocrine cells may be present in both types of tumor.[105]

Mucinous adenocarcinoma is defined as having > 50% extracellular mucin. The mucin may distend large glands or may surround floating clusters of tumor cells. These tumors may contain a nondominant component of signet ring cells. They resemble mucinous carcinomas occurring at other locations, especially the colon.

Clear cell adenocarcinoma is composed predominantly of glycogen-rich clear cells that have well-defined cytoplasmic borders and hyperchromatic nuclei[2,106] (Fig. 13–11). The cytoplasmic clearing is usually supranuclear but may be subnuclear. The cells are arranged in nests, sheets, cords, or trabeculae, but tubular or papillary structures are usually present focally. Some cells may possess eosinophilic granular cytoplasm. This tumor must be distinguished from metastatic renal cell carcinoma, which is rare in the gallbladder or bile ducts, and from the clear cell variant of squamous cell carcinoma. Foci of mucin-producing cells are usually present and assist in the diagnosis of an entopic tumor. Renal cell carcinoma is positive for both cytokeratin and vimentin, but clear cell carcinoma is negative for vimentin, as is squamous cell carcinoma.

Adenosquamous carcinoma contains two malignant elements, glandular and squamous, and accounts for about 3% to 4% of carcinomas.

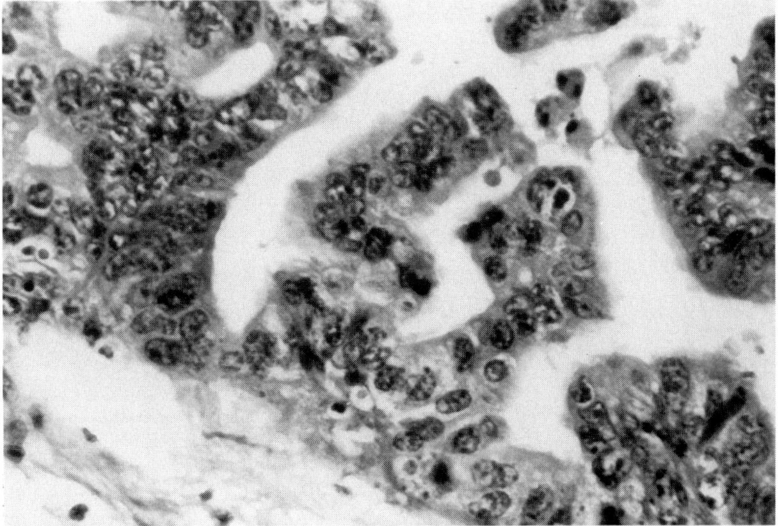

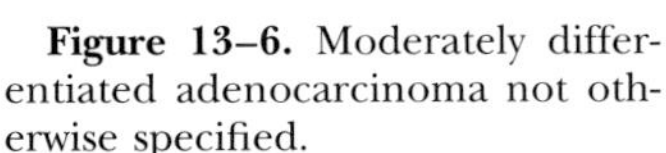

Figure 13–6. Moderately differentiated adenocarcinoma not otherwise specified.

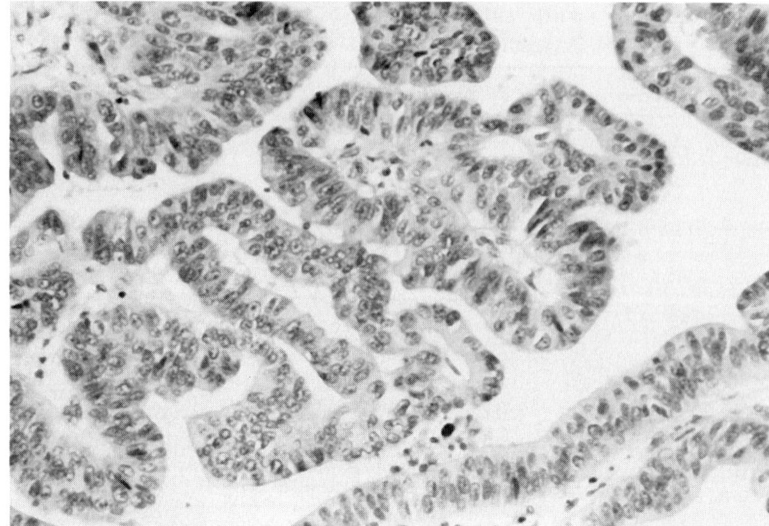

Figure 13–7. Papillary adenocarcinoma. This represents the surface noninvasive component.

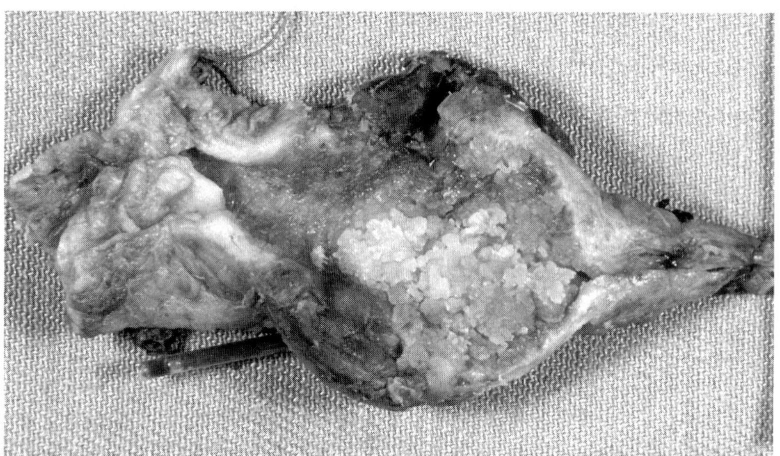

Figure 13–8. Papillary adenocarcinoma growing as an exophytic mass on the mucosal surface of the gallbladder.

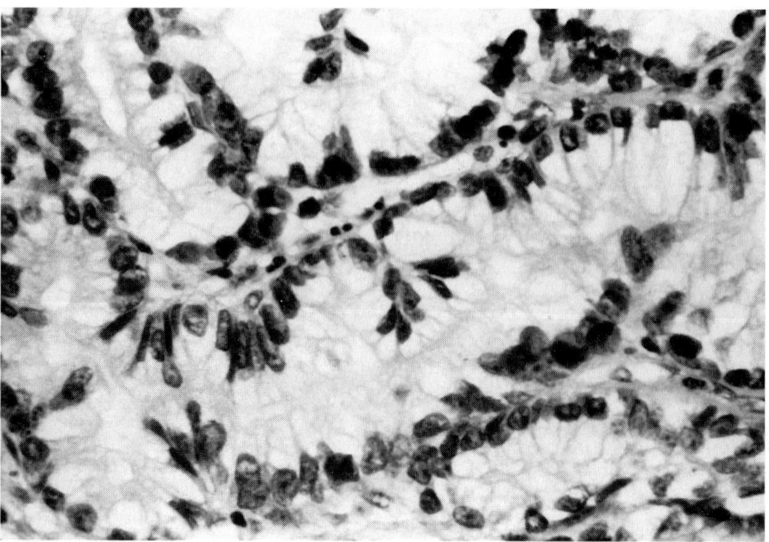

Figure 13–9. Intestinal-type adenocarcinoma with predominance of goblet cells.

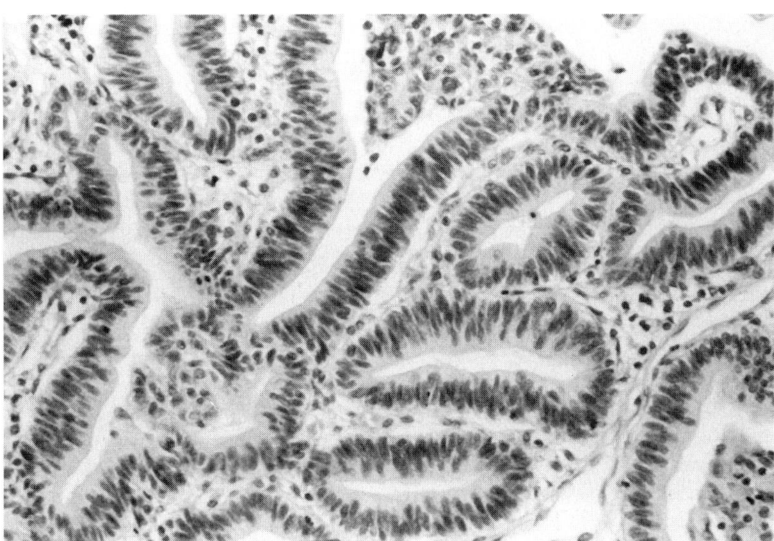

Figure 13–10. Very well differentiated intestinal-type adenocarcinoma with glands lined by bland columnar cells.

Squamous cell carcinoma requires no special description; neither does small cell undifferentiated carcinoma, which resembles its counterpart in the lung. Squamous cell carcinomas account for about 2% of gallbladder carcinomas. A rare clear cell variant shows a predominance of clear cells with foci of squamous differentiation.[106] The majority of patients with small cell carcinoma are women with gallstones. The tumors may be associated with mucosal dysplasia, adenocarcinoma, or squamous cell carcinoma. The small cell tumors may give positive immunostaining for neuron specific enolase, chromogranin, or synaptophysin. Rarely, ectopic hormone production may occur, giving rise to, for example, Cushing's syndrome. The natural course of this cancer is death within 6 months. The appropriate treatment is the chemotherapy regimen that is used for small cell carcinomas of lung. Survival time is increasing on this regimen and therefore it is important to make the diagnosis.

Undifferentiated non–small cell carcinoma (pleomorphic spindle cell and giant cell carcinoma, sarcomatoid carcinoma, or carcinosarcoma) consists of spindle cells, polygonal cells,

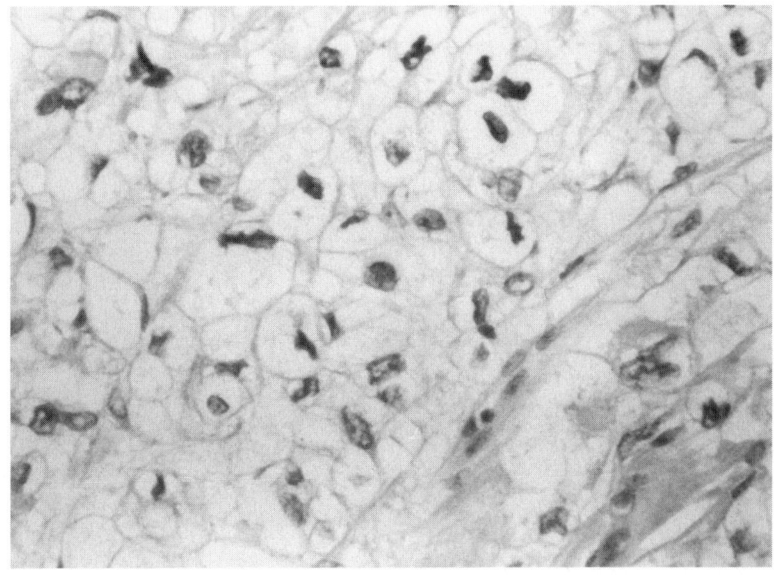

Figure 13–11. Clear cell adenocarcinoma of the gallbladder with an appearance that may easily be confused with that of metastatic renal carcinoma.

and giant cells and may resemble a sarcoma (Fig. 13–12). Small foci of glandular or squamous differentiation may be found after extensive sampling. The sarcomatoid and spindle cells are now regarded as a form of metaplasia, albeit a dominant one.[107] The total number of cases reported to 1993 was < 30.[108] The mean age was 72 years (range, 45 to 91 years). These tumors are similar to carcinomas of the gallbladder in sex distribution, the female-to-male ratio being almost 4 : 1, and gallstones were associated with 14 of 17 patients (82%).[109] Patients with these tumors present with abdominal pain, jaundice, and a right upper quadrant mass. Grossly, most undifferentiated carcinomas are polypoid masses that grow into the lumen of the gallbladder and distend it or form a plaquelike mural infiltrate.[107,108] They range in size from 2 to 15 cm. Microscopically, the carcinomatous element in these tumors is usually a minor one. The dominant sarcomatoid component consists of stellate and spindle-shaped cells and may be admixed with foci of metaplastic osteosarcoma, chondrosarcoma, or rhabdomyosarcoma.[108,110] Immunostaining demonstrates reactivity for cytokeratin, epithelial membrane antigen, and CEA in the carcinomatous component but not in the spindle cells, which are positive for vimentin. Rhabdomyoblastic cells may be reactive for myoglobin.[111] The average survival is 2.9 months after diagnosis.[109] There is an occasional long-term survivor, probably related to early tumor stage. The metastatic pattern is similar to that of conventional carcinomas.[108] The differential diagnosis is from true sarcoma and from the spindle cell variant of malignant melanoma metastatic to gallbladder. Extensive sampling and cytokeratin stains help to distinguish the former and S100 and HMB45 immunostains the latter.

Table 13–4 shows the histologic types of gallbladder cancer reported by the SEER Program and patient survival. In brief, 76% were designated adenocarcinomas NOS and 7.6% were designated carcinoma NOS; 5.8% were papillary adenocarcinomas. Not included in the table were data on 14 patients with signet ring cell carcinoma, 11 with carcinosarcoma, 3 with leiomyosarcoma, 2 with sarcoma NOS, 1 with giant and spindle cell carcinoma, 1 with melanoma, and 28 with malignant neoplasm NOS. These figures differ from those in other series in proportions of cases but reflect the diagnoses rendered in the community. For example, Laitio found adenocarcinoma in 52.5%, papillary carcinoma in 19.4%, mucinous carcinoma in 10.8%, adenosquamous carcinoma in 10.8%, and anaplastic carcinoma in 4.8%.[112]

Histologic Grade

The grading of carcinoma of the gallbladder is subjective, the grading criteria used in reports are often not clearly stated, and interobserver variability has not been studied. As with other adenocarcinomas, the grading is based mainly on gland formation (architectural features). Many studies have clearly shown a better prognosis for papillary and well-differentiated tu-

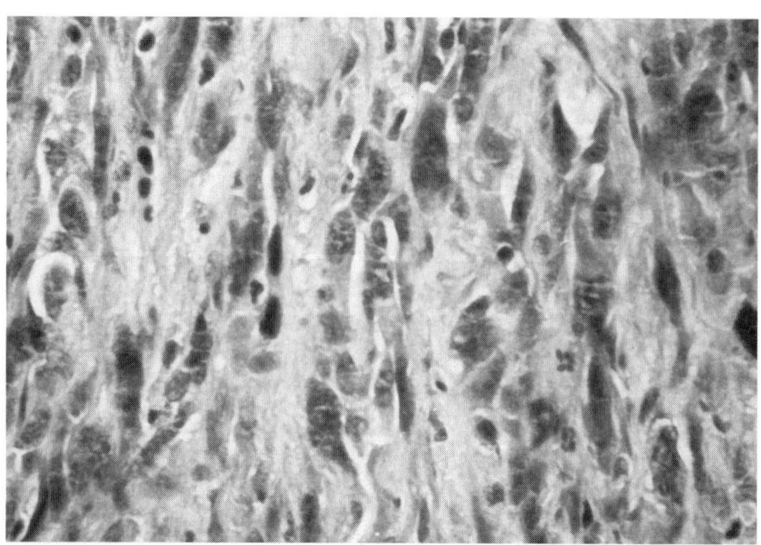

Figure 13–12. Pleomorphic spindle cell carcinoma of the gallbladder.

mors.[107,113–117] Forty-seven percent of the adenocarcinomas NOS of SEER patients (1,442) were graded and 1,295 of these patients had follow-up care. There was a highly significant correlation between grade and survival[53] (Table 13–5). The grading assigned in this study was that of the sign-out pathologist, with no attempt at re-review made by the authors. This table also indicates that the most common grades are the intermediate grades 2 and 3.[53] Expression of p53 protein correlates with grade and is found in 25% of well-differentiated carcinomas but in 50% of moderately or poorly differentiated carcinomas.[118] We suggest grading these tumors architecturally, according to the percentage of well-formed glands by analogy with colorectal adenocarcinomas (Table 13–6).

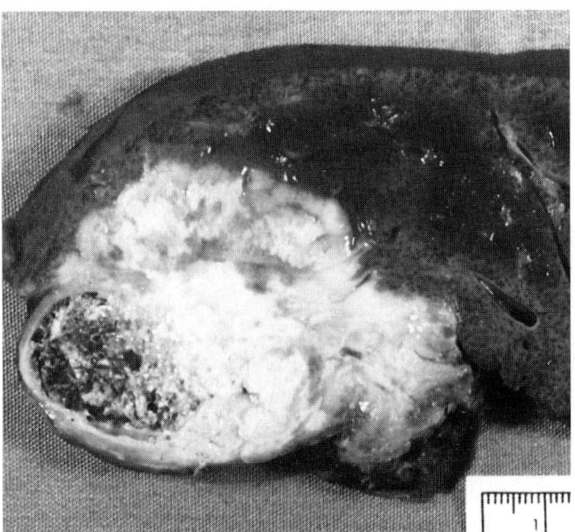

Figure 13–13. Adenocarcinoma of the gallbladder infiltrating the right lobe of the liver.

Spread

The gallbladder wall consists of a thin lamina propria, a single layer of muscle, and loose perimuscular connective tissue. Thus, the barrier to spread is weak. Carcinoma of the gallbladder may grow directly into the liver. It may metastasize transperitoneally, to lymph nodes and hematogenously.[119] Perineural invasion is reported in 71% of cases and has an adverse influence on survival.[120] Gallbladder lymph drains primarily to the cystic duct node and common bile duct node. When the latter node is enlarged by metastatic cancer, it can cause obstructive jaundice. The secondary nodes are the peripancreatic lymph nodes and the tertiary nodes are more distal. Tsukada and colleagues, in a study of radically resected cases, found no nodal metastases in 15 carcinomas that invaded lamina propria or muscle coat but had not penetrated through the muscle coat (pT1 tumors).[121] However, 60 of 96 (62.5%) patients with pT2 to pT4 tumors had lymph node metastasis. At tumor diagnosis, about 50% of patients have nodal metastasis. The frequency of metastasis to secondary nodes was > 15% overall. The more advanced the local stage, the higher the risk of nodal metastasis.[121] Late-stage tumors that involve the serosa or invade adjacent organs have lymph node involvement in 72% and 74.4% of patients, respectively.[122]

Table 13–6. Proposed Histologic Grading of Gallbladder Carcinoma

Grade	Description
X	Grade cannot be assessed
1	Well differentiated (> 95% of tumor composed of glands)
2	Moderately differentiated (50%–95% of tumor composed of glands)
3	Poorly differentiated (5%–50% of tumor composed of glands)
4	Undifferentiated (< 5% of tumor composed of glands)

Liver involvement is usually by direct infiltration forming a single mass in the gallbladder bed (Fig. 13–13) but may be combined with multiple intrahepatic metastases. The mode of spread of gallbladder cancer in the liver was studied in 85 patients who underwent radical cholecystectomy in Japan.[123] Of 20 with liver involvement, 12 had microscopic angiolymphatic portal tract involvement, with or without direct liver invasion; 4 had direct invasion alone, and 3 had distant hepatic nodules. Ninety percent had lymph node metastases.[123] The extent of microscopic angiolymphatic portal tract invasion correlated well with the gross depth of direct invasion of the liver.[123]

Disseminated peritoneal metastases are not common at the time of surgery.[119] Rarely, Krukenberg tumors of the ovary are due to gallbladder carcinoma. Widespread peritoneal and omental metastases and ascites are seen at autopsy. Hematogenous metastases are a late event. Lung metastases are usually solid, but metastases are also described in which the cells have a lepidic growth pattern and, rarely, lymphangitis carcinomatosa.[124] Lung metastases in the absence of liver metastases have been ascribed to lymphatic spread retroperitoneally. Distant metastases to many individual organs, including ovaries, skin, and meninges, have been described.

Staging

The staging by the tumor, node, and metastasis (TNM) system is summarized in Table 13–7. Nevin's staging,[116] now of historical interest, is given in Table 13–8. Other proposed staging schemes include that of Yamaguchi and Enjoji.[9] Stage of disease has a clear prognostic effect. There is a highly significant ($p < 0.00001$) linear association between stage of disease and survival time in the SEER data.[53] As stage increases, survival time decreases (Table 13–9). Nevin staging also shows a direct correlation between stage and survival[116,125,126] (Tables 13–8, 13–9). Radical surgery may provide a small margin of survival benefit.[121]

Table 13–8. Nevin Staging of Gallbladder Cancer

Stage	Description
1	Intramucosal involvement only
2	Involvement of mucosa and muscularis propria
3	Involvement of all three layers
4	Involvement of all three layers and the cystic duct lymph node
5	Involvement of the liver by direct extension or metastasis or the presence of metastases to other organs

Adapted from Nevin JE, Moran TJ, Kay S, et al.: Carcinoma of the gallbladder: Staging, treatment, and prognosis. Cancer 37:141–148, 1976. Copyright © 1976 American Cancer Society. Reprinted by permission of Wiley-Liss, Inc., a subsidiary of John Wiley & Sons, Inc.

Preoperative staging by real-time ultrasonography is accurate in staging the disease in only 38% of patients.[127] The majority of patients are understaged, owing to missed distant metastasis and missed advanced local infiltration. The sensitivity of ultrasound in detecting liver infiltration is 50%; lymph node metastasis, 50%; and

Table 13–7. The Tumor-Node Metastasis Classification for Gallbladder Cancer

Symbol	Description		
Primary tumor (t)			
TX	Primary tumor cannot be assessed		
T0	No evidence of primary tumor		
Tis	Carcinoma in situ		
T1	Tumor invades lamina propria or muscle layer		
T1a	Tumor invades lamina propria		
T1b	Tumor invades muscle layer		
T2	Tumor invades perimuscular connective tissue; no extension beyond serosa or into liver		
T3	Tumor perforates serosa (visceral peritoneum) or directly invades into one adjacent organ or both (extension ≤ 2 cm into liver)		
T4	Tumor extends > 2 cm into liver and/or into two or more adjacent organs (stomach, duodenum, colon, pancreas, omentum, extrahepatic bile ducts, any involvement of liver)		
Regional lymph nodes (N)			
NX	Regional lymph nodes cannot be assessed		
N0	No regional lymph node metastasis		
N1	Regional lymph node metastasis		
N1a	Metastasis in cystic duct, pericholedochal, and/or hilar lymph nodes (i.e., in the hepatoduodenal ligament)		
N1b	Metastasis in peripancreatic (head only), periduodenal, periportal, coeliac, and/or superior mesenteric lymph nodes		
Stage Groupings			
Stage 0	Tis	N0	M0
Stage I	T1	N0	M0
Stage II	T2	N0	M0
Stage III	T1	N1	M0
	T2	N1	M0
	T3	N0, N1	M0
Stage IVA	T4	N0, N1	M0
Stage IVB	Any T	N2	M0
	Any T	Any N	M1

Adapted from Hermanek P, Hutter RVP, Sobin LH, et al.: TNM Atlas; 4th ed. Berlin; Springer-Verlag, 1997, pp 124–130.

Table 13–9. Five-Year Survival By Nevin Stage[125,126] and Tumor-Node-Metastasis Stage[137] After Radical Surgery

Stage	% Survival[125]	% Survival[126]	% Survival[137]
I	100	59	91
II	51	40	85
III	12	9	40
IV	10	7	19
V	0	1	

liver metastasis, 8%. Computed tomography (CT) evaluation gives somewhat better results.[128] The sensitivity of CT in detection of N1 nodal involvement is 36% and of N2 nodal involvement is 47%. Positive predictive values are 94% and 92%, respectively. The sensitivity of CT for detection of direct spread to the liver of < 2 cm is 65%, of > 2 cm is 100%, to the extrahepatic bile duct is 50%, and to the gastrointestinal tract or pancreas is 57%. The respective positive predictive values are 77%, 100%, 90%, and 100%. The sensitivity in detection of liver metastasis is 75% and involvement of aortocaval nodes is 21%.[128]

Prognosis

The prognosis for gallbladder cancer is bleak because there are no early signs or symptoms and the disease is advanced at discovery in most patients. The majority of patients are dead within 1 year of disease diagnosis.[35,53,113,129] Among 6,222 patients whose cases were reviewed in 1978, the 1-year survival was 11.8% and the 5-year survival was 4.1%.[113] Patients with unsuspected carcinomas that were discovered by the pathologist in the gallbladders removed for gallstones did better; the 5-year survival of this subgroup of 215 patients was 14.9%.[113] Stage and grade (discussed above) are the main prognostic factors. Once a tumor has penetrated through the muscle coat, only a loose connective-tissue plane separates it from the peritoneum or from the liver in the gallbladder bed. Thus, there is often direct invasion of the liver or peritoneal dissemination. Prolonged survival is achieved only when tumors are found at an early stage by chance.[117,129,130] A review of 3,000 autopsies in Japan revealed 15 asymptomatic carcinomas of the gallbladder that were all at an early stage: stage 0, 13.3%; stage I, 20.0%; or stage II, 46.7%. By comparison, symptomatic carcinomas were late stage: stage III, 9.3%, or stage IV, 90.7%. Among the symptomatic patients, lymphatic and hematogenous metastasis were found in 94.4% and 64.8%, respectively, whereas the comparable figures for asymptomatic patients were 13.3% and 0%, respectively.[131]

Ouchi and colleagues, confirming and extending the conclusions of Appelman et al., identified five factors that correlate with long survival: absence of spread beyond the perimuscular connective tissue, absence of hepatic infiltration, papillary morphology, well-differentiated histology, and low incidence of lymphatic or blood vessel invasion.[117,132] The first two are clearly stage indicators, and the second two are grade indicators, and as mentioned above, stage and grade are the major prognostic indicators.

If the tumor is confined to the gallbladder, the prognosis is much better than if it has extended to liver or lymph nodes.[53,133] By definition, there are no lymph node metastases in patients in TNM stage I, and these are truly early cancers for which there is a good outlook after cholecystectomy alone.[133,134] Shirai and colleagues confirmed that most pT1 tumors are curable by local surgery and emphasized that the main determinant of prognosis in these cases is the presence of tumor at the margin of resection.[135]

There is controversy about the value of radical surgery for advanced-stage disease. Foster believed that even extended surgery for advanced carcinoma did not improve survival or quality of life.[136] However, Tsukada and colleagues, reporting the outcome of radical surgery for gallbladder cancer in 106 patients, concluded that radical excision yielded statistically significant improvements in 5-year survival rates over noncurative operations.[137] They verified that the depth of invasion correlated well with the presence of lymph node metastasis. Lymph node metastasis was not identified in any patient with pT1 tumor but was identified in 48% of patients with pT2 tumors, in 72% of patients with pT3 tumors, and in 80% of patients with pT4 tumors. There were 35 5-year survivors, including 11 patients with nodal involvement, 10 patients with stage I tumors, 13 with stage II tumors, 10 with stage III tumors, and 2 with stage IV tumors. The cumulative 5-year survival rates are listed in Table 13–9 and are better than in other series, although the patient selection is different, too. Benoist et al. decided that in patients with stage II to stage IV disease, radical resection should be considered only in the absence of lymph node metastasis.[134] Pradeep and colleagues performed a multivariate analysis of data for 87 patients who had undergone surgical treatment and a subset of 55 patients with TNM stage IV disease. The three clinical factors that were significant predictors of survival were the presence of a palpable mass, the type of surgical excision, and the age of the patient.[138] They concluded, not surprisingly, that resectional surgery was associated with better survival than was biliary or gastric bypass or laparotomy alone.[138]

Table 13–10 shows survival by histologic type from the SEER program.[53] Papillary carcinomas have the best survival: a median of 20 months, a 2-year survival of 47%, and a 5-year survival of 32%. This advantage in survival of papillary carcinomas correlates with an earlier stage, as 62% of patients with papillary carcinomas have stage I disease (confined to the gallbladder), compared to 26.4% for all other histologic types. The other main histologic types have very short median survivals and 5-year survivals of < 10% because they present as advanced disease.[53,129]

Vascular invasion has an adverse influence on survival, the 5-year survival for patients with vascular invasion being 13%, compared with 31% for patients without.[53]

CARCINOID TUMORS

Carcinoids are rare primary neoplasms of the gallbladder. About 30 cases have been reported. These tumors tend to be incidental findings at surgery or autopsy. They may present with liver metastases but rarely manifest carcinoid syndrome.[139,140] Carcinoid syndrome has, however, been recorded in patients who had simultaneous carcinoids in the intestine and gallbladder. Adrenocorticotropic hormone secretion has been documented in one case, both clinically and by immunohistochemical methods.[141] We have seen one gallbladder carcinoid that was immunopositive for somatostatin. Carcinoid tumors vary from small yellowish nodules or polyps to infiltrative tumors that extend into the adjacent liver.[142–144] Histologically, they show the typical zellballen (cell clusters) of small cells with regular nuclei and indistinct cytoplasm. The tumor has been reported to produce an associated proliferation of the adjacent epithelium that was ascribed to a paracrine effect.[145] Some cases are concurrent with conventional adenocarcinomas and arise from metaplastic mucosa.[146]

SECONDARY TUMORS

Metastasis to the gallbladder is not often clinically important but is documented at autopsy as a manifestation of wide tumor dissemination, either by hematogenous or transcoelomic spread.[147–150] Malignant melanoma is the most common metastatic tumor, followed by carcinomas of lung, kidney, breast, large bowel, esophagus, stomach, ovary, and pancreas.[148] Individual examples of metastasis from other primary sites have also been described. Willis has stated that gastrointestinal metastasis often accompanies gallbladder metastasis.[147] Hematogenous metastases usually form small mucosal nodules or polyps, whereas transperitoneal spread produces serosal nodules or seedlings.[147,149]

MALIGNANT MELANOMA

Metastatic malignant melanoma to the gallbladder, an uncommon entity, often presents with signs and symptoms compatible with cholecystitis, and one or more polypoid masses within the lumen of the gallbladder are found on ultrasound examination.[151,152] The polyps may be black or may be amelanotic and often distend and enlarge the gallbladder. Typically, the patient has a prior history of melanoma and there

Table 13–10. Stage of Gallbladder Carcinomas and Survival, SEER Program

Stage	No. of Patients	% of Patients	Median Survival (Mo)	2-Year Survival Rate
I	621	26.4	19	0.45
II	117	5	7	0.15
III	678	28.8	4	0.04
IV	936	39.8	2	0.02

Key: SEER, Surveillance, Epidemiology, and End Results (National Cancer Institute).

From Henson DE, Albores-Saavedra J, Corle D: Carcinoma of the gallbladder. Histologic types, stage of disease, grade, and survival data. Cancer 70:1493–1497, 1992.

are other systemic metastases. Rarely, metastasis is isolated to the gallbladder, and after cholecystectomy, there have been long survivals.[153] Malignant melanomas that have no known primary tumor outside the biliary tree have been described as presumed primary malignant melanomas of the gallbladder or biliary tree, although some of these tumors were associated with disseminated disease at the time of diagnosis, suggesting that regression of an occult primary tumor of the skin might be the best explanation. Heath and Womack suggested that three criteria be fulfilled before a primary gallbladder melanoma is diagnosed: (1) tumors must be solitary and arise from the mucosal surface of the gallbladder; (2) they must be papillary or polypoid; and (3) they must either display junctional activity or have any other primary sites excluded by medical history taking, physical examination, and investigation.[154] These criteria are flawed, insofar as most metastatic melanomas to the gallbladder are mucosal lesions that are polypoid, and junctional activity has been described adjacent to metastatic melanomas.[155] Furthermore, melanocytes are not native to the gallbladder and there is a dearth of reports of benign melanocytic nevi, melanomas in situ, or small or early primary melanomas, despite the huge number of cholecystectomies that are performed. For many years, it was believed that the finding of junctional activity beside a malignant melanoma was an incontrovertible sign of primary origin, but even this change can be due to colonization of the epithelium by metastases.[155] We subscribe to the view of Murphy et al.[155] that most, if not all, melanomas of the gallbladder are metastatic deposits from a known, undetected, or regressed primary locus elsewhere.

Table 13–11. Classification of Nonepithelial Tumors of the Gallbladder

Benign
Granular cell tumor
Ganglioneurofibromatosis
Leiomyoma
Lipoma
Hemangioma
Lymphangioma
Neurofibroma
Malignant
Rhabdomyosarcoma
Kaposi's sarcoma
Leiomyosarcoma
Malignant fibrous histiocytoma
Angiosarcoma
Miscellaneous tumors
Carcinosarcoma
Malignant melanoma
Malignant lymphoma

From Albores-Saavedra J, Henson DE, Sobin LH: Histological Typing of Tumors of the Gallbladder and Extrahepatic Bile Ducts, 2nd ed. Berlin: Springer-Verlag, 1991.

MESENCHYMAL AND OTHER NEOPLASMS OF THE GALLBLADDER

Table 13–11 lists nonepithelial tumors of the gallbladder.

Granular cell tumor is much less common in the gallbladder than in the bile ducts. Only 4% of granular cell tumors of the biliary tree are located in gallbladder[156] (see Chapter 16).

Ganglioneurofibroma of the gallbladder can be a manifestation of multiple endocrine neoplasia type 2b.[157] The histologic features are proliferation of nerve sheath cells and ganglion cells in the lamina propria and enlargement of nerve trunks in the muscle coat and serosa. Ganglion cells tend to be scattered more or less randomly in the nerve trunks.

Uncommonly, the gallbladder is the seat of leiomyoma, hemangioma, lipoma, or other benign tumors of soft tissue.[6,158] Leiomyomas have been described in patients with human immunodeficiency virus.[159] A solitary neurofibroma of the gallbladder in a man without neurofibromatosis has been described[160] and another case with many tactile, corpuscle-like structures has been recorded.[161]

Cavernous hemangioma can cause a voluminous enlargement of the gallbladder, creating the clinical impression of a cystic mesenteric tumor.[158,162] A cystic lymphangioma involving the serosa has been described.[163]

A case of infantile myofibromatosis involving the gallbladder has been recounted.[164] On rare occasions, paraganglioma is found incidentally in the gallbladder as a serosal nodule[165] and in the hepatic duct.[166] This tumor shows nests of regular granular cells that are chromogranin positive and a rim of sustentacular cells that are positive for S100 protein. It must be distinguished from carcinoid tumor, which originates in the mucosa, probably in metaplastic intestinal mucosa, and has similar architecture and cytologic features. Either may obstruct the duct.

Primary sarcomas of the gallbladder arise from the muscle coat and other connective tissues. A small number of rhabdomyosarcomas have arisen in the adult gallbladder. They are about evenly distributed between alveolar and embryonal types.[167–169] Most such tumors are seen in the elderly. These tend to be large tumors showing extensive necrosis and hemorrhage. The differential diagnosis is from carcinosarcoma (malignant mixed tumor or sarcomatoid carcinoma). In children, rhabdomyosarcoma of the biliary tree is well known, if uncommon, but very few rhabdomyosarcomas arise in the gallbladder. One such tumor that did was grossly botryoid.[170] Kaposi's sarcoma of the gallbladder is described on rare occasions in patients with disseminated Kaposi's sarcoma, secondary to acquired immunodeficiency syndrome.[171,172] Leiomyosarcoma of the gallbladder is the subject of several case reports.[173–176] Sporadic cases of malignant fibrous histiocytoma[177–180] and angiosarcoma[181] are also documented. Some examples of angiosarcoma are epithelioid in type.[182,183]

Lymphoma of the gallbladder is a very rare primary tumor, with only nine cases being described in the English literature.[184] Most of these are of MALT (mucosa-associated lymphoid tissue) type,[185–188] although Hodgkin's disease,[189] angiotrophic lymphoma,[190] and mycosis fungoides[191] have also been described.

REFERENCES

1. Albores-Saavedra J, Henson DE, Sobin LH: Histological Typing of Tumors of the Gallbladder and Extrahepatic Bile Ducts, 2nd ed. Berlin: Springer-Verlag, 1991.
2. Yamamoto M, Nakajo S, Tahara E: Histological classification of epithelial polypoid lesions of the gallbladder. Acta Pathol Jpn 38:181–192, 1988.
3. Christensen AH, Ishak KG: Benign tumors and pseudotumors of the gallbladder. Report of 180 cases. Arch Pathol 90:423–432, 1970.
4. Tantachamrun T, Borvonsombat S, Theetranont C: Gardner's syndrome associated with adenomatous polyp of the gallbladder. J Med Assoc Thai 62:441–447, 1979.
5. Foster DR, Foster DBE: Gallbladder polyps in Peutz–Jeghers syndrome. Postgrad Med J 56:373–376, 1980.
6. Arbab AA, Brasfield R: Benign tumors of the gallbladder. Surgery 61:535–540, 1967.
7. Hultén J, Johannson H, Olding L: Adenomas of the gallbladder and extrahepatic bile ducts. Acta Chir Scand 136:203–207, 1970.
8. Kerr AB, Lendrum AC: A chloride-secreting papilloma in the gallbladder. A tumor of heterotopic intestinal epithelium containing Paneth's cells and enterochromaffine cells associated with massive chloride loss: With critical review of papilloma of the gallbladder. Br J Surg 23:615–639, 1936.
9. Yamaguchi K, Enjoji M: Gallbladder polyps: Inflammatory, hyperplastic and neoplastic types. Surg Pathol 1:203–213, 1988.
10. Kijima H, Watanabe H, Iwafuchi M, et al.: Histogenesis of gallbladder carcinoma from investigation of early carcinoma and microcarcinoma. Acta Pathol Jpn 39:235–244, 1989.
11. Nishihara K, Yamaguchi K, Hashimoto H, et al.: Tubular adenoma of the gallbladder with squamoid spindle cell metaplasia. Acta Pathol Jpn 41:41–45, 1991.
12. Wistuba II, Miquel JF, Gazdar AF, et al.: Gallbladder adenomas have molecular abnormalities different from those present in gallbladder carcinomas. Hum Pathol 30:21–25, 1999.
13. Sato H, Mizushima M, Ito J, et al.: Sessile adenoma of the gallbladder. Reappraisal of its importance as a precancerous lesion. Arch Pathol Lab Med 109:65–69, 1985.
14. Lin G, Hagerstrand I: Multiple adenomas of the gallbladder. Acta Path Microbiol Scand A 91:475–476, 1983.
15. Mogilner JG, Dharan M, Siplovich L: Adenoma of the gallbladder in childhood. J Pediatr Surg 26:223–224, 1991.
16. Yamamoto M, Murakami H, Ito M, et al.: Ectopic gastric mucosa of the gallbladder: Comparison with metaplastic polyp of the gallbladder. Am J Gastroenterol 84:1423–1426, 1989.
17. Almagro UA: Diffuse papillomatosis of the gallbladder. Am J Gastroenterol 80:274–278, 1985.
18. Thompson LDR, Becker RC, Przygodzki RM, et al.: Mucinous cystic neoplasm (Mucinous cystadenocarcinoma of low-grade malignant potential) of the pancreas. A clinicopathologic study of 130 cases. Am J Surg Pathol 23:1–16, 1999.
19. Buestow PC, Buck JL, Pantongrag-Brown L, et al.: Biliary cystadenoma and cystadenocarcinoma: Clinical-imaging-pathologic correlation with emphasis on the importance of ovarian stroma. Radiology 196:805–810, 1995.
20. Devaney K, Goodman ZD, Ishak KG: Hepatobiliary cystadenoma and cystadenocarcinoma: A light microscopic and immunohistochemical study of 70 patients. Am J Surg Pathol 18:1078–1091, 1994.
21. Warfel KA, Hull MT: Villous papilloma of the gallbladder in association with leukodystrophy. Hum Pathol 15:1192–1194, 1984.
22. Higgins GA, Turner JA: Mixed tumor of the gallbladder. Arch Surg 78:173–176, 1959.
23. Yamaguchi K, Maeda S, Kitamura K: Papillary adenoma of the gallbladder associated with regurgitation of pancreatic juice through abnormally-shaped union. Acta Chir Scand 155:549–552, 1989.
24. Laitio M: Histogenesis of epithelial neoplasms of human gallbladder. I. Dysplasia. Pathol Res Pract 178:51–56, 1983.
25. Albores-Saavedra J, Alcantra-Vazquez A, Cruz-Ortiz H, et al.: The precursor lesions of invasive gallbladder carcinoma. Hyperplasia, atypical hyperplasia and carcinoma-in-situ. Cancer 45:919–927, 1980.
26. Dowling GP, Kelly JK: The histogenesis of carcinoma of the gallbladder. Cancer 58:1702–1708, 1986.
27. Yamagiwa H: Mucosal dysplasia of gallbladder: Isolated and adjacent lesions to carcinomas. Jpn J Cancer Res 80:238–243, 1989.
28. Ojeda VJ, Shilkin KB, Walters MN-I: Premalignant epithelial lesions of the gallbladder: A prospective study of 120 cholecystectomy specimens. Pathology 17:451–454, 1985.
29. De Boer WGRM, Nairn RC: Intestinal metaplasia in gallbladder: An immunohistochemical study. Pathology 4:129–132, 1972.

30. De Boer WGRM, Ma J, Rees JW, et al.: Inappropriate mucin production in gallbladder metaplasia and neoplasia—an immunological study. Histopathology 5:295–303, 1981.
31. Tatematsu M, Ichinose M, Miki K, et al.: Gastric phenotypic expression in human gallbladder cancers revealed by pepsinogen immunohistochemistry and mucin histochemistry. Virchows Archiv A Pathol Anat 413:25–32, 1988.
32. Kushima R, Lohr B, Borchard F: Differentiation towards gastric foveolar, mucopeptic and intestinal goblet cells in gallbladder adenocarcinomas. Histopathology 29:443–448, 1996.
33. Kozuka S, Tsubone M, Yasui A, et al.: Relation of adenoma to carcinoma in the gallbladder. Cancer 50:2226–2234, 1982.
34. Albores-Saavedra J, de Jesus Manrique J, Angeles-Angeles A, et al.: Carcinoma in situ of the gallbladder. A clinicopathologic study of 18 cases. Am J Surg Pathol 8:323–333, 1984.
35. Black WC: The morphogenesis of gallbladder carcinoma. *In:* Progress in Surgical Pathology, Vol II. New York: Masson Publishing, 1980, pp 207–223.
36. Black WC, Key CR, Carmany TB, et al.: Carcinoma of the gallbladder in a population of Southwestern American Indians. Cancer 39:1267–1279, 1977.
37. Jarvi O, Lauren P: Intestinal metaplasia on the mucosa of the gallbladder and common bile duct. Ann Med Exp Fenn 45:213–223, 1967.
38. Laitio M: Goblet cells, enterochromaffin cells, superficial gastric-type epithelium and antral-type glands in the gallbladder. Beitr Path Bd 156:343–358, 1975.
39. Kozuka S, Hachisuka K: Incidence by age and sex of intestinal metaplasia in the gallbladder. Hum Pathol 15:779–784, 1984.
40. Kozuka S, Kurashina M, Tsubone M, et al.: Significance of intestinal metaplasia for evolution of cancer in the biliary tract. Cancer 54:2277–2285, 1984.
41. Tsutsumi Y, Nagura H, Osamura Y, et al.: Histochemical studies of metaplastic lesions in the human gallbladder. Arch Pathol Lab Med 108:917–921, 1984.
42. Laitio M: Intestinal, gastric body- and antral-type mucosal metaplasia in the gallbladder. Beitr Path Bd 159:271–279, 1976.
43. Duarte I, Llanos O, Domke H, et al.: Metaplasia and precursor lesions of gallbladder carcinoma. Frequency, distribution, and probability of detection in routine histologic samples. Cancer 72:1878–1784, 1993.
44. Elfving G, Lehtonen T, Teir H: Clinical significance of primary hyperplasia of gallbladder mucosa. Ann Surg 165:61–69, 1967.
45. Elfving G, Palmu A: Hyperplasia of the gallbladder mucosa as the cause of biliary distress in children. Ann Paediatr Fenn 13:100–103, 1967.
46. Elfving G, Palmu A, Teir H: Cholesterolosis and mucosal hyperplasia of the gallbladder. Ann Chir Gynaec Fenn 57:28–30, 1968.
47. Elfving G, Silvonen E, Teir H: Mucosal hyperplasia of the gallbladder in cases of cholecystolithiasis. Acta Surg Scand 135:519–522, 1969.
48. Hanada K, Itoh M, Fujii K, et al.: Pathology and cellular kinetics of gallbladder with an anomalous junction of the pancreaticobiliary duct. Am J Gastroenterol 91:1007–1011, 1996.
49. Yamamoto M, Nakajo S, Tahara T, et al.: Mucosal changes of the gallbladder in anomalous union with the pancreaticobiliary duct system. Pathol Res Pract 187:241–246, 1991.
50. Tanno S, Obara T, Fujii T, et al.: Proliferative potential and K-*ras* mutation in epithelial hyperplasia of the gallbladder in patients with anomalous pancreaticobiliary ductal union. Cancer 83:267–275, 1998.
51. Feldman M, Feldman M: Cholesterolosis of the gallbladder. An autopsy study of 165 cases. Gastroenterology 27:641–648, 1954.
52. Albores-Saavedra J, Alcantra-Vasquez A, Cruz-Ortiz H, et al.: The precursor lesions of invasive gallbladder carcinoma. Hyperplasia, atypical hyperplasia, and carcinoma in situ. Cancer 45:919–927, 1980.
53. Henson DE, Albores-Saavedra J, Corle D: Carcinoma of the gallbladder. Histologic types, stage of disease, grade, and survival data. Cancer 70:1493–1497, 1992.
54. Warren KW, Hardy, O'Rourke MG: Primary neoplasia of the gallbladder. Surg Gynecol Obstet 126:1036–1040, 1968.
55. Solan MJ, Jackson BT: Carcinoma of the gallbladder. A clinical appraisal and review of 57 cases. Br J Surg 58:593–597, 1971.
56. Keill RH, DeWeese MS: Primary carcinoma of the gallbladder. Am J Surg 125:726–729, 1973.
57. Pemberton LB, Diffenbaugh WF, Strohl EL: The surgical significance of carcinoma of the gallbladder. Am J Surg 122:381–383, 1971.
58. Arnaud JP, Casa C, Georgeac C, et al.: Primary carcinoma of the gallbladder—review of 143 cases. Hepatogastroenterol 42:811–815, 1995.
59. Kotorac V: Biliary peritonitis resulting from a perforated carcinomatous gallbladder. Gastroenterology 63:328–330, 1972.
60. Yoshida S, Todoroki T, Ichikawa Y, et al.: Mutations of p16Ink4/CDKN2 and p15Ink/4B/MTS2 genes in biliary tract cancers. Cancer Res 55:2756–2760, 1995.
61. Hanada K, Itoh M, Fujii K, et al.: TP53 mutations in stage I gallbladder carcinoma with special attention to growth patterns. Eur J Cancer 33:1136–1140, 1997.
62. Wistuba II, Sugio KHJ, Kishimoto Y, et al.: Allele-specific mutations involved in the pathogenesis of endemic gallbladder carcinoma in Chile. Cancer Res 55:2511–2515, 1995.
63. Yukawa M, Fujimori T, Hirayama D, et al.: Expression of oncogene products and growth factors in early gallbladder cancer, advanced gallbladder cancer, and chronic cholecystitis. Hum Pathol 24:37–40, 1993.
64. Diehl AK: Epidemiology of gallbladder cancer: A synthesis of recent data. JNCI 65:1209–1214, 1980.
65. Hart J, Modan B, Shani M: Cholelithiasis in the etiology of gallbladder neoplasms. Lancet 1:1151–1153, 1971.
66. Maram ES, Ludwig J, Kurland LT, et al.: Carcinoma of the gallbladder and extrahepatic bile ducts in Rochester, Minnesota, 1935–1971. Am J Epidemiol 109:152–157, 1979.
67. Lowenfels AB, Lindström CG, Conway MJ, et al.: Gallstones and risk of gallbladder cancer. JNCI 75:77–80, 1985.
68. Lowenfels AB, Walker AM, Althaus DP, et al.: Gallstone growth, size, and risk of gallbladder cancer: An interracial study. Int J Epidemiol 18:50–54, 1989.
69. Sampliner R, Bennett P, Comess L, Rose et al.: Gallbladder disease in Pima Indians: Demonstration of high prevalence and early onset by cholecystography. N Engl J Med 283:1358–1364, 1970.
70. Serra J, Calvo A, Maturana M, et al.: Biliary tract cancer in Chile. Int J Cancer 46:965–971, 1990.

71. Strom BL, Soloway RD, Rios-Dalenz JL, et al.: Risk factors for gallbladder cancer. An international collaborative case-control study. Cancer 76:1747–1756, 1995.
72. Lowenfels AB, Maisonneuve P, Boyle P, et al.: Epidemiology of gallbladder cancer. Hepatogastroenterol 46:1529–1532, 1999.
73. Ghadirian P, Simard A, Baillargeon J: A population-based case-control study of cancer of the bile ducts and gallbladder in Quebec, Canada. Rev Epidemiol Sante Publique 41:107–112, 1993.
74. Babbitt DP, Starshak RJ, Clemett AR: Choledochal cyst: A concept of etiology. Am J Roentgenol 119:57–62, 1973.
75. Kinoshita H, Nagata E, Hirohashi K, et al.: Carcinoma of the gallbladder with an anomalous connection between the choledochus and the pancreatic duct. Cancer 54:762–769, 1984.
76. Mori K, Nagakawa T, Ohta T, et al.: Association between gallbladder cancer and anomalous union of the pancreaticobiliary ductal system. Hepatogastroenterol 40:56–60, 1993.
77. Suda K, Miyano T: Bile pancreatitis. Arch Pathol Lab Med 109:433–436, 1985.
78. Kimura K, Ohto M, Saisho H, et al.: Association of gallbladder carcinoma and anomalous pancreatobiliary ductal union. Gastroenterology 89:1258–1265, 1985.
79. Sugiyama M, Atomi Y: Anomalous pancreatobiliary junction without congenital choledochal cyst. Br J Surg 85:911–916, 1998.
80. Aoki H, Sugaya H, Shimazu M: A clinical study on cancer of the bile duct associated with anomalous arrangements of the pancreaticobiliary ductal system. Analysis of 569 cases collected in Japan. J Bil Tract Pancreas 8:1539–1551, 1987.
81. Tanaka K, Nishimura A, Yamada K, et al.: Cancer of the gallbladder associated with anomalous junction of the pancreaticobiliary duct system without bile duct dilatation. Br J Surg 80:622–624, 1993.
82. Morohoshi T, Kunimura T, Kanda M, et al.: Multiple carcinomata associated with anomalous arrangement of the biliary and pancreatic duct system. Acta Pathol Jpn 40:755–763, 1990.
83. Tokiwa K, Iwai N: Early mucosal changes of the gallbladder in patients with anomalous arrangement of the pancreaticobiliary duct. Gastroenterology 110:1614–1618, 1996.
84. Hanada K, Itoh M, Fujii K, et al.: K-*ras* and p53 mutations in stage I gallbladder carcinoma with an anomalous junction of the pancreaticobiliary duct. Cancer 77:452–458, 1996.
85. Kozu T, Suda K, Toki F: Pancreatic development and anatomical variation. Gastrointest Endosc Clin N Am 5:1–30, 1995.
86. Welton C, Marr JS, Friedman SM: Association between hepatobiliary cancer and typhoid carrier state. Lancet 1:791–794, 1979.
87. Marr JS, Friedman S, Welton J: Clues concerning the etiology of carcinoma of the gallbladder. Gastroenterology 79:400, 1980.
88. Caygill CP, Hill MJ, Braddick M, et al.: Cancer mortality in chronic typhoid and paratyphoid carriers. Lancet 343:83–84, 1994.
89. Nath G, Singh H, Shukla VK: Chronic typhoid carriage and carcinoma of the gallbladder. Eur J Cancer Prev 6:557–559, 1997.
90. Mallory TB, Lawson GM Jr. Chronic typhoid cholecystitis. Am J Pathol 7:71–75, 1931.
91. Fox JG, Dewhirst FE, Shen Z, et al.: Hepatic *Helicobacter* species identified in bile and gallbladder tissue from Chileans with chronic cholecystitis. Gastroenterology 114:755–763, 1998.
92. Ootani T, Shirai Y, Tsukada K, et al.: Relationship between gallbladder carcinoma and the segmental type of adenomyomatosis of the gallbladder. Cancer 69:2647–2652, 1992.
93. Lauwers GY, Wahl SJ, Scott V, et al.: Papillary mucinous adenoma arising in adenomyomatous hyperplasia of the gallbladder. J Clin Pathol 48:965–967, 1995.
94. Albores-Saavedra J, Henson DE: Adenomyomatous hyperplasia of the gallbladder with perineural invasion. Arch Pathol Lab Med 119:1173–1176, 1995.
95. Chijiiwa K, Tanaka M: Polypoid lesions of the gallbladder: Indications of carcinoma and outcome after surgery for malignant polypoid lesion. Int Surg 79:106–109, 1994.
96. Bombi JA, Rives A, Astudillo E, et al.: Polyposis coli associated with adenocarcinoma of the gallbladder. Cancer 53:2561–2563, 1984.
97. Bergquist A, Glaumann H, Persson B, et al.: Risk factors and clinical presentation of hepatobiliary carcinoma in patients with primary sclerosing cholangitis: A case-control study. Hepatology 27:311–316, 1998.
98. Wee A, Ludwig J, Coffee RJ, et al.: Hepatobiliary carcinoma associated with primary sclerosing cholangitis and chronic ulcerative colitis. Hum Pathol 16:719–726, 1985.
99. Brandt DJ, MacCarty RL, Charboneau JW, et al.: Gallbladder disease in patients with primary sclerosing cholangitis. Am J Roentgenol 150:571–574, 1988.
100. Dorudi S, Chapman RW, Kettlewell MG: Carcinoma of the gallbladder in ulcerative colitis and primary sclerosing cholangitis. Report of two cases. Dis Colon Rectum 34:827–828, 1991.
101. Washburn WK, Lewis WD, Jenkins RL: Liver transplantation with incidental gallbladder carcinoma in the recipient hepatectomy. HPB Surg 8:147–149, 1994.
102. Herzog K, Goldblum JR: Gallbladder adenocarcinoma and acalculous chronic lymphoplasmacytic cholecystitis associated with ulcerative colitis. Mod Pathol 9:194–198, 1996.
103. Campbell WL, Ferris JV, Holbert BL, et al.: Biliary tract carcinoma complicating primary sclerosing cholangitis: Evaluation with CT, cholangiography, US, and MR imaging. Radiology 207:41–50, 1998.
104. Albores-Saavedra J, Nadji M, Morales AR, et al.: Carcinoembryonic antigen in normal, preneoplastic and neoplastic gallbladder epithelium. Cancer 52:1069–1072, 1983.
105. Albores-Saavedra J, Nadji M, Henson DE: Intestinal-type adenocarcinoma of the gallbladder. A clinicopathological study of seven cases. Am J Surg Pathol 10:19–25, 1986.
106. Vardaman C, Albores-Saavedra J: Clear cell carcinoma of the gallbladder and extrahepatic bile ducts. Am J Surg Pathol 19:91–99, 1995.
107. Appelman HD, Coopersmith N: Pleomorphic spindle-cell carcinoma of the gallbladder. Cancer 25:535–541, 1970.
108. Iezzoni JC, Mills SE: Sarcomatoid carcinomas (carcinosarcoma) of the gastrointestinal tract: A review. Semin Diag Pathol 10:176–187, 1993.

109. Born MW, Ramey WG, Ryan SF, et al.: Carcinosarcoma and carcinoma of the gallbladder. Cancer 53:2171–2177, 1984.
110. Ishihara T, Kawano H, Takahashi M, et al.: Carcinosarcoma of the gallbladder. A case report with immunohistochemical and ultrastructural studies. Cancer 66:992–997, 1990.
111. Inoshita S, Iwashita A, Enjoji M: Carcinosarcoma of the gallbladder. Report of a case and review of the literature. Acta Pathol Jpn 36:913–920, 1986.
112. Laitio M: Histogenesis of epithelial neoplasms of human gallbladder. II. Carcinoma. Pathol Res Pract 178:57–66, 1983.
113. Piehler JM, Crichlow RW: Primary carcinoma of the gallbladder. Surg Gynecol Obstet 147:929–942, 1978.
114. Beltz WR, Condon RE: Primary carcinoma of the gallbladder. Ann Surg 180:180–184, 1974.
115. Hart J, Modan B: Factors affecting survival of patients with gallbladder neoplasms. Arch Intern Med 129:931–934, 1972.
116. Nevin JE, Moran TJ, Kay S, et al.: Carcinoma of the gallbladder: Staging, treatment, and prognosis. Cancer 37:141–148, 1976.
117. Ouchi K, Matsuno S, Sato T: Long-term survival in carcinoma of the biliary tract. Analysis of prognostic factors in 146 resections. Arch Surg 124:248–252, 1989.
118. Roa I, Villaseca M, Araya J, et al.: p53 tumour suppressor gene protein expression in early and advanced gallbladder carcinoma. Histopathology 31:226–230, 1997.
119. Fahim RB, McDonald JR, Richards JC, et al.: Carcinoma of the gallbladder: A study of its modes of spread. Ann Surg 156:114–124, 1962.
120. Nagakawa T, Mori K, Nakano T, et al.: Perineural invasion of carcinoma of the pancreas and biliary tract. Br J Surg 80:619–621, 1993.
121. Tsukada K, Kurosaki I, Uchida K, et al.: Lymph node spread from carcinoma of the gallbladder. Cancer 80:661–667, 1997.
122. Ogura Y, Mizumoto R, Isaji S, et al.: Radical operations for carcinoma of the gallbladder: Present status in Japan. World J Surg 15:337–343, 1991.
123. Shirai Y, Tsukada K, Ohtani T, et al.: Hepatic metastases from carcinoma of the gallbladder. Cancer 75:2063–2068, 1995.
124. Baba K, Hattori T, Koishikawa I, et al.: Cavitary pulmonary metastases of gallbaldder cancer. Respiration 65:219–222, 1998.
125. Frezza EE, Mezghebe H: Gallbladder carcinoma: A 28-year experience. Int Surg 82:295–300, 1997.
126. Gagner M, Rossi RL: Radical operations for carcinoma of the gallbladder: Present status in North America. World J Surg 15:344–347, 1991.
127. Haribhakti SP, Kapoor VK, Gujral RB, et al.: Staging of carcinoma of the gallbladder—an ultrasonographic evaluation. Hepatogastroenterol 44:1240–1245, 1997.
128. Ohtani T, Shirai Y, Tsukada K, Muto, et al.: Spread of gallbladder carcinoma: CT evaluation with pathological correlation. Abdom Imaging 21:195–201, 1996.
129. Shieh CJ, Dunn E, Standard JE: Primary carcinoma of the gallbladder: A review of a 16-year experience at the Waterbury Hospital Health Center. Cancer 47:996–1004, 1981.
130. Bergdahl L: Gallbladder carcinoma first diagnosed at microscopic examination of gallbladders removed for presumed benign disease. Ann Surg 191:19–22, 1980.
131. Kimura W, Nagai H, Kuroda A, et al.: Clinicopathologic study of asymptomatic gallbladder carcinoma found at autopsy. Cancer 64:98–103, 1989.
132. Appelman RM, Morlock CG, Dahlin DC, et al.: Long-term survival in carcinoma of the gallbladder. Surg Gynecol Obstet 117:459–464, 1963.
133. Yamaguchi K, Enjoji M: Carcinoma of the gallbladder. A clinicopathology of 103 patients and a newly proposed staging. Cancer 62:1425–1432, 1988.
134. Benoist S, Panis Y, Fagniez PL: Long-term results after curative resection for carcinoma of the gallbladder. Am J Surg 175:118–122, 1998.
135. Shirai Y, Yoshida K, Tsukada K, et al.: Early carcinoma of the gallbladder. Eur J Surg 158:545–548, 1992.
136. Foster J: Carcinoma of the gallbladder. *In* Way, LW, Pellegrini CA (eds): Surgery of the Gallbladder and Bile Ducts. Philadelphia: WB Saunders, 1987, pp 471–485.
137. Tsukada K, Hatakeyama K, Kurosaki I, et al.: Outcome of radical surgery for carcinoma of the gallbladder according to the TNM stage. Surgery 120:816–821, 1996.
138. Pradeep R, Kaushik SP, Sikora SS, et al.: Predictors of survival in patients with carcinoma of the gallbladder. Cancer 76:1145–1149, 1995.
139. Khetan N, Bose NC, Arya SV, et al.: Carcinoid tumor of the gallbladder: Report of a case. Surg Today 25:1047–1049, 1995.
140. Psathakis D, Wenk H, Muller G, et al.: Primary carcinoid of the gallbladder. Hepatogastroenterol 43:167–168, 1996.
141. Spence RW, Burns-Cox CJ: ACTH-secreting "apudoma" of gallbaldder. Gut 16:473–476, 1975.
142. Bosse MD: Carcinoid tumor of the gallbladder. Arch Pathol 35:898–899, 1943.
143. Barnes TG: Argentaffinoma (carcinoid) of the gallbladder. Surgery 32:723–727, 1952.
144. Gaffney PR, Coyle LJ: Carcinoid tumor of the gallbladder associated with a meningioma. Ir J Med Sci 147:318–321, 1978.
145. Dirschmid K: Generalized blastomatosis (carcinoidomatosis) of the "Helle Zellen" system. Beitr Pathol Anat 139:187–198, 1969.
146. Yamamoto M, Nakajo S, Miyoshi N, et al.: Endocrine cell carcinoma (carcinoid) of the gallbladder. Am J Surg Pathol 13:292–302, 1989.
147. Willis RA: The Spread of Tumours in the Human Body, 2nd Ed. London: Butterworths, 1952, pp 218–219.
148. Weedon D: Pathology of the Gallbaldder. New York: Masson Publishing, 1984, pp 259–262.
149. Botting AJ, Harrison EG Jr, Black BM: Metastatic hypernephroma masquerading as a polypoid tumor of the gallbladder and review of metastatic tumors of the gallbladder. Proc Mayo Clin 38:225–232, 1963.
150. Abrams HL, Spiro R, Goldstein N: Metastases in carcinoma. Analysis of 1000 autopsied cases. Cancer 3:74–85, 1950.
151. Ostick DG, Haqqani MT: Obstructive cholecystitis due to metastatic malignant melanoma. Postgrad Med J 52:710–712, 1976.
152. Mc Fadden PM, Krementz ET, McKinnon WMP, et al.: Metastatic melanoma of the gallbladder. Cancer 44:1802–1808, 1979.
153. Bugnon PY, Servais B, Boulenger-Bugnon F, et al.: Five year survival after treatment of gallbladder metastasis of malignant melanoma. Bulletin du Cancer 78:169–172, 1991.

154. Heath DI, Womack C: Primary malignant melanoma of the gallbladder. J Clin Pathol 41:1073–1077, 1988.
155. Murphy MN, Lorimer SM, Glennon PE: Metastatic melanoma of the gallbladder: A case report and review of the literature. J Surg Oncol 34:68–72, 1987.
156. Sanchez JA, Nanta RJ: Resection of a granular cell tumor at the hepatic confluence. A precarious location for a benign tumor. Ann Surg 57:446–450, 1991.
157. Carney JA, Sizemore W, Hayles AM: Multiple endocrine neoplasia, type 2b. Pathobiol Annu 8:105–153, 1978.
158. Sewell JH, Miron MA: Benign cavernous hemangioma of the gallbladder. Arch Pathol 88:30–31, 1969.
159. Toma P, Loy A, Pastorino C, et al.: Leiomyomas of the gallbladder and splenic calcifications in an HIV-infected child. Pediatr Radiol 27:92–94, 1997.
160. Acebo E, Fernandez FA, Val-Bernal JF: Solitary neurofibroma of the gallbladder. A case report and review of the literature. Gen Diagn Pathol 143:337–340, 1998.
161. Morizumi H, Sano T, Hirose T, et al.: Neurofibroma of the gallbladder seen as a papillary polyp. Acta Pathol Jpn 38:259–268, 1988.
162. Mayorga H, Hernando M, Val-Bernal JF: Diffuse expansive cavernous hemangioma of the gallbladder. Gen Diagn Pathol 142:211–215, 1997.
163. Ohba K, Sugauchi F, Orito E, et al.: Cystic lymphangioma of the gallbladder: A case report. J Gastroenterol Hepatol 10:693–696, 1995.
164. Goldberg NS, Bauer BS, Kraus H, et al.: Infantile myofibromatosis: A review of clinicopathology with perspectives on new treatment choices. Pediatr Dermatol 5:37–46, 1988.
165. Miller TA, Webber TR, Appelman HD: Paraganglioma of the gallbladder. Arch Surg 105:637–639, 1972.
166. Sarma DP, Rodriguez FH Jr, Hoffman EO: Paraganglioma of the hepatic duct. South J Med 73:1677–1678, 1980.
167. Al-Jaberi TM, al-Masri N, Tbukhi A: Adult rhabdomyosarcoma of the gallbladder: Case report and review of published works. Gut 35:854–856, 1994.
168. Ben Rejeb A, Jabbes H, Essoussi M, et al.: Localisation exceptionnelle du rhabdomyosarcome embryonnaire a la vesicule biliarie. Ann Pathol 14:163–167, 1994.
169. Aldabagh SM, Shibata CS, Taxy JB: Rhabdomyosarcoma of the common bile duct in an adult. Arch Pathol Lab Med 110:547–550, 1986.
170. Mihara S, Matsumoto H, Tokunaga F, et al.: Botryoid rhabdosarcoma of the gallbladder in a child. Cancer 49:812–818, 1982.
171. Enad JG, Lapa JC, Jaklie B, et al.: Kaposi's sarcoma of the gallbladder. Mil Med 157:559–561, 1992.
172. French AL, Beaudet LM, Benator DA, et al.: Cholecystectomy in patients with AIDS: Clinicopathologic correlations in 107 cases. Clin Infect Dis 21:852–858, 1995.
173. Kumar S, Gupta A, Shrivastava UK, et al.: Leiomyosarcoma of gallbladder: A case report. Indian J Pathol Microbiol 36:78–80, 1993.
174. Willen R, Willen H: Primary sarcoma of the gallbladder. A light and electron microscopical study. Virchows Arch Pathol Anat 396:91–102, 1982.
175. Fotiadis C, Gugulakis A, Nakopoulou L, et al.: Primary leiomyosarcoma of the gallbladder. Case report and review of the literature. HPB Surg 2:211–214, 1990.
176. Zeig DA, Memon MA, Kennedy DR, et al.: Leiomyosarcoma of the gallbladder—a case report and review of the literature. Acta Oncol 37:212–214, 1998.
177. Sasada A, Yanagawa M, Hayashi S, et al.: Primary malignant fibrous histiocytoma of the gallbladder: A case report. Nippon Geka Gakkai Zasshi 89:1306–1309, 1988.
178. Tomono H, Fujioka S, Kato K, et al.: Malignant fibrous histiocytoma of the gallbladder. Hepatogastroenterol 45:1468–1472, 1998.
179. Kristofferson AO, Domellof L, Emdin SO, et al.: Malignant fibrous histiocytoma of the gallbladder: A case report. J Surg Oncol 23:56–59, 1983.
180. Sreekantaiah C, Rao UN, Karakousis CP, et al.: Cytogenetic findings in malignant fibrous histiocytoma of the gallbladder. Cancer Genet Cytogenet 59:30–34, 1992.
181. Kumar A, Lal BK, Singh MK, et al.: Angiosarcoma of the gallbladder. Am J Gastroenterol 84:1431–1433, 1989.
182. Byers RJ, McMahon RF: Epithelioid angiosarcoma of the gallbladder. Histopathology 25:502–503, 1994.
183. White J, Chan YF: Epithelioid angiosarcoma of the gallbladder. Histopathology 24:269–271, 1994.
184. Chatila R, Fiedler PN, Vender RJ: Primary lymphoma of the gallbladder: Case report and review of the literature. Am J Gastroenterol 91:2242–2244, 1996.
185. Mosnier JF, Brousse N, Sevestre C, et al.: Primary low-grade B-cell lymphoma of the mucosa-associated lymphoid tissue arising within the gallbladder. Histopathology 20:273–275, 1992.
186. McCluggage WG, Mackel E, McCusker G: Primary low grade malignant lymphoma of mucosa-associated lymphoid tissue of the gallbladder. Histopathology 29:285–287, 1996.
187. Abe Y, Takatsuki H, Okada Y, et al.: Mucosa-associated lymphoid tissue type lymphoma of the gallbladder associated with acute myeloid leukemia. Intern Med 38:442–444, 1999.
188. Bickel A, Eitan A, Tsilman B, et al.: Low grade B-cell lymphoma of mucosa associated lymphoid tissue (MALT) arising in the gallbladder. Hepatogastroenterol 46:1643–1646, 1999.
189. Orton DF, Saigh JA: CT of Hodgkin's lymphoma limited to the gallbladder. Abdom Imaging 21:238–239, 1996.
190. Laurino L, Melato M: Malignant angioendotheliomatosis (angiotrophic lymphoma) limited to the gallbladder. Wirchows Arch A Pathol Anat Histopathol 417:243–246, 1990.
191. Madsen JA, Tallini G, Glusae EJ, et al.: Biliary tract obstruction secondary to mycosis fungoides: A case report. J Clin Gastroenterol 28:56–80, 1999.

Chapter

14

BILE DUCTS: EMBRYOLOGY, ANATOMY, HISTOLOGY, AND DEVELOPMENTAL ANOMALIES

EMBRYOLOGY

The bile ducts are derived from a midgut diverticulum of the duodenum. As this grows into mesoderm, the cranial end forms the left and right lobes of the liver and the caudal end forms the extrahepatic bile ducts, the cystic duct, and the gallbladder. With rotation of the duodenum, the origin of the bile duct at the ampulla of Vater lies to the left and the bile duct passes posterior to the duodenum to the porta hepatis.

ANATOMY

The left and right hepatic ducts emerge from the liver and extend for approximately 1.0 cm before they fuse to form the common hepatic duct. Occasionally, two right segmental ducts fuse in an extrahepatic location to form the right hepatic duct. The common hepatic duct extends down in the porta hepatis for an average of 2.0 cm (range, 0.8 to 5.2 cm), before it joins the cystic duct.[1] The cystic duct is present in the free edge of the lesser omentum. Typically, it is 3.0 cm in length (range, 0.4 to 6.5 cm), with a diameter of 0.4 cm. There is some variability in the manner in which the cystic duct unites with the hepatic duct, a factor of considerable importance in biliary surgery. In the majority of instances, the junction is an acute angle with the right side of the hepatic duct. However, in 10% of instances, the junction occurs on either the anterior or posterior aspect of the hepatic duct. Furthermore, in an additional 15% of cases, the cystic duct runs alongside the hepatic duct in the same connective-tissue sheath, before anastomosing with it.[2] If this variant is not correctly identified at the time of surgery, it may result in ligation and cutting of the common sheath. The damage will not become apparent until several days after surgery, when profound obstructive jaundice develops. Surgical repair of the severed bile duct may prove difficult. Rarely, the hepatic duct–cystic duct junction may be higher up the porta hepatis, at the level of the right and left hepatic duct anastomosis.

The common bile duct is formed by anastomosis of the cystic duct and the common hepatic duct. Its course may be divided into supraduodenal, retroduodenal, pancreatic, and intraduodenal segments. It is usually 0.4 to 1.3 cm in diameter and 5.0 cm long (range, 1.5 to 9.0 cm). At its lower end, it runs alongside—and, in most cases, unites with—the main pancreatic duct of Wirsung before emptying into the duodenum at the papilla.

The anatomy of the ampullary region is complex and is subject to a number of anatomic variations (Fig. 14–1). In 74% of individuals, the ducts fuse to form a common channel before entering the duodenum; however, in 19%

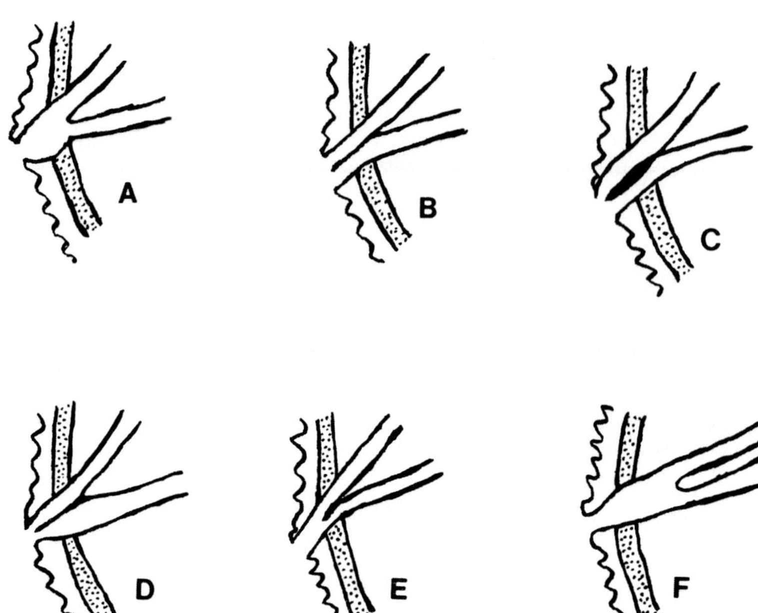

Figure 14–1. Variations of anatomy in the periampullory region: *A,* normal arrangement with ampulla of Vater; *B,* interposed septum; *C,* separate openings; *D,* short common channel; *E,* short common channel; *F,* long common channel with fusion outside of the duodenal wall. (From Frierson HF, Jr: Gallbladder and extraheptic biliary system. *In* Sternberg SS (ed): Histology for Pathologists, 2nd ed., Philadelphia: Lippincott-Raven, 1997, pp 593–611.)

of individuals, the ducts run alongside each other without uniting, to form adjacent but separate openings at the duodenum. In this situation, the bile duct opening is cranial and medial to the orifice of the duct of Wirsung. In the remaining 7% of individuals, the ducts unite but the lumina remain separated by a septum.[3] Not all individuals have a well-defined ampulla of Vater (dilated portion of distal duct). This is only found in 25% of persons who have a common distal pancreaticobiliary channel. The remaining persons have either a short (31%) or long (18%) segment common channel without ampullary dilation. The common channel may extend up to 33 mm (average, 22 mm) from the duodenal orifice.[4] Anastomosing ducts that occur outside of the duodenal wall are beyond the influence of the sphincter of Oddi.[5] This anatomic arrangement allows for the possibility of pancreatic reflux into the bile ducts or gallbladder and may be a factor in the later development of gallbladder cancer.[4,5]

The duodenal papilla is located 8 to 10 cm distal to the pylorus and generally projects for a little way into the lumen of second portion of the duodenum. Its mean length is 11 mm and its diameter is 5 mm.[6,7] Mucosal folds, or flaps, ranging from 1 to 5 mm in length are present within the terminal common portion of bile and pancreatic ducts and ampulla of >90% of normal individuals. It seems likely that these folds function as valves, flattening out during periods of secretion and becoming elevated at other times to prevent duodenal fluid regurgitation.[8]

The duodenal mucosa covering the papilla may form a series of small folds and flaps. Surrounding the papilla are the muscular fibers of the sphincter of Oddi, which are derived from the hepatic bud but are attached to, and held in place by, the muscularis propria of the duodenal wall. This sphincter controls the flow of bile and pancreatic juice into the duodenum and also prevents reflux of duodenal contents. The arrangement of muscle and collagen fibers is highly complex and may vary considerably from person to person. It is probable that in most individuals, fibers of the sphincter of Oddi extend along the duct of Wirsung and the common bile duct, proximal to their junction.[9] This implies an element of independent sphincteric control of the separate ducts.

HISTOLOGY

All extrahepatic bile ducts are lined by a single layer of columnar epithelium. The cells have rounded, basally located nuclei, with evenly distributed chromatin and tiny nucleoli (Fig. 14–2). The cytoplasm contains small amounts of mucin, predominately sulfomucin. These cells are positive when immunostained for low-molecular-weight keratin CAM 5.2.[10] No goblet

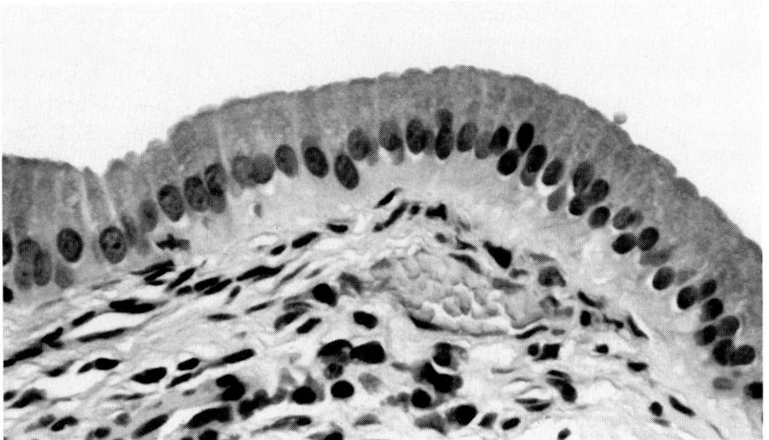

Figure 14–2. Bile duct epithelial lining cells. These are columnar with basal nuclei containing tiny nucleoli.

cells are present outside the region of the ampulla, but throughout the bile ducts there are scattered endocrine cells immunopositive for somatostatin.

The surface epithelium of the hepatic and common bile duct is not smooth but contains numerous regular depressions, or pits, referred to as the sacculi of Beale. In tangential sections, these sacculi may appear to be isolated from the surface. Surrounding the sacculi and emptying into them are numerous mucus-secreting glands that are lobulated and may be surrounded by a dense stroma (Fig. 14–3). These glands are found throughout the bile duct system but are most numerous around the proximal and distal portions. Each gland consists of 5 to 20 ductlike structures that may be branched but are generally circular in cross-section. The glands are lined by a single layer of low columnar mucus-secreting cells, with a flattened nucleus, located just superior to the basement membrane. These glands may show weak immunopositivity for pancreatic enzymes, such as amylase, lipase, and trypsin. In instances of chronic periductal inflammation and fibrosis, difficulties may arise on biopsy in distinguishing mucus glands from a low-grade sclerosing adenocarcinoma. However, even in extreme reactive situations, mucus glands retain their lobular arrangement. Furthermore, perineural infiltration by benign glands has not been reported at this location.[10] Consideration of these two

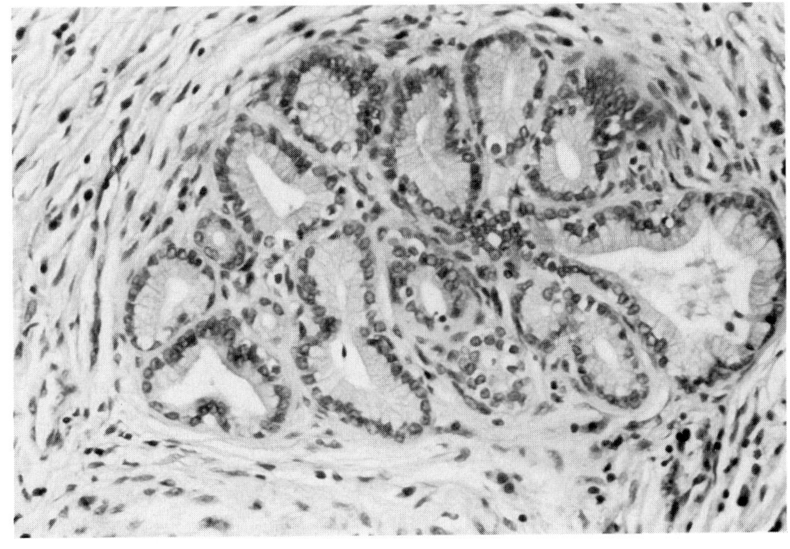

Figure 14–3. Mucus-secreting glands found surrounding the main bile ducts.

points can be most useful in interpreting the small and often distorted biopsies obtained from fibrous strictures of the bile ducts.

Within the ampulla and distal common bile duct, the lining epithelium is thrown into a series of slender folds, with delicate fibrovascular cores (Fig. 14–4). The epithelium itself is similar to that found elsewhere in the bile duct and major pancreatic ducts. However, in addition, the surface mucosa contains scattered mucus-secreting goblet cells. A large number of mucus-secreting glands surround the terminal portions of the bile duct, the pancreatic duct, and the ampulla. These are structurally similar to the mucus glands of the more proximal portions of the bile duct but are larger and contain more ductules. In addition, small accessory pancreatic ducts, which drain acini in the head of the pancreas, also empty into the ampulla.

ARTERY AND NERVE SUPPLY, AND VENOUS LYMPHATIC DRAINAGE

A variety of arterial branches supply the bile duct throughout its length. These include the common hepatic arteries; the right and left hepatic arteries; and the retroduodenal, cystic, gastroduodenal, and retroportal arteries.[11] The location of these vessels, in relation to the duct, are subject to considerable individual variation. In most instances, however, the right hepatic artery is behind (i.e., dorsal to) the common hepatic and right hepatic ducts. The left hepatic artery lies to the left of the extrahepatic ducts.

The portal and hepatic veins are usually located dorsal to the bile duct system. Veins, draining the proximal portions of the extrahepatic bile ducts, may drain directly into the liver. The veins from the distal ducts drain into the hepatic and portal veins. Lymphatic channels generally follow the veins. Nodes are present alongside the duct, in the porta hepatis, and along the superior border of the pancreas.

The bile ducts receive both sympathetic and parasympathetic nerves. Sympathetic fibers derive from the celiac ganglia, whereas the parasympathetic fibers are branches of the vagus.

DEVELOPMENTAL ABNORMALITIES

Atresia

The most important bile duct abnormality is extrahepatic biliary atresia, in which the normal ducts are partly or completely destroyed by a sclerosing inflammatory process.[12] Histologic findings in the most severe cases include dense porta hepatis fibrous tissue, containing a few inflammatory cells. In intermediate cases, bile ducts may be identified, either as fibrous cords or with incomplete small lumina, lined by cuboidal or stratified squamous epithelium. The mildest affected cases involve narrowed, residual bile ducts measuring <150 μm in diameter. These cases have been termed hypoplasia[13,14] and may represent an early stage of atresia.

Histologic changes within the liver are variable. In the early pretreatment phase, the classi-

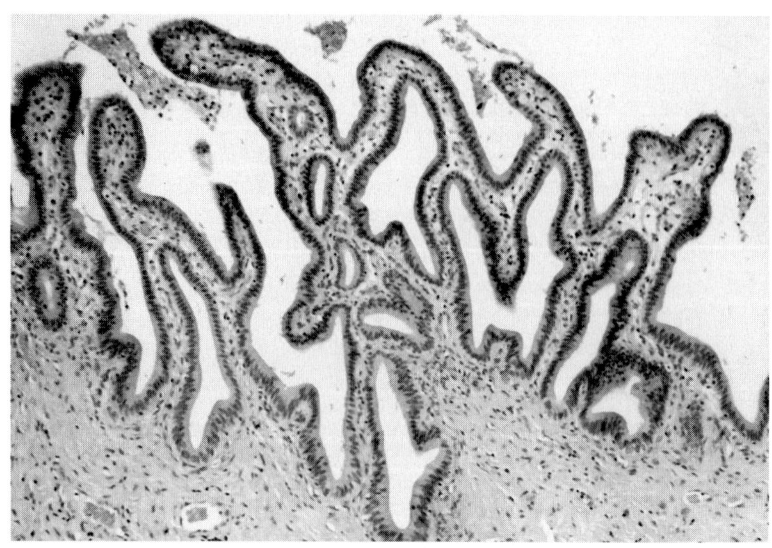

Figure 14–4. Mucosal folds in the ampulla of Vater.

cal changes of extrahepatic obstruction may be identified (portal edema and bile ductular proliferation), along with giant cell transformation of hepatocytes. If no treatment is carried out, biliary cirrhosis develops, usually within the first year of life. Treatment consists of some form of portoenterostomy (Kasai operation) and, in the majority of cases, is initially successful in relieving obstructive jaundice. Ultimately, however, jaundice recurs after ongoing damage to intrahepatic ducts and the development of cirrhosis. At this stage, liver transplantation offers the only hope for a cure. The reasons for this progressive intrahepatic duct damage are controversial. Some authors consider it to be a consequence of recurrent ascending cholangitis, whereas others believe that the primary disease is manifested at both extra- and intrahepatic locations. Recent work suggests that the intrahepatic duct obliteration is a consequence of duct reobstruction occurring at the portoenterostomy site, as wound healing and scarring takes place.[15]

Patients with bile duct atresia present as neonates with a profound obstructive jaundice. The incidence is about 1 in 8,000 to 12,000 live births, with girls slightly more commonly affected than boys.[16] In the United States, between 400 and 600 new diagnoses are made each year.[17] Atresia occurs in two clinical forms, an embryonic (or fetal) form and a perinatal form. The perinatal form is the most common and accounts for approximately 65% of cases. The underlying cause of both forms is an obliterative cholangiopathy. A wide variety of possible causes have been considered, including exposure to intrauterine toxins, occult viral infection, and immunologic and vascular disorders. At present, it is considered that the key abnormality is a failure of normal remodeling of bile ducts at the hepatic hilum, with persistence of fetal bile ducts, poorly supported by mesenchymal tissues.[16] This abnormality becomes manifest in the perinatal period as bile flow increases, leading to bile leakage, with the creation of an intense inflammatory reaction. The underlying abnormality(ies) causing failure of remodeling is unknown, but it is likely that a variety of factors are responsible.[16]

In the majority of cases, biliary atresia is an isolated abnormality. However, in 10% to 25% of patients, there may be associated abnormalities. These include ventricular septal defect; portal vein or vena cava malformation; intestinal malrotation; solitary kidney; polysplenia; or asplenia and trisomies 17, 18, or 21.[18]

Biliary atresia has to be distinguished from the much rarer condition of agenesis of extrahepatic bile ducts.[19] Either the duct is completely absent or the proximal portion is missing. Jaundice in patients with biliary agenesis usually develops much earlier than it does with atresia. Unlike atresia, individuals with biliary agenesis do not have a fibrotic mass in the porta hepatis.

Strictures, Duplications, and Abnormal Anatomy

These abnormalities are all exceedingly rare. Congenital stricture formation has been described in a patient in whom it was discovered incidentally and was not accompanied by obstructive jaundice.[20] Duplications of the bile duct may be complete[21] or partial[22] and there may or may not be anastomoses between the duplicated ducts. Some so-called duplications may actually represent the presence of accessory ducts, arising from the left or right hepatic ducts and emptying separately into the duodenum.[21]

Anomalous course and insertion of the bile duct may have many variations. The duct may occasionally empty into the stomach, either at the pylorus or at a prepyloric location,[23] or, in cases of atresia of the second part of the duodenum, the bile duct may pass anterior to the duodenum.[24]

Choledochal Cysts

A variety of bile duct cysts (choledochal cysts) have been described. These are classified according to their shape and location[25] and are illustrated diagrammatically in Fig. 14–5. Type I is a fusiform dilation of the common bile duct. Type II is a supraduodenal diverticulum of the common bile duct with a narrow neck, communicating with a normal biliary tree. Type III is an isolated intraduodenal diverticulum. Type IV has two subvariants: In type A, there are multiple fusiform dilations of extra- and intrahepatic bile ducts; type B is similar but has only an extrahepatic component. In Type V, there are multiple dilated intrahepatic bile ducts. This form is also referred to as Caroli's syndrome.[26,27] These cysts may be combined with other developmental abnormalities, such as absence, duplication, or hypoplasia of the gallbladder. There is also an association with extra-

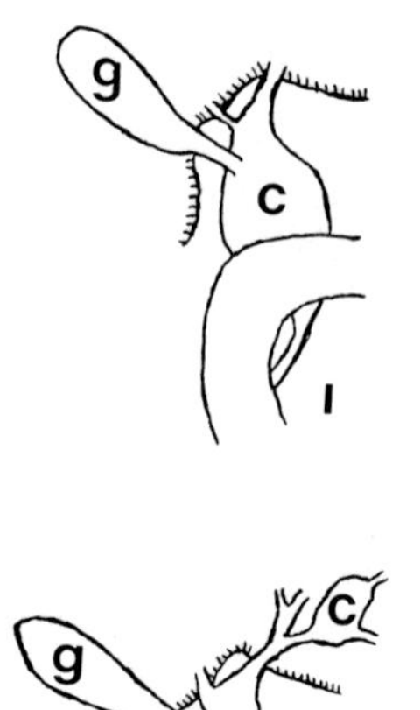

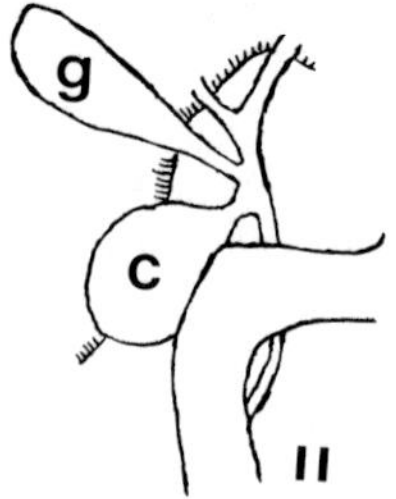

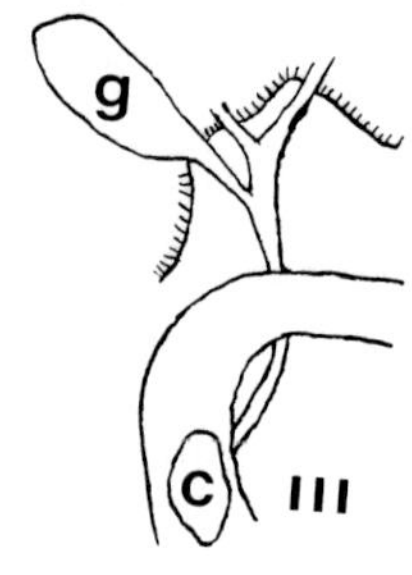

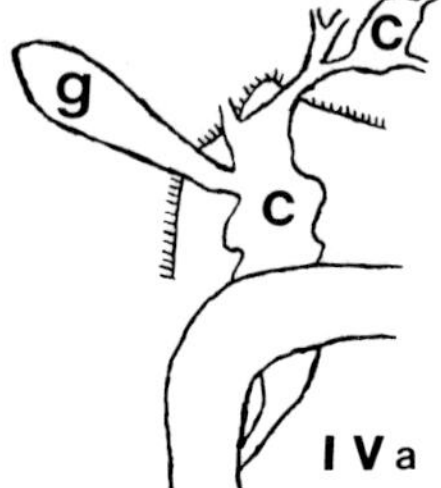

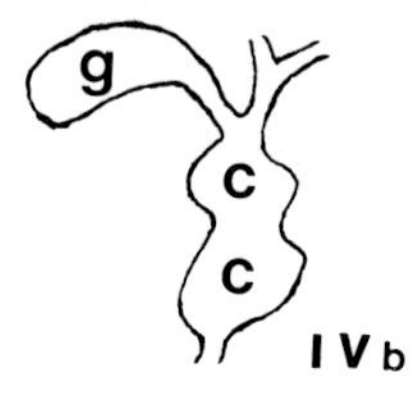

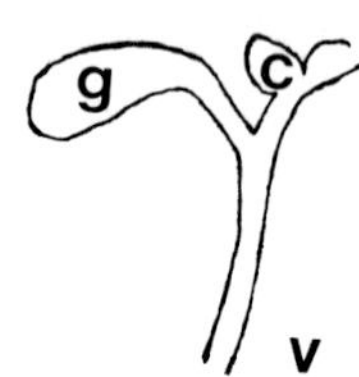

Figure 14–5. Various types of choledochal cyst. g, gallbladder; c, cyst. (From Weedon D: Pathology of the Gallbladder. New York: Masson Publishing, 1984, pp 266–269.)

hepatic cystic disease, especially in the kidney.[28] A percentage of patients with cysts, especially type V cysts, may also develop congenital hepatic fibrosis.[29] The complex interrelationships of these anomalies and the genetic abnormalities underlying them are, at present, ill understood.

Choledochal cysts are more common in females and in the United States occur in 1 in 13,000 live births.[30] For unexplained reasons, they seem particularly common in Japan.[31] Surprisingly, not all cysts are evident in the neonatal period, although most become manifest in the first decade of life. Abdominal pain and jaundice are the most common symptoms and a mass may be felt on examination.[32]

By gross examination, most cysts are roughly spherical in shape. They vary considerably in size and may contain between 30 and 5,000 mL of bile.[33] The wall varies in thickness from 2 to 10 mm. Histologically, the cysts are lined by the usual columnar epithelium and the wall is composed of dense fibrous tissue, with variable amounts of smooth muscle and a chronic inflammatory infiltrate. The epithelium may show hyperplasia, metaplasia, and even dysplasia.

Complications of choledochal cysts are common. Stones are present in up to 30% of patients.[32,34] Spontaneous perforation,[35] cholangitis,[36] and obstructive jaundice[37] have also been described. Carcinoma of the bile duct may complicate biliary cysts in up to 30% of patients,[38] and the risk of carcinoma developing is up to 20 times that of the general population, increasing gradually with age.[39] About one half of the carcinomas arise within the cysts themselves,[40,41] with the remainder occurring in either the gallbladder[42,43] or the noncystic bile ducts.[44] As would be expected, most of these tumors are well-differentiated adenocarcinomas. Benign tumors, such as biliary papillomatosis, have also been recognized.[45]

The origin of choledochal cysts is a matter of some debate. It seems likely that a minority of cysts are truly congenital in origin and arise as a consequence of disordered proliferation of hepatic bud cells during the phase of embryogenesis, when the buds are solid structures.[46] Many more cysts arise as a consequence of reflux of pancreatic juice into the biliary tree. This mechanism may occur in individuals with a normal biliary tract anatomy but is particularly frequent in people with anomalous pancreaticobiliary duct junctions.[47]

REFERENCES

1. Dowdy GS Jr, Waldron GW, Brown WG: Surgical anatomy of the pancreaticobiliary system. Arch Surg 84:229–246, 1962.
2. Berci G: Biliary ductal anatomy and anomalies. The role of intraoperative cholangiography during laparoscopic cholecystectomy. Surg Clin North Am 72:1069–1075, 1992.
3. DiMagno EP, Shorter RG, Taylor WF, et al.: Relationships between pancreaticobiliary ductal anatomy and

pancreatic ductal and parenchymal histology. Cancer 49:361–368, 1982.

4. Suda K, Matsumoto Y, Miyano T: An extended common channel in patients with biliary tract carcinoma and congenital biliary dilatation. Surg Pathol 1:65–69, 1988.
5. Kimura K, Ohto M, Saisho H, et al.: Association of gallbladder carcinoma and anomalous pancreatobiliary duct union. Gastroenterology 89:1258–1265, 1985.
6. Newman HF, Weinberg SB, Newman EB, et al.: The papilla of Vater and distal portions of the common bile duct and duct of Wirsung. Surg Gynecol Obstet 106:687–694, 1958.
7. Hand BH: Anatomy and function of the extrahepatic biliary system. Clin Gastroenterol 2:3–29, 1973.
8. Brown JO, Echenberg RJ: Mucosal reduplications associated with the ampullary portion of the major duodenal papilla in humans. Anat Rec 150:293–302, 1964.
9. Goff JS: The human sphincter of Oddi. Physiology and pathophysiology. Arch Intern Med 148:2673–2677, 1988.
10. Frierson HF, Jr: Gall bladder and extrahepatic biliary system. *In* Sternberg SS (ed): Histology for Pathologists, 2nd ed. Philadelphia: Lippincott-Raven, 1997, pp 593–611.
11. Northover JM, Terblanche J: A new look at the arterial supply of the bile duct in man and its surgical implications. Br J Surg 66:379–384, 1979.
12. Mieli-Vergani G, Howard ER, Mowat AP: Liver disease in infancy: A 20 year perspective. Gut(suppl) S123–S128, 1991.
13. Witzleben CL: Extrahepatic biliary atresia: Concepts of cause, diagnosis and management. Perspect Pediatr Pathol 5:41–62, 1979.
14. Psacharopoulos HT, Howard ER, Portman B, et al.: Extrahepatic biliary atresia. Preoperative assessment and surgical results in 47 consecutive cases. Arch Dis Child 55:851–856, 1980.
15. Nietgen GW, Vacanti JP, Pérez-Atayde AR: Intrahepatic bile duct loss in biliary atresia despite portoenterostomy: A consequence of ongoing obstruction? Gastroenterology 102:2126–2133, 1992.
16. Balistreri WF, Grand R, Hoofnagle JH, et al.: Biliary atresia: Current concepts and research directions. Summary of a symposium. Hepatology 23:1682–1692, 1996.
17. Lefkowitch JH: Biliary atresia. Mayo Clin Proc 73:90–95, 1998.
18. Carmi R, Magee CA, Neil CA, et al.: Extrahepatic biliary atresia and associated anomalies: Etiologic heterogeneity suggested by distinctive patterns of associations. Am J Med Genet 45:683–693, 1993.
19. Schwartz MZ, Hall RJ, Reubner B, et al.: Agenesis of the extrahepatic bile ducts: Report of five cases. J Pediatr Surg 25:805–807, 1990.
20. Chapoy PR, Kendall RS, Foukalsrud E, et al.: Congenital stricture of the common hepatic duct: An unusual case without jaundice. Gastroenterology 80:380–383, 1981.
21. Kodama T, Iseki J, Murata N, et al.: Duplication of common bile duct—A case report. Jpn J Surg 10:67–71, 1980.
22. Loria LE, Yamamoto K, Eto T, et al.: A case of a rare anomaly of the common bile duct associated with an abnormal arrangement of the pancreaticobiliary ductal union. Jpn J Surg 18:718–724, 1988.
23. Sites EG, Lauridsen J: Anomalous opening of the common bile duct into the stomach. Report of a case. J Int Coll Surg 14:420–424, 1950.
24. Patti G, Marrocco G, Mazzoni G, et al.: Esophageal and duodenal atresia with preduodenal common bile duct and portal vein in a new born. J Pediatr Surg 20:167–168, 1985.
25. Todani T, Watanabe Y, Narusue M, et al.: Congenital bile duct cysts: Classification, operative procedures and review of thirty-seven cases, including cancer arising from choledochal cyst. Am J Surg 134:263–269, 1977.
26. Caroli J: Diseases of the intrahepatic biliary tree. Clin Gastroenterol 2:147–161, 1973.
27. Thung SN, Gerber MA: Caroli's disease. A rarely recognised entity. Arch Pathol Lab Med 103:650–652, 1979.
28. Gagnadoux MF, Habib R, Levy M, et al.: Cystic renal diseases in children. Adv Nephrol 18:33–57, 1989.
29. Nakanuma Y, Terada T, Ohta G, et al.: Caroli's disease in congenital hepatic fibrosis and infantile polycystic disease. Liver 2:346–354, 1982.
30. Ryckman FC, Noseworthy J: Neonatal cholestatic conditions requiring surgical reconstruction. Semin Liver Dis 7:134–154, 1987.
31. Iwata F, Uchida A, Miyaki T, et al.: Familial occurrence of congenital bile duct cysts. J Gastroenterol Hepatol 13:316–319, 1998.
32. Flanigan DP: Biliary cysts. Ann Surg 182:635–643, 1975.
33. Dickinson EH, Spencer FC: Choledochal cyst. Report of a case with unusual features. J Pediatr 41:462–466, 1952.
34. Tajiri H: Choledochocele-containing stones. Am J Gastroenterol 91:1046–1048, 1996.
35. Ando K, Miyano T, Kohno S, et al.: Spontaneous perforation of choledochal cyst: A study of 13 cases. Eur J Pediatr Surg 8:23–25, 1998.
36. Katyal D, Lees GM: Choledochal cysts: A retrospective review of 28 patients and a review of the literature. Can J Surg 35:584–588, 1992.
37. Patel S, Sterkin L, Donahue PE, et al.: Congenital cyst of common bile duct: An unusual cause of obstructive jaundice. Surgery 109:333–335, 1991.
38. Flanigan DP: Biliary carcinoma associated with biliary cysts. Cancer 40:880–883, 1977.
39. Voyles CR, Smadja C, Shands C, et al.: Carcinoma in choledochal cysts. Age-related incidence. Arch Surg 118:986–988, 1983.
40. Tajiri K, Takenawa A, Yamaoka K, et al.: Choledochal cyst with adenocarcinoma in the cystically dilated intrahepatic duct. Abdom Imag 22:190–193, 1997.
41. Holzinger F, Baer HU, Schilling M, et al.: Congenital bile duct cyst: A premalignant lesion of the biliary tract associated with adenocarcinoma: A case report. Z Gastroenterol 34:382–385, 1996.
42. Chao TC, Jan YY, Chen MF: Primary carcinoma of the gallbladder associated with anomalous pancreatobiliary duct junction. J Clin Gastroenterol 21:306–308, 1995.
43. Tonfecq Khan TF, Sherazi ZA, Tan YY: Gallbladder tumor, choledochal cyst and anomalous pancreaticobiliary junction. HPB Surgery 8:185–186, 1995.
44. Bloustein PA: Association of carcinoma with congenital cystic conditions of the liver and bile ducts. Am J Gastroenterol 67:40–46, 1977.
45. Ohita H, Yamaguchi Y, Yamakawa O, et al.: Biliary papillomatosis with point mutation of k-*ras* gene arising in congenital choledochal cyst. Gastroenterology 105:1209–1212, 1993.
46. Fonkalsrud EW: Choledochal cysts. Surg Clin North Am 53:1275–1281, 1973.
47. O'Neill JA Jr: Choledochal cyst. Curr Probl Surg 29:361–410, 1992.

Chapter

15

ACQUIRED NONNEOPLASTIC BILE DUCT DISEASES

Inflammatory disease of the common bile duct and hepatic ducts is termed *cholangitis.* This designation is also applied to inflammation affecting the intrahepatic bile ducts and bile ductules. Broadly speaking, intrahepatic ducts demonstrate a range of disease and morphologic abnormalities similar to those encountered in the larger extrahepatic ducts. Various causes of inflammation have been identified with a variety of clinical associations (Table 15–1). There is, however, overlapping terminology by which a single disease may be labeled according to either its origins or its morphologic appearances. Chronic cholangitis is frequently associated with stricture formation and may be labeled sclerosing cholangitis. Secondary sclerosing cholangitis, therefore, forms a heterogeneous group of conditions with a variety of causes and must be distinguished from primary sclerosing cholangitis, a disease in which the inflammation and scarring is considered to be autoimmune in origin.

BILE DUCT INJURY

Most bile duct injuries (Table 15–2) are not primarily inflammatory in origin. Nevertheless, the injury is frequently persistent and exerts its clinical effect by causing a chronic inflammatory response. This secondary inflammation may occur with or without stricture formation.

The vast majority of bile duct injuries are iatrogenic and occur at the time of cholecystectomy.[1] As a general rule, laparascopic surgery is approximately twice as likely to result in injury as open cholecystectomy.[2] The magnitude of the risk of complication in laparascopic cholecystectomy is approximately 1%, although this figure includes bile duct injuries, major bile leaks, and injuries to bowel or vascular structures.[2]

One common problem in cholecystectomy surgery occurs after a failure to recognize variants of the normal cystic duct–bile duct architecture (see Chapter 14). In most instances, the cystic duct unites with the hepatic duct at a right angle. However, in approximately 15% of normal individuals, the cystic duct runs for a short distance alongside the hepatic duct in the same fibrous sheath before anastomosing with it. If this anatomic variant is not recognized, it may result in ligation and transection of both ducts. This will inevitably result in obstructive jaundice. Subsequent surgical repair of the defect is always difficult and is frequently complicated by stricture formation with ascending cholangitis.

Nonsurgical trauma to the extrahepatic bile ducts is rare. Both penetrating and nonpenetrating (blunt) injuries may be responsible.[3,4] These may be extensive and life-threatening and may be accompanied by large bile leaks. In a majority of patients, there is associated liver injury and the bile duct damage may consist of lacerations, transections, and avulsions.[3]

Gallstones entering the common bile duct may impact at its lower end and cause obstructive jaundice. If not removed, these stones may eventually erode into the wall of the ampulla of Vater. Gallstones impacted in the neck of the gallbladder may, by virtue of their size, im-

Table 15–1. Primary Inflammatory Conditions of the Extrahepatic Bile Ducts

Bacterial
Ascending (obstructive) cholangitis
Fungal
Candidiasis
Cryptococcosis
Protozoal
Cryptosporidiosis
Microsporidiosis
Viral
Cytomegalovirus
Helminthic
Clonorchiasis
Fascioliasis
Ascariasis
Schistosomiasis
Oriental cholangiohepatitis
Primary sclerosing cholangitis
Cystic fibrosis

pinge on the common hepatic duct at the cystic duct–hepatic duct junction and also cause obstructive jaundice. Persistence of impaction may lead to erosion of the stone through the wall of the gallbladder, with damage to the wall of the common bile duct. A cholecystocholedochal fistula may become established. Eventually, the stone may erode the wall of the duodenum, producing a cholecystoduodenal fistula. This complex of impacted and eroding gallstones at the gallbladder neck that produces jaundice has been termed *Mirizzi syndrome.*[5–9] Although it represents only approximately 1% to 2% of acquired biliary tract abnormalities, in patients undergoing cholecystectomy, it is important for surgeons to recognize Mirizzi syndrome and treat appropriately.[9] Various groups of surgeons have devised classification schemes of Mirizzi syndrome based on the extent of the erosion and disordered anatomy.[5,8,9] The details of these schemes are not particularly relevant to pathologists, although it is important to distinguish an impacted but nonerosive stone (Mirizzi syndrome type I) from a stone associated with fistula formation (Mirizzi syndrome type II).[9]

The clinical presentation of Mirizzi syndrome invariably includes upper abdominal pain and obstructive jaundice. Particularly when a fistula is present, secondary ascending cholangitis may develop.[10] At surgery, the gallbladder is usually small and contracted. There are no known factors predisposing patients with gallstones to Mirizzi syndrome.

Rarer examples of acquired structural damage to the extrahepatic biliary tree have been described in a case of necrosis secondary to chemoradiotherapy[11] and in a case of acute pancreatitis with subsequent pseudocyst formation, leading to a fistula between the pseudocyst and the common bile duct.[12]

ASCENDING CHOLANGITIS

Ascending cholangitis (bacterial cholangitis) may occur following partial or complete obstruction of the common bile duct. In 80% to 90% of instances, obstruction is the sequel of choledocholithiasis. A smaller number of cases become obstructed after stent placement, neoplastic obstruction, or fibrous stricture formation. Rarer causes of obstruction include parasitic diseases, congenital anomalies, primary sclerosing cholangitis, and the protein bile plug syndrome. Various normal defense systems exist that prevent bacteria present within the duodenum from entering the biliary system.[13] Spread from the portal vein via the liver is prevented by the presence of Kupffer cells and tight junctions between hepatocytes. Spread via the biliary system is primarily prevented by the sphincter of Oddi, which forms an important mechanical barrier to reflux of duodenal contents. The sphincter also maintains the intraductal bile at a higher pressure than the duodenal lumen contents. In addition, the continuous flushing action of bile, together with the bacteriostatic effects of bile salts, keeps the biliary tract sterile under normal conditions. An additional important bacteriocidal mechanism is the presence of secretory immunoglobulin A, which is found in mucus secreted by the biliary epithelium. This functions as an antiadherence factor preventing bacterial colonization. As might be anticipated, cholangitis occurs more frequently where the obstruction is intermittent and incomplete than it does with complete obstruction. Infection is therefore most common in individuals with a stricture or biliary stent and least common in persons with a malignancy.[14]

Table 15–2. Causes of Bile Duct Injury

Iatrogenic (surgical)
Nonsurgical trauma
Gallstones, Mirizzi syndrome
Radiotherapy and chemotherapy
Pancreatitis
Endoscopic retrograde cholangiopancreatography

The clinical presentation of ascending cholangitis is variable. Seventy percent of patients have Charcot's triad: pain, jaundice, and fever. If these are not all present, the condition may be difficult to diagnose.[14,15] Fever is present in 95% of patients, pain in 90%, and jaundice in 80%.[15] Commonly, the febrile illness consists of transient self-limited chills, with a fever spike. However, in a smaller number of patients, there is onset of septicemia and shock. This severe form of the disease may be immediately fatal or may result in the development of intrahepatic abscesses.

Blood cultures, taken during the fever spike, are usually positive. The organisms most commonly recovered include *Escherichia coli, Klebsiella, Pseudomonas, Proteus,* and enterococci.[14,15] Infection with *E. coli* may be accompanied by infection with anaerobic organisms in about 15% of patients. These organisms include *Bacterioides fragilis* and *Clostridium perfringens.*[17]

In patients with ascending cholangitis, biopsy material from the extrahepatic biliary tree is rarely available for study. Liver biopsies, however, are occasionally obtained and may demonstrate portal edema with infiltration by neutrophils (Fig. 15–1). Neutrophils are encountered in the periductal tissues, in the ductal epithelium, and within the bile duct lumen. In severe infections, there is damage to the epithelial cells and microabscesses may form. In examples of recurrent cholangitis, there may be periportal fibrosis and concentric periductal fibrosis. It is most important to realize that simply finding neutrophils in and around bile ductules does not mean that the patient has an ascending infection. A similar statement is also true when neutrophils are encountered in biopsies of extrahepatic ducts. Histologic evidence of acute inflammation may be encountered in a wide variety of noninfectious conditions, including simple extrahepatic bile duct destruction and in relation to strictures. In these circumstances, inflammation is probably secondary to the irritative effects of inspissated bile. Some clinicians tend to equate a diagnosis of acute cholangitis with the presence of infection. To avoid this misinterpretation, the pathologist should indicate that acute cholangitis may be infectious or noninfectious and that culture of tissues or bile is required to establish an infectious component of the disease.

FUNGAL INFECTIONS

Fungal infections of the bile ducts may occur in individuals with[18] and without[19–21] preexistent biliary abnormalities and in instances in which there is no obvious predisposing cause. Manipulation of the bile ducts occurring during endoscopic retrograde cholangiopancreatography (ERCP) may give rise to systemic fungal infections, particularly candidiasis.[22] This may occur in patients without an obvious preexistent biliary fungal infection. Fungal infection may also be confined to the biliary tract. Organisms identified have included *Candida*[19–22] and *Cryptococcus neoformans.*[18] Some patients present with obstructive jaundice and examination of the bile

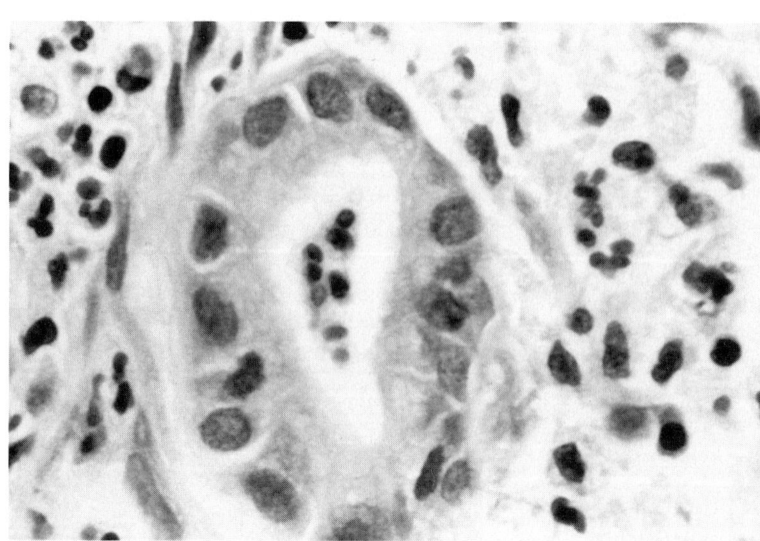

Figure 15–1. Liver biopsy from a patient with ascending cholangitis. The duct lumen is full of pus.

ducts reveals the presence of fungus balls, which presumably are the cause of the obstruction.[20,21] In other patients, the fungal infection occurs in association with a biliary stricture.[18,19] Occasionally, it is evident that the obstruction and stricture formation antedated the presence of fungal infection,[18] but in other instances, it seems possible that fungal infection was primary and actually caused a fibrous stricture.[19]

Fungal infection of the biliary tract may also occur as part of a generalized fungemia. Most of these patients are immunosuppressed. Death occurs as a consequence of a severe septic illness and the biliary involvement is not usually clinically significant.

PROTOZOAL AND VIRAL INFECTIONS

Protozoal and viral infections of the bile ducts often occur together, although they can also be encountered as separate infections. Many patients are immunosuppressed either because of acquired immunodeficiency syndrome (AIDS)[23–26] or as a result of transplant rejection therapy.[27] AIDS-associated cholangiopathy may be subdivided into two groups, depending on the type of cholangiographic abnormality present. All such patients have gradual and regular stenosis of the distal common bile duct, with dilation of intrahepatic bile ducts. However, in approximately 75% of patients, there is an associated diffuse irregularity in the caliber of intrahepatic ducts. This radiologic abnormality resembles idiopathic sclerosing cholangitis. In the remaining 25% of individuals, stenosis and dilation are not accompanied by intrahepatic duct irregularity.[23]

Organisms thought to be responsible for AIDS cholangiopathy include cytomegalovirus (CMV),[23] *Cryptosporidium* species,[23,24] and the *Microsporida* species *Enterocytozoon bieneusi*[25] or *Encephalitozoon* (*Septata*) *intestinalis*.[26] All these organisms are regarded as potential causes of fibrous bile duct strictures. Patients with AIDS cholangiopathy typically present with upper abdominal pain, developing in association with elevations of alkaline phosphatase, bilirubin, aspartate transaminase, and alanine aminotransferase. Patients do not usually have clinical jaundice at the time of presentation, although a low-grade fever may be encountered.[26] Initial treatment is by sphincterotomy to correct the bile duct stenosis and to relieve the obstruction.

Other biliary tract diseases encountered in patients with AIDS include primary lymphoma[28,29] and bacillary angiomatosis.[30]

HELMINTHIC INFECTIONS

Helminthic infections of the bile ducts may be caused by liver flukes, particularly *Clonorchis* (*Opisthorchis*) *sinensis, Opisthorchis viverrini, Opisthorchus felineus,* and *Fasciola hepatica.* Occasionally, roundworms, such as *Ascaris lumbricoides,* may migrate from the duodenum into the bile ducts and cause obstructive jaundice.

Clonorchiasis is endemic in southeast Asia, including southern China, Taiwan, Japan, Korea, Hong Kong, and Vietnam, where it has been estimated to infect 19 million people. *O. viverrini* is endemic in Thailand, Laos, and Cambodia and may infect as many as 7 million people. *O. felineus* is endemic in Russia, eastern Europe, Turkey, and western Siberia. Worldwide, it may infect several million individuals.[31] All these organisms have virtually identical life cycles and produce similar clinical features. There are only minor morphologic differences between species, so all are discussed together here. The parasites are acquired by eating raw or undercooked fish or crawfish. Freshwater fish of the carp species are primarily responsible for spread of the disease. Snails ingest eggs of the parasite, which are present in the water of ponds contaminated by human or animal feces. The eggs hatch within the snails and form cercariae, which escape from the host, swim in water, and penetrate the skin of susceptible fish, forming encysted metacercariae. When humans ingest metacercariae, they pass to the duodenum, excyst, and migrate up the bile ducts. Adult worms are mature in 3 to 4 weeks, undergo a sexual cycle, and produce eggs, which are ultimately shed in the feces. Cats, dogs, and pigs may also be infected.[31]

The clinical signs and symptoms of clonorchiasis vary, depending on the number of flukes present. Small numbers are asymptomatic. Moderate numbers may cause fatigue, anorexia, diarrhea, and right upper quadrant pain or discomfort. Infested children may have growth retardation. Heavy fluke burdens may result in bile duct obstruction, ascending cholangitis, and jaundice. Blood eosinophilia is not a constant feature of infection.

Eggs may be detected by examination of the feces. They are ovoid, measuring on average 29 by 16 μm, and are operculated with prominent shoulders (Fig. 15–2). Adult worms may be recovered from the bile duct at the time of surgery or at autopsy. These measure on average 10 to 25 mm in length and 3 to 5 mm in width. They are dark brown or black in color (Fig. 15–3). When individual flukes are transilluminated, details of their internal structure may be visible with low-power dissecting microscope examination[31] (Fig. 15–4).

In mild infestations, the liver at autopsy may appear unremarkable. In heavy infestations, the intrahepatic bile ducts are dilated. The ducts themselves appear prominent and thick walled. Adult worms are usually easily identified and may be motile, if the autopsy examination is performed soon after death. In uncomplicated infestations, the gallbladder and extrahepatic ducts are usually unremarkable. Microscopic examination of the bile duct system shows cross-sections of flukes (Fig. 15–5). The biliary epithelium demonstrates progressive abnormalities that may be grouped into four stages: desquamation of epithelial cells, hyperplasia of surviving cells, periductal proliferation of small glands (Fig. 15–6), and periductal fibrosis.[32,33] Goblet cell metaplasia may also been seen.[31]

Complications of clonorchis infection include Oriental cholangiohepatitis (discussed in the next section) and cholangiocarcinoma.[34–36] Cholangiocarcinoma may occur particularly in the larger intrahepatic ducts and extrahepatic ducts at the hilum of the liver. The frequency of this complication is not known. Histologically, the neoplasm is a mucus-secreting adeno-

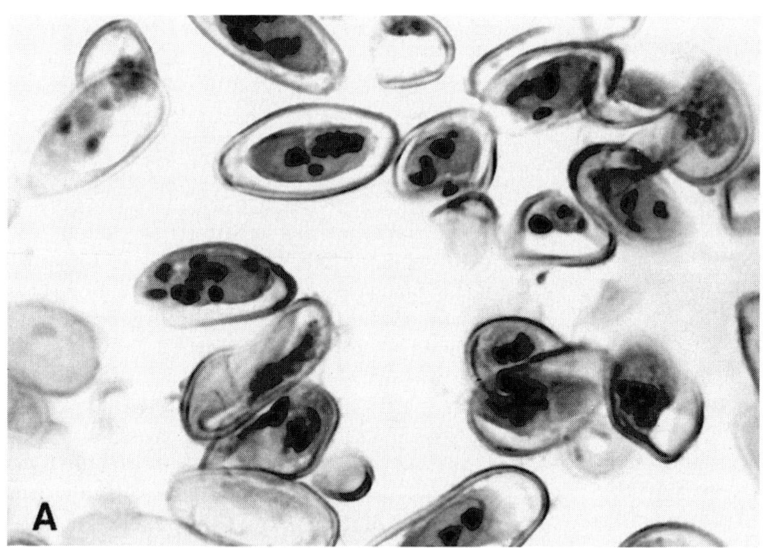

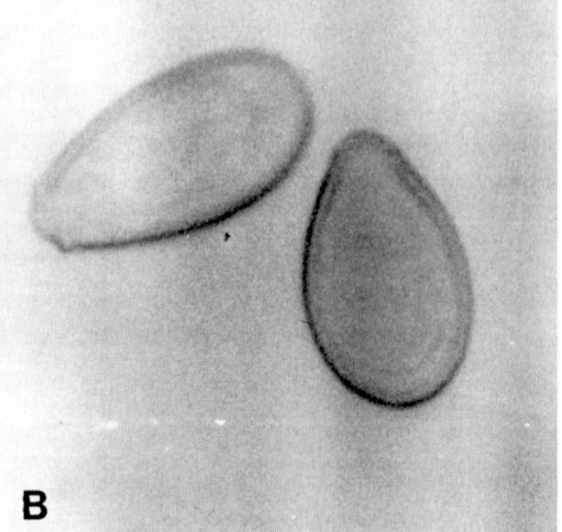

Figure 15–2. Eggs of *Clonorchis sinensis* as they appear in tissue sections (*A*) and stool samples (*B*).

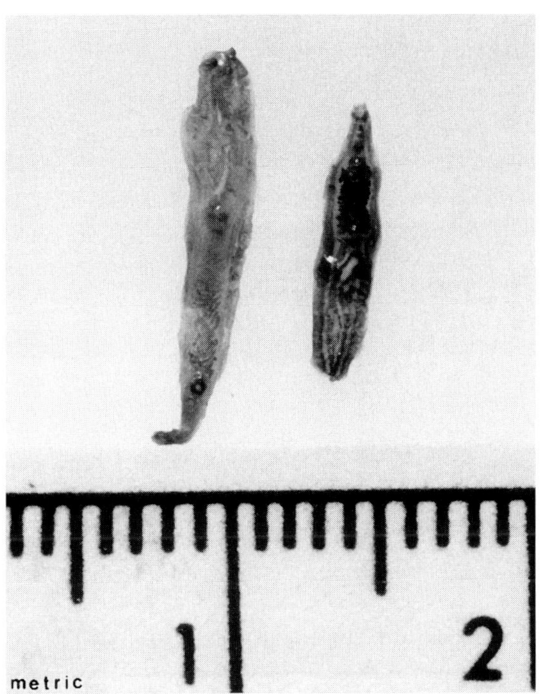

Figure 15–3. Adult *Clonorchis* extracted from the main bile duct.

carcinoma, frequently multifocal in distribution. Intraductal neoplasms have also been described in individuals with long-standing *Clonorchis* infections.[37,38] These tumors morphologically resemble diffuse biliary papillary adenomatosis but may also show areas of intraductal carcinoma.

Fascioliasis is common in farm animals, particularly cattle and sheep, but only rarely affects humans. Most infections are acquired from eating watercress grown in water contaminated by feces and containing certain species of snail. Metacercariae attached to water plants are ingested, pass to the duodenum, excyst, and penetrate the bowel wall. From within the peritoneal cavity, they penetrate the capsule of the liver and pass into the bile ductular system, where they mature into adults. Light infections are asymptomatic. Moderate or heavy infections result in an acute illness, characterized by fever, hepatomegaly, and blood eosinophilia, as the immature flukes pass through the liver.[39] The acute phase may last up to 11 weeks, by which time the flukes become established within the bile ducts, resulting in a chronic illness characterized by dyspepsia, diarrhea, jaundice, cholecystitis, and biliary colic.[39]

As the migrating flukes pass through the liver, they cause tissue damage, characterized by coagulative necrosis, hemorrhage, and abscess formation. In the chronic stage of the disease, flukes present within the bile ducts cause chronic inflammation and periductal fibrosis. The epithelium becomes hyperplastic, with proliferation of periductal glandular elements similar to the changes encountered in clonorchiasis. Occasionally, the flukes cause obstruction, with the possible occurrence of secondary bacterial infection and increased periductal fibrosis. No association with cholangiocarcinoma has been described.

Ascariasis is a nemotodal infection that is common in tropical countries but rare in North America and Europe. About 25% of the world's population is infected. Adult worms, which may measure up to 350 mm in length and between 3 to 6 mm in diameter, live in the duodenum and upper small bowel, where they may be present in sufficient numbers to cause intestinal obstruction. More serious, however, is the ectopic migration of worms, especially into the pancreatic duct and common bile ducts. Unmated female worms are mainly responsible and migration occurs when they become

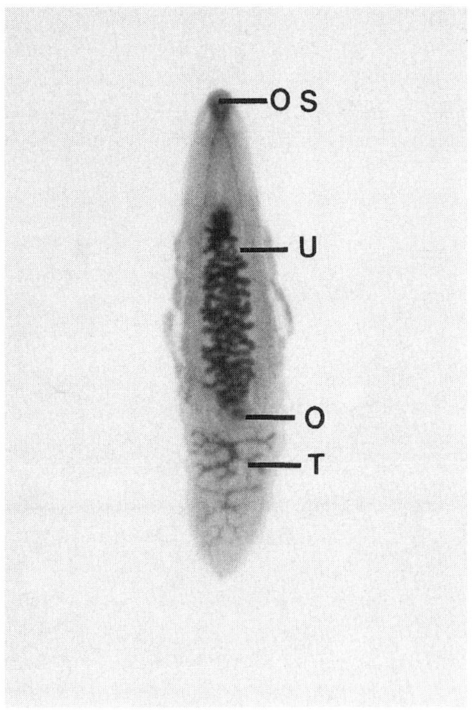

Figure 15–4. Adult *Clonorchis sinensis.* Note the oral sucker (OS), uterus (U), ovaries (O), and testes (T).

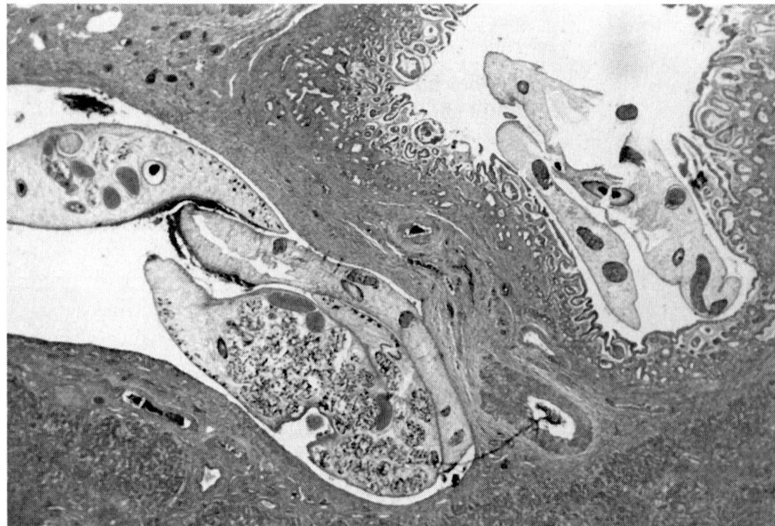

Figure 15–5. Flukes within intrahepatic bile ducts.

stressed by an unusually spicy diet or by certain antihelminthic drugs. When worms enter the bile duct, there may be a sudden onset of severe right upper quadrant pain radiating through to the back region. This may last for up to 20 minutes. Worms entering the pancreatic duct may cause a hemorrhagic pancreatitis. In histologic cross-section, *Ascaris* have the following features: an outer cuticle, which is supported by a thin hypodermis; a layer of subcuticular somatic muscle; lateral cords representing extensions of the hypodermis; and a central intestine. Ovaries, oviducts, and uteri are present in the posterior two thirds of the female body.

Schistosomiasis, particularly due to *Schistosoma mansoni* and *S. japonicum,* commonly involves both intra- and extrahepatic bile ductules. Adult worms, living in small tributaries of the portal vein, lay eggs that normally pass through the walls of the venules and into the bowel lumen. Eggs may, however, get carried into the main portal vein and become lodged in branches at the liver hilum, where they penetrate the vein wall. As eggs become trapped in the perivenular connective tissues, they may become nonviable. Dead eggs set up a vigorous inflammatory reaction and cause extensive fibrosis, which entraps both veins and bile ducts.

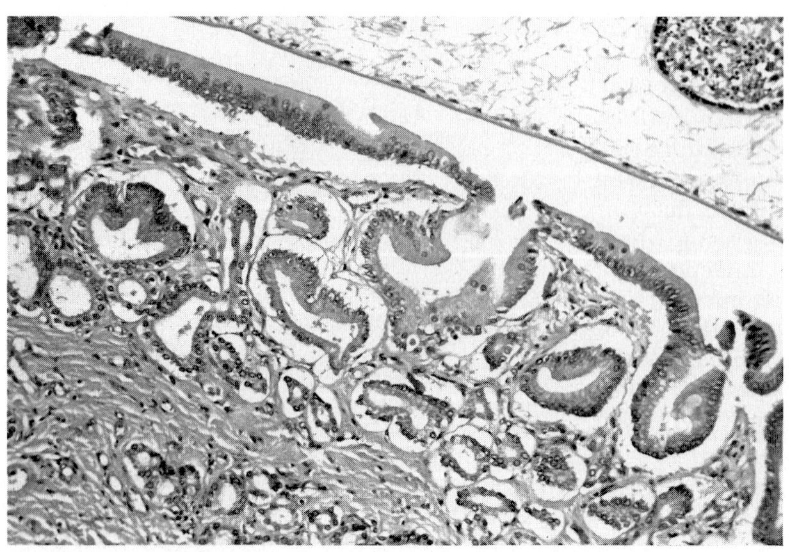

Figure 15–6. Proliferation of periductular mucus glands. Even if flukes are not encountered, this is presumptive evidence of present or recent infection.

This extensive and florid reaction, which has been termed pipestem fibrosis, results in noncirrhotic portal hypertension as it destroys the vascular bed. Obstructive jaundice, cholangitis, and cholelithiasis are not features of schistosomiasis. Vein involvement always predominates over bile duct involvement. Viable and nonviable eggs may be present in fibrous tissue, adjacent to intra- and extrahepatic ducts. However, eggs are not usually seen within the ductal system.

ORIENTAL CHOLANGIOHEPATITIS

Oriental cholangiohepatitis is also called recurrent pyogenic cholangitis. Many of the features of this condition are entirely similar to bacterial (ascending) cholangitis, which was described earlier. However, there are some unique findings that serve to distinguish it as a separate syndrome. As the name suggests, Oriental cholangiohepatitis is endemic to countries of southeast Asia, particularly China, Hong Kong, Taiwan, Vietnam, the Philippines, Singapore, Malaysia, Korea, and Japan.[40–43] When the disease occurs in North America, Europe, and Australia, it usually affects immigrants from southeast Asia, although there are rare accounts of the disease affecting whites.[44] It is generally agreed that the cholangitis occurs secondary to bacterial infection, which reaches the biliary system from the bowel via the portal vein. *E. coli* is the most commonly isolated organism, but *Klebsiella, Proteus,* and *Pseudomonas,* as well as anaerobic organisms, have also been isolated. A mixed infection is not uncommon.

An underlying abnormality is thought to be present within the biliary system that prevents the clearing of bacterial organisms from the bile, although in most instances the nature of this abnormality remains unknown. It is, however, speculated that parasites, especially *Clonorchis,* but also possibly roundworms, may be the initiating factor. This would explain the preponderance of the disease in southeast Asia. The rare occurrence of the condition outside this geographic location may be initiated by the presence of *Ascaris* in the biliary system. This theory does not, however, explain why only a small percentage of patients infected by biliary helminths develop cholangiohepatitis.[45] An alternative explanation for the disease onset is that it occurs as a result of malnutrition.[46] Malnutrition may act independently of or in conjunction with helminth infection. It has been suggested that a low-protein diet may produce a relative deficiency in the bile of glucaro-1:4-lactone, which is an inhibitor of the enzyme β-glucouronidase.[47] According to this theory, uninhibited β-glucouronidase activity in bile has the ability to deconjugate water-soluble bilirubin, resulting in bile precipitation and, ultimately, stone formation. Once stone formation occurs, it is impossible to eliminate the infection and a self-repeating cycle is initiated.

Autopsies of patients with cholangiohepatitis reveal dilated bile ducts, containing numerous pigment stones and sludge.[43,45] Stones are present in both intra- and extrahepatic locations. Typically, these are brown stones and consist of calcium bilirubinate, calcium palmitate, and cholesterol. Unlike black pigment stones, they are soft with a flaky consistency and often contain eggs or fragments of fluke. The affected ducts are surrounded by dense fibrous tissue, containing a variety of acute and chronic inflammatory cells. Granuloma formation is not, however, a feature. Obviously, the extent of fibrosis and inflammation depends on the number of previous attacks of cholangitis. In the later stages of the disease, the liver becomes shrunken and extensively scarred, with numerous capsular adhesions. The cut surface may reveal the presence of abscesses (Fig. 15–7).

Imaging investigations in patients with cholangiohepatitis may include ultrasound, cholangiography, and contrast-enhanced computed tomography (CT).[43] Ultrasound examination will show duct dilation. Stones are identified in up to 90% of patients and are visible by ultrasound. In the remaining 10% of patients, the ducts contain sludge, which is not usually appreciated using this technique. Cholangiography is usually performed by the endoscopic route (ERCP). It may reveal the presence of bile duct stones; disproportionately severe dilation of extrahepatic ducts, with mild or no dilation of intrahepatic ducts; and/or focal strictures and acute peripheral tapering, straightening, rigidity, decreased arborization, and increased branching angle of the intrahepatic ducts.[43] CT examination can visualize ducts that are not filled by cholangiography.[42,43] Often, there are dilated central intrahepatic ducts with acute tapering of peripheral ducts. Stones, bilomas, and abscesses are all best diagnosed by CT examination.

Typically, cholangiohepatitis is a disease of middle-aged and elderly adults,[42,43] who present with Charcot's triad.[15] Fifteen percent to 30% of patients present with an initial attack, but in

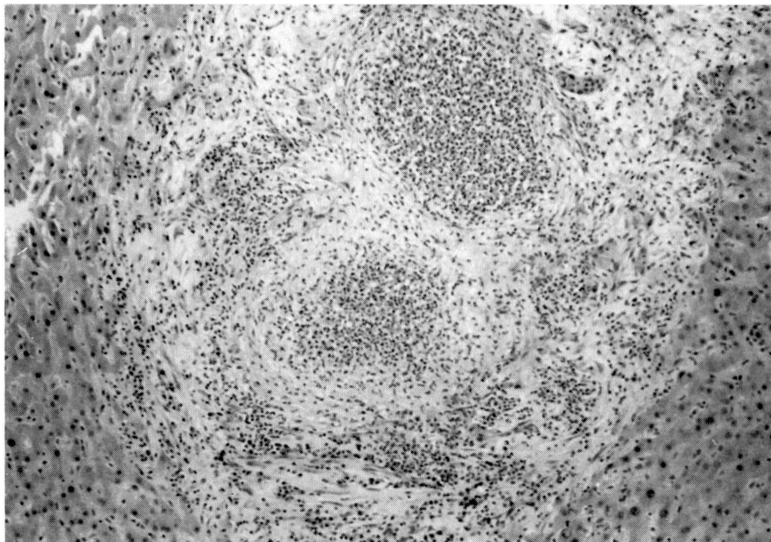

Figure 15–7. Hepatic abscess formation in a case of Oriental cholangiohepatitis.

the remainder, there is a history of previous episodes, extending back several years and occurring at the rate of one to two per year. Physical examination reveals jaundice and upper abdominal tenderness. In about 30% of patients, an enlarged gallbladder is palpable. Systemic complications of the disease include gram-negative septicemia and shock. Local complications include abscess formation, peritonitis, portal vein thrombosis, and hemobilia.

SCLEROSING CHOLANGITIS

Sclerosing cholangitis is a common sequel of chronic inflammation of the biliary tract. Inflammation is accompanied by fibrosis, which is typically patchy, resulting in focal stricture formation. As the disease progresses, the patient may ultimately develop secondary biliary cirrhosis, with portal hypertension and liver failure.

Sclerosing cholangitis has a large number of causes (Table 15–3). Common causes include secondary obstruction, immunodeficiency, infiltrative diseases, and certain neoplasms. The term *primary sclerosing cholangitis* (PSC) is used to refer to disease for which there is no known cause or when the patient has either inflammatory bowel disease, autoimmune disease, or idiopathic fibrosis. In most cases of obstructive, toxic, or ischemic injury, secondary bacterial infections may be responsible for ongoing damage. Sclerosis in immunodeficient states may be secondary to bacterial, viral, or parasitic infection. Identifying the cause of sclerosing cholangitis from biopsy appearances or cholangiographic findings is usually impossible and reliance has to be placed on medical history or ancillary investigations.

Table 15–3. Causes of Sclerosing Cholangitis

Obstruction of bile ducts
Choledocholithiasis
Surgical or nonsurgical trauma
Parasites or fungus balls
Cystic fibrosis
Choledochal cysts
Toxic
Misplaced alcohol or sclerosant injections
Chemotherapeutic drugs
Ischemic
Trauma
Emboli
Vasculitis
Neoplastic
Low-grade cholangiocarcinoma
Infiltrative diseases
Sarcoidosis
Langerhans cell histiocytosis
Immunodeficiency diseases
Congenital
Acquired
Associated with transplantation or graft-versus-host disease
Primary sclerosing cholangitis
Inflammatory bowel disease
Idiopathic fibrosis
Autoimmune disease

PRIMARY SCLEROSING CHOLANGITIS

PSC occurs most frequently in association with ulcerative colitis. Cholangiographic abnormalities typical of PSC occur in 2.4% to 4.0% of all patients with ulcerative colitis and in up to 5.5% of patients with pancolitis.[48,49] In individuals with ulcerative colitis confined to the distal colon, the prevalence is considerably less (approximately 0.5%).[49] There is, however, no relationship between PSC and the severity of the colitis. Colectomy does not cure PSC. It is now appreciated that many patients with ulcerative colitis who have abnormal liver function test results and nonspecific inflammatory changes, including pericholangitis on liver biopsy, will be found to have PSC if cholangiography is performed.[50,51] The percentage of patients with Crohn's disease with PSC is lower and has been estimated at approximately 1.5%.[52] Conversely, idiopathic inflammatory bowel disease is present in about 65% of patients with PSC, with most individuals having ulcerative colitis. Other clinical conditions occurring in association with PSC include a group with a presumed autoimmune etiology, such as Sjögren's syndrome,[53] celiac disease,[54] type I diabetes mellitus,[55,56] and systemic lupus erythematosus,[56] and a group characterized by idiopathic fibrosis, including retroperitoneal fibrosis,[57] Riedel's thyroiditis,[57,58] and Peyronie's disease.[59]

The pathogenetic mechanisms underlying PSC remain unknown. Currently, it is supposed that both PSC and idiopathic inflammatory bowel disease represent variable organ responses to a common cause. Genetic, immunologic, and infectious factors may play a role. There is a highly consistent association between PSC and human leukocyte antigen (HLA) B8 DR3 and DR2 haplotypes.[60] Interestingly, no association exists between ulcerative colitis unaccompanied by PSC and these HLA types, although HLA B8 DR3/DR2 is associated with other autoimmune diseases, such as type I diabetes mellitus, celiac disease, and myasthenia gravis.[53] This HLA type is linked to disordered Fc-receptor function on T lymphocytes and defective clearing of immune complexes.[61] Immunologic factors of possible relevance in the pathogenesis of PSC include activation of the complement system via the classic pathway,[62] the presence in two thirds of PSC patients of antineutrophil cytoplasmic antibodies,[63] expression on bile ductular epithelial cells of aberrant HLA class II antigens (including DR3) to which an immune attack may be directed,[64] and an absolute decline in numbers of CD8-positive T lymphocytes.[65] Possible relevant toxic and infectious factors include bacterial products or toxic bile acids present within bile[66] and CMV or reovirus type 3, which are trophic for biliary epithelium.[67,68]

The pathologic findings in PSC may be subdivided into those affecting intrahepatic ducts and those affecting extrahepatic ducts. Grossly, the extrahepatic ducts are thickened and hardened, resembling a thrombosed vessel.[69] The ducts may be surrounded by adhesions and there may be local lymphadenopathy.[69] Within the duct lumen, biliary sludge is commonly present. By microscopic examination, the duct walls are extensively fibrotic, with fibrosis extending into the periadventitial fat. Nonspecific inflammatory changes are noted, with a predominance of lymphocytes.[69,70] Without knowledge of the clinical situation, it is impossible to make a diagnosis of PSC. Intrahepatic bile duct abnormalities may be identified by liver biopsy or in explanted livers removed at the time of transplantation.[71] Major intrahepatic ducts may show either dilation, fibrosis, or fibrous obliteration. The obliterated ducts are transformed into fibrous cords. The fibrosed ducts show a characteristic concentric periductal distribution of fibrous tissue. The dilated ducts may have either a tubular or a saccular configuration. In the portal tracts present within a liver biopsy, concentric periductal fibrous distribution (onionskinning) is found in 50% of patients (Fig. 15–8). Fibrotic obliteration of ductules may also be encountered but is present in <10% of biopsies[72] (Fig. 15–9).

Cholangiography, usually performed endoscopically, is the gold standard for the diagnosis of PSC. In addition, the technique provides information about the distribution of the disease and the presence of dominant strictures that may be amenable to surgical correction. In 15% to 20% of patients, the changes affect only intrahepatic ducts.[48,49] In <10% of patients, extrahepatic ducts are involved in isolation.[73] The major abnormalities encountered consist of diffusely distributed multifocal strictures. These are typically short segments, measuring 2 to 20 mm in length. Between the strictures, the ducts may show a slight dilation, giving rise to a beaded appearance (Fig. 15–10). Occasional diverticulum-like outpouchings may occur. Most strictures are concentric, but there can be mural filling defects, producing a shaggy appearance to the wall of the bile duct. Within the liver,

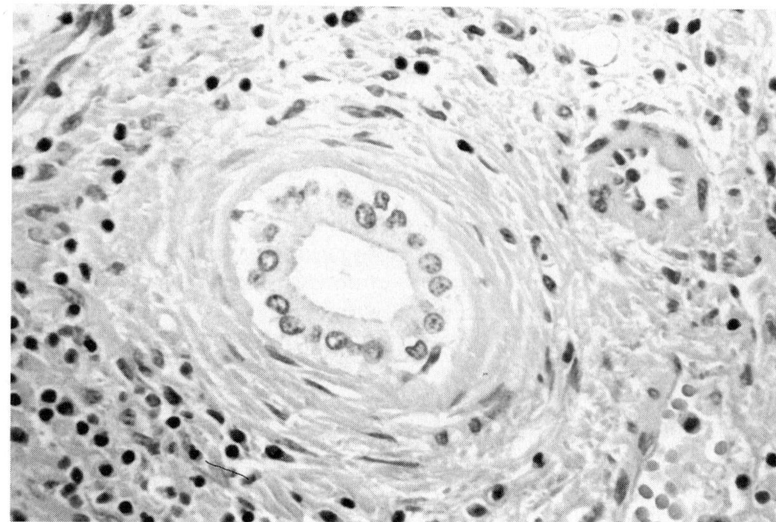

Figure 15–8. Liver biopsy from a patient with primary sclerosing cholangitis showing concentric fibrous distribution around bile ductules.

the distal smaller ducts are commonly difficult to fill, giving rise to a truncated appearance of the biliary tree. The cholangiographic changes in PSC are usually distinct from those encountered in secondary sclerosing cholangitis. In particular, secondary disease gives rise to focal strictures, with a more general dilation of the portion of the duct proximal to the dominant stricture.[74]

PSC is most commonly diagnosed in young adults between the ages of 24 and 45.[49,59] However, occasional examples are encountered in the very young or the very old. Men are affected up to two times as frequently as women,[49,58,59] but this is the case only with patients who have PSC in combination with ulcerative colitis. In persons without ulcerative colitis, the disease is equally common in men and women. Most patients present with right upper quadrant abdominal pain, which may be accompanied by jaundice and pruritus. Fatigue and weight loss, occurring as a consequence to malabsorption, are also often encountered. Rarely, there may be fever and evidence of cholangitis. Asymptomatic patients may be detected if individuals with ulcerative colitis are screened for PSC. In some series of patients with ulcerative colitis, up to 30% have asymptomatic cholangiographic

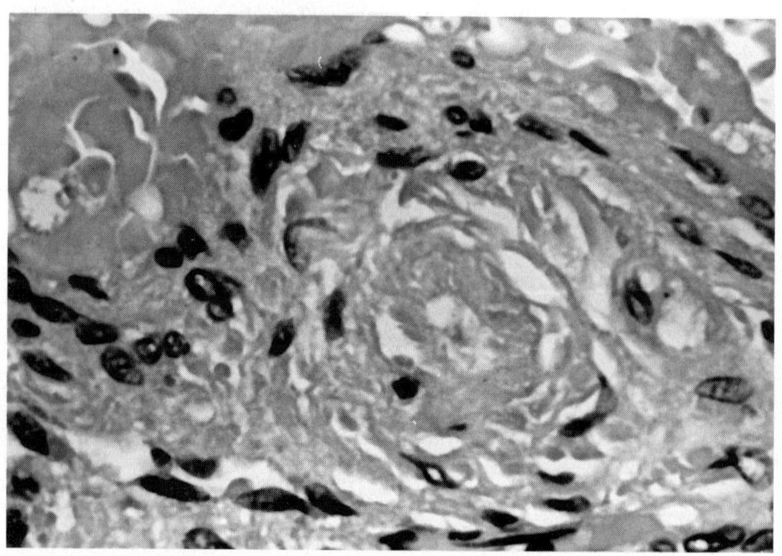

Figure 15–9. Fibrous obliteration of a bile ductule in a patient with primary sclerosing cholangitis. The outline of the destroyed duct is barely discernable (*arrows*).

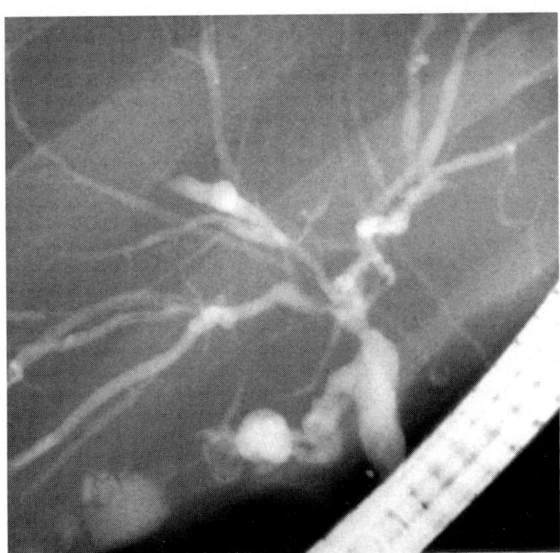

Figure 15–10. Endoscopic retrograde cholangiopancreatographic appearances in sclerosing cholangitis. Note the strictures and beaded appearance. (Radiograph courtesy of S. Ho, MD, Vancouver General Hospital.)

abnormalities.[52,75] Laboratory investigation reveals that PSC patients may have a three- to fivefold increase in alkaline phosphatase and γ-glutamyl transpeptidase. Serum transaminases are generally only mildly elevated. Antinuclear and anti–smooth muscle antibodies may be present at a low titer, but mitochondrial antibodies are not detected.[76]

Complications of PSC include deficiencies of fat-soluble vitamins A, D, K, and E occurring secondary to malabsorption, secondary biliary cirrhosis, gallstones, pancreatic disease, and cholangiocarcinoma. Pancreatic abnormalities include chronic pancreatitis[77] and strictures with beadlike dilation of the main pancreatic duct resembling the appearances of the bile ducts in PSC.[78] Abnormal pancreatograms may be found in up to 77% of patients with PSC. In a large majority of individuals with PSC affecting the pancreatic ducts, there are no clinical consequences. Occasional patients might have mild exocrine insufficiency, which may contribute to malabsorption. Rare examples of acute pancreatitis have also been recorded.

Cholangiocarcinoma is now a well-recognized complication of PSC. Its prevalence in clinical series of PSC is between 4% and 9%.[59,79,80] Its incidence in autopsy cases of PSC is much higher and, in some series, is up to 40%.[79,80] In most instances, cholangiocarcinoma is a late complication of PSC, arising many years after the initial diagnosis. In a small number of cases, cholangiocarcinoma is diagnosed either at the same time as sclerosing cholangitis or a few months later. In these circumstances, it is not possible to be sure whether the sclerosing cholangitis existed previously and was asymptomatic or instead whether cholangiocarcinoma was the primary disease and was responsible for a secondary sclerosing cholangitis. In the context of PSC, most cholangiocarcinomas arise at an extrahepatic location, usually in the region of the bifurcation of the common, hepatic duct.[81] Histologically, these tumors are predominantly glandular in type but may also have a papillary or cystic configuration. Multicentricity is common, and between macroscopic deposits of neoplasm, the intervening bile ducts may demonstrate dysplasia or carcinoma in situ. One case has been described that arose in a patient with biliary cirrhosis in whom there was intrahepatic mixed cholangiocarcinoma and hepatocellular carcinoma.[81] Early diagnosis of cholangiocarcinoma by cholangiography and CT scan may be difficult. Attention should be paid to the presence of a marked and progressive duct dilation and progressive eccentric stricture formation.[82]

CYSTIC FIBROSIS

Approximately 25% of adults with cystic fibrosis (CF) have abnormal liver function.[83–85] Morphologic abnormalities of the biliary tract are numerous in CF and include "microgallbladders,"[86] choledocholithiasis, distal strictures with proximal dilation,[86] and intrahepatic bile duct changes resembling sclerosing cholangitis.[83–85] Unlike with the bronchi and pancreatic ducts, mucus plugging is not observed in the biliary tract. In the majority of instances, bile duct abnormalities are encountered only in individuals with abnormal liver function.[86] Visualization of the duct system by cholangiography is the best method for demonstrating these morphologic abnormalities.[87,88]

REFERENCES

1. De Wit LT, Rauws EA, Gouma DJ: Surgical management of iatrogenic bile duct injury. Scand J Gastroenterol 230(suppl):89–94, 1999.
2. Fletcher DR, Hobbs MS, Tan P, et al.: Complications of cholecystectomy: Risks of the laparascopic approach and protective effects of operative cholangiography: A population based study. Ann Surg 229:449–457, 1999.

3. Feliciano DV: Biliary injuries as a result of blunt and penetrating trauma. Surg Clin North Am 74:897–907, 1994.
4. Parks RW, Diamond T: Non-surgical trauma to the extrahepatic biliary tract. Br J Surg 82:1303–1310, 1995.
5. Csendes A, Diaz JC, Burdiles P, et al.: Mirizzi syndrome and cholecystobiliary fistula: A unifying classification. Br J Surg 76:1139–1143, 1989.
6. Mishra MC, Vashishtha S, Tandon R: Biliobiliary fistula: Preoperative diagnosis and management implications. Surgery 108:1139–1143, 1990.
7. Pemberton M, Wells AD: The Mirizzi syndrome. Postgrad Med J 73:487–490, 1997.
8. Nagakawa T, Ohta T, Kayahara M, et al.: A new classification of Mirizzi syndrome from diagnostic and therapeutic viewpoints. Hepatogastroenterology 44:63–67, 1997.
9. Dorrance HR, Lingam MK, Hair A, et al.: Acquired abnormalities of the biliary tract from chronic gallstone disease. J Am Coll Surg 189:269–273, 1999.
10. Ibrarullah M, Saxena R, Sikora SS, et al.: Mirizzi's syndrome: Identification and management strategy. Aust N Z J Surg 63:802–806, 1993.
11. Wiig JN, Telhang R, Odegaard A, et al.: Isolated necrosis of the common bile duct subsequent to irradiation and chemotherapy. Case report. Acta Chir Scand 153:701–703, 1987.
12. Raimondo M, Ashby AM, York EA, et al.: Pancreatic pseudocyst with fistula to the common bile duct presenting with gastrointestinal bleeding. Dig Dis Sci 43:2622–2626, 1998.
13. Sung JY, Costerton JW, Shaffer EA: Defense system in the biliary tract against bacterial infection. Dig Dis Sci 37:689–696, 1992.
14. Boey JH, Way LW: Acute cholangitis. Ann Surg 191:264–270, 1980.
15. O'Connor MJ, Schwartz LM, McQuarrie DG, et al.: Acute bacterial cholangitis. An analysis of clinical manifestations. Arch Surg 117:437–441, 1982.
16. Kinoshita H, Hirohashi K, Igawa S, et al.: Cholangitis. World J Surg 8:963–969, 1984.
17. Shimada K, Noro T, Inamatsu T, et al.: Bacteriology of acute obstructive suppurative cholangitis of the aged. J Clin Microbiol 14:522–526, 1981.
18. Nucuvalas JC, Bore KE, Kaufman RA, et al.: Cholangitis associated with *Cryptococcus neoformans.* Gastroenterology 88:1055–1059, 1985.
19. Irani M, Truong LD: Candidiasis of the extrahepatic biliary tract. Arch Pathol Lab Med 110:1087–1090, 1986.
20. Ho F, Snape WJ Jr, Venegas R, et al.: Choledochal fungal ball. An unusual cause of biliary obstruction. Dig Dis Sci 33:1030–1034, 1988.
21. Wig JD, Singh K, Chawla YK, et al.: Cholangitis due to candidiasis of the extrahepatic biliary tract. HPB Surg 11:51–54, 1998.
22. Ojeas H, Hu HC, Greenberg SB: Candidemia after endoscopic retrograde cholangiopancreatography. South J Med 88:465–466, 1995.
23. Benhamou Y, Caumes E, Gerosa Y, et al.: AIDS-related cholangiopathy. Critical analysis of a prospective series of 26 patients. Dig Dis Sci 38:1113–1118, 1993.
24. Dowsett JF, Miller R, Davidson R, et al.: Sclerosing cholangitis in acquired immunodeficiency syndrome. Case reports and review of the literature. Scand J Gastroenterol 23:1267–1274, 1988.
25. Pol S, Romana CA, Richard S, et al.: Microsporidia infection in patients with the human immunodeficiency virus and unexplained cholangitis. N Engl J Med 328:95–99, 1993.
26. Liberman E, Yen TS: Foamy macrophages in acquired immunodeficiency syndrome cholangiopathy with *Encephalitozoon intestinalis.* Arch Pathol Lab Med 121:985–988, 1997.
27. Kowdley KV, Fawaz KA, Kaplan MM: Extrahepatic biliary stricture associated with cytomegalovirus in a liver transplant recipient. Transpl Int 9:161–163, 1996.
28. Kaplan LD, Kahn J, Jacobson M, et al.: Bile duct lymphoma and the acquired immunodeficiency syndrome (AIDS). Ann Intern Med 110:161–162, 1989.
29. Podbielski FJ, Pearsall GF Jr, Nelson DG, et al.: Lymphoma of the extrahepatic biliary ducts in acquired immunodeficiency syndrome. Ann Surg 63:807–810, 1997.
30. Krekorian TD, Radner AB, Alcorn JM, et al.: Biliary obstruction caused by bacillary angiomatosis in a patients with AIDS. Am J Med 89:820–822, 1990.
31. Sun T: Clonorchiasis and opisthorchiasis. *In* Connor DH, Chandler FW, Schwartz DA, Manz HJ, Lack EE (eds): Pathology of Infectious Diseases. Stamford, CT: Appleton & Lange, 1997, pp 1351–1360.
32. Hon PC: The pathology of *Clonorchis sinensis* infestation of the liver. J Pathol Bacteriol 70:53–64, 1955.
33. Min HK: Clonorchis sinensis: Pathogenesis and clinical features of infection. Arzneimittelforschung 34:1131–1133, 1984.
34. Belmaric J: Intrahepatic bile duct carcinoma and *C. sinensis* infection in Hong Kong. Cancer 31:468–473, 1973.
35. Schwartz DA: Cholangiocarcinoma associated with liver fluke infection: A preventable source of morbidity in Asian immigrants. Am J Gastroenterol 81:76–79, 1986.
36. Ona FV, Dytoc JN: *Clonorchis*-associated cholangiocarcinoma: A report of two cases with unusual manifestations. Gastroenterology 101:831–839, 1991.
37. Kim YL, Yu ES, Kim ST: Intraductal variant of peripheral cholangiocarcinoma of the liver with *Clonorchis sinensis* infection. Cancer 63:1562–1566, 1989.
38. Kim KH, Kim CD, Lee HS, et al.: Biliary papillary hyperplasia with *clonorchis* resembling cholangiocarcinoma. Am J Gastroenterol 94:514–517, 1999.
39. Lopez P, Gonzalez P, Tunon MJ, et al.: The effects of experimental fasciolosis on bilirubin metabolism in the rat. Exp Parasitol 78:386–393, 1994.
40. Lam SK, Wong KP, Chan PK, et al.: Recurrent pyogenic cholangitis: A study by retrograde cholangiography. Gastroenterology 74:1196–1203, 1978.
41. Turner WW Jr, Cramer CR: Recurrent oriental cholangiohepatitis. Surgery 93:397–401, 1983.
42. Carmona RH, Crass RA, Lim RC, et al.: Oriental cholangitis. Am J Surg 148:117–124, 1984.
43. Lim JH: Oriental cholangiohepatitis: Pathologic, clinical and radiologic features. AJR 157:1–8, 1991.
44. Wilson MK, Stephen MS, Mathur M, et al.: Recurrent pyogenic cholangitis or "oriental cholangiohepatitis" in occidentals: Case report of four patients. Aust N Z J Surg 66:649–652, 1996.
45. Chou S-T, Chan CW: Recurrent pyogenic cholangitis: A necropsy study. Pathology 12:415–428, 1980.
46. Ong GB: A study of recurrent pyogenic cholangitis. Arch Surg 84:199–225, 1962.
47. Maki T: Pathogenesis of calcium bilirubinate gallstones: Role of *E. coli,* beta-glucouronidase and coagulation by inorganic ions, polyelectrolytes and agitation. Ann Surg 164:90–100, 1966.
48. Schrumpf E, Elgjo K, Fausa O, et al.: Sclerosing cholangitis in ulcerative colitis. Scand J Gastroenterol 15:689–697, 1980.

49. Olsson R, Danielsson A, Järnerot G, et al.: Prevalence of primary sclerosing cholangitis in patients with ulcerative colitis. Gastroenterology 100:1319–1323, 1991.
50. Dordal E, Glagov S, Kirsner JB: Hepatic lesions in chronic inflammatory bowel disease. I. Clinical correlation with liver biopsy diagnosis in 103 patients. Gastroenterology 52:239–253, 1967.
51. Dew MJ, Thompson H, Allan RN: The spectrum of hepatic dysfunction in inflammatory bowel disease. Q J Med 48:113–135, 1979.
52. Tobias R, Wright JP, Kottler RE, et al.: Primary sclerosing cholangitis associated with inflammatory bowel disease in Cape Town 1975–1981. S Afr Med J 63:229–235, 1983.
53. Jorge AD, Esley C, Ahumada J: Family incidence of primary sclerosing cholangitis associated with immunologic diseases. Endoscopy 19:114–117, 1987.
54. Hay JE, Wiesner RH, Shorter RG, et al.: Primary sclerosing cholangitis and celiac disease. A novel association. Ann Int Med 109:713–717, 1988.
55. Smith MP, Loe RH: Sclerosing cholangitis. Review of recent case reports and associated diseases and four new cases. Am J Surg 110:239–246, 1965.
56. Alberti-Flor JJ, Jeffers L, Schiff ER: Primary sclerosing cholangitis occurring in a patient with systemic lupus erythematosus and diabetes mellitus. Am J Gastroenterol 79:889–891, 1984.
57. Bartholomew LG, Cain JC, Woolner LB, et al.: Sclerosing cholangitis. Its possible association with Riedel's struma and fibrous retroperitonitis—Report of two cases. N Engl J Med 269:8–12, 1963.
58. Wiesner RH, La Russo NF: Clinicopathologic features of the syndrome of primary sclerosing cholangitis. Gastroenterology 79:200–206, 1980.
59. Farrant JM, Hayllar KM, Wilkinson ML, et al.: Natural history and prognostic variables in primary sclerosing cholangitis. Gastroenterology 100:1710–1717, 1991.
60. Donaldson PT, Farrant JM, Wilkinson ML, et al.: Dual association of HLA DR2 and DR3 with primary sclerosing cholangitis. Hepatology 13:129–133, 1991.
61. Fraile G, Rodriguez-Garcia JL, Moreno A: Primary sclerosing cholangitis associated with systemic sclerosis. Postgrad Med J 67:189–192, 1991.
62. Senaldi G, Donaldson PT, Magrin S, et al.: Activation of complement system in primary sclerosing cholangitis. Gastroenterology 97:1430–1434, 1989.
63. Duerr RH, Targan SR, Landers CJ, et al.: Neutrophil cytoplasmic antibodies: A link between primary sclerosing cholangitis and ulcerative colitis. Gastroenterology 100:1385–1391, 1991.
64. Broomé U, Glaumann H, Hultcrantz R, et al.: Distribution of HLA-DR, HLA-DP, HLA-DQ antigens in liver tissue from patients with primary sclerosing cholangitis. Scand J Gastroenterol 25:54–58, 1990.
65. Snook JA, Chapman RW, Sachder GK, et al.: Peripheral blood and portal tract lymphocyte populations in primary sclerosing cholangitis. J Hepatol 9:36–41, 1989.
66. Sherlock S: Pathogenesis of sclerosing cholangitis: The role of non-immune factors. Semin Liv Dis 11:5–10, 1991.
67. Morecki R, Glaser JH, Cho S, et al.: Biliary atresia and rheovirus type 3 infection. N Engl J Med 307:481–484, 1982.
68. Lurie M, Elmalach I, Schuger L, et al.: Liver findings in infantile cytomegalovirus infection: Similarity to extrahepatic biliary obstruction. Histopathology 11:1171–1180, 1987.
69. Lefkowitch JH: Primary sclerosing cholangitis. Arch Intern Med 142:1157–1160, 1982.
70. Ludwig J: Surgical pathology of the syndrome of primary sclerosing cholangitis. Am J Surg Pathol 13(suppl):43–49, 1989.
71. Ludwig J, MacCarty RL, La Russo NF, et al.: Intrahepatic cholangiectasis and large duct obliteration in primary sclerosing cholangitis. Hepatology 6:560–568, 1986.
72. Ludwig J, Czaja AJ, Dickson ER, et al.: Manifestations of non-suppurative cholangitis in chronic hepatobiliary disorders. Morphologic spectrum, clinical correlations and terminology. Liver 4:105–116, 1984.
73. Porayko MK, Wiesner RH, La Russo NF, et al.: Patients with asymptomatic primary sclerosing cholangitis frequently have progressive disease. Gastroenterology 98:1594–1602, 1990.
74. Longmire WP: When is cholangitis sclerosing? Am J Surg 135:312–330, 1978.
75. Chapman RWG, Burroughs AK, Bass NM, et al.: Longstanding asymptomatic primary sclerosing cholangitis. A report of 3 cases. Dig Dis Sci 26:778–782, 1981.
76. Helzberg JH, Petersen JH, Boyer JL: Improved survival with primary sclerosing cholangitis. A review of clinicopathologic features and comparison of symptomatic and asymptomatic patients. Gastroenterology 92:1869–1875, 1987.
77. Whelton MJ: Sclerosing cholangitis. Clin Gastroenterol 2:163–173, 1973.
78. Epstein O, Chapman RWG, Lake-Bakaar G, et al.: The pancreas in primary biliary cirrhosis and primary sclerosing cholangitis. Gastroenterology 83:1177–1182, 1982.
79. Aadland E, Schrumpf E, Fausa O, et al.: Primary sclerosing cholangitis. A long-term follow-up study. Scand J Gastroenterol 22:655–664, 1987.
80. Rosen CB, Nagorney DM, Wiesner RH, et al.: Cholangiocarcinoma complicating primary sclerosing cholangitis. Ann Surg 213:21–25, 1991.
81. Wee A, Ludwig J, Coffey RJ Jr, et al.: Hepatobiliary carcinoma associated with primary sclerosing cholangitis and chronic ulcerative colitis. Hum Pathol 16:719–726, 1985.
82. MacCarty RL, La Russo NF, May GR, et al.: Cholangiocarcinoma complicating primary sclerosing cholangitis. Cholangiographic appearances. Radiology 156:43–46, 1985.
83. Nagel RA, Westaby D, Javaid A, et al.: Liver disease and bile duct abnormalities in adults with cystic fibrosis. Lancet 2:1422–1425, 1989.
84. O'Brien S, Keogan M, Casey M, et al.: Biliary complications of cystic fibrosis. Gut 33:387–391, 1992.
85. Colombo C, Battezzati PM, Strazzabosco M, et al.: Liver and biliary problems in cystic fibrosis. Semin Liver Dis 18:227–235, 1998.
86. Gaskin KJ, Waters DL, Howman-Giles R, et al.: Liver disease and common bile duct stenosis in cystic fibrosis. N Engl J Med 318:340–346, 1988.
87. Bass S, Cannon J, Ho C: Biliary tree in cystic fibrosis. Biliary tract abnormalities in cystic fibrosis demonstrated by endoscopic retrograde cholangiography. Gastroenterology 84:1592–1596, 1983.
88. Strandvik B, Hjelte L, Gabrielsson N, et al.: Sclerosing cholangitis in cystic fibrosis. Scand J Gastroenterol 143(suppl):121–124, 1988.

Chapter

16

NEOPLASMS OF THE EXTRAHEPATIC BILE DUCTS

ADENOMAS OF THE LARGE BILE DUCTS

A classification of neoplasms of the extrahepatic bile ducts is given in Table 16–1.[1] The term *bile duct adenoma* is most often used to describe a rare benign liver lesion that is now recognized to be a hamartoma of the peribiliary glands.[2,3] Adenomas of the extrahepatic bile ducts are a different entity. These rare neoplasms are referred to as papillomas in older literature.[4,5] Two thirds of adenomas are located in the common bile duct and the remainder in the common hepatic, cystic, and left and right hepatic ducts.[5] The main clinical symptoms and signs are jaundice (which may be intermittent), pruritus, right upper quadrant abdominal pain, and hepatomegaly.[4–6] Ulceration and bleeding, sometimes massive, has been recorded. Adenomas of the bile ducts are histologically similar to adenomas of the colon. They show glandular proliferation; epithelial dysplasia; and tubular, villous, or tubulovillous morphology. They may contain metaplastic goblet cells, Paneth's cells, and endocrine cells. The preferred treatment is complete removal or ablation of the tumor as local removal or curettage are generally followed by recurrence.[6]

Multiple Biliary Papillomatosis

The designation *biliary papillomatosis* refers to multiple or extensive villous adenomas of the bile ducts. It resembles the intraductal papillary-mucinous tumor of the pancreas and rarely occurs in association with it. Typically, the bile ducts are distended by soft, gray-white or tan friable, sessile cauliflower-like masses that tend to extend circumferentially. Microscopically, the polyps are villous or tubulovillous adenomas. This rare condition, first described by Caroli in 1958, presents with progressive jaundice.[7,8] The male-to-female ratio is 1.7:1.[9] Most patients are in the sixth or seventh decade, but the age range is from 19 to 89 years.[9] A minority of cases are associated with familial adenomatous polyposis,[10] idiopathic ulcerative colitis,[11] or congenital choledochal cyst.[12] Rarely, biliary papillomatosis is confined to intrahepatic bile ducts,[5,13,14] and involvement of the gallbladder and proximal pancreatic duct has been recorded.[11] One review of 30 villous neoplasms of the biliary tract excluding the ampulla of Vater found that 22 were multicentric in the biliary tract, 6 had lesions isolated to one hepatic duct, and 3 had diffuse papillomatosis. Overall, 50% of patients died of their disease.[15] Malignant change ultimately supervenes in many cases, and once this occurs, the prognosis is very poor.[11,16,17]

The treatment of multiple papillomas is a challenge. Only radical excision will produce cure, but the surgery required for radical excision is formidable. Curettage and drainage are temporary solutions, and ultimately, recurrent cholangitis or malignancy, resulting in biliary obstruction, supervenes. Chemotherapy has been tried.[18] Laser therapy via the choledochoscope is a recent and promising modality.[19] Mean survival after diagnosis is 36 months.[9]

Table 16–1. Neoplasms of the Extrahepatic Ducts

Epithelial tumors
- Benign
  - Adenoma, tubular and papillary
  - Cystadenoma
  - Papillomatosis
- Malignant
  - Adenocarcinoma not otherwise specified
  - Papillary adenocarcinoma
  - Adenocarcinoma, intestinal type
  - Mucinous (colloid) adenocarcinoma
  - Clear cell adenocarcinoma
  - Signet ring cell adenocarcinoma
  - Adenosquamous and pure squamous carcinoma
  - Small cell carcinoma

Endocrine tumors
- Carcinoid tumor
- Mixed carcinoid-adenocarcinoma
- Paraganglioma

Nonepithelial tumors
- Benign
  - Granular cell tumor
  - Ganglioneurofibroma/neurofibroma
  - Leiomyoma
  - Lipoma
  - Vascular tumor
- Malignant
  - Rhabdomyosarcoma
  - Leiomyosarcoma
  - Kaposi's sarcoma
  - Malignant fibrous histiocytoma
  - Vascular tumor

Lymphoma

Metastatic tumors
- Malignant melanoma
- Adenocarcinoma

Modified from Albores-Saavedra J, Henson DE, Sobin LH: Histological Typing of Tumors of the Gallbladder and Extrahepatic Bile Ducts, 2nd ed. Berlin: Springer-Verlag, 1991, pp 7–21.

Biliary Granular Cell Tumor

Granular cell tumors of the bile ducts are rare benign tumors that mainly affect young black women.[20–25] These tumors may be discovered by chance or may present with biliary obstruction. Cholangiographically, they demonstrate concentric narrowing of the bile duct, mimicking cholangiocarcinoma. Up to 1988, the total number reported was 39,[20] affecting 24 (61%) black women, 2 Oriental women, 7 white women, and 2 males, 1 an 11-year-old boy.[26] The mean age of patients is 34.7 years (range 11 to 61 years). According to Butterly et al., the majority of tumors occurred at or near the junction of the cystic, hepatic, and common bile ducts, thus making them amenable to relatively simple procedures for excision and reanastomosis.[20] Fifty percent involve the common bile duct, 37% the cystic duct, 15% the hepatic ducts, and 4% the gallbladder.[27] The case of one patient has been described who had multiple granular cell tumors involving the gallbladder, cystic duct, and common bile duct.[21] Granular cell tumors may also be simultaneously present at locations elsewhere in the body.[22] When they are located in the common bile duct or common hepatic duct, granular cell tumors present with obstructive jaundice, hepatomegaly, and right upper quadrant pain. If they are located in the cystic duct, right upper quadrant pain is the most common presenting feature.

Grossly, granular cell tumors are firm or hard, yellowish, ill-defined nodules < 3 cm in diameter that in most instances grow concentrically around the duct, compressing the lumen. Microscopically they are composed of sheets of cells with small hyperchromatic nuclei and abundant granular cytoplasm. Collagenous bands may intersect the tumor and can be a prominent feature in mature tumors. Spindled granular cells may be seen. Rarely, there is glandular atypia of the biliary glands that are surrounded by the tumor.[25] The tumors stain positively with Periodic acid–Schiff (PAS) stain and with immunostains for S100, neuron-specific enolase, myelin basic protein, laminin, Leu 7, and cathepsin B.[25] Malignant granular cell tumors have occasionally been documented at extrabiliary locations but never in the biliary tract.

Carcinoid Tumors of the Bile Ducts

Carcinoid tumors are rare and are the subject of individual case reports. In one review, reports of 11 cases were collected from the literature[28] and several more cases have been published since then. The average age of patients is 40 years and the sex ratio is equal. The presenting symptoms are jaundice and abdominal pain, although occasionally, a tumor is an incidental discovery.[29] In the review cited, 6 patients had no metastasis, 3 had liver metastasis (1 of these also had lymph node metastasis), and 1 had portal vein invasion, indicating that about 40% of those tumors are malignant and 60% are benign.[28] Grossly, most carcinoid tumors are circumscribed nodules. In one instance, the carcinoid tumor arose within a choledochal cyst.[30] Treatment is by surgical excision.

The origin of carcinoids in the bile ducts is likely from the rare endocrine cells that have been described in the epithelium of the hepatic ducts, which have undergone metaplasia.[31] These endocrine cells may be immunoreactive for somatostatin.[32]

Hepatobiliary Cystadenoma

Hepatobiliary cystadenoma is a rare tumor that may occur in the liver or extrahepatic bile ducts. Only about 100 cases have been reported in the English literature.[33,34] The mean age of the patients at presentation is 45 years, the median age is 46 years, and the range is 2 to 87 years. Ninety-six percent of patients with cystadenomas are women, and no racial predilection is observed. The malignant counterpart of this neoplasm, cystadenocarcinoma, presents at a mean age of 59 years (median, 61 years). Most hepatobiliary cystadenomas are intrahepatic and only a minority arise in the extrahepatic bile ducts—7 of 52 patients (13%) in the largest series reported to date.[33] These tumors are the equivalent of pancreatic mucinous cystic neoplasms and share the same female predominance, ovarian-type stroma, and variable epithelial dysplasia (see Chapter 8).

Grossly, cystadenomas are multilocular cystic tumors that range in size from 2.5 to 28 cm (mean, 15 cm). Microscopically, they consist of cellular septa lined by simple columnar epithelium of biliary type. Foci of intestinal goblet cell metaplasia and Paneth's cell metaplasia are found in about one fifth of neoplasms. Foci of atypical or dysplastic epithelium will show multilayering, tufting, nuclear enlargement and hyperchromasia. The stroma in the majority of cases, particularly in women, consists of a densely cellular layer beneath the epithelium, with a hyalinized stromal layer on the outer aspect. The cellular layer is composed of spindle cells, reminiscent of ovarian stroma or primitive mesenchyme. In about 14% of patients, this specialized stroma is absent. Nonspecific reactive stromal changes are seen occasionally, such as aggregates of foamy histiocytes, lipofuscin-laden macrophages, hemosiderin deposits, cholesterol clefts, or multinucleate giant cells associated with foci of hemorrhage.[33] The differential diagnosis includes endometriosis, but the lining epithelium is biliary rather than endometrial. Cystadenomas can undergo malignant change to cystadenocarcinomas and therefore complete excision is the preferred treatment.

Paraganglioma

A paraganglioma that obstructed the left and right hepatic ducts near their confluence has been reported.[35] This is a rare tumor at this site.

Other Benign Tumors and Tumorlike Lesions

Fibroma, leiomyoma, lipoma, adenomyoma, adenofibroma, and hamartoma have been described in the bile ducts.[4,5]

Traumatic (amputation) neuroma of the bile ducts usually follows cholecystectomy and is an incidental finding at subsequent surgery or autopsy. Because the outer walls of the bile ducts contain abundant nerves, the amputated cystic duct is a frequent site of traumatic neuromas. No clear relationship has been established between such neuromas and post-cholecystectomy pain. Rarely, neuromas cause jaundice many years after cholecystectomy, when they arise in the common hepatic duct or common bile duct that was injured during surgery. The neuroma protrudes through the wall of the bile duct and eventually causes partial or complete duct obstruction, mimicking a true neoplasm.[36]

Heterotopic pancreas, gastric mucosa, and duodenal mucosa are rarely found in the extrahepatic bile ducts or at the ampulla of Vater.[37–40]

CLASSIFICATION OF CARCINOMAS OF THE BILIARY TREE

Carcinomas of the biliary tract can be divided into five groups: (1) cholangiocarcinoma arising in an intrahepatic bile duct beyond the first bifurcation of the right and left hepatic ducts (peripheral type), (2) hilar cholangiocarcinoma arising in the right or left hepatic ducts or in the common hepatic duct (hilar type or upper third tumor, Klatskin tumor), (3) carcinoma of the middle third of the extrahepatic bile duct (the common bile duct from its origin to the border of pancreas), (4) carcinoma of the distal third or intrapancreatic common bile duct, and (5) carcinoma of the ampulla of Vater. Types 2, 3, and 4 are generally considered carcinomas of the extrahepatic bile ducts.[41,42] Some authors merge middle-third and lower-third tumors into one group.[41,43] Bismuth et al. further subdivided the hilar carcinomas as follows: Type I are tumors below the confluence of the left and right hepatic ducts; type II are tumors that reach the confluence; types IIIa and IIIb occlude the common hepatic duct and either the right or left hepatic duct, respectively.[44]

Carcinoma of the Extrahepatic Bile Ducts

Carcinoma of the extrahepatic bile ducts is mainly a tumor of older people, three exceptions being those carcinomas that complicate primary sclerosing cholangitis, choledochal cyst, or pancreatobiliary maljunction in young adults. Carcinoma of the extrahepatic bile ducts is about half as frequent as carcinoma of the gallbladder. Therefore, at present there are approximately 5,000 gallbladder cancers and 2,500 bile duct cancers diagnosed annually in the United States.[45–48] In populations that have a high risk of gallbladder cancer, the ratio of gallbladder to bile duct cancers is higher. The Surveillance, Epidemiology, and End Results (SEER) Program of the National Cancer Institute identified 1,766 patients with carcinoma of the extrahepatic bile ducts and 3,038 patients with carcinoma of gallbladder, a ratio of 1:1.7.[47,48] A British study found extrahepatic bile duct carcinomas were more numerous than gallbladder carcinomas. The incidence per million population per year was estimated at 8.0 for gallbladder carcinoma, 2.9 for ampullary carcinoma, and 11.6 for carcinoma of the extrahepatic bile ducts.[43] Similarly, a Japanese study also found an excess of bile duct cancers over gallbladder cancers.[49]

The frequency of extrahepatic bile duct cancers increases with age. The average age at diagnosis in men is 68.4 years (range, 22 to 98 years) and in women is 72.7 years (range, 28 to 104 years).[47] The sex incidence is approximately equal in North America,[47] but there is a male excess in Japanese series in a ratio of 1.9:1.[31]

Despite their strategic location, bile duct tumors do not usually present early enough to facilitate curative resection. Obstructive jaundice is the most frequent presenting feature. About one quarter of all patients are not clinically icteric, though most have elevated serum bilirubin.[43] Weight loss, pain in the right upper quadrant, and pruritus are each present in one third of patients.[50] The gallbladder may be enlarged and palpable if the tumor involves the cystic duct or common bile duct. Serum alkaline phosphatase and γ-glutamyl transferase are moderately increased. CA 19–9 levels are elevated in most cases and this serum test is useful to detect cholangiocarcinoma in patients with primary sclerosing cholangitis.[51]

Diagnostic imaging of the biliary tract begins with ultrasonography, which has sensitivity of about 75% for detecting choledocholithiasis in dilated bile ducts and 50% in nondilated ducts.[52,53] Its use is limited by gas in the bowel masking the tissues, as tumors tend to have ill-defined outlines. Computed tomography (CT) provides a more comprehensive imaging of the liver, bile ducts, pancreas, lymph nodes, and blood vessels[53] and can confirm the sonographic findings. However, CT has similar sensitivity to ultrasound and therefore direct cholangiography is required in many cases. Endoscopic retrograde cholangiopancreatography (ERCP) can identify the site of bile duct obstruction and also allows inspection of the papilla, brush cytology of the bile ducts, papillotomy, stone extraction, and biopsy as required by the findings. An abrupt stricture is more likely to be a carcinoma, whereas a tapering stricture is likely to be benign. Percutaneous transhepatic cholangiography may be used for proximal tumors. Both the proximal and the distal ends of the tumor must be visualized to help the surgeon plan treatment. Direct cholangiographic examinations are the most important for determining the resectability of a tumor.[54] Three-dimensional magnetic resonance imaging with contrast is an excellent modality for imaging not only the bile ducts but the blood vessels and soft tissues as well. It may replace CT and angiography for the preoperative evaluation of biliary cancers.[54] This technique has a high sensitivity for detecting calculi.[55] Endoscopic ultrasonography is also a reasonably accurate way to measure tumor depth and stage cancer of the extrahepatic bile ducts, although for detection of distant metastasis, additional transcutaneous ultrasonography or CT is necessary.[56]

Morphologic confirmation of malignancy by cytology or biopsy establishes the diagnosis. Cytology preparations can be made from retrieved stents, stent removers, and bile, although the best preparations are obtained by brushing the biliary stricture.[57] Brush cytology is useful for separating benign from malignant bile duct strictures.[58–60] The overall assessment of malignancy in cytology shows good reproducibility between pathologists and is the best criterion of malignancy.[60] The reproducible criteria of malignancy are chromatin clumping, increased nuclear-to-cytoplasmic ratio, and either nuclear molding (including cell-in-cell arrangement) or loss of honeycombing.[60] In practice, the sensitivity of bile duct brushings for diagnosis of carcinoma may be as low as 36% or as high as 75%, but the specificity is 97% to 100%.[57,60–62] Endoscopic biopsies are limited by their small size but can be diagnostic. In these biopsies, the normal glands present in the walls of the extrahepatic bile ducts, the sacculi of Beale, must not be mistaken for neoplasm. They typically show a lobular pattern and benign cytology, whereas carcinomas show the cytologic features of malignancy and often an infiltrative pattern and stromal desmoplasia.

Risk Factors for Bile Duct Carcinoma

Risk factors for carcinoma of the large bile ducts are listed in Table 16–2. About 5% to 6% of carcinomas of the extrahepatic bile ducts are secondary to primary sclerosing cholangitis.[43,63–65] Conversely, 10% to 20% of all patients with primary sclerosing cholangitis develop cholangiocarcinoma.[66,67] In most patients, primary sclerosing cholangitis complicates idiopathic ulcerative colitis; mainly men are affected. The mean duration from onset of ulcerative colitis to development of symptoms of biliary duct carcinoma is 19 years and from colectomy to onset of biliary cancer is an average of 9.4 years.[68] The mean age of patients at onset of symptoms of biliary duct cancer is 38 years (range, 23 to 62 years). The risk of hepatobiliary carcinoma in patients with primary sclerosing cholangitis is significantly increased if there is a history of cigarette smoking.[69]

Congenital cystic disease of the biliary tree is occasionally complicated by carcinoma. The spectrum of cystic disease includes choledochal cysts, Caroli's disease, congenital hepatic fibrosis, and von Meyenburg complexes.[70–74] Precancerous lesions, such as dysplasia or atypical hyperplasia, appear to precede the development of carcinoma.[70,75,76] Carcinoma is a well-recognized complication of choledochal cyst, occurs in 2.5% of cases, and usually arises many years after drainage by enteric anastomosis.[77–82] The patients tend to be younger than the average for biliary carcinoma, the mean age being 32 years.[31,32] The mucosa lining the cysts becomes chronically inflamed and neoplasia develops in this background of chronic inflammation. Type I and type IV cysts are those mainly at risk of malignant complications. Type I cysts involve the common bile duct or hepatic duct in a localized, segmental, or diffuse pattern. Type IV consists of multiple cysts along the extrahepatic ducts or both extrahepatic and intrahepatic ducts. The risk of developing cancer is one reason why the preferred treatment for choledochal cyst is complete excision. Stones are present in about 25% of these cysts that develop carcinoma and may also play a role in carcinogenesis. The carcinomas that arise in choledochal cysts are mainly adenocarcinomas, but adenosquamous carcinomas, or pure squamous carcinomas, have been described.

Table 16–2. Risk Factors for Carcinoma of the Bile Ducts

Primary sclerosing cholangitis
Choledochal cysts
Pancreaticobiliary maljunction and reflux of pancreatic juice
Gallstones
Carcinoma of the gallbladder
Oral contraceptives
Cigarette smoking
Bilioenteric anastomosis

Choledochal cysts are now recognized to be secondary to pancreaticobiliary maljunction, especially the type in which there is a long common channel, which permits reflux of pancreatic juice into the bile duct. There is growing evidence that bile duct and gallbladder cancers arise more frequently in patients with maljunction, even without choledochal cyst. Suda and Miyano found pancreaticobiliary maljunction in 16.4% of their biliary tract carcinomas (12 cases, including 8 carcinomas of the common bile duct and 4 carcinomas of the gallbladder).[83] Other isolated cases have been reported, including cases involving combined bile duct and pancreatic ductal carcinoma.[84–87]

About one third of patients with extrahepatic bile duct carcinoma either have or have had gallstones.[43,63] and the evidence that gallstones play a causative role in carcinogenesis in the bile ducts is growing. Case-control studies have implicated gallstones,[88,89] and a large Swedish study concluded that gallstones probably play a causal role in the pathogenesis of bile duct cancer.[90]

Carcinoma of the gallbladder is associated with carcinoma of the biliary tree in about 7% of patients, suggesting that some carcinogenic factors act on both epithelia.[31] In addition to gallstones, these influences may include pancreaticobiliary maljunction and primary sclerosing cholangitis (PSC). The pathway to both begins with mucosal intestinal metaplasia.[91]

Two risk factors for peripheral (intrahepatic) cholangiocarcinoma could be viewed as chronic irritants of the biliary epithelium—parasites and stones. In Asian countries, where the prevalence is high, cholangiocarcinoma is associated with parasitic infestations by *Clonorchis sinensis* and *Opisthorchis viverrini.* These flukes parasitize the biliary tree and induce adenomatous proliferation of the paraductal glands, a proliferation that precedes and predisposes to carcinoma, via atypical hyperplasia and dysplasia.[92–94] Hepatolithiasis is common in southeast Asia and in many cases is an end stage of parasitic infestation, the stone entombing the dead parasite. Cholangiocarcinoma develops in 5% to 10% of patients with hepatolithiasis.[95,96] Chronic proliferative cholangitis is found both with hepatolithiasis alone and when lithiasis is complicated by cancer. Simple proliferative cholangitis may be complicated by atypical hyperplasia and dysplasia, both putative precancerous lesions.[95] In all of these conditions, there is likely to be recurrent ulceration and regeneration of the biliary epithelium and possibly superimposed bacterial infection,[95] a sequence that has been demonstrated experimentally.[97]

Chemical agents that have been linked to cholangiocarcinoma include Thorotrast and cigarette smoking. Thorotrast, an obsolete angiographic contrast medium that contains the radioactive element thorium, has been associated uncommonly with angiosarcoma of the liver or spleen, hepatocellular carcinoma, and cholangiocarcinoma.[97–99] Cigarette smoking was found to be positively associated with bile duct cancer in one study[100] but negatively associated in another.[88] In patients with PSC, as mentioned above, smoking has been associated with cancer. The use of oral contraceptives has been significantly associated with cholangiocarcinoma in women younger than age 60 years.[88] Rare cases of intrahepatic cholangiocarcinoma have arisen in persons taking anabolic androgens, but a causal connection has not been established.[101]

Bile duct carcinoma may occur many years after bilioenteric anastomosis.[102] This raises the question as to whether the procedure, most often performed for complications of cholecystectomy, may predispose to cancer. Ascending bacterial cholangitis and choledocholithiasis are known to complicate choledochoenterostomy, and this may be a causal link.[103]

Precancerous Lesions of the Bile Ducts

Adenoma and dysplasia are the precursors of carcinoma in the bile ducts.[31,103,104] Residual adenoma or dysplasia is found in about 20% of patients, especially in polypoid and villous lesions.[31] A computer-assisted three-dimensional reconstruction study of hepatohilar bile duct carcinomas confirmed a dysplasia–carcinoma sequence, with dysplasia surrounding the carcinoma. Multiple foci of carcinoma, arising from the dysplasia, have also been found in 42% of patients, and some of the foci were independent without any intervening dysplasia.[105] Laitio studied the borders of 15 carcinomas of the extrahepatic bile ducts and found metaplasia in 12 (80%), antral type in 9, intestinal in 2, and combined in 1. All of these specimens had dysplastic changes in superficial epithelium.[106] This confirms that metaplasia is a common precursor of dysplasia in the extrahepatic bile ducts, just as it is in the gallbladder. Metaplasia is thus the first recognizable morphologic change along the pathway to cancer.

Gross Features of Bile Duct Cancer

Cancers of the bile ducts may be papillary, nodular, constricting, or diffusely infiltrating.[31,107,108] The most common tumors are small and constricting. They are grayish white in color and firm in consistency, with ill-defined margins at the periphery. The mucosa overlying the tumor is granular and roughened. The bile duct shows proximal dilation. Most nonpapillary carcinomas have a scirrhous stroma. Diffusely infiltrating carcinomas spread along the bile ducts for considerable distances and into surrounding tissues. The rare giant cell carcinomas, or oat cell carcinomas, may be large masses with necrosis and hemorrhage. Tumor location is variously categorized, but the system popularized by Longmire and others divides the extrahepatic bile ducts into thirds. The upper third includes the left and right hepatic ducts and the common hepatic duct down to the usual point of entry of the cystic duct. The middle third is from the cystic duct to the upper border of pancreas, and the distal third is the intrapancreatic portion.[42] The proportion of tumors in

Table 16–3. Histologic Grade and Survival for Adenocarcinoma Not Otherwise Specified, SEER Program data

Grade	No. of Patients	% of Patients Graded	Median Survival (mo)	2-Year Survival Rate
1	221	32.5	10	0.24
2	241	35.4	8	0.16
3	212	31.2	4	0.07
4	6	0.9	2	0.0

Key: SEER, Surveillance, Epidemiology, and End Results (National Cancer Institute).
Data from Henson DE, Albores-Saavedra J, Corle, D: Carcinoma of the extrahepatic bile ducts. Histologic types, stage of disease, grade, and survival rates. Cancer 70:1498–1501, 1992.

each third is variable, but in a large French series was found to be as follows: upper third, 56%; middle third, 13%; lower third, 18%; and diffuse tumors, 10%.[109] Similar proportions have been reported by other authors, over half of the tumors being located in the hilum.[43,110–112]

Microscopic Findings in Bile Duct Carcinoma

Papillary and nodular tumors tend to be well differentiated, whereas flat or ulcerated tumors tend to be poorly differentiated.[31] The grossly polypoid, nodular, or papillary tumors often have a superficial component of adenoma or dysplasia, from which the carcinoma arises. Resected papillary tumors of the bile ducts that appear noninvasive should be totally submitted so that a small invasive focus is not missed. The grossly flat or ulcerated tumors are tubular adenocarcinomas or poorly differentiated carcinomas and, rarely, adenosquamous carcinomas.[111] The proportion of poorly differentiated carcinomas was 40% in one series,[111] but only 18% in another.[113] The SEER Program study found approximately equal numbers of patients with tumors in grades 1, 2, and 3 with very few in grade 4 (Table 16–3).[47] Laitio found 36% of cases to involve papillary carcinomas and 64% to involve gland-forming tumors. His series did not include any mucoid, squamous, or adenosquamous carcinomas.[106] The SEER data for carcinoma subtypes are given in Table 16–4. A majority of the adenocarcinomas are of intestinal type and contain goblet cells, whereas some resemble pancreatic or gallbladder carcinomas.[106] Mucinous (colloid) carcinomas are uncommon in the bile duct and are identical to mucinous carcinomas from other locations. By definition, they must have > 50% of extracellular mucin and typically show nests of tumor cells floating in a pool of mucus. Adenosquamous carcinomas occur occasionally, but pure squamous carcinomas are rare and are found mainly in choledochal cysts.[114] An unusual example of clear cell carcinoma has recently been described consisting of cords, sheets, nests, papillae, and trabeculae of clear cells, with well-defined cytoplasmic borders.[115] This glycogen-rich carcinoma may be distinguished from metastatic renal cell carcinoma by the

Table 16–4. Histologic Types of and Survival for Cancers of the Extrahepatic Bile Ducts, SEER Program Data

Histologic Type	No. of Patients	% of Total	2-Year Survival Rate	Median Survival (mo)
Adenocarcinoma NOS	1,133	70.9	0.15	6
Carcinoma NOS	267	16.7	0.09	3
Papillary adenocarcinoma	108	6.8	0.33	15
Mucinous	68	4.3	0.07	4
Adenosquamous	9	0.6	0	4
Squamous	8	0.5	0	2
Oat cell	5	0.3	0	2

Key: NOS, not otherwise specified; SEER, Surveillance, Epidemiology, and End Results (National Cancer Institute).
Data from Henson DE, Albores-Saavedra J, Corle D: Carcinoma of the extrahepatic bile ducts. Histologic types, stage of disease, grade, and rates. Cancer 70:1498–1501, 1992.

presence of small foci of conventional adenocarcinoma, with or without squamous differentiation. Immmunohistochemical findings are identical in both primary and metastatic clear cell carcinomas.[115] Another variant of well-differentiated carcinoma resembles gastric foveolar epithelium but may show less-differentiated areas and perineural invasion in the deep portions of the tumor. The cells of this variant are positive for alcian blue, PAS, cytokeratins 8 and 20, cathepsin D, and p53.[116]

Perineural invasion is as prominent a feature of invasion in carcinomas of the common bile duct as it is in pancreatic carcinomas. It is present in 85% of patients and extends to the extramural biliary or pancreatic nerve plexuses in 60% of patients.[117] Three-dimensional reconstructions have shown that the tumor in perineural spaces is in continuity with the main tumor mass, via a complex branching network of tumor cells.[118] The tumor may follow a path of least resistance, or it may be attracted by neural factors, such as transforming growth factor-α.[119] At this location, perineural invasion is a powerful adverse prognostic factor.[117]

Mucins and cytoplasmic carcinoembryonic antigen (CEA) are almost always present in bile duct carcinoma.[1,50] Immunoreactivity for p53 is not found in adenocarcinomas of the common bile duct, though it may be seen in poorly differentiated carcinomas of the gallbladder.[120] Immunostaining reveals pancreatic digestive enzymes in some of these tumors and also in normal extrahepatic bile duct epithelium.[121]

The incidence and significance of endocrine differentiation in carcinomas of the extrahepatic biliary tract were studied by Hsu et al., who divided the tumors into five categories on the basis of immunostaining for neuroendocrine differentiation markers (Table 16–5). The survival time of patients with any of the two neuroendocrine carcinomas and five predominantly neuroendocrine carcinomas was significantly less than the survival times of patients from the other groups (2.6 versus 13.5 months; $p = 0.015$).[122]

Table 16–5. Endocrine Differentiation in Carcinomas of the Biliary Tract*

Carcinoma Type	*n*
Pure adenocarcinoma	8
Predominantly adenocarcinoma with occasional neuroendocrine cells	9
Mixed adenoneuroendocrine carcinoma	4
Pure neuroendocrine	2
Predominantly neuroendocrine with occasional exocrine cells	5

* $n = 28$: 15 gallbladder, 13 bile duct.

Adapted from Hsu W, Deziel DJ, Gould VE, et al.: Neuroendocrine differentiation and prognosis of extrahepatic biliary tract carcinomas. Surgery 110:604–610, 1991.

Staging of Carcinomas of the Extrahepatic Bile Ducts

The staging recommended is the TNM (tumor-node-metastasis) system (Table 16–6) and is complemented by assessing residual tumor and classifying it according to the R classification: R_0 resection, no residual tumor (resection margins clear); R_1, microscopic residual tumor; and R_2, macroscopic residual tumor.

In the SEER study, stage of disease is less formally defined than in the TNM system but did show significant correlation with survival.[48] In 28% of patients, the tumor was confined to the bile ducts, but the 5-year survival for these patients was only 11%.

Differential Diagnosis of Bile Duct Carcinoma

There may be a problem in deciding on the origin of larger tumors—whether from bile duct, pancreas, ampulla, or liver. Gross appearances usually permit this distinction. Carcinoma in situ is the best microscopic indicator of site of origin but is present within the excised material in only a low proportion of patients, (10% in one series).[1] Sometimes the origin cannot be determined with certainty. The second problem is distinguishing well-differentiated carcinoma from PSC or secondary sclerosing cholangitis, particularly on small biopsies that are artifactually distorted. The normal glandular lobules in the wall of the bile ducts, the sacculi of Beale, may show cytologic reactive changes or distortion in cholangitis and must not be overdiagnosed as carcinoma. Infiltration, high-grade cytologic atypia, and perineural invasion are features that have been found helpful in making a definite diagnosis on small biopsies. Reactive glands retain a lobular arrangement, even though the cytologic features may be difficult to distinguish from carcinoma. Stents may also cause marked reactive epithelial changes and inflammation that makes diagnosis of carcinoma difficult.[123]

Table 16–6. The Tumor-Node-Metastasis Staging of Bile Duct Carcinomas

Symbol	Description
Primary tumor (T)	
Tx	Primary tumor cannot be assessed
T0	No evidence of primary tumor
Tis	Carcinoma in situ
T1	Tumor invades subepithelial connective tissue or fibromuscular layer
T1a	Tumor invades subepithelial connective tissue
T1b	Tumor invades fibromuscular layer
T2	Tumor invades perifibromuscular connective tissue
T3	Tumor invades adjacent structures: liver, pancreas, duodenum, gallbladder, colon, stomach
Regional Lymph Nodes (N)	
NX	Regional lymph nodes cannot be assessed
N0	No regional lymph node metastasis
N1	Metastasis in cystic duct, pericholedochal, and/or hilar lymph nodes (i.e., in the hepatoduodenal ligament)
N2	Metastasis in peripancreatic (head only), periduodenal, periportal, coeliac, superior mesenteric, posterior peripancreaticoduodenal lymph nodes
Distant Metastasis (M)	
MX	Distant metastasis cannot be assessed
M0	No distant metastasis
M1	Distant metastasis

Stage Groupings

Stage 0	Tis	N0	M0
Stage I	T1	N0	M0
Stage II	T2	N0	M0
Stage III	T1	N1, N2	M0
	T2	N1, N2	M0
Stage IVA	T3	Any N	M0
Stage IVB	Any T	Any N	M1

Modified from Albores-Saavedra J, Henson DE, Sobin LH: Histological Typing of Tumors of the Gallbladder and Extrahepatic Bile Ducts, 2nd ed. Berlin: Springer-Verlag, 1991, pp 23–28.

Treatment and Prognosis of Bile Duct Cancer

Carcinomas of the bile ducts are treated by local resection, wide local excision, liver transplantation, or by stenting and radiation. Complications include recurrent cholangitis and liver abscess, bleeding, and bowel obstruction.[123] Despite the fact that it produces biliary obstruction early in the course of the disease, the prognosis of carcinoma of the extrahepatic bile ducts is still extremely poor. The overall 5-year survival is only between 10% and 12.7%,[43,124,125] and the majority of patients are dead within 1 year. This is due to infiltration of the tumor into surrounding connective tissues that are rich in nerves and vessels and have no natural barriers to spread. The average survival of surgically treated patients is about 16 months. Even 5-year survival does not necessarily mean cure of the disease, and late recurrence is not uncommon. There is a low rate of resectability (about 15% in most series) and a high local recurrence rate after resection.[63]

Hilar carcinoma at the confluence of the right and left hepatic ducts is sometimes termed Klatskin's tumor, after Gerald Klatskin, the hepatologist who described its distinctive clinical features.[126] Carcinoma of the bifurcation is a technical therapeutic challenge, requiring a skilled specialist surgeon. It is treated by resection and/or liver transplantation, when feasible. The resectability rate is 50% or slightly greater if liver transplantation is included.[125] The 5-year survival rate overall is 9.4% and survivors are nearly all survivors of surgery or liver transplantation.[125] Multivariate analysis has shown that long-term survival after resection is negatively correlated with lymph node involvement, residual tumor (involved margins), and advanced tumor stage.[125,127] Intraluminal brachytherapy may prolong survival.[128]

Tumors of the middle third of the bile duct are strongly associated with perineural invasion. Connective tissue margins near the adjacent major vessels are often involved and make curative resection difficult. The 5-year survival rate is only 12.5% for tumors of the middle third that are treated by local resection and choledochoenterostomy.[110] Most long-term survivors have papillary or nodular tumors, whereas most short-term survivors have infiltrative tumors.[49]

Tumors of the distal third that are treated by pancreatoduodenectomy have the most favorable outlook and a 5-year survival of 28% to 32%.[110,129] The prognosis depends on whether lymph node metastasis; venous, lymphatic, or perineural invasion; or residual tumor are present.[49,129] The survival of patients with a tumor classified as R_0 is approximately 25% at 5 years, but for R_1 patients, it falls to only 6%, and for patients with a tumor classified as R_2, it falls to zero.[129] In the R_0 group, the incidence of liver recurrence was similar to that in the R_1 group, but the incidence of lymph node and peritoneal metastasis was less. Microscopic vascular involvement is a high-risk factor for liver recurrence and is also the only independent factor for survival in the R_0 group.[129] Stenting is a common palliative procedure and is quite effective in diminishing the incidence of recurrent pyogenic cholangitis and biliary obstruction that formerly characterized this disease.

Unusual and Metastatic Tumors of the Extrahepatic Bile Ducts

Malignant melanoma of the bile ducts is a rare occurrence and is usually secondary, although occasional primary tumors are described.[130] Melanoma tends to grow intraluminally as a polypoid mass. As elsewhere, the tumor is immunopositive for S100 protein and HMB45. The comments on gallbladder melanomas apply equally to biliary melanomas (see Chapter 13).

Metastatic colonic adenocarcinoma may grow intraluminally within the biliary system in the liver and extrahepatic bile ducts, simulating primary cholangiocarcinoma.[131] Indeed, rarely, this tumor can replace the biliary epithelium, grow along the basement membrane, and mimic dysplasia of the bile ducts.

CHOLANGIOCARCINOMA OF THE LIVER (PERIPHERAL CHOLANGIOCARCINOMA)

Intrahepatic cholangiocarcinoma is defined by the Japanese Liver Study Group as cholangiocarcinoma arising in a segmental duct (the first major branches of each hepatic duct) or a more peripheral duct. Intrahepatic cholangiocarcinoma is a disease of older people, affects the sexes equally, arises in noncirrhotic livers, and affects the right lobe mainly. It is about one fifth as prevalent as hepatocellular carcinoma in Western countries but constitutes a smaller proportion of primary liver tumors in most Asian and African countries, where hepatocellular carcinoma is more prevalent.[132] The average age of patients is 62.2 years.[132,133] There is usually no history of chronic liver disease.

Abdominal pain and malaise are the most common presenting features, although occasionally an abdominal mass is present. Jaundice is an uncommon presenting feature but occurs eventually in one third of cases.[132] Laboratory features are nonspecific. The alphafetoprotein level is not elevated in peripheral blood. Causative factors are shared with extrahepatic bile duct carcinomas and the histopathology is similar.

The gross types of cholangiocarcinoma are massive, nodular, and diffuse, and to these, annular sclerosing and intraluminal spongy types were recently added.[134] Two thirds of intrahepatic cholangiocarcinomas are solitary tumors and one third are multiple or multicentric tumors. They are usually hard, scirrhous masses, with a gray-white color and irregular margins. Calcification is uncommonly present. Cholangiocarcinoma, arising in association with intrahepatic lithiasis, can be either of periductal spreading type or of massive type.[134] The periductal spreading type extends along the biliary tree, with variable invasion of the surrounding parenchyma, whereas the massive type forms one large expanding mass. Stones may be embedded in the cancer. Cholangiocarcinoma shows gland (tubule) formation, papillary structures, and less differentiated cords and sheets in an abundant desmoplastic stroma. The epithelial elements may be widely separated from one another by the stroma, and this form of tumor must be distinguished from sclerosing hemangioendothelioma. Intracellular and intraluminal mucin is a helpful feature in the distinction from liver cell carcinoma but not from metastatic carcinoma. Only a minority of tumors are rich in extracellular mucin or of signet ring cell type.[133] Uncommon histologic variants include adenosquamous, squamous, and spindle cell carcinomas (carcinosarcomas or metaplastic carcinomas).[134,135] Mixed or combined liver cell carcinoma with cholangiocarcinoma is rare, and entrapped liver cells should not be confused with mixed tumors. The well-differentiated form of intrahepatic cholangiocarcinoma is composed of anastomosing tubules set in a fibrous stroma. It displays an infiltrative pattern and often extends along the portal tracts. The tumor cells are cuboidal and the nuclei are ovoid and uniform, without pleomorphism or prominent mitoses. Rarely, the cytoplasm may be eosinophilic and abundant. A clear cell papillary variant of peripheral cholangiocarcinoma has been described.[136]

Distinguishing intrahepatic bile duct cancer from bile duct adenomas can be difficult. Adenomas generally show well-defined individual tubules, not anastomosing tubules, and they are solitary lesions that rarely exceed 2 cm in diameter. If the cells of cholangiocarcinoma have eosinophilic cytoplasm, the pseudoglandular form of hepatocellular carcinoma must be confirmed or excluded. In this tumor, there are usually zones of conventional liver cell carcinoma with a trabecular and sinusoidal pattern, and in the acinar areas, there are pleomorphic nuclei. The alcian blue stain is negative for epithelial mucin, but bilirubin is sometimes present. Benign fibrosing disease at the hepatic confluence can mimic Klatskin's tumor and accounted for 11 of 82 resections performed for lesions presumed to be cancers.[137] The outlook for peripheral cholangiocarcinomas is poor, with a median survival of about 6 months from diagnosis. Metastases are seen in lymph nodes, lung, and peritoneum.

TUMORS OF AMPULLA OF VATER

The term *periampullary tumor* is best confined to tumors that involve the duodenal mucosa around the ampulla. This term has sometimes been applied to all of the tumors that can arise near the ampulla—from the periampullary duodenal mucosa, the ampulla itself, the common bile duct, or the main pancreatic duct. The distinction of one of these tumors from another is not always clear-cut; general diagnostic guidelines are given in Table 16–7. Benign tumors of the ampulla include adenoma, granular cell tumor, leiomyoma, hemangioma, and neurofibroma. Adenomyoma is a hamartoma, not a neoplasm.

Most adenomas are sporadic; a minority are associated with familial adenomatous polyposis (FAP). In FAP, the incidence of periampullary neoplasms is about 75%.[138] They present with abdominal pain and laboratory evidence of biliary obstruction, but rarely produce obstructive jaundice unless complicated by invasive carcinoma. Adenomas may be tubular, villous or tubulovillous and resemble colonic adenomas, showing a range of dysplasia, but often containing many Paneth cells. The adenoma–carcinoma sequence is operative at the ampulla and residual benign adenomas are found in 20% to 90% of carcinomas.[139–142] The risk of malignancy complicating ampullary adenomas is far greater than in adenomas elsewhere in the duodenum.[142] The mean age of patients with a final diagnosis of adenoma is 65.2 years and of those with carcinoma is 73 years,[140] figures that suggest an 8-year duration for the adenoma-to-carcinoma conversion. The frequency of residual adenoma in carcinomas decreases significantly with increasing T stage,[14] a finding that suggests replacement of adenoma by carcinoma as the lesion enlarges. Adenomas of the ampulla are being diagnosed more frequently, owing to the ease of endoscopy. Adenomas rarely produce jaundice, unless a carci-

Table 16–7. Periampullary Adenocarcinomas—Comparative Features

	Ampulla	Bile Duct	Duodenum	Head of Pancreas
Incidence	Uncommon	Occasional	Rare	Common
Size	Very small	Small	Medium	Large
Associations	FAP	Ulcerative colitis, anomalous union of the pancreaticobiliary duct	FAP HNPCC	Chronic pancreatitis
Gross	Villous tumor	Stricture	Villous or ulcerative	Scirrhous tumor
Associated adenoma	Frequent	Rare	Frequent	No
Resectability	High	Medium	Medium	Low
Prognosis if resectable	50% 5-y if node negative	25% 5-y	25% 5-y	10% 5-y

Key: FAP, familial adenomatous polyposis.

noma has developed. Local excision of adenomas with double-duct sphincteroplasty is a successful method of treatment, but some tumors may require radical surgery.[143] The final diagnosis of adenoma can be confirmed only when the entire lesion has been examined histologically.

Adenocarcinoma, the most common malignancy of the ampulla, resembles carcinoma of large bowel in most instances.[144] It is recognized by the combination of invasion and high-grade cytologic dysplasia. Over 40% of patients show residual adenoma and another 30% show flat dysplasia of the adjacent biliary or pancreatic duct epithelium.[144] The mean age of patients was 73 years in the series of Stolte et al. and 65 years in the series of Talamini at al.[140,145] The sex ratio is even.[144,145] Jaundice (71%), weight loss (61%), and abdominal or back pain (46%) are the most common symptoms.[145] Serum amylase is elevated in 30% of patients, but pancreatitis is uncommon. Hypoalbuminemia is found in 28% of patients.[145]

Clinical Findings and Diagnostic Techniques in Ampullary Neoplasms

The main clinical presenting features of ampullary tumors are jaundice, abdominal pain, weight loss, intestinal bleeding, anemia, and, uncommonly, pancreatitis. These features occur in different combinations.[146] Diagnostic imaging of the biliary tract begins with ultrasonography and/or CT. These images can establish the location of obstruction or lithiasis and the presence of proximal biliary dilatation. Magnetic resonance cholangiopancreatography is emerging as a useful modality for bile duct imaging. ERCP can identify the site of obstruction and allows inspection of the papilla, with sampling by biopsy or brush cytology. If there is a tumor at the ampulla, endoscopic ultrasonography may help to delineate tumor extent and depth of penetration.[147–149] When multiple biopsies are taken by an experienced operator, the diagnostic yield is good. Initial endoscopic biopsies may be negative for carcinoma in 15% to 25% of patients who ultimately prove to have either in situ or invasive carcinoma.[150,151] If initial biopsies are negative but clinical and endoscopic suspicion of malignancy persists, rebiopsy should be performed. Carcinomas typically display severe dysplasia, nuclear features of malignancy, desmoplastic stroma, infiltrative growth, and sometimes lymphatic invasion. The diagnosis of carcinoma on endoscopic biopsy is limited by the size and depth of the biopsy and by biopsy artifact, so there is a significant false negative rate, but when multiple and repeated biopsies are obtained and stepsectioned, the diagnostic reliability in patients with tumor and carcinoma is > 90%.[151] Large-particle biopsy, using a snare cautery, provides excellent tissue samples.[152,153] Biopsies performed after papillotomy have a higher yield, but biopsy that is performed at an interval of a few days after papillotomy may show only reactive cellular atypia.[154] Brush cytology is a useful adjunct to biopsy.[155,156] Brush cytology and fine-needle aspiration cytology can be employed for lesions of the ampulla and bile ducts, and the usual criteria of malignancy—high cellularity, dyscohesion, nuclear pleomorphism, nuclear enlargement (four times normal diameter), nuclear molding, irregular cell placement, and macronucleoli—may be relied on to establish a diagnosis.

Gross and Microscopic Pathology of Ampullary Carcinoma

Grossly and endoscopically, ampullary tumors may be polypoid, ulcerating (Fig. 16–1), or infiltrating.[157] The tumor may expand the papilla from within and be visible only after endoscopic papillotomy. Adenomas are usually polypoid tumors and may be lobulated or villous, whereas ulcerating and infiltrating tumors are usually carcinomas (Fig. 16–2). Superficial biopsies of ampullary carcinomas may reveal only fragments of adenomatous epithelium, with no invasion present (Fig. 16–3). However, if the patient has obstructive jaundice, an underlying carcinoma is almost always present. The gross appearance of an ampullary carcinoma predicts lymph node involvement—protruding tumors are associated with only 22% of involved lymph nodes, with 42% of mixed type, and with 100% of ulcerating type.[158]

Histologically, ampullary carcinomas resemble intestinal or pancreatobiliary carcinomas and mixed forms occur. Mucinous carcinomas are also seen.

Gastric cancer occasionally coexists with ampullary cancer,[159] but there is no greater risk of other subsequent primary cancers in patients who have ampullary cancer than in the general population.[160] The majority of carcinomas (16 of 17 in one series) give positive immunostaining for p53.[161]

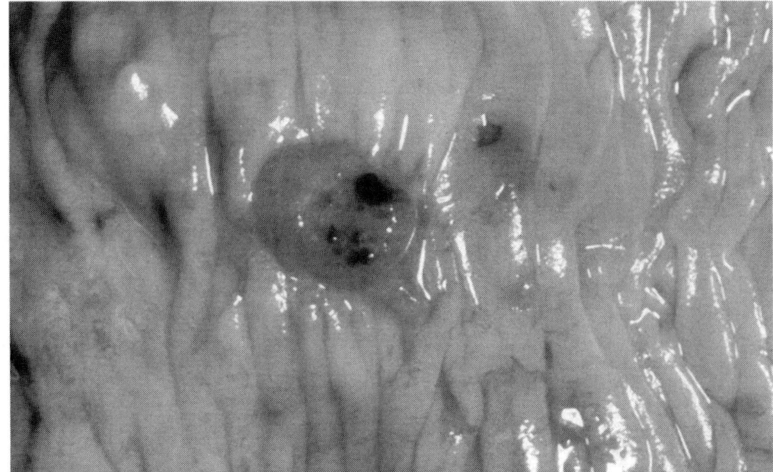

Figure 16–1. Ampullary carcinoma presenting as an ulcer within the duodenum.

The TNM system is used as the basis of staging of ampullary carcinomas. (Table 16–8).[162] The influence of extent of spread is well documented by Yamaguchi and Enjoji, whose staging system differs slightly from the TNM system.[139] Ampullary cancer spreads through the muscle coat of the sphincter or duodenum into pancreas and periduodenal connective tissue and along the common bile duct (Fig. 16–4). Lymph-borne spread is first to the pancreaticoduodenal nodes and less frequently to superior mesenteric, pericholedochal, retroportal, and paraaortic nodes.[163]

Treatment and Prognosis of Ampullary Carcinoma

Early carcinomas are confined to the ampulla or the muscle of the sphincter of Oddi (pT1), are well-differentiated, and measure < 6 mm in diameter. They can be resected locally.[139,164,165] Despite the potential curability of ampullary tumors, many patients are not suitable candidates for curative surgery on grounds of age, poor health, or advanced disease. In one series, only half of those with potentially curable disease underwent poten-

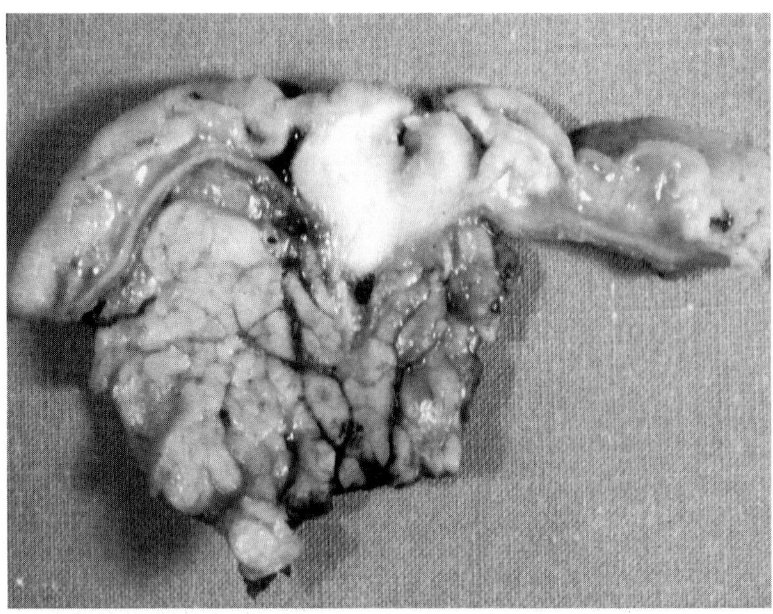

Figure 16–2. Ampullary carcinoma that has destroyed the muscularis of the bowel and is infiltrating into the head of the pancreas.

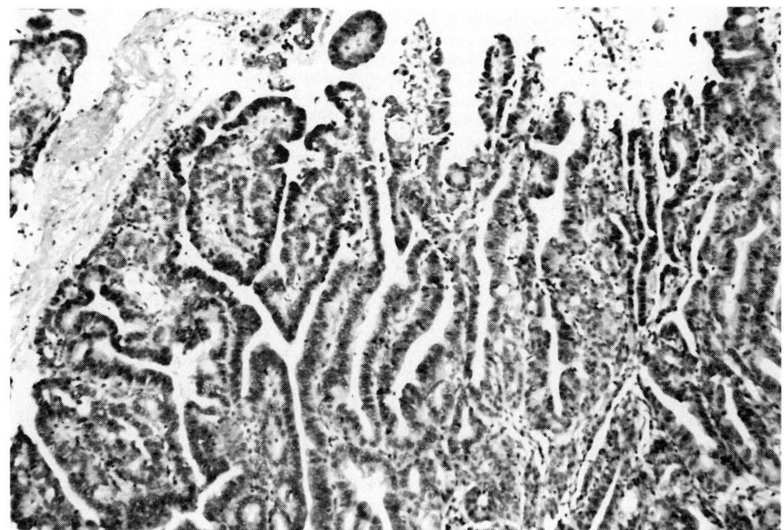

Figure 16–3. Superficial portion of a papillary carcinoma of the ampulla. Biopsies taken at the surface may not demonstrate the invasive component.

Table 16–8. The Tumor-Node-Metastasis Staging of Tumors of the Ampulla of Vater

Symbol	Description
Primary tumor (T)	
Tx	Primary tumor cannot be assessed
T0	No evidence of primary tumor
Tis	Carcinoma in situ
T1	Tumor limited to ampulla of Vater or sphincter of Oddi
T2	Tumor invades duodenal wall
T3	Tumor invades ≤ 2 cm into pancreas
T4	Tumor invades > 2 cm into pancreas and/or into other adjacent organs
Regional lymph nodes (N)*	
NX	Regional lymph nodes cannot be assessed
N0	No regional lymph node metastasis
N1	Regional lymph node metastasis
Distant metastasis (M)	
MX	Distant metastasis cannot be assessed
M0	No distant metastasis
M1	Distant metastasis

Stage Groupings

Stage 0	Tis	N0	M0
Stage I	T1	N0	M0
Stage II	T2	N0	M0
	T3	N0	M0
Stage III	T1	N1	M0
	T2	N1	M0
	T3	N1	M0
Stage IV	T4	Any N	M0
	Any T	Any N	M1

* Regarding pN0: histologic examination of a regional lymphadenectomy specimen will ordinarily include ≥ 10 lymph nodes.

Adapted from Sobin LH, Wittekind Ch. (eds): TNM Classification of Malignant Tumours, 5th ed. New York: John Wiley & Sons, 1997, p 136–143.

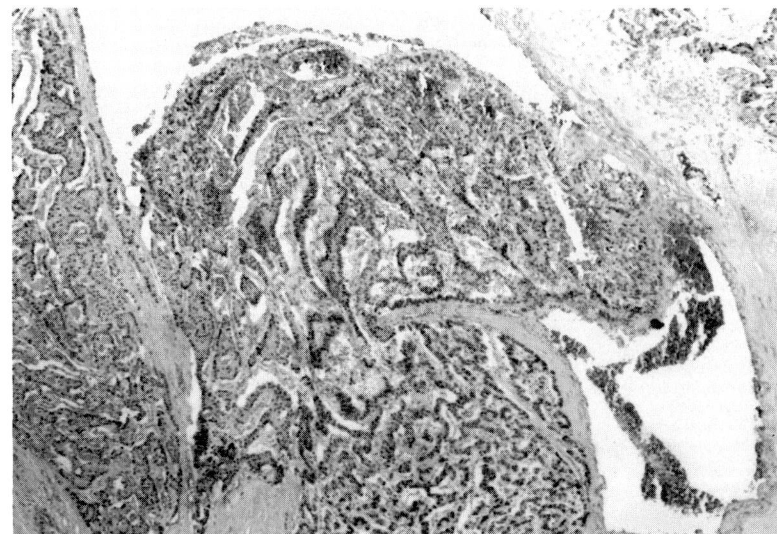

Figure 16–4. Carcinoma filling up the ampulla and invading the muscular wall.

tially curative surgery.[166] Whipple's operation, or pylorus-preserving pancreatoduodenectomy, is the operation mainly used for curative surgery.[145,163] Local excision is employed for adenomas, for carcinomas that are thought not to penetrate the muscle of Oddi, and for palliation of larger tumors in patients who are not candidates for resection. Other patients unsuited for resection are treated by stenting alone or by adjuvant chemo- and radiotherapy. The survival of patients treated by stenting is not significantly different from those treated by Whipple's operation.[166] The latter surgery still bears a significant morbidity rate, even though the surgical mortality rate is now quite low. Photodynamic therapy has also been used for palliation.

Prognosis relates to extent of spread, involvement of lymph nodes, and tumor differentiation. There is suggestive evidence that earlier diagnosis and better surgical technique, better anesthesia, and better critical care may be giving longer survivals. The 5-year survival in a large series studied from 1949 to 1974 was 6%,[167] as compared with a single-institution rate of 33% in a series studied between 1969 and 1996[145] and 16% to 52% in other later series.[168–171]

Carcinomas confined within the muscle of Oddi carry an excellent prognosis with 100% 5-year survival, whereas tumor extension into the muscle coat or beyond lowers the 5-year survival rate to 25%.[139] The 5-year survival for all radically excised cases is 35% to 62.7%,[145,164,171,172] with an actuarial survival of 44% for all surgically treated patients.[173] Penetration of the muscularis propria of the duodenum is an adverse prognostic finding; the 5-year survival of patients with penetration through the muscle coat was 28% as compared with 59% for patients with tumors with no penetration.[174] Invasion of the pancreatic parenchyma is associated with a particularly poor prognosis.[171]

Lymph node involvement is a significant adverse prognostic factor for ampullary cancer.[145,164] The lymph nodes with the highest metastatic rate are the inferior pancreaticoduodenal nodes (#13b) and the superior mesenteric nodes (#14).[158,163] Patients without nodal disease have a 5-year survival rate of between 74% and 81%, whereas those with positive superior mesenteric nodes have only a 27% 5-year survival and those with four or more involved nodes have a 0% 5-year survival.[158,163]

Tumor differentiation has a significant influence on prognosis; the 5-year survival of patients with poorly differentiated tumors was 18% versus 49% for the combined class of well-differentiated and moderately differentiated tumors ($p < 0.01$).[145]

Molecular Biology of Ampullary Carcinoma

Loss of heterozygosity at 5q is found in 50% of ampullary neoplasms, APC mutations in 17%, and K-*ras* mutations in 55%.[175] Overexpression of c-*erb*-B2 antigen correlates with Ki-

67 positivity and poor clinical outcome.[176] Expression of the mucin core protein antigen DF3 associated with the MUC 1 gene is found in 61% of carcinomas and is associated with deep invasion of pancreas and poor clinical prognosis.[177] Conversely, patients in whom the MUC 2 gene product is expressed show longer survival than do those without expression of the product, and expression correlates with minimal invasion.[177]

Rare and Unusual Tumors of the Ampulla

Before an unusual tumor is accepted as a primary arising within the ampulla, it is necessary to have an excision specimen or autopsy to confirm the nature, type, and extent of the tumor. A biopsy may not be enough, because it may not be representative of the entire lesion. For example, a biopsy showing squamous cell carcinoma of the ampulla could represent the squamous element of an adenosquamous carcinoma or a pure squamous carcinoma, but this decision would require the entire specimen to be examined. Rare tumors reported in the ampulla include small cell undifferentiated carcinoma,[178–180] follicular center cell lymphoma,[181] metastatic renal cell carcinoma[182] and sarcomatoid carcinoma.[183]

REFERENCES

1. Albores-Saavedra J, Henson DE, Sobin LH: Histological Typing of Tumors of the Gallbladder and Extrahepatic Bile Ducts, 2nd ed. Berlin: Springer-Verlag, 1991.
2. Allaire GS, Rabin L, Ishak KG, et al.: Bile duct adenoma. A study of 152 cases. Am J Surg Pathol 12:708–715, 1988.
3. Bhathal PS, Hughes NR, Goodman ZD: The so-called bile duct adenoma is a peribiliary gland hamartoma. Am J Surg Pathol 20:858–864, 1996.
4. Chu PT: Benign neoplasms of the extrahepatic biliary ducts. Arch Pathol Lab Med 50:84–97, 1950.
5. Burhans R, Myers RT: Benign neoplasms of the extrahepatic biliary ducts. Am Surg 37:161–166, 1971.
6. Roberts JW: Carcinoma of the extrahepatic bile ducts. Surg Clin N Am 66:751–756, 1986.
7. Caroli J, Soupault R, Champeau M, et al.: Papillomes et papillomatose de la voie biliaire principale. Rev Med Chir Mal Foie 34:191–230, 1959.
8. Eiss S, DiMaio D, Caedo JP: Multiple papillomas of the entire biliary tract: Case report. Ann Surg 132:320–324, 1960.
9. Hubens G, Delvaux G, Willem G, et al.: Papillomatosis of the intra- and extrahepatic bile ducts with involvement of the pancreatic duct. Hepatogastroenterol 38:413–418, 1991.
10. Jarvinen HJ, Nyberg M, Peltokallio P: Biliary involvement in familial adenomatosis coli. Dis Colon Rectum 26:525–528, 1983.
11. Neumann R, Livolsi V, Rosenthal N, et al.: Adenocarcinoma in biliary papillomatosis. Gastroenterology 70:779–782, 1976.
12. Ohita H, Yamaguchi Y, Yamakawa O, et al.: Biliary papillomatosis with the point mutation of K-*ras* gene arising in congenital choledochal cyst. Gastroenterology 105:1209–1212, 1993.
13. Okulski EG, Dolin BJ, Kandawalla NM: Intrahepatic biliary papillomatosis. Arch Pathol Lab Med 103:647–649, 1979.
14. Terada T, Mitsui T, Nakanuma Y, et al.: Intrahepatic biliary papillomatosis arising in nonobstructive intrahepatic biliary dilatations confined to the hepatic left lobe. Am J Gastroenterol 86:1523–1526, 1991.
15. Helling TS, Strobach RS: The surgical challenge of papillary neoplasia of the biliary tract. Liver Transpl Surg 2:290–298, 1996.
16. Marchal G, Vernette M, Roustan J, et al.: Papillomatose biliaire cancérisée avec atteinte de l'ampoule de Vater et de canal de Wirsung. J Chir (Paris) 107:555–578, 1974.
17. Helpap B: Malignant papillomatosis of the intrahepatic bile ducts. Acta Hepatogastroenterol (Stuttg) 24:419–425, 1977.
18. Madden JJ, Smith GW: Multiple biliary papillomatosis. Cancer 34:1316–1320, 1974.
19. Meng WC, Lau WY, Choi CL, et al.: Laser therapy for multiple biliary papillomatosis via choledochoscopy. Aust N Z J Surg 67:664–666, 1997.
20. Butterly LF, Schapiro RH, LaMuraglia GM, et al.: Biliary granular cell tumor: A little-known curable bile duct neoplasm of young people. Surgery 103:328–334, 1988.
21. Aisner SC, Khaneja S, Ramirez O: Multiple granular cell tumors of the gallbladder and biliary tree. Arch Pathol Lab Med 106:470–471, 1982.
22. Assor D: Granular cell myoblastoma involving the common bile duct. Am J Surg 137:673–675, 1979.
23. Farris KB, Faust BF: Granular cell tumors of biliary ducts. Arch Pathol Lab Med 103:510–512, 1979.
24. LiVolsi VA, Perzin KH, Badder EM, et al.: Granular cell tumors of the biliary tract. Arch Pathol 95:13–17, 1973.
25. Eisen RN, Kirby WM, O'Quinn JL: Granular cell tumor of the biliary tree. A report of two cases and a review of the literature. Am J Surg Pathol 15:460–465, 1991.
26. Zvargulis JE, Keating JP, Askin FB, et al.: Granular cell myoblastoma: A cause of biliary obstruction. Am J Dis Child 132:68–70, 1978.
27. Sanchez JA, Nauta RJ: Resection of a granular cell tumor at the hepatic confluence. A precarious location for a benign tumor. Am Surg 57:446–450, 1991.
28. Rugge M, Sonego F, Militello C, et al.: Primary carcinoid tumor of the cystic and common bile ducts. Am J Surg Pathol 16:802–807, 1992.
29. Hao L, Friedman AL, Navarro VJ, et al.: Carcinoid tumor of the common bile duct producing gastrin and serotonin. J Clin Gastroenterol 23:63–65, 1996.
30. Ueyama T, Ding J, Hashimoto H, et al.: Carcinoid tumor arising in the wall of a congenital bile duct cyst. Arch Pathol Lab Med 116:291–293, 1992.
31. Kozuka S, Tsubone M, Hachisuka K: Evolution of carcinoma in the extrahepatic bile ducts. Cancer 54:65–72, 1984.
32. Dancygier H, Klein U, Hubner K, et al.: Somatostatin-containing cells in the extrahepatic biliary tract of human. Gastroenterology 86:892–896, 1984.

33. Devaney K, Goodman ZD, Ishak KG: Hepatobiliary cystadenoma and cystadenocarcinoma: A light microscopic and immunohistochemical study of 70 patients. Am J Surg Pathol 18:1078–1091, 1994.
34. Buestow PC, Buck JL, Pantongrag-Brown L, et al.: Biliary cystadenoma and cystadenocarcinoma: Clinical-imaging-pathologic correlation with emphasis on the importance of ovarian stroma. Radiology 196:805–810, 1995.
35. Sarma DP, Rodriguez FH, Hoffman EO: Paraganglioma of the hepatic duct. South Med J 73:1677–1678, 1980.
36. Larson DM, Storsteen KA: Traumatic neuroma of the bile ducts with intrahepatic extension causing obstructive jaundice. Hum Pathol 15:287–290, 1984.
37. Sabini AM, Baden JP, Norman JD, et al.: Heterotopic pancreatic tissue in the common bile duct or ampulla of Vater. Am Surg 36:662–666, 1970.
38. Dolan RV, Remine WH, Dockerty MB: The fate of heterotopic pancreatic tissue. Arch Surg 109:762–765, 1974.
39. Blundell CR, Kanum CS, Earnest DL: Biliary obstruction by heterotopic gastric mucosa at the ampulla of Vater. Am J Gastroenterol 77:111–114, 1982.
40. Galloway PG: Heterotopic duodenum in the cystic duct. Arch Pathol Lab Med 108:666–668, 1984.
41. Okuda K, Kubo Y, Okazaki N, et al.: Clinical aspects of intrahepatic bile duct carcinoma including hilar carcinoma. A study of 57 autopsy-proven cases. Cancer 39:232–246, 1977.
42. Longmire WP, Mc Arthur MS, Bastounis EA, et al.: Carcinoma of the extrahepatic biliary tract. Ann Surg 178:333–345, 1973.
43. Anderson JB, Cooper MJ, Williamson RCN: Adenocarcinoma of the extrahepatic biliary tree. Ann Roy Coll Surg 67:139–143, 1985.
44. Bismuth H, Nakache R, Diamond T: Management strategies in resection for hilar cholangiocarcinoma. Ann Surg 215:31–38, 1992.
45. Landis SH, Murray T, Bolden S, et al.: Cancer statistics 1998. CA Cancer J Clin 48:6–29 (errata pp 192, 329), 1998.
46. Krain LS: Gallbladder and extrahepatic bile duct carcinoma. Geriatrics 27:111–117, 1972.
47. Henson DE, Albores-Saavedra J, Corle D: Carcinoma of the extrahepatic bile ducts. Histologic types, stage of disease, grade, and survival rates. Cancer 70:1498–1501, 1992.
48. Henson DE, Albores-Saavedra J, Corle D: Carcinoma of the gallbaldder. Histologic types, stage of disease, grade, and survival rates. Cancer 70:1493–1497, 1992.
49. Ouchi K, Matsuno S, Sato T: Long-term survival in carcinoma of the biliary tract. Analysis of prognostic factors in 146 resections. Arch Surg 124:248–252, 1989.
50. Davis RI, Sloan JM, Hood JM, et al.: Carcinoma of the extrahepatic biliary tract: A clinicopathological and immunohistochemical study. Histopathology 12:623–631, 1988.
51. Nichols JC, Gores GJ, LaRusso NF, et al.: Diagnostic role of serum CA 19-9 for cholangiocarcinoma in patients with primary sclerosing cholangitis. Mayo Clin Proc 68:874–879, 1993.
52. Laing FC, Jeffrey RB, Wing VW: Improved visualization of choledocholithiasis by sonography. Am J Roentgenol 143:949–952, 1984.
53. Saini S: Imaging of the hepatobiliary tract. N Engl J Med 336:1889–1894, 1997.
54. De Groen PC, Gores GJ, LaRusso NF, et al.: Biliary tract cancers. N Engl J Med 341:1368–1378, 1999.
55. Chan Y-L, Chan ACW, Lam WWM, et al.: Choledocholithiasis: Comparison of MR cholangiography and endoscopic retrograde cholangiography. Radiology 200:85–89, 1996.
56. Tio TL, Cheng J, Wijers OB, et al.: Endosonograpic TNM staging of extrahepatic bile duct cancer: Comparison with pathological staging. Gastroenterology 100:1351–1361, 1991.
57. Mansfield JC, Griffin SM, Wahedra V, et al.: A prospective evaluation of cytology from biliary strictures. Gut 40:671–677, 1997.
58. Nakajima T, Tajima Y, Sugano I, et al.: Multivariate statistical analysis of bile cytology. Acta Cytol 38:51–55, 1994.
59. Cohen MB, Wittchow RJ, Johlin FC, et al.: Brush cytology of the extrahepatic biliary tract: Comparison of cytologic features of adenocarcinoma and benign biliary strictures. Mod Pathol 8:498–502, 1995.
60. Renshaw AA, Madge R, Jiroutec M, et al.: Bile duct brushing cytology. Statistical analysis of proposed diagnostic criteria. Am J Clin Pathol 110:635–640, 1998.
61. Kocjan G, Smith AN: Bile duct brushings cytology: Potential pitfalls in diagnosis. Diag Cytopathol 16:358–363, 1997.
62. Kurzawinski T, Deery A, Davidson BR: Diagnostic value of cytology for biliary strictures. Br J Surg 80:414–421, 1993.
63. Braasch JW: Carcinoma of the bile duct. Surg Clin North Am 53:1217–1227, 1973.
64. Ritchie JK, Allan RN, Macartney J, et al.: Biliary tract carcinoma associated with ulcerative colitis. Q J Med 43:263–279, 1974.
65. Wee A, Ludwig J, Coffee RJ, et al.: Hepatobiliary carcinoma associated with primary sclerosing cholangitis and chronic ulcerative colitis. Hum Pathol 16:719–726, 1985.
66. Weisner RH, Ludwig J, LaRusso NF, et al.: Diagnosis and treatment of primary sclerosing cholangitis. Semin Liv Dis 5:241–253, 1985.
67. Kornfeld D, Ekbom A, Ihre T: Survival and risk of cholangiocarcinoma in patients with primary sclerosing cholangitis. A population-based study. Scand J Gastroenterol 32:1042–1045, 1997.
68. Akwari OE, VanHeerden JA, Foulk WT, et al.: Cancer of the bile ducts associated with ulcerative colitis. Ann Surg 181:303–309, 1975.
69. Bergquist A, Glaumann H, Persson B, et al.: Risk factors and clinical presentation of hepatobiliary carcinoma in patients with primary sclerosing cholangitis: A clinicopathological study. Hepatology 27:311–316, 1998.
70. Phinney PR, Austin GE, Kadell BM: Cholangiocarcinoma arising in Caroli's disease. Arch Pathol Lab Med 105:194–197, 1981.
71. Daroca PJ, Tuthill R, Reed RJ: Cholangiocarcinoma arising in congenital hepatic fibrosis. Arch Pathol 99:592–595, 1975.
72. Burns CD, Kuhns JG, Wieman TJ: Cholangiocarcinoma in association with multiple biliary microhamartomas. Arch Pathol Lab Med 114:1287–1289, 1990.
73. Imamura M, Miyashita T, Tani T, et al.: Cholangiocellular carcinoma associated with multiple liver cysts. Am J Gastroenterol 79:790–795, 1984.
74. Honda N, Cobb C, Lechago J: Bile duct carcinoma associated with multiple von Meyenburg complexes in the liver. Hum Pathol 17:1287–1290, 1986.

75. Gallagher PJ, Millis RR, Mitchison MJ: Congenital dilatation of the intrahepatic bile ducts with cholangiocarcinoma. J Clin Pathol 25:804–808, 1972.
76. Jones AW, Shreeve DR: Congenital dilatation of the intrahepatic bile ducts with cholangiocarcinoma. Br Med J 2:277–278, 1970.
77. Bloustein PA: Association of carcinoma with congenital cystic conditions of the liver and bile ducts. Am J Gastroenterol 67:40–46, 1977.
78. Todani T, Tabuchi K, Watanabe Y, et al.: Carcinoma arising in the wall of congenital bile duct cysts. Cancer 44:1134–1141, 1979.
79. Tsuchiya R, Harada N, Ito T, et al.: Malignant tumors in choledochal cysts Ann Surg 186:22–28, 1977.
80. Kagawa Y, Kashihara S, Kuramoto S, et al.: Carcinoma arising in a congenitally dilated biliary tree. Gastroenterology 72:1286–1294, 1978.
81. Rossi RL, Silverman ML, Braasch JW, et al.: Carcinoma arising in cystic conditions of the bile ducts: A clinical and pathologic study. Ann Surg 205:377–384, 1987.
82. Flanigan DP: Biliary carcinoma associated with biliary cysts. Cancer 40:880–883, 1977.
83. Suda K, Miyano T: Bile pancreatitis. Arch Pathol Lab Med 109:433–436, 1985.
84. Morohoshi T, Kunimura T, Kanda M, et al.: Multiple carcinomata associated with anomalous arrangement of the biliary and pancreatic duct system. Acta Pathol Jpn 40:755–763, 1990.
85. Kimura K, Ohto M, Saisho H, et al.: Association of gallbladder carcinoma and anomalous pancreatobiliary ductal union. Gastroenterology 89:1258–1265, 1985.
86. Sugiyama M, Atomi Y: Anomalous pancreatobiliary junction without congenital choledochal cyst. Br J Surg 85:911–916, 1998.
87. Sharma SS: Pancreaticobiliary ductal union in cholangiocarcinoma. Gastrointest Endosc 40:171–173, 1994.
88. Yen S, Hsieh C-C, MacMahon B: Extrahepatic bile duct cancer and smoking, beverage consumption, past medical history, and oral contraceptive use. Cancer 59:2112–2116, 1987.
89. Kato K, Akai S, Tominaga S, et al.: A case-control study of biliary tract cancer in Niigata prefecture, Japan. Jpn J Cancer Res 80:932–938, 1989.
90. Ekbom A, Hsieh C-C, Yuen J, et al.: Risk of extrahepatic bile duct cancer after cholecystectomy. Lancet 342:1262–1265, 1993.
91. Jarvi O, Lauren P: Intestinal metaplasia on the mucosa of the gallbladder and common bile duct. Ann Med Exp Fenn 45:213–223, 1967.
92. Hou PC: The relationship between primary carcinoma of the liver and infestation with *Clonorchis sinensis.* J Pathol Bacteriol 72:239–246, 1956.
93. Ona FV, Dytoc JN: *Clonorchis*-associated cholangiocarcinoma: A report of two cases with unusual manifestations. Gastroenterology 101:831–839, 1991.
94. Kurathong S, Lerdveresirikul P, Wongpaitoon V, et al.: *Opisthorchis viverrini* infection and cholangiocarcinoma: A prospective, case-controlled study. Gastroenterology 89:151–156, 1985.
95. Nakanuma Y, Tereda T, Tanaka Y, et al.: Are hepatolithiasis and cholangiocarcinoma etiologically related? A morphological study of twelve cases of hepatolithiasis associated with cholangiocarcinoma. Virchows Arch A Pathol Anat 406:45–58, 1985.
96. Koga A, Ichimiya H, Yamaguchi K, et al.: Hepatolithiasis associated with cholangiocarcinoma: Possible etiologic significance. Cancer 55:2826–2829, 1985.
97. Hou PC: Primary carcinoma of bile ducts of the liver of the cat (felis catus) infested with *Clonorchis sinensis.* J Pathol Bacteriol 87:239–244, 1964.
98. Dahlgren S: Thorotrast tumors: A review of the literature and report of two cases. Arch Pathol Microbiol Scand 53:147–161, 1961.
99. Rubel LR, Ishak KG: Thorotrast-associated cholangiocarcinoma: An epidemiologic and clinicopathologic study. Cancer 50:1408–1415, 1982.
100. Ghadirian P, Simard A, Baillargeon J: A population-based case-control study of cancer of the bile ducts and gallbladder in Quebec, Canada. Rev Epidemiol Sante Publique 41:107–112, 1993.
101. Stromeyer FW, Smith DH, Ishak KG: Anabolic steroid therapy and intrahepatic cholangiocarcinoma. Cancer 43:440–443, 1979.
102. Perez Ruiz L, Gabarrell Oto A, Vinas Salas J, et al.: Biliary tract cancer following bilioenteric anastomosis. Rev Esp Enferm Dig 86:853–855, 1994.
103. Schumacher G, Bechstein WD, Kling N, et al.: Bile duct carcinoma in an adenoma in the anastomotic area after hepaticojejunostomy—A case report. Z Gastroenterol 35:1081–1086, 1997.
104. Harvath AC, Manley BN, Groll A, et al.: Bile duct and biliary tract dysplasia in chronic ulcerative colitis. Arch Pathol Lab Med 113:434–436, 1989.
105. Suzuki M, Takahashi T, Ouchi K, et al.: The development and extension of hepatohilar bile duct carcinoma: A three-dimensional tumor mapping in the intrahepatic biliary tree visualized with the aid of a graphics computer system. Cancer 64:658–666, 1989.
106. Laitio M: Carcinoma of extrahepatic bile ducts. A histopathologic study. Path Res Pract 178:67–72, 1983.
107. Sako K, Seitzinger GL, Garside E: Carcinoma of the extrahepatic bile ducts: Review of the literature and report of six cases. Surgery 41:416–437, 1957.
108. Todoroki RK, Okamura T, Fukao K, et al.: Gross appearance of carcinoma of the main hepatic duct and its prognosis. Surg Gynecol Obstet 150:33–40, 1980.
109. Reding R, Buard J-L, Lebeau G, et al.: Surgical management of 552 carcinomas of the extrahepatic bile ducts (gallbladder and periampullary tumors excluded). Ann Surg 213:236–241, 1991.
110. Tompkins RK, Saunders K, Roslyn JJ, et al.: Changing patterns in diagnosis and management of bile duct cancer. Ann Surg 21:614–621, 1990.
111. Alexander F, Rossi RL, O'Bryan M, et al.: Biliary carcinoma. A review of 109 cases. Am J Surg 147:503–509, 1984.
112. Nakeeb A, Pitt HA, Sohn TA, et al.: Cholangiocarcinoma: A spectrum of intrahepatic, perihilar and distal tumors. Ann Surg 224:463–475, 1996.
113. Albores-Saavedra J, Henson DE: Tumors of the gallbladder and extrahepatic bile ducts. Atlas of Tumor Pathology, second series, fascicle 22. Washington, DC: Armed Forces Institute of Pathology, 1986, pp 164–181.
114. Aranha GV, Reyes CV, Greenlee HB, et al.: Squamous cell carcinoma of the proximal bile ducts: A case report. J Surg Oncol 15:29–35, 1980.
115. Vardaman C, Albores-Saavedra J: Clear cell carcinomas of the gallbladder and extrahepatic bile ducts. Am J Surg Pathol 19:91–99, 1995.
116. Albores-Saavedra J, Delgado R, Henson DE: Well-differentiated adenocarcinoma, foveolar type, of the extrahepatic bile ducts: A previously unrecognised and distinctive morphologic variant of bile duct carcinoma. Ann Diagn Pathol 3:75–80, 1999.

117. Nagakawa T, Mori K, Nakano T, et al.: Perineural invasion of carcinoma of the pancreas and biliary tract. Br J Surg 80:619–621, 1993.
118. Maxwell P, Hamilton PW, Sloan JM: Three-dimensional reconstruction of perineural invasion in carcinoma of the extrahepatic bile ducts. J Pathol 180:142–145, 1996.
119. Bockman DE, Buchler M, Beger HG: Interaction of pancreatic ductal carcinoma with nerves leads to nerve damage. Gastroenterology 107:219–230, 1994.
120. Lee CS, Pirdas A: p53 protein immunoreactivity in cancers of the gallbladder, extrahepatic bile ducts and ampulla of Vater. Pathology 27:117–120, 1995.
121. Terada T, Kitimura Y, Ashida K, et al.: Expression of pancreatic digestive enzymes in normal and pathologic epithelial cells of the human gastrointestinal system. Virchows Archiv 431:195–203, 1997.
122. Hsu W, Deziel DJ, Gould VE, et al.: Neuroendocrine differentiation and prognosis of extrahepatic biliary tract carcinomas. Surgery 110:604–610, 1991.
123. Qualman SJ, Haupt HM, Bauer TM, et al.: Adenocarcinoma of the hepatic duct junction. A reappraisal of the histologic features of malignancy. Cancer 53:1545–1551, 1984.
124. Carriaga MT, Henson DE: Liver, gallbladder, extrahepatic bile ducts, and pancreas. Cancer 75:(suppl 1):171–190, 1995.
125. Klempnauer J, Ridder GJ, Werner M, et al.: What constitutes long-term survival after surgery for hilar cholangiocarcinoma? Cancer 79:26–34, 1997.
126. Klatskin G: Adenocarcinoma of the hepatic duct at its bifurcation within the porta hepatis: An unusual tumor with distinctive clinical and pathological features. Am J Med 38:241–256, 1965.
127. Bengmark S, Ekberg H, Evander A, et al.: Major liver resection for hilar cholangiocarcinoma. Ann Surg 207:120–125, 1988.
128. Montemaggi P, Costamagna G, Dobelbower RR, et al.: Intraluminal brachytherapy in the treatment of pancreas and bile duct carcinoma. Int J Rad Oncol Biol Phys 32:437–443, 1995.
129. Takao S, Shinchi K, Uchikura M, et al.: Liver metastases after curative resection in patients with distal bile duct cancer. Br J Surg 86:327–331, 1999.
130. Deugnier Y, Turlin B, Lehry D, et al.: Malignant melanoma of the hepatic and common bile ducts. A case report and review of the literature. Arch Pathol Lab Med 115:915–917, 1991.
131. Riopel MA, Klimstra DS, Godellas CV, et al.: Intrabiliary growth of metastatic colonic adenocarcinoma. A pattern of intrahepatic spread easily confused with primary neoplasia of the biliary tract. Am J Surg Pathol 21:1030–1036, 1997.
132. Okuda K, Kubo Y, Okazaki N, et al.: Clinical aspects of intrahepatic bile duct carcinoma. Cancer 39:232–246, 1977.
133. Nakajima T, Kondo Y, Miyazaki M, et al.: A histopathologic study of 102 cases of intrahepatic cholangiocarcinoma: Histologic classification and mode of spreading. Hum Pathol 19:1228–1234, 1988.
134. Nakajima K, Tajima Y, Sugano I, et al.: Intrahepatic cholangiocarcinoma with sarcomatous change. Clinicopathologic and immunohistochemical evaluation of seven cases. Cancer 15:1872–1877, 1993.
135. Nakajima T, Kondo Y: A clinicopathologic study of intrahepatic cholangiocarcinoma containing a component of squamous cell carcinoma. Cancer 65:1401–1404, 1990.
136. Tihan T, Blumgart L, Klimstra DS: Clear cell papillary carcinoma of the liver: An unusual variant of peripheral cholangiocarcinoma. Hum Pathol 29:196–200, 1998.
137. Verbeek PCM, van Leeuwen DJ, deWit L Th, et al.: Benign fibrosing disease at the hepatic confluence mimicking Klatskin tumors. Surgery 112:866–871, 1992.
138. Noda Y, Watanabe H, Iida M et al.: Histologic follow-up of ampullary adenomas in patients with familial adenomatosis coli. Cancer 70:1847–1856, 1992.
139. Yamaguchi K, Enjoji M: Carcinoma of the ampulla of Vater: A clinicopathologic study and pathologic staging of 109 cases of carcinoma and 5 cases of adenomas. Cancer 59:506–515, 1981.
140. Stolte M, Pscherer C: Adenoma-carcinoma sequence in the papilla of Vater. Scand J Gastroenterol 31:376–382, 1996.
141. Baczako K, Buchler M, Beger H-G, et al.: Morphogenesis and possible precursor lesions of invasive carcinoma of the papilla of Vater: Epithelial dysplasia and adenoma. Hum Pathol 16:305–310, 1985.
142. Seifert E, Schulte F, Stolte M: Adenoma and carcinoma of the duodenum and papilla of Vater: A clinicopathologic study. Am J Gastrol 87:37–41, 1992.
143. Rosenberg J, Welch JP, Pyrtek LJ, et al.: Benign villous adenoma of the ampulla of Vater. Cancer 58:1563–1568, 1986.
144. Talbot IC, Neoptolomos JP, Shaw DE, et al.: The histopathology and staging of carcinoma of the ampulla of Vater. Histopathology 12:155–165, 1988.
145. Talamini MA Moesinger RC, Pitt HA, et al.: Adenocarcinoma of the ampulla of Vater. A 28 year experience. Ann Surg 225:590–600, 1997.
146. Sticca RP, Weatherford DA, McAlhany JC Jr: Carcinoma of the ampulla of Vater: A community hospital experience. Am Surg 62:197–202, 1996.
147. Zhang Q, Nian W, Zhang L, Liang J: Endoscopic ultrasonography assessment in preoperative staging for carcinoma of ampulla of Vater and extrahepatic bile duct. Chinese Med J 109:622–625, 1996.
148. Rösch T, Braig C, Gain T, et al.: Staging of pancreatic and ampullary carcinoma by endoscopic ultrasonography. Gastroenterology 102:188–199, 1992.
149. Menzel, Hoepffner N, Sulkowski U, et al.: Polypoid tumors of the major duodenal papilla: Preoperative staging with intraductal US, EUS, and CT—a prospective, histopathologically-controlled study. Gastrointest Endosc 49:349–357, 1999.
150. Blackman E, Nash SV: Diagnosis of duodenal and ampullary epithelial neoplasms by endoscopic biopsy: A clinicopathologic and immunohistological study. Hum Pathol 16:901–910, 1985.
151. Komorowski RA, Beggs BK, Geenan JE, et al.: Assessment of ampulla of Vater pathology. An endoscopic approach. Am J Surg Pathol 15:1188–1196, 1991.
152. Rosch W: Endoscopic sphincterotomy in carcinoma of the ampulla of Vater. Gastrointest Endosc 28:203–204, 1982.
153. Nakao NL, Siegel JH, Stenger RJ, et al.: Tumors of the ampulla of Vater: Early diagnosis by intraampullary biopsy during endoscopic cannulation. Two case presentations and a review of the literature. Gastroenterology 83:459–464, 1982.
154. Bourgeois N, Dunham F, Verhest A, et al.: Endoscopic biopsies of the papilla of Vater at the time of endoscopic sphincterotomy: Difficulties in interpretation. Gastrointest Endosc 30:163–166, 1984.

155. Bardales RH, Stanley MW, Simpson DD, et al.: Diagnostic value of brush cytology in the diagnosis of duodenal, biliary, and ampullary neoplasms. Am J Clin Pathol 109:540–548, 1998.
156. Witte S: Brush cytology of the papilla of Vater. Scand J Gastroenterol 54(suppl):55–58, 1979.
157. Ponchon T, Berger F, Chavaillon A, et al.: Contribution of endoscopy to diagnosis and treatment of tumors of the ampulla of Vater. Cancer 64:161–167, 1989.
158. Kayahara M, Nagakawa T, Ohta T, et al.: Surgical strategy for carcinoma of the papilla of Vater on the basis of lymphatic spread and mode of recurrence. Surgery 121:611–617, 1997.
159. Shirai Y, Tsukada K, Ohtani T, et al.: Carcinoma of the ampulla of Vater: Histopathologic analysis of tumor spread in Whipple pancreatectomy specimens. World J Surg 19:102–107, 1995.
160. Moran A, Collins S, Evans DG, et al.: Risk of subsequent primary cancers in patients with carcinoma of the ampulla of Vater. Br J Cancer 76:1232–1233, 1997.
161. Younes M, Riley S, Genta RM, et al.: p53 protein accumulation in tumors of the ampulla of Vater. Cancer 76:1150–1154, 1995.
162. Sobin LH, Wittekind Ch. (eds): TNM Classification of Malignant Tumours, 5th ed. New York: John Wiley & Sons, 1997.
163. Shirai Y, Ohtani T, Tsukada K, et al.: Patterns of lymphatic spread of carcinoma of the ampulla of Vater. Br J Surg 84:1012–1016, 1997.
164. Bottger TC, Boddin J, Heintz A, et al.: Clinicopathologic study for the assessment of resection for ampullary carcinoma. World J Surg 21:379–383, 1997.
165. Klein P, Reingruber B, Kastl S, et al.: Is local excision of pT1-ampullary carcinomas justified? Eur J Surg Oncol 22:366–371, 1996.
166. Farrell RJ, Noonan N, Khan IM, et al.: Carcinoma of the ampulla of Vater: A tumor with a poor prognosis? Eur J Gastroenterol Hepatol 8:139–144, 1996.
167. Nakase A, Matsumoto Y, Uchida K, et al.: Surgical treatment of cancer of the pancreas and the periampullary region: Cumulative results in 57 institutions in Japan. Ann Surg 183:341–344, 1976.
168. Matory YL, Gaynor J, Brennan M: Carcinoma of the ampulla of Vater. Surg Gynecol Obstet 177:366–370, 1993.
169. Walsh DB, Eckhauser FE, Cronenwett JL, et al.: Adenocarcinoma of the ampulla of Vater. Ann Surg 195:152–157, 1982.
170. Willet CG, Warshaw AL, Convery K, et al.: Patterns of failure after pancreatoduodenectomy for ampullary carcinoma. Surg Gynecol Obstet 176:33–38, 1993.
171. Nakao A, Harada A, Nonami T, et al.: Prognosis of cancer of the duodenal papilla of Vater in relation to clinicopathological tumor extension. Hepatogastroenterol 41:73–78, 1994.
172. Roder JD, Schneider PM, Stein HJ, et al.: Number of lymph node metastases is significantly associated with survival in patients with radically resected carcinoma of the ampulla of Vater. Br J Surg 82:1693–1696, 1995.
173. Dorandeu A, Raoul JL, Siriser F, et al.: Carcinoma of the ampulla of Vater: Prognostic factors after curative surgery: A series of 45 cases. Gut 40:350–355, 1997.
174. Shirai Y, Tsukada K, Ohtani T, et al.: Carcinoma of the ampulla of Vater: Is radical lymphadenectomy beneficial to patients with nodal disease? J Surg Oncol 61:190–194, 1996.
175. Achille A, Scupoli MT, Magalini AR, et al.: APC gene mutations and allelic losses in sporadic ampullary tumours: Evidence of genetic difference from tumors associated with familial adenomatous polyposis. Int J Cancer 68:305–312, 1996.
176. Vaidya P, Kawarada Y, Higashiguchi T, et al.: Overexpression of different members of the type 1 growth factor receptor family and their association with cell proliferation in pariampullary carcinoma. J Pathol 178:140–145, 1996.
177. Kitamura H, Yonezawa S, Tanaka S, et al.: Expression of mucin carbohydrates and core proteins in carcinoma of the ampulla of vater: their relationship to prognosis. Jpn J Cancer Res 87:631–640, 1996.
178. Sato T, Yamamoto K, Ouchi A, et al.: Undifferentiated carcinoma of the duodenal ampulla. J Gastroenterol 30:517–519, 1995.
179. Soon Lee C, Machet D, Rode J: Small cell carcinoma of the ampulla of Vater. Cancer 70:1502–1504, 1992.
180. Zamboni G, Franzin G, Bonetti F, et al.: Small-cell neuroendocrine carcinoma of the ampullary region. A clinicopathologic, immunohistochemical, and ultrastructural study of three cases. Am J Surg Pathol 14:703–713, 1990.
181. Misdraji J, Fernandez del Castillo C, Ferry JA: Follicle centre lymphoma of the ampulla of Vater presenting with jaundice. Am J Surg Pathol 21:484–488, 1997.
182. Janzen BM, Ramj AS, Flint JD, et al.: Obscure gastrointestinal bleeding from an ampullary tumour in a patient with a remote history of renal cell carcinoma: A diagnostic conundrum. Can J Gastroenterol 12:75–78, 1998.
183. Kench JG, Frommer DJ: Sarcomatoid carcinoma of the ampulla of Vater. Pathology 29:89–91, 1997.

Index

Note: Page numbers in *italics* indicate figures; those followed by t indicate tables.

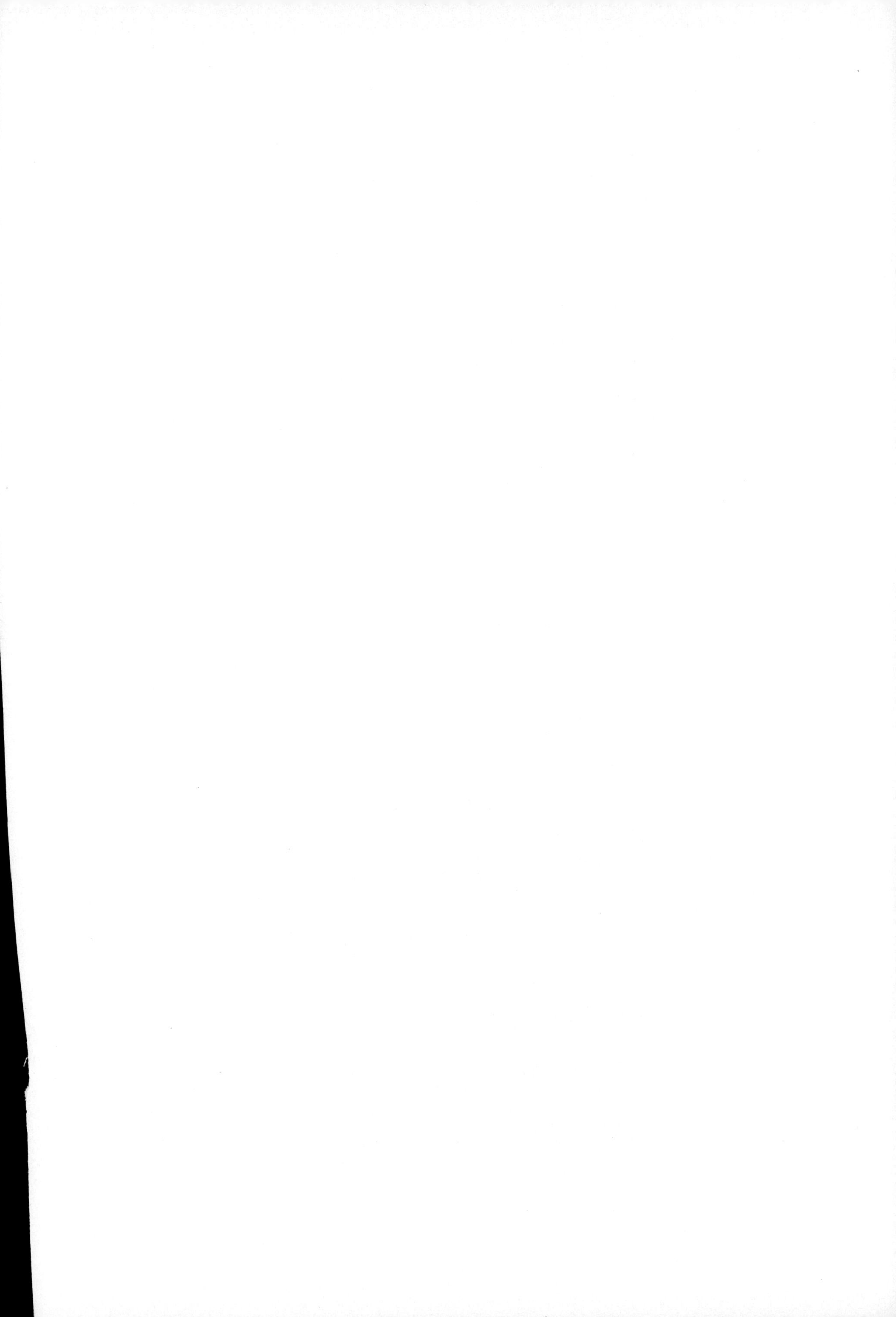

9 780721 619101 90038

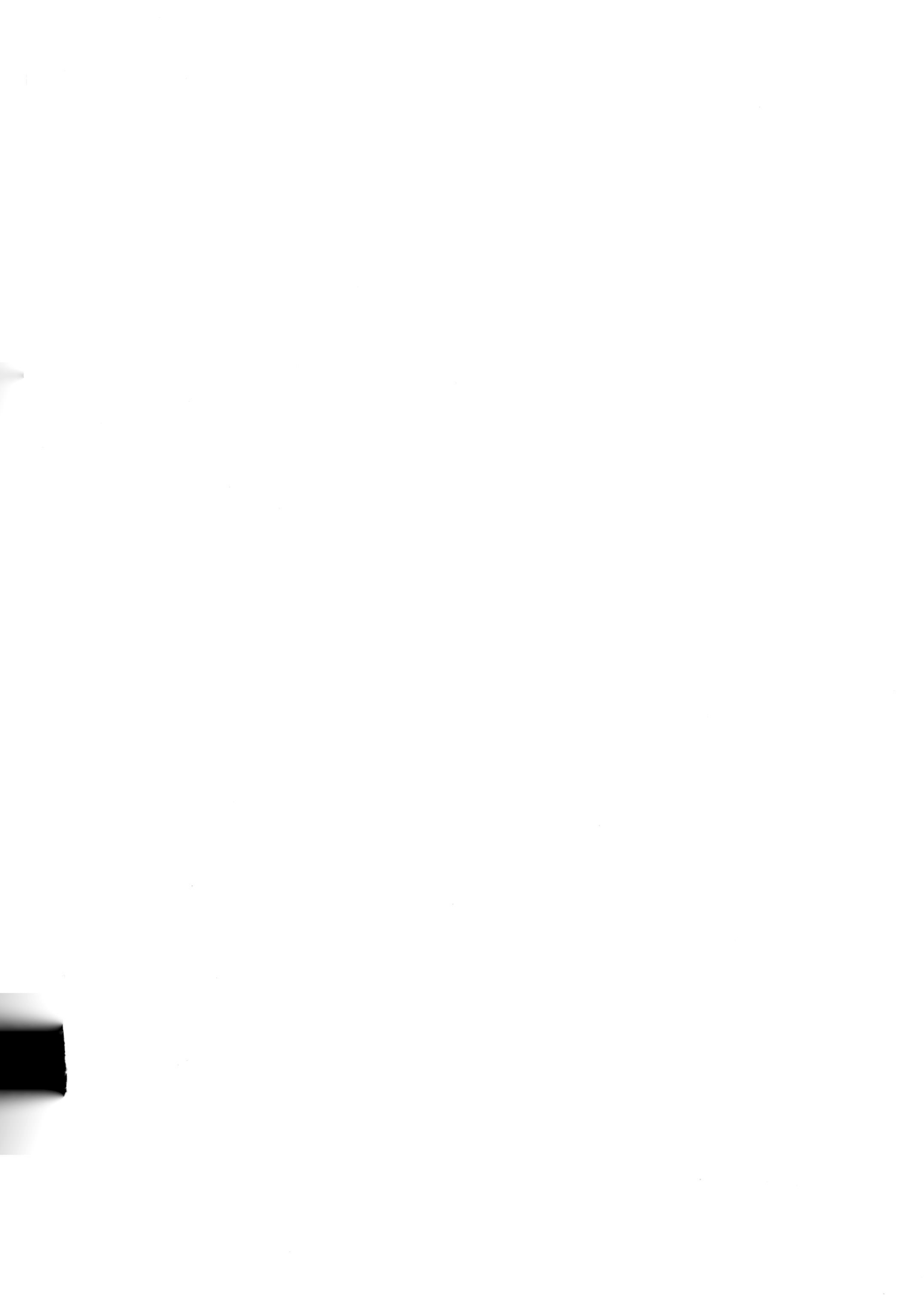